Mosby's
Comprehensive Review of Practical Nursing

Mosby's Comprehensive Review of Practical Nursing

EDITOR

Mary Yannes-Eyles, *RN, MA*

Director, Education Department
Kessler Institute for Rehabilitation, Inc.
West Orange, New Jersey

Instructor, LPN Review Course
Rockland Community College
Suffern, New York

(formerly) Director of Continuing Education
National Association for Practical Nurse Education and Service, Inc. (NAPNES)

ELEVENTH EDITION
with 117 illustrations

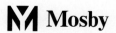 Mosby

St. Louis Baltimore Boston Chicago London Madrid Philadelphia Sydney Toronto

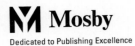

Mosby
Dedicated to Publishing Excellence

Editor: Susan Epstein
Developmental Editor: Beverly Copland
Project Manager: Gayle May Morris
Production Editor: Lisa Nomura
Manufacturing Supervisor: Betty Richmond
Designer: Susan Lane

ELEVENTH EDITION

Printed in the United States of America

Previous editions copyrighted 1956, 1957, 1961, 1966, 1970, 1974, 1978, 1982, 1986, 1990

Composition by Graphic World
Printing/binding by Maple-Vail Book Mfg. Group

Mosby–Year Book, Inc.
11830 Westline Industrial Drive
St. Louis, Missouri 63146

Library of Congress Cataloging-in-Publication Data

Mosby's comprehensive review of practical nursing/editor, Mary Yannes-Eyles.—11th ed.
　　p.　cm.
　　Includes bibliographical references and index.
　　ISBN 0-8016-7006-3
　　1. Practical nursing—Examinations, questions, etc.　I. Yannes-Eyles, Mary.
　　II. Title: Comprehensive review of practical nursing.
　　[DNLM:　1. Nursing, Practical—examination questions.　2. Nursing, Practical—outlines.
WY 18 M8939 1993]
RT62.M62　1993
610.73′076—dc20
DNLM/DLC
for Library of Congress
93-25174
CIP

93　94　95　96　97　/　9　8　7　6　5　4　3　2　1

This text is dedicated to all individuals and organizations
involved in the profession of practical/vocational nursing
for their knowledge, skills, and abilities
in promoting and providing excellence in patient care
within the United States and Canada.

Editorial Panel

CONTRIBUTING AUTHORS

Carol Anderson, RN, BSN, MEd

Coordinator, New York City Campus
Practical Nursing Program
Iona College
New Rochelle, New York

Dawn E. Bleau, RN, BSN

Director
Knoedler School of Practical Nurse Education
Jefferson, Ohio

Mary G. Kawamura Chapus, RN, BSN, MPH, ACCE, CPHN

Adjunct Faculty Member
School of Practical Nursing
Iona College
New Rochelle, New York

Kathryn Koppen Clark, BSN, RN, PHN, CPN

Assistant Director of Patient Care Services/Director of Staff
  Development
Shriners Hospital for Crippled Children
Chicago, Illinois

Norma J. Jones, RN, MPH

President and Chief Executive Officer
Casa Loma College
Sylmar, California

Marjorie Knox, BSN, MA, MPA

Professor of Nursing
Community College of Rhode Island Nursing Program
Warwick, Rhode Island

Vicky Mack, RN, BSEd

Practical Nurse Instructor
Flint River Technical Institute
Thomaston, Georgia

Mary Miller-Werlinger, RN, MS, CNS

Director of Quality Assurance and Education
Goodall-Witcher Hospital Foundation
Clifton, Texas

Suzanne M. Philip, RN, BScNE, BEd, MA

Professor, Health Sciences Division
Humber College
Toronto, Ontario

Martha Phillips, RN, MA

Associate Professor of Nursing
Iona College
New Rochelle, New York

Gary W. Stogsdill, RN, MA

Assistant Professor of Vocational Nursing
Alamo Community College District
San Antonio, Texas

REVIEWERS

Catherine Burke, BSN, MS

Nursing Instructor
Kankakee Community College
Kankakee, Illinois

Mary Ann Cosgarea, RN, BA, BSN

Coordinator, Portage Lakes Career Center
W. Howard Nicol School of Practical Nursing
Greensburg, Ohio

Carolyn Dean, LPN, BSN

Coordinator Practical Nursing Program
North Central Missouri College
Trenton, Missouri

Margaret L. Denton, ADAS, BSPA, MSCE

Division Chair, Nursing and Allied Health
Hobson State Technical College
Thomasville, Alabama

Preface

Mosby's Comprehensive Review of Practical Nursing has been developed to provide individuals preparing for entry or reentry into nursing at the practical/vocational nurse level with a dependable source of information as they prepare to become valued members of today's health care team. The most current, up-to-date developments in health care today in the field of practical/vocational nursing are incorporated in the text, as each contributor has recently been or is currently active in practical/vocational nursing education.

In this eleventh edition of *Mosby's Comprehensive Review of Practical Nursing*, the basic practical/vocational nursing curriculum is addressed, from concepts basic to all levels of nursing to the complexities of specialty areas, while incorporating the nursing process throughout. This text also refers to the 1992 approved listing of NANDA nursing diagnoses (see Appendix A for a complete listing). Although the LP/VN is not responsible for the formulation of a nursing diagnosis, the practical nurse does assist the registered professional nurse by collecting data essential to formulating a nursing diagnosis.

The text contains 12 chapters: Chapter 1 serves as an introduction to the use of the text and its contents; Chapters 2 through 5 deal with the basic sciences and the fundamental nursing concepts of the practical/vocational nursing curriculum; Chapters 6 through 11 cover the more complex nursing concepts encountered in the various specialty areas of nursing, such as medical-surgical nursing, obstetrics, pediatrics, gerontology, and emergency nursing; and Chapter 12 covers today's trends in nursing and health care in the United States and Canada.

In addition, each chapter (except Chapter 1) contains a set of questions that will help you determine how much you have learned in that particular area before you advance to the next chapter. A unique feature of this text is that rationales for both correct and incorrect answers are presented at the end of this book.

Two comprehensive tests are included in the text. Each contains 250 questions similar in style to those on the National Council Licensure Examination for Practical Nurses (NCLEX-PN). The correct answer and rationale for both the correct and incorrect answers are also given for these questions.

To make this text a truly complete and comprehensive review tool, we have included over 100 illustrations. The index permits easy location of specific information. Should you still feel the need to refer back to a text for further study, a bibliography is provided at the end of each chapter.

Although every effort was made to minimize duplication of material, the nature of some chapters required overlap. The focus of these topics, however, will differ based on the content.

For the sake of clarity and consistency the word *nurse* is used to indicate a practical/vocational nurse, and the feminine pronoun is used. The recipient of care is termed the *patient* to provide consistency as well, although we acknowledge that the term *client* may be preferred and has been used in some cases within this text.

The editor and constributors of this text have the utmost respect for and recognize the LP/VN as a valued member of today's health care team providing quality nursing care to patients nationwide. It is because of this respect and recognition that this text has been developed, with the hope that individuals preparing for entry or reentry into nursing at the practical/vocational nursing level will find a dependable source by which to prepare to become that valued member of today's health care team.

As coordinating editor, I would like to thank all those individuals who have worked so diligently in the preparation of this text, that is, all the contributors and consultants, as well as all those at Mosby, especially Susan Epstein, without whom this text would not have been possible. I would also like to extend a special note of thanks to my husband, Robert, for being so supportive of our efforts during the revision of this text.

To those who will use the text, we wish the very best as you enter into a service that will offer you the greatest satisfaction of all, the satisfaction of extending your hand to those in need.

Welcome to the caring profession—
welcome to nursing.

Mary Yannes-Eyles

Contents

Mosby's
Comprehensive Review of Practical Nursing

CHAPTER 1

Introduction for Students Preparing for the Licensure Examination

The practice of nursing is regulated by law in each state, the District of Columbia, Guam, Puerto Rico, and the Virgin Islands for the express purpose of public protection. The state board of nursing in each of the above is charged with upholding the regulation of such law. To do so each state board requires that qualified individuals take a licensing examination prepared by the National Council of State Boards of Nursing (NCSBN). Puerto Rico has developed its own licensing examination and does not use the one prepared by the NCSBN. However, content covered in its examination closely parallels that in the National Council Licensure Examination for Practical Nurses (NCLEX-PN). This book provides a valuable review tool regardless of the licensure examination taken. A special note appears at the end of this chapter for Canadian readers.

The NCLEX-PN covers all areas of the practical/vocational nursing curriculum and has been designed to test your nursing knowledge, including your ability to apply the principles of that knowledge to given clinical situations in a safe and effective manner. Periodic revision of the NCLEX-PN test plan can be expected because of the continually changing face of nursing. Nevertheless, such changes do not compromise your use of this text as you prepare for the licensing examination.

WHY REVIEW?

The purpose of this text is threefold: (1) to assist you in determining the extent of your nursing knowledge relative to your areas of specific strengths and weaknesses, (2) to increase your understanding of nursing knowledge through additional study, and (3) to increase your familiarity with and ability to respond to written test questions and corresponding clinical situations similar to those presented in the NCLEX-PN licensing examination.

The NCSBN's test plan for the NCLEX-PN encompasses two major components in which the practical/vocational nurse must participate to provide safe as well as quality care. Each component is vital to ensure the final intent of the examination: to protect the public through safe practitioners. The components as given in the actual test plan, including the percentage of questions allocated to the broad categories of each component, are provided later in this chapter.

EFFECTIVE STUDY

The key to effective study and the use of this text can only be determined by you. The review is presented in a manner that is easily adaptable to various forms of study habits, in addition to familiarizing you with timed tests/examinations.

Each chapter outlines a specific content area within the practical/vocational nurse curriculum, followed by a set of questions relative to that particular content area. The correct answers and the rationales for both the correct and incorrect

responses for each chapter are found in the rear of the text. In addition, each question is coded according to cognitive level, phase of the nursing process, client need, and level of difficulty.

You may want to start with the questions to determine areas in which you need more study and then return to review the outline of that particular chapter. Concentrate study efforts on those areas in which you scored low (i.e., less than 80% to 85% of the questions answered correctly). Should you need more in-depth study, you may refer to texts from the bibliography found at the end of each chapter, your own nursing texts, or current nursing journals.

Once you have completed the review and corresponding questions of all chapters, you are ready to take the two comprehensive examinations. Each comprehensive examination contains 125 questions and should take 2 hours to complete. Time yourself with your alarm clock or have someone else monitor your time.

As of April 1994, the NCLEX-PN examination will be administered via computerized adaptive testing (CAT), a change from the traditional paper-and-pencil method of testing. To effectively use this text in preparation for CAT, we suggest that you darken your answer choice on the chapter review questions and the comprehensive examination questions. Marking your answers in this manner permits you to focus all your concentration on answering the questions.

Candidates will be able to take the examination at their own pace. There is no set minimum amount of time for the examination; however, there is a maximum time of 5 hours. In addition to the questions at the end of each chapter, this review book contains two examinations, each having two parts, simulating the NCLEX-PN examination content. Each part of the examinations contains 125 questions, which should be completed in 2 hours. Even though time may no longer be a major concern during the examination, becoming more proficient in time-management skills will be to your advantage during the actual examination. Proper use of this text not only increases your nursing knowledge but also increases your self-confidence in your test-taking abilities.

Remember, intelligence plays a vital role in your ability to learn. However, being "smart" involves more than just intelligence. *Being practical and applying common sense* are also part of the learning experience.

Regardless of how you choose to study, following simple study guides may be helpful:
1. Establish priorities and the goals by which to achieve those priorities
2. Enhance organizational skills by developing a checklist and creating ways to improve your ability to retain information (e.g., index cards, which are easy to carry)
3. Enhance time-management abilities by designing a study schedule that best suits your needs, considering:
   - Amount of time needed
   - Amount of time available
   - "Best" time to study
   - Allowance for emergencies/free time
4. Prepare for study by considering:
   - Conducive environment
   - Appropriate study material
   - Planned study sessions alone or with friend/group
   - Formal review course

A note of warning: do not expect to achieve the maximum benefits of this text by cramming a few days before the examination. It doesn't work. Instead, organize planned study sessions, by yourself or with others, over a reasonable period of time in an environment that you find relaxing and conducive to learning.

TEST-TAKING SKILLS

By now you more than likely have been exposed to a variety of testing in both the objective and subjective forms. The licensing examination, however, deals only with the objective type and more precisely with the objective multiple choice form of testing. Although this form of testing may be familiar to you, let's take a look at how you can avoid some common test-taking errors:
1. Answer the question that is asked. To do so you need to read, not scan, the situation and the question carefully, looking for key words or phrases. Do not read anything into the question or apply what you did in a similar situation during one of your clinical experiences. Think of each question as pertaining to an ideal situation. No one is trying to trick you. Each question contains a stem (the main intent of the question), followed by four plausible answers or alternatives that either complete a statement or answer the question presented. Only one of the alternatives is the *best* answer; the remaining three alternatives are known as distractors, so named because they are written in such a way that they could be the correct answer and so distract you to a certain degree. However, your nursing knowledge will lead you to the correct answer.

For example:
   Which of the following hormones is secreted only during early pregnancy?
   - Estrogen
   - Progesterone
   - Human chorionic gonadotropin (HCG)
   - Follicle-stimulating hormone (FSH)

The correct answer is HCG. The alternatives are female hormones and are intended to distract you; however, the key phrase, "only during early pregnancy," is the clue to the correct answer.
2. Listen to the examiner and follow directions carefully. All candidates will be given a short training session, which includes a keyboard tutorial complete with a practice session. No prior computer experience is necessary. Should you have any question regarding the directions, ask the examiner for clarification.
3. Have confidence in your response to a question, because it probably is the correct answer. If you are unable to answer immediately, eliminate the alternatives you know are incorrect and proceed from there. Remember, although a time factor is not involved, don't spend an excessive amount of time on any one question. One minute is the recommended time allotted to any question. Not all questions consume a full minute; some may take only 20 or 30 seconds to read and answer. With CAT, skipping questions or going back to review and/or change responses is not possible. In fact, you must answer the question because you will not be able to continue with the examination until you do so.
4. Taking a wild guess at an answer should be avoided at all costs; however, should you feel insecure about a question, eliminate the alternatives you believe are definitely incorrect. This approach increases your chances of randomly selecting the correct answer. While there is no penalty for guessing on the NCLEX-PN examination, the subsequent question will be based, to an extent, on the response to a given question; that is, if you answer a question incorrectly, the computer will adapt the next question accordingly based on your knowledge/skill performance on the examination to that point.
5. Above all, begin with a positive attitude about yourself, your nursing knowledge, and your test-taking abilities. A positive attitude is achieved through self-confidence gained by studying effectively. Stated simply this means (a) answering questions (assessment), (b) organizing study time (planning), (c) reading and further study (implementation), and (d) again answering questions (evaluation).

Being emotionally prepared for an examination is also a key factor to your success; however, proper use of this text over an extended period ensures your understanding of the mechanics of the examination as well as increases your confidence about your nursing knowledge. Practicing a few relaxation techniques may also prove helpful, especially on the day of the examination.

Some additional advice before you begin your review sessions or take the licensing examination:
- Many times the correct answer is the longest alternative given; however, don't count on it. Individuals who prepare the examination are also aware of this fact and attempt to avoid offering you any such "helpful hints."
- Avoid looking for an answer pattern or code. Many times

four or five consecutive questions have the same letter or number for the correct answer.

- Key words or phrases in the stem of the question, such as *first, primary, early,* or *best,* are also important. Likewise, words such as *only, always, never,* and *all* in the alternatives are frequently evidence of a wrong response; as in life, there are no real absolutes in nursing. Of course, there are exceptions to every rule, so answer with care.
- Be alert for grammatical inconsistencies. If the response is intended to complete the stem (an incomplete sentence) but makes no grammatical sense to you, it could be a distractor rather than the correct answer. However, test developers try to eliminate such inconsistencies.
- Answering questions. You have at least a 25% chance of selecting the correct answer. Should you feel uncertain about a question, eliminate those choices you think are wrong and then call on your knowledge, skills, and abilities to choose from the remaining responses.
- The night before the examination you may wish to review some material, but then relax and get a good night's sleep. Remember to set your alarm or to have someone wake you. In the morning allow yourself plenty of time to dress comfortably, have breakfast, and arrive at the testing site a few minutes early. Be sure you know where to park and where the test will be given. Also, remember to take eyeglasses (if needed), your admission card, and second proof of identity. Being prepared will reduce your stress/tension level. Remember that *positive attitude.*

NCLEX-PN

The number of questions will vary in CAT and will be based on the candidate's performance, which measures knowledge, skills, and abilities. All successful candidates will answer no fewer than 75 questions or a maximum of approximately 195 questions within the 5-hour time frame. Rest periods (one mandatory after the first 2 hours of testing and one optional following the next 90 minutes of testing) and the computer tutorial are included as part of the 5-hour testing session. Tests are scored to determine the number of correct answers (raw score). The raw score is then equated to a standard score, which simply indicates where a candidate stands relative to the minimum passing score set by his or her particular state board of nursing. Scores reflect the "pass" or "fail" status of the candidate, with the majority of the boards using the same pass/fail score as determined via a statistical analysis by the NCSBN.

A candidate who fails will receive a diagnostic profile, which will assist in focusing further study efforts for retaking the examination.

The examination has been developed with the basic knowledge necessary for the practice of practical/vocational nursing, and contains test items reflecting the cognitive levels of knowledge, comprehension, and application.

The two major components of the test plan are (1) the phases of the nursing process and (2) client needs. Keep in mind that the elements of accountability, nutrition, anatomy and physiology, growth and development, documentation, communication, fundamentals, and patient education are included throughout the examination.

Please note that the NCLEX-PN examination may contain test items (questions) that are being validated for future NCLEX-PN examinations, which are not identifiable to the test taker. Whether you answer these questions correctly or

---

Test Plan for the National Council Licensure Examination for Practical Nurses

Percentage of items relative to the phases of the nursing process

Data collection (assessment) (30%)
Collects data in clients with predictable outcomes, which contributes to a data base as well as assists in the formulation of a nursing diagnosis
Planning (20%)
Contributes to the nursing care plan by assisting in setting of goals, identifying client needs (some of which may require a change in the plan of care), and communicating with all those involved in the client's care
Implementation (30%)
Covers performing of basic therapeutic and preventive nursing measures in a safe and effective environment that follow a prescribed plan to achieve established goals, which includes appropriate reporting and documenting of data, as well as assisting client, family, and other members of the health team in understanding the plan of care
Evaluation (20%)
Participates in evaluating effectiveness of care, observing and documenting client response to care and how/if identified outcomes have been realized

Percentage of items relative to client needs

Safe, effective care environment (24% to 30%)
Includes coordinated care; standards of care; goal-oriented care; environmental safety; preparation for treatment/procedures; safe and effective treatments/procedures
Physiologic integrity (42% to 48%)
Includes physiological adaptation; reduction of risk potential; mobility; comfort; and provisions of basic care
Psychosocial integrity (7% to 13%)
Includes psychosocial adaptation and coping skills
Health promotion/maintenance (15% to 21%)
Includes continued growth and development; self-care; integrity of support system; and prevention and early treatment of disease

Adapted from NCLEX-PN Test Plan for National Council Licensure Examination for Practical Nurses, 1989. Printed with the permission of the National Council of State Boards of Nursing, Chicago.

---

incorrectly, you *do not* gain or lose points. As already stated, these test items are being validated (tested) for use in future NCLEX-PN examinations.

In all likelihood, no two candidates will be given the same questions to answer, because the examination is individualized according to the candidate's knowledge and skills while meeting test plan requirements.

A SPECIAL NOTE FOR CANADIAN CANDIDATES

Nursing is regulated by law in each province in Canada. A designated body of nurses in each province has the responsibility for ensuring minimum standards of safe practice for nurses and practical/vocational nurses and thus ensuring the patient and the public a consistent standard of nursing care in any health care agency. To be allowed to practice as a practical/vocational nurse in Canada, qualified individuals are required to take a registration/licensing examination before receiving a certificate of competence. All provinces except Quebec use the examinations prepared by the Canadian

Nurses Association (CNA). Quebec uses its own examination. Examinations are available in both English and French.

The examination prepared by the CNA is given in two parts on 1 day. The examination is integrated and comprehensive. Each part consists of 120 to 130 multiple choice questions presented in situations and is timed at 2½ hours. Questions require either a single choice answer as used in this book, a multiple option, or a combination-response answer. The total examination is planned to test knowledge of safe practice, covering all areas of practical nursing across the life span. Your knowledge of the biologic, psychologic, and social sciences is tested, as well as your knowledge of nursing and your ability to apply principles from any area to given clinical situations. Most situations on the examination are based on situations similar to those encountered during your educational program. However, because of the diversity of nursing practice, you may come across situations with which you have had little if any opportunity for actual "hands on" experience. In these situations you must apply basic knowledge and principles. All participating provinces and territories have had opportunity for input into the preparation of the examinations; thus, they reflect common health problems encountered across the life span that are representative of practical/vocational nursing curricula across the country.

The CNA Blueprint for a Comprehensive Examination for Practical/Vocational Nurse Registration/Licensure identifies major concepts and content areas to be covered in the examination, as well as the use of all steps in the nursing process. In your review, study all areas covered in the examination and budget your time appropriately. This text has three main purposes: (1) to assist you in determining the extent of your nursing knowledge relative to your specific areas of strengths and weaknesses, (2) to increase the understanding of your nursing knowledge through additional study, and (3) to increase your familiarity with, and ability to respond to, written test questions and corresponding clinical situations. Although the situations in this text are geared to the American NCLEX-PN examination and therefore include questions on areas such as medication administration, intravenous infusion, and other therapeutic interventions that are not performed by all Canadian practical/vocational nurses, the majority of the situations and questions are directly applicable to all Canadian practical/vocational nurses. Using this text with your notes and other texts will focus your attention on the material applicable to your program, which is the bulk of the text. This text should not be used for last minute cramming but rather should be used as an adjunct to planned study and for practicing examination questions with instant feedback. Refer to sections on effective study and test-taking skills earlier in the chapter.

The following is adapted from the blueprint used for the practical/vocational nurse registration examination with permission from the Canadian Nurses Association, Ottawa, Canada.

Framework for the Development of Situations

1. Needs: this dimension is not weighted. Knowledge of all needs must be tested. Needs identified for the blueprint include

   a. Physiologic (primary) needs: oxygen, food/fluid, elimination, activity, sleep/rest, safety/comfort, sexuality
   b. Psychosocial (higher-level) needs: security, love and belonging, self-esteem
2. Factors affecting health: this dimension is not weighted. All categories affecting health must be tested in relation to common health problems. (Factors relating to common health problems include biologic, psychologic, sociocultural, mechanical, chemical, and thermal.)
3. Developmental stages: The weights assigned to the developmental stages are intended to reflect current practice of the practical/vocational nurse. Knowledge about each developmental stage must be tested.

Developmental stages	Percent of questions
Fetal (conception to birth)	
Infancy (birth to 1 year)	
Toddler (1 to 3 years)	
Preschool (3 to 5 years)	20%
School age (5 to 12 years)	
Adolescent (12 to 18 years)	
Early adult (18 to 30 years)	
Middle adult (30 to 65 years)	40%
Elderly adult (65 years and over)	40%

Content	
1. Professional aspects of nursing including professional responsibilities (legal and ethical), relationships, and communication.	5% to 10%
2. Body of nursing knowledge including principles and concepts from selected areas and nursing measures and the underlying rationale.	90% to 95%

Framework for development of objectives	Percent of questions
1. Nursing process: this dimension is not weighted. However, all steps of the nursing process should be reflected in the examination.	
2. Types of nursing care: this dimension is not weighted. However, both types of nursing care (preventive and therapeutic) should be reflected in the examination.	
3. Cognitive level	
Recall	5% to 10%
Comprehension	25% to 30%
Application	55% to 60%
Analysis	3% to 5%
Evaluation	

CONCLUSION

You started preparation for the licensing examination the first day you began your nursing program. Every lecture, quiz, examination, term paper, and clinical experience had definite purpose and meaning. This eleventh edition of *Mosby's Comprehensive Review of Practical Nursing* has been developed as a culmination of this preparation process. It is now in your hands, for only your initiative and dedication to achieving a long-awaited goal will be rewarded with success.

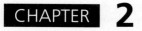

Basic Nursing Concepts and the Nursing Process

Nursing is an ongoing relationship with patients (clients) in various stages of the health-illness continuum and growth and development. Basic to nursing are knowledge of the patient as a person, factors contributing to health and illness, ability to use problem-solving techniques, and ability to perform nursing skills.

This chapter reviews the concepts basic to effective bedside care.

HEALTH-ILLNESS
Health Defined

A. According to the World Health Organization (WHO), health is "a state of complete physical, mental, and social well-being and not merely an absence of disease or infirmity"
B. According to Abraham H. Maslow, health exists when all human needs are satisfied
C. According to Hans Selye, health exists when an individual is in a relative state of adaptation to his or her environment

Illness Defined

A. No one definition
B. Illness exists when disease is present, when an individual believes he or she is ill, or when signs of illness are detected by the individual or the professional
C. Illness exists when all basic human needs are not satisfied
D. Illness is a state of disturbance of body structure or function or emotional or sociologic functioning

Health-Illness Continuum

A. An individual is rarely either totally healthy or totally ill
B. The individual's position is constantly changing in the balance between health and illness
C. The individual's position on the continuum is determined by need satisfaction, the stage of disease progression, and his or her perception of relative health or illness

FACTORS INFLUENCING HEALTH-ILLNESS
Growth and Development of the Adult

A. Growth is change in physical size and functioning
B. Development is change in psychosocial functioning
C. Growth and development progress from the simple to the complex and in orderly sequences
D. Individuals grow and develop at different rates
E. Most growth has occurred by adulthood
F. Certain tasks must be accomplished in each stage of development

G. Stages cannot be skipped; each must be accomplished before the next
H. Stages and tasks of adult development
   1. Young adulthood (18 to 40 years)
      a. Characteristics
         (1) The "prime" of biologic life
         (2) Reproductive capacity is at its height
         (3) A generally healthy period of life
      b. Tasks
         (1) Developing a set of personal moral values
         (2) Establishing a personal identity and lifestyle
         (3) Establishing intimate relationships outside the family
         (4) Establishing own family/support unit
         (5) Establishing a career: a field of work
         (6) Achieving independence
   2. Middle adulthood (40 to 65 years)
      a. Characteristics
         (1) Physical changes develop gradually: diminishing strength, energy, and endurance, wrinkles, graying and loss of hair, changes in vision, menopause, and weight increases
         (2) Beginning of chronic illnesses: cancer and heart disease
         (3) Decreased demands of parenthood, with children achieving independence
         (4) Increased demands of aged parents
         (5) Expected period of work and financial success
         (6) A period sometimes involving crisis: the "empty nest," realization that lifelong dreams are yet unmet
      b. Tasks
         (1) Adjusting to changes: physical, family, and social
         (2) Recognizing own mortality
         (3) Developing concern beyond the family: future generations and society in general

3. Older adulthood (over 65 years)
   a. Characteristics
      (1) Much variation in levels of functioning and health
      (2) Retirement often brings fixed income
      (3) Most are undergoing the normal physical changes of the aging process
      (4) Most maintain active lifestyles
   b. Tasks
      (1) Adjusting to loss of friends and family members
      (2) Adapting to the physical changes of the aging process
      (3) Adapting to psychosocial changes: relationships with children, retirement, housing
      (4) Review life and prepare for death
4. Development of the family
   a. Understanding the patient's role in the family, the influence of the family on the patient, and the developmental stage of the family helps to better understand the patient and his or her feelings and needs
   b. Characteristics
      (1) Traditional: wife, husband, and perhaps children
      (2) Nontraditional but common
         (a) Single parent (usually the mother) as a result of death, divorce, or never having been married
         (b) Communal: unrelated adults with or without children in a group setting
   c. Stages and tasks
      (1) Marriage stage
         (a) Establishing a home
         (b) Establishing individual responsibilities
         (c) Establishing a gratifying sexual relationship
         (d) Establishing good communication
      (2) Child-rearing stage
         (a) Taking on new responsibilities: financial and maintaining an optimal atmosphere for growth and development
         (b) Continuing efforts to maintain communication between all family members
         (c) Adapting to changes that occur as children become independent
      (3) Postparental stage
         (a) A crisis period caused by lifestyle changes, or
         (b) A relaxed period with fewer parental demands
         (c) More time available for hobbies and personal pleasures

Environmental Factors

A. Physical agents
   1. Heat: may lead to heat exhaustion or heat stroke
   2. Ultraviolet rays of the sun: produce sunburn

3. Cold: may cause hypothermia, frostbite, or even death, especially in the very young or very old
   4. Electric current: may cause shock, burns, or death
B. Chemical agents
   1. Taken accidentally or intentionally
   2. Taken by ingestion, such as medicine overdose
   3. Inhaled, such as gases, insecticidal sprays, and factory emissions
C. Infectious agents
   1. Microorganisms: small living organisms that can only be seen with a microscope
      a. Pathogens: disease-producing organisms
      b. Nonpathogens: organisms that do not usually cause disease
      c. Normal flora: microorganisms that normally live on or in an individual's body
   2. Types of microorganisms
      a. Bacteria
      b. Viruses
      c. Fungi
      d. Protozoa
D. Socioeconomic level
   1. Economic level may influence accessibility of health care
   2. Lack of social and economic resources may contribute to disturbed mental health
   3. Substandard living accomodations and sanitation may predispose to diseases such as tuberculosis
E. Cultural background: the beliefs and practices common to a group of people and passed down from generation to generation
   1. Cultural practices influence food habits, reactions to illness, family interactions, and health practices
   2. The nurse needs to be aware of patient's cultural practices and beliefs to meet needs in a way most beneficial to the patient
F. Religious background
   1. Religious practices may affect health practices
   2. Complying with a patient's religious practices may help reduce anxiety during illness
   3. Must be aware of the patient: may follow all, some, or none of the religion's practices; may turn to or completely away from them while ill
   4. The nurse must know the practices of the major religions and learn about others when the occasion arises to best meet the patient's needs (Table 2-1)

Internal Factors

A. Congenital factors
   1. Defined as being present at birth
   2. Defects may be hereditary, caused by malformation during intrauterine life, or a result of birth injuries
   3. Maternal contraction of German measles during the first trimester of pregnancy often results in congenital defects
   4. Certain drugs, including alcohol, are implicated in congenital defects
B. Hereditary factors
   1. Defined as being transmitted via the genes from parents to offspring
   2. Can produce conditions such as phenylketonuria (PKU), hemophilia, or sickle cell disease

Table 2-1. Common religious practices

Religion	Clergy	Sabbath	Practices
Judaism Reform Conservative Orthodox	Rabbi	Sundown Friday to sundown Saturday	Observation of Kosher laws Meat and dairy products not served at the same meal No pork products Only fish with scales may be eaten Circumcision of male child Are excused from dietary practices when ill
Protestantism Episcopal Methodist Presbyterian Baptist Others	Priest Minister	Sunday	Sacraments of baptism and communion
Catholicism Roman Others	Priest	Sunday	Sacraments of baptism, confession, communion, anointing of the sick (last rites) Critially ill infants may be baptized by the nurse Abstention from meat on Ash Wednesday and on Fridays during Lent (40 days from Ash Wednesday to Easter) Some still abstain from meat on all Fridays Many feel they must attend Mass each week—can be performed at the bedside
Jehovah's Witnesses	Every member is a minister	Sunday	Do not accept blood products
Seventh Day Adventists	Elder	Sundown Friday to sundown Saturday	Abstain from pork and pork products
Islam	Imam	Friday	Alcohol and pork and pork products are forbidden
The Church of Jesus Christ of Latter-day Saints (Mormons)	Elder	Sunday	Abstain from tobacco, coffee, tea, colas, alcohol

C. Body defense mechanisms
   1. Methods used by the body to protect itself from invasion by disease-producing substances
   2. First barriers are unbroken skin and mucous membranes
   3. Tears wash foreign particles including some microorganisms from the eyes
   4. The normally acid secretions of the vagina usually destroy pathogens
   5. Cilia (hairlike projections) in the nose, trachea, and bronchi sweep pathogens out of the respiratory tract
   6. Reflexes such as coughing and sneezing rid the body of pathogens
   7. Inflammatory reaction
      a. A local reaction that occurs when tissue is injured by physical agents, chemical agents, or microorganisms
      b. Signs: redness, heat, pain, swelling, and limited movement
      c. After an injury the inflammatory process begins: there is increased blood flow to the area; leukocytes move out of capillaries to the area; phagocytes begin to engulf and digest bacteria; pus forms from dead pathogens and dead tissue; healing begins
      d. Conditions caused by inflammation commonly end with the suffix *itis,* (e.g., vaginitis and cystitis)
   8. Immune response
      a. The body's response to the invasion of foreign protein substances: bacteria, viruses, foods, chemicals, and tissue
      b. Antigen: any invading substance that can trigger the immune response
      c. Antibody: proteins (gamma globulins) produced by the body to defend against the invading antigen

D. Immunity
   1. The state of being resistant to a particular pathogen
   2. Active immunity: occurs when the individual produces his or her own antibodies
      a. Results naturally after having had a specific disease such as chickenpox, or
      b. Acquired after the administration of
         (1) Vaccines made up of living or killed organisms such as the measles vaccine
         (2) Toxoids made up of neutralized toxins (poisons) produced by bacteria such as tetanus
   3. Passive immunity: results from receiving antibodies developed by another source (animal or human)
      a. Received naturally by fetus from mother: lasts only about 6 months
      b. Acquired from the administration of
         (1) Immune serum, usually from animals: provides short-term immunity to a specific organism such as that causing rabies
         (2) Gamma globulin, usually from humans: also provides short-term immunity to a specific organism such as hepatitis

4. Autoimmunity
   a. Antibodies are produced by the body against its own tissues
   b. Thought to be a factor in diseases such as rheumatoid arthritis and rheumatic fever
E. Fluid and electrolyte balance
   1. 50% to 60% of adult body weight is body fluid
   2. 75% to 80% of a young child's weight is body fluid
   3. Body fluids consist mostly of water
   4. Electrolytes are substances that when dissolved in water become electrically charged ions (Table 2-2)
   5. Amounts of fluid and electrolytes must be normal at all times for the body to be in homeostasis (a state of equilibrium)
   6. Fluids and electrolytes are present in "compartments" but constantly flow between the compartments to maintain balance (Fig. 2-1)
F. Tissue and wound healing
   1. Healing is affected by a person's general condition, age, nutritional status, the blood supply to the area, and extent of the injury
   2. Many injured tissues are repaired by cell regeneration: cells replaced by identical or similar cells
      a. Tissues of the skin, digestive and respiratory tracts, and bone regenerate well
      b. Nervous, muscle, and elastic tissues have little ability to regenerate
   3. When regeneration cannot take place, granulation tissue is formed, which eventually becomes a scar

4. Formation of scar tissue often leaves disfigurement, such as after burns, or diminished function, such as in heart tissue after myocardial infarction
5. Types of wounds
   a. Incision: clean wound made by sharp instrument
   b. Contusion: closed wound; bruise: made with blunt force; underlying tissue is damaged
   c. Abrasion: rubbed or scraped off skin or mucous membrane
   d. Puncture: small opening or hole made by a pointed instrument
   e. Laceration: tear or rip leaving jagged edges
6. Wound healing is classified by first, second, or third intention (Table 2-3)

CONCEPTS BASIC TO NURSING
Body Mechanics
A. Defined as efficient use of the body's structure and muscles
B. Applies to patients as well as nurses
C. Use of good body mechanics helps to prevent injuries, conserve energy, and prevent fatigue
D. Principles of good body mechanics
   1. Maintain proper alignment (posture): head, neck, and spine should be in a straight line with feet 10 to 12 inches (25 to 31 cm) apart and pointed straight ahead and knees slightly flexed (Fig. 2-2)
   2. Maintain a wide base of support: keep feet separated to provide balance (Fig. 2-2)

Table 2-2. Principal electrolytes

Principal electrolytes	Normal serum value	Problems associated with excess	Problems associated with deficit
Na⁺ (sodium)	135-145 mEq/L	Dry mucous membranes, thirst, restlessness (hypernatremia)	Confusion, weakness, coma (hyponatremia)
K⁺ (potassium)	3.6-5 mEq/L	Nausea, vomiting, diarrhea, irritability, cardiac standstill (hyperkalemia)	Weakness, cardiac arrhythmias (hypokalemia)
Ca⁺⁺ (calcium)	9-11 mg/dl	Nausea, vomiting, muscle weakness, death (hypercalcemia)	Muscle cramps, tetany, convulsions (hypocalcemia)

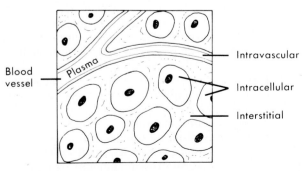

FIG. 2-1. Body fluid compartments. Intracellular, inside the cells; extracellular, outside the cells. Extracellular compartments may be either interstitial, between the cells, or intravascular, in the vessels.

Table 2-3. Wound healing

Healing by	Type of wound	How it heals
First intention	Minimal tissue damage / Simple incision	Without infection / No separation of wound edges / Results in minimal scar
Second intention	Decubitus ulcer / Severe burn	Wound edges do not join / Spaces between wound edges fill with granulation tissue / Results in scar
Third intention	Dehisced suture line	Wound edges come together at first, then reopen / Results in scar and possibly contraction of surrounding tissue

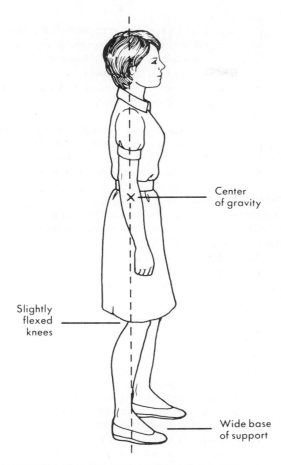

FIG. 2-2. Body alignment. Lateral view of adult with alignment of head, neck, spine, slightly flexed knees, and wide base of support. (Adapted from Sorrentino SA: *Textbook for nursing assistants,* ed 3, St Louis, 1992, Mosby.)

3. Keep center of gravity directly above the base of support (Fig. 2-3)

E. Points to remember
   1. Use largest and strongest muscles (legs, arms, and shoulders) when moving or lifting heavy objects (Fig. 2-3)
   2. Do not let your back do the work
   3. Roll, slide, push, or pull an object rather than lift it
   4. Keep objects close to your body when lifting or moving; avoid reaching, twisting or bending unnecessarily
   5. Point feet in the direction of movement
   6. Use devices whenever possible: patient lifters, trapeze, turning sheets, and rolling carts
   7. Get assistance when necessary
   8. Have the patient help as much as possible when being moved or lifted

Reducing the Spread of Microorganisms

A. Infectious disease chain
   1. Presence of pathogenic organisms
   2. A susceptible host: susceptibility affected by
      a. Nutritional status
      b. Age
      c. Personal health habits
      d. Medical treatments in progress (radiation therapy and bone marrow–depressing drugs)
      e. Trauma
      f. Chronic illness
      g. Stress
      h. Fatigue
   3. Portal of entry to the body: break in skin or mucous membrane, vaginal opening, or blood
   4. Reservoir: bladder, lungs, or throat

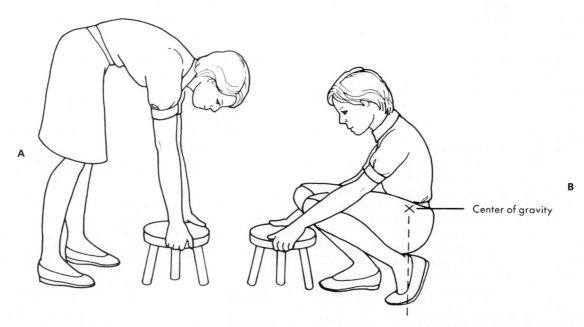

FIG. 2-3. A, Lifting with poor body mechanics: using back muscles. **B,** Lifting with good body mechanics: using leg muscles with object close to body. (Adapted from Sorrentino SA: *Textbook for nursing assistants,* ed 3, St Louis, 1992, Mosby.)

5. Modes of transmission (movement/spread) of microorganisms
   a. By contact (excreta or used tissues)
   b. By air, on droplets (sneezing and coughing)
   c. On fomites (books and stethoscopes)
   d. In food or water
   e. By vectors (animals and insects)
6. Portal of exit from the body: mouth, nose, rectum, skin, blood, or reproductive tract
B. Measures to reduce the spread by breaking the chain (interrupting the process)
   1. Hand washing: most important measure
   2. Medical asepsis: practices that limit the numbers, growth, and spread of microorganisms (clean technique)
      a. Linens: no shaking or holding against uniform
      b. Use of antiseptics and disinfectants
      c. Anything touching the floor is not to be used
   3. Surgical asepsis: practices that eliminate microorganisms and their spores from sterile items or areas (sterile technique)
      a. Used in operative procedures, delivery room, and caring for patients with breaks in skin and for procedures that enter sterile body cavities (e.g., bladder, lung, and vein)
      b. General principles
         (1) Sterile items become nonsterile (contaminated) when touched by anything that is not sterile
         (2) Sterile field that becomes wet is considered nonsterile
         (3) Sterile items out of eyesight or below waist level are considered nonsterile
         (4) Nurses need to develop a sterile conscience (self-judgment of whether aseptic practices have been broken) and act accordingly
      c. Means of sterilization
         (1) Steam under pressure: autoclave
         (2) Boiling
         (3) Liquid chemicals
         (4) Gas
   4. Isolation and barrier techniques (protective asepsis): practices that limit the transfer of microorganisms either from the infected person or to a highly susceptible person
      a. Category-specific isolation
         (1) Enteric: to reduce spread of pathogens via feces (e.g., hepatitis A)
         (2) Respiratory: to reduce spread of pathogens through the air (e.g., tuberculosis)
         (3) Strict: to reduce spread of pathogens by air or contact (e.g., chickenpox)
         (4) Drainage/secretion: to reduce spread of pathogens by contact with the infected person or contaminated articles (linens) (e.g., draining wounds)
         (5) Universal blood and body fluid: to protect from transmission by direct or indirect contact with infective blood or body fluids (e.g., AIDS)
         (6) Care of severely compromised patients: to protect a highly susceptible person (with lowered resistance) from becoming infected (e.g., leukemia)
      b. Disease-specific isolation: each disease receives its specific protective measures
C. Types of infections
   1. Nosocomial: acquired as a result of hospitalization
   2. Local: confined to a relatively small, specific area (e.g., a wound)
   3. Systemic: infection spreads throughout body

Communication

A. Definition: exchange of messages between two or more people, including information, thoughts, and feelings
B. Purposes in nursing
   1. To establish a meaningful, helping relationship between nurse and patient
   2. To transmit information between health care workers
C. Means
   1. Verbal
   2. Written
   3. Nonverbal
D. Guidelines
   1. Verbal communication
      a. Introduce self, stating name and title
      b. Be sincerely interested in the patient
      c. Be an attentive, active listener
      d. Stand or sit close to the patient
      e. Allow the patient to express thoughts and feelings freely without fear of being judged
      f. Clarify what has been said to ensure understanding
      g. Ask open-ended questions rather than questions resulting in yes or no answers: "what has happened to change your mind?"
      h. Use incomplete sentences: "you are afraid that . . ."
      i. Report information accurately and thoroughly
      j. Report abnormal findings immediately
      k. Maintain confidentiality
   2. Written communication
      a. Record information clearly, concisely, and accurately
      b. Nurses' notes are part of a legal document
         (1) Use pen
         (2) Use only standard abbreviations
         (3) Do not erase or obliterate errors (Fig. 2-4)
         (4) Leave no blank spaces
         (5) Sign the note at the time it is written
         (6) Date and time each entry
      c. Formats for nurses' notes
         (1) Narrative—in paragraph form

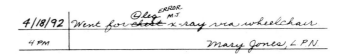

FIG. 2-4. Correcting an error in a nurse's note.

4/18/92	PROBLEM #6 — Drainage on Cast, Ⓛ
4 PM	lateral aspect of knee
	S — "I have no pain or numbness."
	O — Toes pink, warm, mobile. VS stable.
	A — Normal postoperative drainage.
	P — Mark area of drainage. Reassess
	patient and cast q ½ hr.
	Elaine Stevens, L.P.N.

FIG. 2-5. Nurse's note in SOAP format.

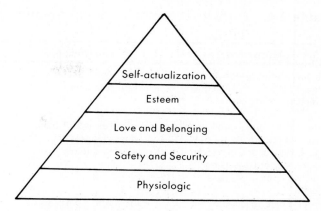

FIG. 2-6. Hierarchy of basic human needs as described by Maslow.

(2) SOAP: **S**ubjective data, **O**bjective data, **A**ssessment, **P**lan (Fig. 2-5)

(3) PIE: **P**roblem, **I**ntervention, **E**valuation

3. Nonverbal communication
   a. Exchanging messages by body posture, movements, gestures, and touch
   b. Often a more accurate expression of what is being thought or felt than verbal expression

BASIC HUMAN NEEDS

A. Definition: described by the psychologist Abraham Maslow as those needs that must be met for humans to function at their highest possible level
B. Used by many nurses as a systematic guide for assessment
C. Premises
   1. There is a hierarchy of needs; lower level needs must be met before higher level ones can be addressed
   2. People will usually be able to meet their own needs
   3. When people are unable to meet their own needs, intervention is required
   4. In caring for the whole person, the nurse is involved in helping to meet the basic needs as well as in dealing with signs and symptoms of disease
D. Hierarchy of needs (Fig. 2-6)
   1. Physiologic: oxygen, water, food, elimination, rest and sleep, activity, sexuality, and relief of pain
   2. Safety and security: protection from injury, maintenance of body defenses, structure and order in both the environment and relationships, and freedom from anxiety
   3. Love and belonging: not just romantic love but a feeling of affection (the need for caring relationships)
   4. Esteem: a feeling of worth and value to both self and others
   5. Self-actualization: reaching one's fullest potential

THE NURSING PROCESS

A. Definition: a set of predetermined steps used by nurses to identify and to help solve patient problems
B. Purposes
   1. To provide planned, coordinated, and individualized patient care
   2. To communicate problems and approaches among all those providing patient care

C. The process: names of steps differ slightly according to various sources but include the following
   1. Assessment: gathering and organizing of data; statement of patient problems (unmet needs); the nursing diagnosis
   2. Planning: setting goals to be accomplished and constructing a plan of action to accomplish the goals
   3. Implementation: carrying out the nursing actions to accomplish the goals and solve the problem (meet the need)
   4. Evaluation: determining whether the goal was accomplished and the problem solved
   5. Practical nurses' role in nursing process (Table 2-4)

Assessment: A Continuous Process

A. Sources of data
   1. Patient
   2. Family or significant others
   3. Patient's chart
      a. Physician's order sheet
      b. Nurses' notes
      c. Laboratory reports
         (1) Blood chemistry
            (a) Electrolytes: see fluid and electrolyte balance
            (b) Creatinine: assesses kidney function
         (2) Complete blood count (CBC): assesses adequacy of the various blood cells: red, white, and platelets
         (3) Blood sugar (BS) or glucose: fasting (FBS) or postprandial (after meals)
      d. X-ray reports
         (1) Chest x-ray examination: assesses condition of lungs and size of heart
         (2) Upper gastrointestinal (UGI) series: assesses condition of esophagus, stomach, and duodenum with barium sulfate used as the contrast medium
         (3) Barium enema (BaE): assesses condition of colon with barium sulfate used as the contrast medium
         (4) Gallbladder series (GBS): assesses condition of the gallbladder with radiopaque dye

Table 2-4. Entry level competencies in the use of the nursing process by the practical/vocational nurse

Assessment	Planning	Implementation	Evaluation
Obtains specific information from patients, through goal-directed interviews	Determines priorities and plans care accordingly	Uses basic communication skills in a structured care setting	Evaluates, with guidance if necessary, the care given and makes necessary adjustments
Participates in the identification of physical, emotional, spiritual, cultural and overt learning needs of patients by collecting appropriate data	Formulates and/or collaborates in developing written nursing care plans	Safely performs therapeutic and preventative nursing procedures, incorporating fundamental biologic and psychologic principles in giving individualized care	Records evaluations of the results of nursing actions
Analyzes data collected in relation to patients' pathophysiology	Participates in developing preventative or long-term health plans for patients and/or families	Observes patients and communicates significant findings to the health care team. Does incidental teaching and supports and reinforces the teaching plan for a specific patient and/or family	

Adapted from Statement of practical/vocational nursing entry level competencies prepared by the Education Committee of the National Association for Practical Nurse Education and Service, New York, 1980.

e. Electrocardiogram (ECG) reports: assesses the electrical activity of the heart
f. Biopsy reports: assesses a tissue specimen for cell changes
g. Progress notes of other health care workers
   (1) Physician
   (2) Social Worker
   (3) Dietitian
   (4) Physical therapist
   (5) Occupational therapist
   (6) Respiratory therapist
4. Nursing report
B. Subjective versus objective data
  1. Subjective data
     a. Information reported by the patient
     b. Information that is not observable by another person
     EXAMPLES
     Pain
     Nausea
     Anxiety
     Dizziness
     Ringing in the ears (tinnitus)
     Numbness
  2. Objective data
     a. Information gathered through the senses: sight, hearing, smell, and feel
     b. Information gathered with a measuring instrument: thermometer, sphygmomanometer, and scale
     EXAMPLES
     Vital signs
     Weight, height
     Hematuria
     Wheezing
     Edema
     Cyanosis

C. Methods of gathering data
  1. Formal interviewing (communication with patient or family or significant others): usually on patient's admission to the hospital
     a. Gather data on age, occupation, reason for hospitalization, medications, allergies, previous hospitalizations, previous illnesses, prostheses, valuables, and special diet
     b. Gather data on difficulty with activities of daily living (ADL), sleep, elimination, activity, eating, and any special needs
  2. Listening
  3. Observation of the patient and attached equipment
     a. Use an orderly approach
        (1) Head-to-toe
        (2) System-by-system
        (3) Basic human needs
     b. Look for signs and symptoms of disease or change in disease
  4. Physical examination
     a. Methods
        (1) Inspection
        (2) Palpation
        (3) Percussion
        (4) Auscultation
     b. Assisting with the physical examination
        (1) Be sure that the patient understands the examination and why it is being done
        (2) Gather equipment
        (3) Position patient appropriately (Fig. 2-7)
        (4) Drape covers to provide for privacy
        (5) Assist as necessary
        (6) After the examination make the patient comfortable and safe, following orders, if any
        (7) Chart the procedure and patient's reactions; note specimens obtained

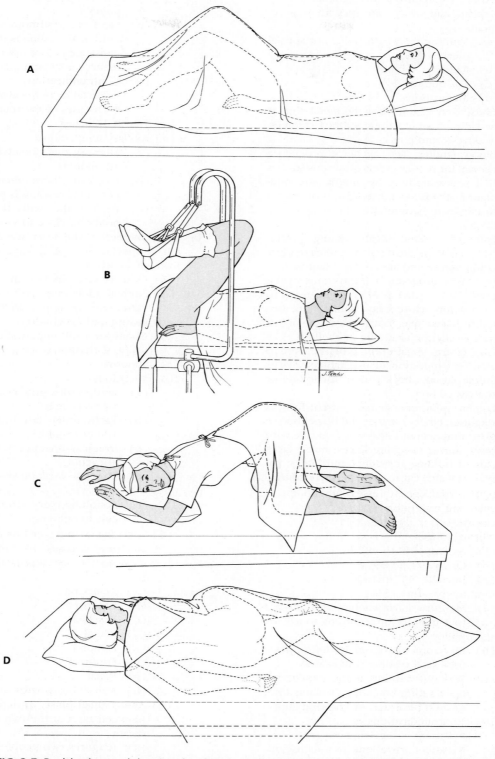

FIG. 2-7. Positioning and draping for the physical examination. **A,** Dorsal recumbent position. **B,** Lithotomy position. **C,** Knee-chest position. **D,** Sims' position. (Adapted from Sorrentino SA: *Textbook for nursing assistants,* ed 3, St Louis, 1992, Mosby.)

c. The practical nurse's role in assisting with diagnostic examinations
   (1) Explain procedure to the patient
   (2) Explain and carry out specific requirements
      (a) Nothing by mouth (NPO) or special meals
      (b) Clothing
      (c) Positioning
      (d) Medications
   (3) Chest x-ray examination: no metal objects in view of x-ray (zippers, bra fastenings, necklaces, and pins)
   (4) Blood studies: see agency's procedure manual for requirements of various studies
   (5) UGI series: nothing by mouth after midnight (NPO p̄ MN), medication or enema to eliminate barium after the x-ray examination
   (6) BaE: low-residue meal evening before, NPO p̄ MN, medications or enema to clear colon before and after x-ray examination
   (7) Excretory urogram or intravenous pyelogram (IVP): NPO p̄ MN, medications to clear colon before x-ray examination; uses iodine-based dye; notify physician if patient is allergic to iodine or shellfish
   (8) GBS: fat-free meal evening before, NPO p̄ MN, oral ingestion of dye tablets; dye is iodine based; check patient for iodine or shellfish allergy
   (9) Lumbar puncture: signed consent form is required; empty bladder and bowel before procedure; patient lies curled on side with head almost touching knees; nurse faces patient holding shoulders and knees; patient remains flat in bed after procedure

5. Measurement of vital signs: to assess functioning of cardiovascular and respiratory systems
   a. Temperature
      (1) Normal ranges
         (a) Axillary: 96° to 98° F
         (b) Orally: 97° to 99° F
         (c) Rectally: 98° to 100° F
      (2) Oral temperature
         (a) Mercury thermometer left in place 2 to 4 minutes or according to agency policy
         (b) Electronic thermometer left in place until final reading is indicated
         (c) Wait 10 minutes if the patient has been eating, smoking, drinking a hot or cold beverage, or chewing gum
         (d) Contraindications
            ■ Patient is receiving oxygen
            ■ Patient is irrational or unconscious
            ■ Patient is under 5 years of age
            ■ Patient is breathing through the mouth
            ■ Patient is prone to seizures
            ■ Patient recently had oral surgery or mouth trauma

      (3) Rectal temperature
         (a) Mercury thermometer held in place 3 to 4 minutes or according to agency policy
         (b) Electronic thermometer held in place until final reading is indicated
         (c) Lubricate before inserting; insert 1½ inches (3.75 cm)
         (d) Contraindications
            ■ Rectal or perineal surgery
            ■ Diseases of the rectum
            ■ Diarrhea
      (4) Axillary temperature
         (a) Mercury thermometer held in place 10 minutes
         (b) Electronic thermometer held in place until final reading is indicated
         (c) Pat dry the axilla before inserting; hold arm close to side
   b. Pulse: the beat of the heart heard at the apex or felt at specific sites as a wave of blood flows through an artery
      (1) Observe rate, rhythm, and strength
      (2) Normal adult range: 60 to 80 beats/min varies greatly among individuals; rate is more rapid for children
      (3) Count for 1 full minute if taking pulse apically, if rhythm is irregular, or if rate is abnormal
      (4) Variations
         (a) Bradycardia: slow heart rate—under 60 beats/min
         (b) Tachycardia: fast heart beat—over 100 beats/min
         (c) Irregular: intervals between beats are uneven
         (d) Thready: weak pulse—easily obliterated
         (e) Bounding: very strong pulse—difficult to obliterate
      (5) Sites: felt with finger tips at places where an artery crosses over muscle or bone close to the skin and at the apex of the heart
         (a) Temporal
         (b) Carotid
         (c) Brachial
         (d) Radial
         (e) Femoral
         (f) Popliteal
         (g) Pedal
         (h) Apical: heard with stethoscope
      (6) Apical-radial pulse: to detect a difference between rates at the two sites (the pulse deficit)
         (a) Requires two people: one taking the radial pulse and one taking the apical pulse
         (b) Must be counted simultaneously for 1 full minute
         (c) Apical rate can never be lower than the radial rate

c. Respiration: the process of inhaling and exhaling air into and out of the lungs; one inhalation plus one exhalation equals one respiration
   (1) Observe rate, rhythm, and depth; normal adult range is 14 to 20 respirations per minute; varies greatly with activity level; rate is higher for children
   (2) Patient must not be aware that respirations are being observed
   (3) Variations
      (a) Apnea: absence of breathing
      (b) Tachypnea: rapid breathing
      (c) Stertorous: noisy breathing—snoring
      (d) Cheyne-Stokes: rhythmic repeated cycles of slow shallow respirations increasing in depth and rate, then gradually becoming slower and more shallow, followed by a period of apnea; often precedes death
      (e) Dyspnea: difficulty breathing
      (f) Orthopnea: breathing is possible only while in an upright position
      (g) Kussmaul's: paroxysms of dyspnea often preceeding diabetic coma
   (4) Count respirations for 1 full minute if rate is abnormal or rhythm is irregular
d. Blood pressure (BP): force exerted by the blood against the walls of the arteries (measured in millimeters [mm] of mercury [Hg])
   (1) Normal adult range is 60 to 80 mm Hg diastolic, 90 to 120 mm Hg systolic, varies among individuals and with activity
   (2) Can be measured at brachial artery or popliteal artery
   (3) Be sure cuff is proper size for the individual
   (4) Terminology
      (a) Systolic: pressure in the arteries during contraction of the heart
      (b) Diastolic: pressure in the arteries during relaxation of the heart
      (c) Hypotension: lower than normal blood pressure—under 100/60
      (d) Hypertension: higher than normal blood pressure—over 140/90
      (e) Pulse pressure: difference between systolic and diastolic pressures

6. Measurement of weight and height
   a. Weight
      (1) Should be done before breakfast
      (2) Should be done in same amount of clothing each day: shoes should be off
      (3) Can use results in establishing medication dosages, gain or loss of body fluid, and nutritional status
      (4) Can use standing, chair, or stretcher scale; be sure scale is balanced
   b. Height
      (1) Have patient be in bare feet, standing on a paper towel
      (2) Have patient stand tall
      (3) Can use in determining some medication dosages and anesthesia requirements

7. Collection of specimens
   a. General guidelines
      (1) Follow your agency's procedure for collection, container, labels, requisitions, and recording
      (2) Label all specimen containers correctly and send with a laboratory requisition
      (3) Send specimens to the laboratory promptly
      (4) Wear protective gloves
      (5) Wash hands thoroughly after handling specimen
   b. Urine specimens
      (1) Urinalysis: routine examination of urine
         (a) Patient and container need only be clean
         (b) Often collected as part of admission procedure
      (2) Culture and sensitivity
         (a) Clean-catch, midstream: genitalia and meatus are cleansed; specimen is taken after stream has started but before voiding is completed
         (b) Catheterized specimen: by using sterile technique and equipment
      (3) 24-hour specimens: first voiding is discarded and time is noted; all urine for the next 24 hours is collected; see agency policy for type of container and storage methods
      (4) Sugar and acetone testing
         (a) Urine should be obtained 30 to 60 minutes before meal or at designated time
         (b) Double-voided specimen gives more accurate results
            ▪ Have patient empty bladder
            ▪ Collect specimen as soon as patient can void again
            ▪ May need additional fluids to produce specimen
         (c) Test specimen with Tes-tape, Clinitest, Clinistix, or Keto-diastix; follow manufacturer's directions precisely for accurate results
         (d) Report results immediately to medication nurse
         (e) Record results in proper place
      (5) Specimens from indwelling catheter
         (a) Closed drainage system must be maintained
         (b) Specimens must be obtained from specimen "port" with needle and syringe by sterile technique
   c. Stool specimens
      (1) Collect in clean bedpan
      (2) Use tongue depressor or wooden spatula to transfer stool to specimen container
      (3) Types of testing
         (a) For blood: occult (guaiac, Hematest); patient may be on a red meat–free diet 3 days before test
         (b) For culture and sensitivity: use sterile container

(c) For ova and parasites: stool must still be warm when it reaches the laboratory

d. Sputum specimens
(1) Best collected in the morning before breakfast
(2) Patient first rinses mouth with water
(3) Instruct patient to take deep breath, cough deeply, and expectorate into container
(4) Specimen must be from the lung, not just mouth saliva

e. Blood specimen: capillary puncture for blood glucose testing—usually requires agency certification
(1) Explain procedure to patient; warn that it does hurt
(2) Assemble equipment: gloves, alcohol swab, lancet, collector, gauze or cotton ball, and adhesive bandage
(3) Wash hands; don gloves
(4) Enhance blood supply to puncture site by "milking" or applying warmth—use finger on nondominant hand when possible
(5) With gloved hands, swab site with alcohol; let alcohol dry
(6) Puncture with lancet; collect blood (some devices require the first drop of blood to be wiped away before collecting sample)
(7) Apply pressure to site; apply adhesive bandage

f. Other specimens
(1) Vomitus: may be tested for blood
(2) Gastric analysis: examination of stomach contents; obtained by aspirating from nasogastric tube
(3) Wound drainage: if infection is suspected

D. Statement of patient problems requiring nursing intervention
1. Identifying unmet basic human needs resulting in a problem for the patient
2. Identifying problems arising from the patient's signs and symptoms
3. Actual problems: those that the patient is currently having
4. Potential problems: those that may develop and need to be prevented from occurring (see the example below)

E. Nursing diagnosis: the practical nurse assists the registered nurse in formulating nursing diagnosis

---

EXAMPLE: Actual and potential unmet basic needs and problems

Situation: At 7 AM, Mrs. Clayton tells the nurse that she has a productive cough. She states that it began at about 3 AM and continues.

Actual problem: productive cough
Actual unmet need: rest and sleep
Potential unmet need: oxygen
Potential problem: decreased oxygen

Planning Patient Care

A. Definition: process of setting priorities, determining patient-centered goals, and deciding on nursing actions to achieve the goals; ends with writing of the nursing care plan

B. Setting priorities
1. Problems that are life threatening are of highest priority
2. When no single problem seems more important than the others, the patient may help determine priorities

C. Determining goals/expected outcomes
1. Stated in terms of patient behavior so that achievement can easily be evaluated
2. Whenever possible patients should be involved in setting goals
3. Long-term goals are those hoped for in the future, usually set by the registered nurse
4. Short-term goals are those sought immediately or in the near future

D. Decisions about which nursing measures to use are based on sound knowledge of current nursing practice, principles, rationales, and judgment

E. Written nursing care plan provides continuity of patient care (see the example below)

Implementation of Nursing Measures

A. Principles
1. Preparation
a. Nurse: must know how, when, and why measure is to be performed, checking for a physician's order when necessary
b. Patient/family/significant others
(1) To reduce anxiety, patients need to know what measure is to be performed and why, as well as what is expected of them
(2) May need special preparation for the specific measure: positioning, medications, attire
c. Have all necessary equipment ready and in working order
2. Performance
a. Nurse must have knowledge of and ability to perform measure and to seek help when necessary
b. Medical asepsis is always followed: surgical asep-

EXAMPLE: Nursing care plan for 39-year-old woman 4 days after cesarean section

Problem	Goal	Nursing actions
Constipation × 4 days	Will have a stool today and at least every other day thereafter	Encourage walking Encourage fluids to at least 2500 ml/day Encourage eating roughage and fruits Give prn laxative Record bowel movements (BMs) in nurses' notes every shift Teach patient relationship of activity, fluids, and fiber to stool elimination

sis and universal precautions are followed as required
   c. Work must be organized to conserve nurse's and patient's energy and to meet patient's need for security
   d. Assessment of patient's response to the measure is ongoing
3. Aftercare
   a. Patient made safe and comfortable
   b. Equipment cleaned and returned to proper place or disposed of
   c. Evaluation of results of the measure and whether it helped achieve the goal
4. Reporting and recording
   a. Significant observations immediately
   b. When the measure was performed and the results

Evaluation of Plan of Care

A. Criteria for evaluation
   1. Has the need been met?
   2. Is the problem solved or being solved?
   3. Has the goal/expected outcome been achieved?
B. Revision of the nursing care plan
   1. Based on evaluation of effectiveness
   2. Practical nurse collaborates with the registered nurse in revising problem list, goals, and nursing measures

MEASURES TO MEET OXYGEN NEEDS

A. Assessment: color, level of consciousness, vital signs, presence of cough (productive or nonproductive), nature of sputum (amount, consistency, and color), and energy level
B. General measures
   1. Encourage exercise and activity to help expand lungs, providing better oxygenation
   2. Bedridden patients must be turned and positioned every 2 hours (q2h) to prevent pooling of secretions in the lungs
   3. Encourage coughing and deep breathing at least q2h for inactive or bedridden patients to help with oxygenation and bringing up secretions
   4. Ensure adequate fluid intake to keep secretions thin, thus easier to expectorate
C. Use of nebulizer (aerosol)
   1. Method of delivering medications directly to the respiratory tract
   2. Nebulizer breaks liquids into a mist of droplets, which are inhaled
D. Incentive spirometer: to improve inspiratory volume
   1. With lips sealed around a mouthpiece, the patient takes a deep breath, holds it for 3 seconds, and slowly exhales
   2. The spirometer indicates with a light or small plastic balls reaching an indicated level whether the patient has inhaled the desired volume
E. Intermittent positive pressure breathing therapy (IPPB)
   1. Forces the patient to inhale more deeply, allowing better oxygenation and loosening of secretions
   2. May be attached to oxygen or compressed air
   3. Humidity is provided, usually by normal saline solution
   4. Medications may be added

5. Patient should be sitting up during treatment and encouraged to cough up secretions after treatment
F. Chest physical therapy
   1. Postural drainage: use of various positions so that gravity can assist in removal of secretions (Fig. 2-8)
   2. Percussion is a manual technique of striking the chest wall over the affected area with cupped hands in a rhythmic motion
   3. Vibration is a manual compression and tremorlike motion with hands or mechanical device against chest wall of affected area done during exhalation
   4. Nurse positions patient so affected areas are vertical and gravity can assist in drainage
   5. Position also depends on diagnosis and condition
   6. Nurse provides emesis basin and tissues and gives oral hygiene after treatment
   7. This therapy is contraindicated in patients with lung abscess or tumors, pneumothorax, and diseases of the chest wall
G. Suctioning: oral, nasopharyngeal, or tracheal
   1. To remove accumulated secretions blocking airway or to obtain sputum specimen
   2. Usually a sterile procedure
   3. Introduce catheter gently; do not apply suction while introducing catheter
   4. Suction intermittently for no more than 10 seconds
   5. Slowly withdraw catheter by rotating motion while suctioning continues
   6. Unless there are copious amounts of secretions, wait 30 seconds between suctionings
   7. Repeat procedure until all excess secretions are removed
   8. Administer oxygen before and between suctionings if needed
H. Administration of oxygen
   1. Safety precautions
      a. Caution patients and visitors that smoking is prohibited
      b. Post warning sign on door or bed: NO SMOKING— OXYGEN IN USE
      c. Do not use heating pads, electric blankets, or electric razors
      d. Do not use woolen blankets
      e. Secure oxygen tanks so they do not tip over
   2. Physician's order is required for method of administration, rate of oxygen flow, or concentration
   3. Oxygen must always be humidified
   4. Nasal cannula; prongs fit into nares
      a. Turn oxygen on and check flow through prongs before positioning on patient
      b. Adjust strap after placing cannula on patient
      c. Periodically check that there is sufficient water in humidity source
      d. Periodically check patient's nares and behind ears for pressure
      e. Periodically assess patient for changes in condition
   5. Oxygen by mask: simple; Venturi (delivers oxygen in precise concentrations)
      a. Proceed as with nasal cannula
      b. Fit mask snugly to face and adjust strap
      c. Periodically assess patient and equipment as with nasal cannula

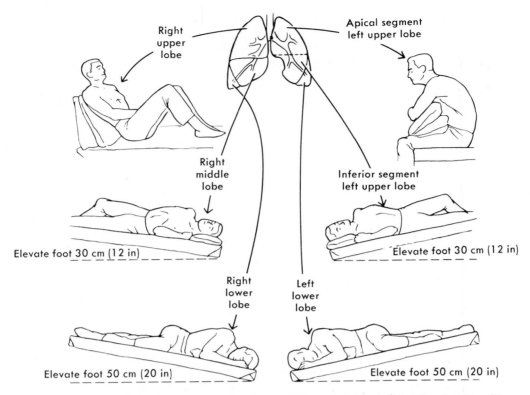

FIG. 2-8. Positions for postural drainage. (From Phipps WJ, Long BC, Woods NF, editors: *Medical-surgical nursing: concepts and clinical practice,* ed 4, St Louis, 1991, Mosby.)

I. Care of patient with a tracheostomy
1. Tracheotomy: opening into the trachea
2. Tracheostomy: tube inserted into tracheal opening
3. Tube is either metal or plastic, which is usually cuffed (Figs. 2-9 and 2-10)
4. Tube is held securely in place with cotton ties around the neck (Fig. 2-11)
5. Ties are changed with extreme caution to prevent patient from coughing out tube
6. A gauze dressing is placed under the tube to absorb secretions and must be changed at least every shift
7. Inner cannula is removed, cleaned with peroxide and pipe cleaners, and rinsed with normal saline at least once a shift by sterile technique; commercially prepared kits are available
8. Skin around stoma is cleansed with peroxide, rinsed with saline, and assessed at least once a shift
9. Patient is often apprehensive and needs frequent reassurance
10. Tube must be suctioned frequently
J. Medication classifications: refer to Chapter 4 for more detailed information on drugs that affect the respiratory system
1. Respiratory stimulants
2. Respiratory depressants
3. Those acting on mucous membranes: administered orally or as spray or vapor
   a. Mucolytics
   b. Expectorants
4. Bronchodilators

MEASURES TO MEET FLUID NEEDS

A. Assessment: daily weights, comparison of intake and output, appearance of urine, presence of edema, fluid preferences, and skin turgor
B. Fluid excess (edema)
1. Associated with heart and kidney disease: body unable to rid itself of excess fluid
2. Can result from excessive intravenous (IV) fluids
3. Observed as edema as well as weight gain and reduced urine output
4. Sites of edema: eyes, fingers, ankles, and sacral area
C. Fluid deficit (dehydration)
1. Associated with inadequate fluid intake, diarrhea, excessive perspiration, vomiting, bleeding, and increased urine output
2. Observed as dry skin and mucous membranes, thick mucus, poor skin turgor, behavioral changes, or changes in vital signs
D. Measuring intake and output
1. Measure all fluids taken in: IV, tube feedings, and obvious fluids such as water, milk, ice cream, gelatin, custard, and soup
2. Measure all fluids leaving the body: urine, vomitus, diarrhea, gastric secretions, and blood
3. Know capacity of agency's fluid containers
4. Set measuring containers on level surface to read measurements accurately
5. Record and total amounts in appropriate places
E. Administering IV fluids
1. Assess site of needle insertion

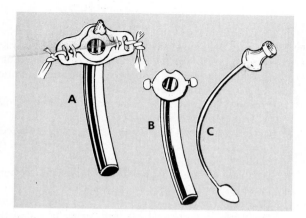

FIG. 2-9. Metal tracheostomy tube. **A,** Outer cannula. **B,** Inner cannula. **C,** Obturator. (From Hood GH, Dincher JR: *Total patient care: foundations and practices,* ed 8, St Louis, 1992, Mosby.)

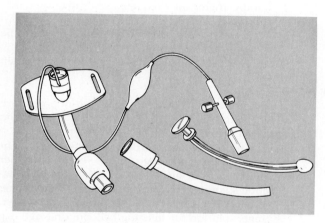

FIG. 2-10. Cuffed tracheostomy tube. (From Hood GH, Dincher JR: *Total patient care: foundations and practices,* ed 8, St Louis, 1992, Mosby.)

a. Infiltration: fluid entering subcutaneous tissues instead of vein; area is pale, cool, and swollen
b. Phlebitis: inflammation of vein; area is red, warm, and swollen
2. Assess tubing: no kinks; no leakage along entire length of tubing; tubing should be changed every 24 hours
3. Assess rate of flow
4. Assess container
a. It must match physician's order
b. Check that the amount absorbed is on schedule
F. Medication classifications—diuretics: refer to Chapter 4 for more detailed information

MEASURES TO MEET NUTRITIONAL NEEDS

A. Assessment: weight/height ratio, weight changes, skin and mucous membranes, food preferences, meal patterns, ability to eat, and appetite
B. Preparing for meals
1. Environment
a. Control odors, noise, and unpleasant sights; remove soiled equipment and linens
b. Avoid stressful situations before and during mealtime
2. Patient
a. Provide oral hygiene and opportunity for elimination and hand washing
b. Position comfortably, preferably in sitting position
3. Meal tray
a. Ensure correct tray for correct patient
b. Arrange tray to be accessible to patient
c. Assist in opening containers, removing covers, and cutting and preparing food
d. Serve trays first to patients able to feed themselves
C. Assisting the patient to eat
1. Place napkin across chest
2. Explain what foods and liquids are on the tray

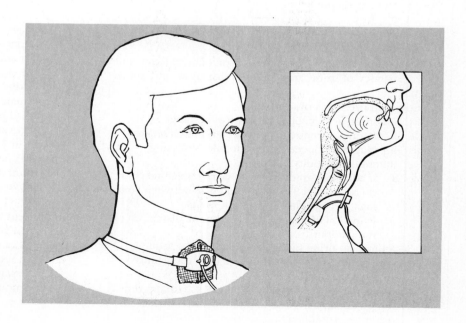

FIG. 2-11. Tracheostomy tube in place. (From Hood GH, Dincher JR: *Total patient care: foundations and practices,* ed 8, St Louis, 1992, Mosby.)

3. Prepare foods and feed in order of patient's preference
4. Encourage the patient to assist as much as possible
5. Do not rush: allow time to chew and swallow
6. Talk with the patient during meal
7. Provide opportunity for handwashing and oral care

D. Gastric gavage (tube feeding)
   1. Used when patient is unable to eat, swallow, or take in adequate quantities of food
   2. Blended foods and fluids (commercially or agency prepared) are passed to the stomach through a nasogastric tube either intermittently or by slow continuous drip
   3. Check amount, frequency, and type ordered by physician
   4. Feeding must be at room temperature before administering
   5. Placement of tube must be checked before feeding begins
      a. By aspirating stomach contents with a syringe
      b. Inject 10 cc of air into tube while simultaneously listening with a stethoscope over the stomach to hear a whooshing sound
   6. Place patient in sitting position
   7. Administer feeding slowly: 200 ml during 30- to 45-minute period
   8. Feeding should be followed by ordered amount of water
   9. Clamp tube after completion of feeding to prevent air entering stomach
   10. If nausea, vomiting, diarrhea, or cramps occur, rate may be too fast or patient may be intolerant of feeding or volume
   11. Tube may be left in place between feedings or removed after each feeding as ordered by physician
   12. Have patient remain in sitting position for 45 minutes to help prevent aspiration

E. Medication classifications: refer to Chapter 4 for more detailed information
   1. Vitamin supplements
   2. Mineral supplements

MEASURES TO MEET URINARY ELIMINATION NEEDS

A. Assessment: intake/output ratio, color, odor, amount, and consistency of urine, frequency of urination, and continence

B. Common problems of urination
   1. Incontinence: inability to control voiding
      a. Requires frequent skin care and linen change
      b. May be reduced with scheduled toileting
   2. Retention: inability to void
      a. If adequate amounts of fluid have been taken in, no more than 8 hours should pass between voidings, except during sleeping hours
      b. Palpation of bladder can determine distention of full bladder
   3. Anuria: no urine being produced by the kidneys
   4. Dysuria: difficult or painful urination ("burning")

C. Assisting with urination
   1. Offer bedpan or urinal at regularly scheduled times
   2. Keep bedpan or urinal and toilet tissue within easy reach for patients who can assist themselves

3. Keep call signal within easy reach
4. Provide privacy
5. Hearing the sound of running water or having warm water poured over the perineum may induce voiding
6. Provide opportunity for hand washing after urination

D. Care of patient with retention catheter
   1. Presence of indwelling catheter greatly predisposes patient to urinary tract infection
   2. Opening a closed urinary system is to be avoided
   3. Drainage container must be kept below level of the bladder but must not touch the floor
   4. Drainage tubing must be free of kinks and catheter taped to patient's leg allowing slack
   5. Drainage container is emptied at end of shift or if container becomes nearly full; urine is measured, assessed, and amount recorded
   6. Catheter care is given at least once per shift
      a. Meatus and catheter are cleansed with soap and water
      b. Removal of crusts and secretions from meatus and catheter may require use of hydrogen peroxide
      c. A bacteriostatic ointment is often ordered to be applied to the meatus
   7. Unless contraindicated, fluid intake should reach 2000 to 3000 ml/24 hr

E. Catheterization
   1. "Straight": catheter is removed at end of procedure
   2. Indwelling, retention or Foley: catheter is left in place in bladder
   3. Assemble equipment: sterile catheterization tray or disposable kit containing catheter, basin, container with lid (for specimen, if ordered), cotton balls, antiseptic solution, lubricant, sterile gloves, and drape
   4. For indwelling catheterization, add Foley catheter, syringe, solution for inflating balloon, drainage bag with tubing, and tape for securing catheter
   5. After explaining procedure to patient and ensuring privacy, place female in dorsal recumbent position and male in supine position
   6. Place equipment between patient's legs; using sterile technique open package, don gloves, and place drapes
   7. For female patient, while holding labia apart, cleanse vulva and meatus well going from front to back toward vagina; use cotton ball for one stroke only before discarding
   8. For male patient, cleanse around penis from meatus toward base using each cotton ball once around
   9. Insert catheter into meatus (3 to 4 inches [7.5 to 10 cm] in female and 6 to 8 inches [15 to 20 cm] in male) until urine flows; drain urine (no more than 750 ml at one time to prevent bleeding or shock); remove catheter ("straight") or inflate balloon and connect drainage tubing (indwelling)

F. Intermittent bladder irrigation (hand bladder irrigation)
   1. To rid bladder and catheter of clots or mucus; to instill antibiotic or other solutions
   2. Open technique
      a. Assemble equipment: sterile solution (type and amount as ordered), sterile container for solution, bulb syringe, and basin for return flow
      b. Disconnect catheter from drainage tube over

empty basin; protect ends from contamination
  c. Allow solution to flow in by gravity or gentle pressure; drain by gravity or gentle suction; repeat until returns are clear or ordered amount of solution has been used
  d. Subtract amount of solution used from amount of returns; record output
3. Closed technique
  a. Assemble equipment: 20- to 30-ml syringe with needle, alcohol swabs, solution ordered, and clamp
  b. Draw solution into syringe by sterile technique
  c. Clamp tubing distal to needle entry port
  d. Cleanse resealable rubber entry port on drainage tubing with alcohol swab
  e. Insert needle into port
  f. Inject fluid into catheter
  g. Remove needle
  h. Release clamp and allow fluid to drain into drainage bag
  i. Observe fluid return
  j. Repeat until ordered amount of solution has been used
  k. Empty drainage bag, subtracting amount of irrigant from total; record urine output
G. Continuous bladder irrigation (through and through or three-way irrigation)
  1. To prevent clot formation; to reduce obstruction of catheter; to circulate antibiotic or other solutions continuously in bladder
  2. Equipment: patient has three-way catheter or needs sterile Y tube connector attached to regular two-way catheter's drainage channel; large bottle or bag of solution, with tubing attached, hanging from IV pole
  3. With three-way catheter: using sterile technique
    a. Remove plug from irrigating channel; protect plug and tubing from contamination
    b. Insert solution tubing into irrigating channel
  4. With two-way catheter: using sterile technique
    a. Attach single end of sterile Y tube connector to catheter
    b. Attach drainage tubing to one end of Y
    c. Attach solution tubing to other end of Y
  5. Start solution flow at rate ordered by physician
  6. Observe fluid return through drainage tubing
  7. Replace solution bottle or bag as it becomes nearly empty
  8. Empty drainage container as it becomes nearly full and when solution container is replaced
  9. Subtract amount of irrigant solution from total amount of drainage to record actual urine output
H. Removal of indwelling catheter
  1. Assemble equipment: syringe without needle, underpad, basin, urinal or bedpan, toilet tissue, and protective gloves
  2. After explaining procedure and ensuring privacy, place pad under patient
  3. Remove tape from catheter and patient's leg
  4. Put on protective gloves
  5. Place basin under patient's meatus
  6. Insert syringe into balloon channel; fluid will return on its own
  7. After all fluid has returned, gently pull on catheter to remove it
  8. If resistance is met, stop and obtain assistance
  9. Assist patient to wash perineum
  10. Teaching
    a. Patient should continue to drink fluids
    b. Burning on urination may occur during first few voidings
    c. Complete continence and normal voiding pattern may take awhile to return
    d. Patient should void into bedpan or urinal so that urine can be assessed
  11. Encourage relaxation: anxiety may inhibit ability to void
  12. Continue to assess bladder distention, intake/output ratio, and patient complaints until normal patterns of elimination are achieved
I. Medication classifications
  1. Cholinergics: to induce bladder contraction (bethanechol [Urecholine] and neostigmine [Prostigmin])
  2. Anticholinergics: to reduce bladder spasms and urinary frequency (methantheline [Banthine] and flavoxate hydrochloride [Urispas])

MEASURES TO MEET BOWEL ELIMINATION NEEDS

A. Assessment: the patient's pattern of elimination; amount, color, consistency, odor, and shape of stool; patient's activity level; amount and type of food and fluid intake; passage of flatus; abdominal distention
B. Common problems of elimination
  1. Constipation: passage of dry, hard feces
  2. Diarrhea: frequent passage of liquid or unformed stools
  3. Impaction: formation of a hardened mass of stool in the lower bowel forming an obstruction to the passage of normal stool; often characterized by the frequent seepage of small amounts of liquid stool
  4. Abdominal distention: swollen abdomen caused by retention of flatus in the intestines
C. General nursing measures
  1. Encourage intake of roughage in the diet: fresh fruits and vegetables and whole grain breads and cereals
  2. Encourage intake of adequate amounts of fluids unless contraindicated: 2000 to 3000 ml/day
  3. Encourage maximum amount of physical activity
  4. Encourage patient to respond to the urge to defecate
  5. Position patient comfortably and provide adequate time and privacy for elimination
  6. Provide access to call signal and toilet tissue
  7. Provide opportunity for handwashing after elimination
D. Rectal tube
  1. To assist in expelling flatus
  2. Assemble equipment: rectal tube with flatus bag or waterproof pad, lubricant, glove, and tape
  3. After explaining procedure and providing privacy, position patient in side-lying (Sims') position
  4. With gloved hand insert lubricated tube 2 to 4 inches (5 to 10 cm) into rectum
  5. Tape tube to patient's buttock and leave in place no longer than 20 to 30 minutes
  6. Note passage of flatus or stool; report and record findings

E. Rectal suppository
1. Purposes
    a. To stimulate peristalsis and stool elimination
    b. To soothe painful rectum or anus
2. Assemble equipment: suppository as ordered, glove, bedpan, and toilet tissue
3. Suppository begins to melt at room temperature, providing its own lubrication
4. Separate buttocks and with gloved index finger insert pointed end of suppository into anus
5. Gently insert 3 to 4 inches (7.5 to 10 cm) into rectum
6. Hold buttocks together until initial urge to defecate has passed
7. Best results occur within 30 minutes
F. Commercially prepared prefilled enema
1. To promote bowel or flatus movement
2. Assemble equipment: enema (usually 120 ml), underpad, bedpan, toilet paper and gloves
3. After explaining procedure and providing privacy, place patient in side-lying (Sims') position
4. With gloved hand insert prelubricated tip of enema to the hub and squeeze container until most of solution is instilled
5. Encourage patient to retain solution until urge to defecate is felt
6. Place call signal, bedpan, and toilet tissue within easy reach
7. If patient uses toilet, instruct not to flush so that results can be assessed
G. Oil-retention enema
1. To soften and lubricate stool, promoting easier passage
2. Often followed by cleansing enema
3. Equipment and administration are the same as for commercially prepared enema above
4. Encourage patient to retain oil 30 to 60 minutes
H. Cleansing enemas
1. To relieve constipation or flatus or to cleanse the bowel before diagnostic procedures, surgery, or childbirth
2. Solutions used as ordered by physician
    a. Tap water: can cause fluid and electrolyte imbalance
    b. Soap solution: 5 ml of liquid soap to 1000 ml of water; can irritate mucous membranes of bowel
    c. Saline solution: can cause fluid and electrolyte imbalance
3. Assemble equipment: disposable enema kit containing enema bag, tubing with clamp, liquid soap, and lubricant; waterproof underpad; solution at a temperature no greater than 105° F; bedpan and toilet tissue; IV pole; protective gloves
4. After explaining procedure and providing privacy, place patient in side-lying (Sims') position (usually left)
5. Put on protective gloves.
6. Insert lubricated tubing about 3 to 5 inches (7.5 to 12.5 cm) into rectum
7. With bottom of enema bag hanging 12 inches (30 cm) above anus or 18 inches (45 cm) above mattress, slowly administer 500 to 1000 ml of solution

8. If patient complains of cramping or has difficulty retaining solution
    a. Slow administration rate, or
    b. Temporarily stop flow
    c. Encourage slow, deep breathing through the mouth
9. After fluid has been administered, assist patient to bathroom or onto bedpan or commode; instruct patient not to flush toilet so that results can be assessed
10. If enemas are ordered "until clear," repeat procedure until returns are clear of stool (or of barium after barium enema)
11. Observe patient during procedure for signs of weakness or fatigue, which would necessitate stopping the procedure to allow rest
I. Digital removal of fecal impaction
1. Breaking up the hard fecal mass and removing it
2. Assemble equipment: gloves, waterproof underpad, lubricant, and bedpan
3. Liberally lubricate gloved index finger
4. With patient in side-lying (Sims') position gently insert finger into hardened mass of stool
5. Gently break off small pieces of the stool, bringing them out and placing them in the bedpan
6. Assess patient for signs of weakness and fatigue; this is an uncomfortable, tiring procedure and may need to be intermittently stopped
7. Assist patient to bedpan: disimpaction may induce defecation
J. Colostomy irrigation
1. To regulate the discharge and drainage of fecal contents and flatus
2. Time of irrigation depends on physician's order and patient's own established routine; when colostomy has become regulated, irrigation may be only done every other day; some patients never irrigate their colostomy
3. Assemble equipment
    a. Irrigating appliance (types vary)
    b. Irrigating container (enema bag)
    c. Tubing and catheter (may be part of enema kit)
    d. Irrigating solution: usually 500 to 1000 ml of tap water or physiologic saline solution at 100° F
    e. Lubricant
    f. Drainage bag (may be part of irrigating appliance) and bedpan if not using on toilet
    g. Waterproof underpad if being performed in bed
    h. Fresh colostomy appliance, dressing, or stoma pad
    i. IV pole
    j. Protective gloves
4. After explaining procedure and ensuring privacy, place patient on toilet (most convenient) or in bed in side-lying (Sims') position
5. Put on protective gloves
6. Raise irrigation container 18 inches (45 cm) above stoma, clear catheter of air, lubricate catheter, introduce catheter through irrigating appliance, and insert catheter into stoma 2 to 6 inches (5 to 15 cm); do not advance if resistance is met
7. Allow solution to flow slowly and remove catheter; return is usually completed within 45 to 60 minutes

8. When return is completed, remove irrigating appliance, wash and dry abdomen, and apply fresh colostomy appliance, dressing, or stoma pad as indicated
9. Record character and amount of returns, patient's tolerance, and degree of assistance provided by patient

K. Medication classifications: refer to Chapter 4 for more detailed information on drugs that affect the gastrointestinal (GI) system
   1. Stool softeners
   2. Laxatives/cathartics
   3. Antidiarrhetics

MEASURES TO MEET REST AND SLEEP NEEDS

Rest and sleep are necessary for restoring physical and mental well-being, reducing stress and anxiety, and maintaining the ability to attend to and concentrate on activities of life

A. Assessment: normal number of hours of sleep, usual bedtime, usual bedtime habits or practices, sleep difficulties, daytime fatigue, usual methods of obtaining rest, and sleep medications being used
B. Physician's orders for rest must be clarified: is bed rest ordered to provide rest for a damaged heart, the entire body, or an injured part such as a foot?
C. Providing for rest and sleep
   1. Promote relaxation: provide diversions, pain relief, clean, wrinkle-free bed, a noise-free and odor-free room, and easy access to bedside equipment and call signal; give a relaxing back rub
   2. Reduce patient's anxiety level by allowing time for the patient to talk about stressful or fear-producing situations
   3. If possible, position patient in usual sleeping position with amount of covers desired
   4. Plan and organize care to allow the patient uninterrupted rest and sleep periods
   5. Give sleeping medication if ordered and if required by the patient
D. Medication classifications: refer to Chapter 4 for more detailed information
   1. Sedatives: to reduce anxiety
   2. Hypnotics: to induce sleep

MEASURES TO MEET ACTIVITY AND EXERCISE NEEDS

Physical activity is necessary for proper functioning of all body systems as well as for promotion of emotional well-being; immobility can lead to physical as well as emotional disability

A. Assessment: posture, ability to walk, ability to turn and move in bed, usual activity level, and skin condition
B. Patient's activity and exercise level is ordered by the physician
   1. Bed rest (BR): patient is confined to bed
   2. Bathroom privileges (BRP): although confined to bed, patient may perform urinary and bowel elimination in the bathroom
   3. May dangle: although confined to bed, patient may sit on edge of bed with legs and feet hanging down over side of bed and supported by footstool

   a. Often accompanied by orders for frequency and duration of dangling time (e.g., dangle every shift for 10 minutes)
   b. Provide footstool
   c. Assess vital signs
   d. Stay with patient to assess tolerance and assist back to bed
   4. Allow to chair: although patient may sit in chair, he or she is not permitted to ambulate any farther
   5. Out of bed (OOB) ad lib: can and should perform as much activity out of bed as desired
   6. Encourage patients to perform as much activity as orders permit
C. Dangers of immobility
   1. Atelectasis: collapse of lung caused by reduced depth and rate of respirations or obstruction of lungs by excessive secretions
   2. Hypostatic pneumonia: caused by pooling of lung secretions and the resulting congestion
   3. Thrombus formation: caused by reduced rate of blood flow through the veins and prolonged coagulation time
   4. Constipation: caused by slowed peristaltic action
   5. Contractures: permanent shortening of muscles leading to joint immobility
   6. Skin breakdown and decubitus ulcer formation caused by prolonged pressure and reduced circulation to an area
   7. Development of urinary tract infections and kidney stones caused by stasis of urine and demineralization of bones
D. Measures to prevent dangers of immobility
   1. Coughing and deep breathing
      a. Performed q2h
      b. Patient should be in semi-Fowler's position and take 10 deep breaths followed by deep cough to raise secretions
   2. Turning and repositioning q2h
   3. Range-of-motion (ROM) exercises: to maintain full range and flexibility of joint movement
      a. Performed 8 to 10 times on each joint at least qd
      b. Passive range-of-motion (PROM): performed for the patient
      c. Active range-of-motion (AROM): performed by the patient
      d. Each joint is put through all its possible movements (Fig. 2-12)
   4. Maintain adequate fluid intake (2000 to 3000 ml/day)
   5. Provide for adequate nutritional intake
   6. Frequent skin care, keeping skin clean, dry, and lubricated
E. Devices used to help prevent dangers of immobility
   1. Footboard: to prevent plantar flexion (footdrop)
      a. Soles of patient's feet are flat against board and in good alignment
      b. Board should be padded
   2. Bed cradle: to keep weight of bed covers off a body part
   3. Alternating pressure mattress: to constantly change pressure on body parts in contact with the mattress

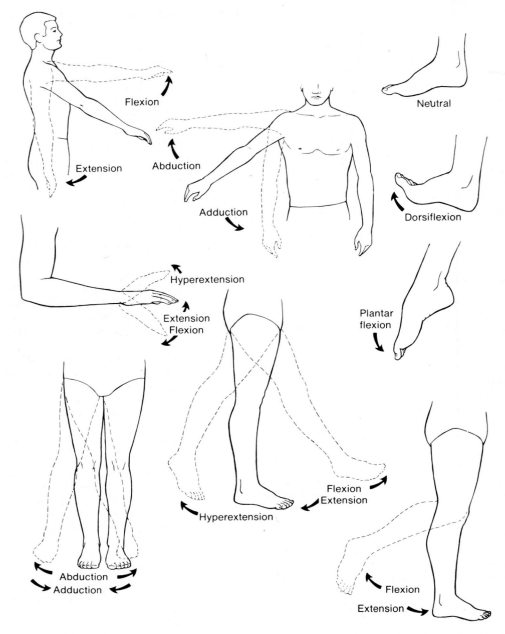

FIG. 2-12. Range-of-joint motions. (From Hood GH, Dincher JR: *Total patient care: foundations and practices*, ed 8, St Louis, 1992, Mosby.)

a. Only one layer of loosely pulled linen should be between mattress and patient
b. Keep pins and other pointed objects away from this mattress
4. Sheepskin: provides a soft surface, reducing skin abrasion
5. Special beds such as the CircOlectric allow patient's position to be changed more readily
6. Venodixie boots: prevent thrombophlebitis

MEASURES TO MEET PAIN RELIEF NEEDS

Individuals (including nurses) vary in their perception of and response to pain. Pain is often intensified in the presence of anxiety and fatigue.

A. Assessment: intensity, onset, duration, quality, and location of pain, patient's nonverbal responses to pain: behavior, change in vital signs, and nausea; factors associated with the pain: activity and visitors; pain relief measures
B. Therapeutic relationship may help reduce anxiety, thus reducing pain level
C. Altering contributing factors: relieving constipation and nausea; eliminating environmental disturbances such as bright lights, odors, and noise
D. Providing diversional activities: television, radio, and visitors
E. Repositioning, back rub, and tightening linens
F. Application of heat or cold if ordered
G. Relaxation
   1. To reduce muscle tension
   2. First need
      a. A comfortable position
      b. A quiet environment
      c. Focus on something outside the body, such as a

word to repeat, an object to look at, or something to imagine

3. Techniques
   a. Exercises in which various muscle groups are alternately tensed and relaxed
   b. Exercises in which various muscle groups are alternately stretched and relaxed
   c. Breathing techniques similar to those used in the Lamaze method of childbirth
   d. Biofeedback: learning to control normally autonomic body functions
      (1) Muscle tension is monitored
      (2) Subject receives feedback as to the success of attempts to control functions

H. Medication classifications: refer to Chapter 4 for more detailed information
   1. Placebo: inactive substance administered to satisfy the patient's need for a drug
      a. Pain relief after administration is probably a result of anxiety reduction
      b. That relief is felt after placebo does not mean there was no pain
   2. Analgesics
      a. Narcotics
      b. Nonnarcotics

MEASURES TO MEET SAFETY AND HYGIENE NEEDS

Individuals are usually capable of meeting these needs themselves, but in strange environments and in times of stress and illness, help is often needed. Individuals need protection from injury, maintenance of intact skin and mucous membranes and of body alignment, and structure and order in their environment

A. Assessment
   1. Protection from injury: level of consciousness, ability to move, knowledge of environment and equipment, and patient's medications
   2. Maintenance of intact skin and mucous membranes and alignment: personal hygiene, condition of skin, mucous membranes, and joints, and posture
   3. Structure and order in the environment: arrangement of personal belongings, cleanliness of patient's unit, environmental conditions, and potential hazards

B. Measures to protect from injury
   1. Bed side rails: use whenever bed is above its lowest level; use for patients who are unconscious, disoriented, or confused or for children
   2. Call signal: should always be within patient's reach; patient should know how to use it
   3. Restraints
      a. Require physician's order to place and remove unless there is an emergency and patient is in immediate need of protection
      b. Used to restrict movement of the individual or of one or more extremities
      c. Explain to patient and family why restraint is being used
      d. Remain quiet and calm while applying restraint to reduce patient's fear and stress
      e. Apply restraint securely enough to provide protection but loosely enough to permit circulation and lung expansion

f. Periodically check pulses and skin integrity
g. Continue to provide patient with all necessary nursing care including turning, fluids, hygiene, and opportunity for elimination
h. Secure restraint to bed frame rather than to bed rail
i. Types of restraints
   (1) Sheet around waist to secure patient in chair
   (2) Jacket or vest, mitts, ankle and wrist restraints
   (3) Safety belts

4. Reduce environmental hazards
   a. Proper care of hospital equipment
      (1) Equipment should be stored properly
      (2) All apparatus, equipment, and furnishings should be kept in good repair
      (3) All equipment, apparatus, and furnishings should be used correctly
   b. Prevention of fire
      (1) Proper care and use of electrical equipment
      (2) Minimization of smoking in bed
      (3) Observance of oxygen safety measures
   c. Prevention of accidents
      (1) Keep floor dry, clean, and free of litter
      (2) Place rubber tips on crutches, canes, and walkers
      (3) Dispose of dressings and needles properly
      (4) Have frequent fire drills
      (5) Lock wheels on beds, wheelchairs, and stretchers
      (6) Maintain good lighting
   d. Protect from microorganisms and pests
      (1) Hand washing and maintenance of medical asepsis
      (2) Proper disinfection and sterilization
      (3) Minimize food storage in patient unit

5. Transferring patient from bed
   a. Protect from falling by using transfer belt and having patient wear sturdy shoes rather than slippers
   b. Two or three people may be required to transfer helpless or heavy patients
   c. Be sure bed and stretcher wheels and wheelchairs are in locked position
   d. Make use of lifting devices such as Hoyer lift
   e. Use good body mechanics

C. Measures to promote and maintain intact skin and mucous membranes
   1. Bed making: dry, tight, wrinkle-free bed helps maintain skin integrity as well as provide for comfort
      a. Assemble equipment: sheets, spread, blanket, pillow, and pillow covering
      b. Care of soiled linens
         (1) Always place on a surface above floor or in individual laundry bags
         (2) Deposit in linen hamper (disposable "linens" are available and are used especially for patients with communicable diseases)
      c. Types of bed making
         (1) Closed bed is made in preparation for new patient

(2) Open bed is occupied but patient is out of bed

(3) Occupied bed is made with patient in it

(4) Fracture or orthopedic bed is made from head to foot

(5) Postanesthetic or recovery bed is made to receive patient easily from stretcher (Fig. 2-13)

d. Bed positions

(1) Low Fowler's: head is raised (gatched) 18 to 20 inches (45 to 50 cm) above flat bed level

(2) Semi-Fowler's: head is raised 45 degrees and knee is gatched 15 degrees

(3) High Fowler's: head of bed is raised to a 90-degree angle

(4) Trendelenburg's: head is lower than the level of the feet (no Gatch)

2. Daily bath

a. Clean, dry, intact, and healthy skin and mucous membranes are first line of defense against microorganisms

b. Bath time is also important for establishing relationship with patient and for assessment

c. Some patients do not desire, need, or require complete bath each day

d. Bed bath: given to patient who is restricted to bed or helpless in bathing self

e. Assisted bath: patient bathes as much of self as possible; may need assistance with back, feet, legs, and perineum

f. Tub bath or shower: for patient who is capable of doing so; must have physician's order

3. Skin care

a. Use soap sparingly; rinse well with warm water; pat skin dry

b. Lotions prevent dry skin

c. Gently massage bony prominences with lotion to promote circulation

d. Use deodorant or antiperspirant as necessary

e. Avoid heavy use of powder, which can cake, causing skin irritation

4. Mouth care

a. Routine mouth care: use of toothbrush, mouthwash, or substitutes

b. Special mouth care: more frequent routine care plus the judicious use of glycerin and lemon swabs or hydrogen peroxide if ordered

c. Care of dentures

(1) Clean dentures over towel-lined basin of water to reduce chance of breakage if dropped

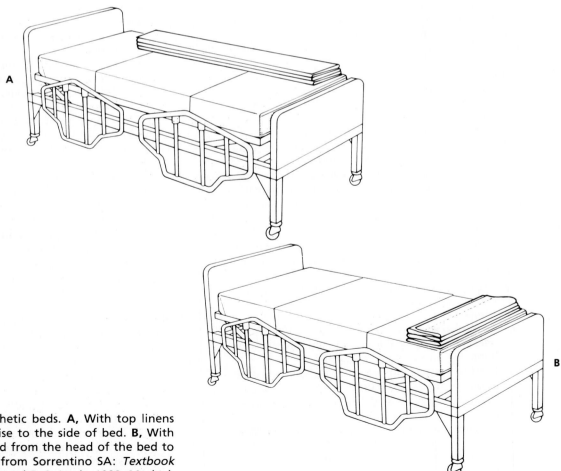

FIG. 2-13. Postanesthetic beds. **A,** With top linens fan folded lengthwise to the side of bed. **B,** With top linens fan folded from the head of the bed to the foot. (Adapted from Sorrentino SA: *Textbook for nursing assistants,* ed 3, St Louis, 1992, Mosby.)

(2) Hold dentures with gauze or cloth to prevent dropping

(3) Clean with tepid water; hot water may change shape

(4) Store dentures in denture cup with tepid water in drawer of bedside stand when not in patient's mouth

5. Hair care
   a. Comb or brush daily; groom as desired
   b. If tangled
      (1) Use 95% alcohol for oily hair
      (2) Use mineral oil for dry hair
      (3) Start at ends working toward scalp
      (4) Hold hair close to head to prevent pulling
   c. Braid long hair if not objectionable to patient
   d. Shampoo as often as necessary and as patient's condition permits
   e. Give pediculosis (lice) treatment as ordered by physician
      (1) Commercial preparations are available
      (2) Use fine-toothed comb to remove nits (eggs)
      (3) Patient may be isolated to avoid spread

6. Nail care: daily and as indicated; must have physician's order to cut nails; extreme care must be used with patients with diabetes or circulatory problems
   a. Scrub under nails as necessary
   b. Cut nails even with tips of fingers and toes
   c. Round fingernails to curve with fingertips
   d. Cut toenails straight across

7. Decubitus (pressure) ulcer care: assess areas over all bony prominences, such as sacrum, heels, elbows, hips and shoulder blades, and along edges of casts and braces
   a. Contributing factors
      (1) Crumbs or food particles in the bed
      (2) Exposure to moisture such as urine
      (3) Wrinkles in sheets
      (4) Unrelieved pressure for longer than 2 hours
      (5) Conditions that restrict movement
      (6) Poor nutritional or fluid balance states
   b. Treatment
      (1) "An ounce of prevention is worth a pound of cure"—turn and reposition q2h
      (2) Identify high-risk patients
      (3) Report and initiate care for beginning signs of redness, whiteness, or breaks in skin
      (4) Use devices such as sheepskin, egg-crate mattress, alternating-pressure mattress, water mattress, or Clinitron bed
      (5) Avoid use of waterproof underpads
      (6) Use special cleansing agents and dressings as ordered by physician or as indicated by agency policy

8. Use turning sheet to move and turn patient with minimum of friction, which may cause abrasions

D. Measures to maintain body alignment
   1. Encourage good posture while sitting, standing, and lying
   2. Bed lying positions
      a. Supine: lying on back
      b. Prone: lying on abdomen with head turned to the side
      c. Side-lying (Sims'): lying on side with upper hip and knee sharply flexed
   3. Reposition patient at least q2h
   4. Guidelines for proper positioning
      a. Normal body curves must be supported by small pillows or pads: use "bridging" techniques
      b. Joints that are normally flexed need support
      c. Bony prominences need to be protected from pressure
      d. Use devices such as sandbags or rolls to keep joints and body parts positioned
      e. Periodically check patient for discomfort or difficulties
      f. Ensure that patient can reach call signal

E. Measures to promote structure and order in the patient's environment
   1. Physical factors
      a. Lighting
         (1) Lighting should be indirect except for reading or for procedures
         (2) General lighting should be diffused
         (3) Sunlight promotes healing and feeling of well-being
      b. Waste disposal: trash, human excretions, and soiled dressings and linens should be discarded according to agency's procedures
   2. Esthetic factors
      a. Sound
         (1) Music therapy promotes rest and relaxation
         (2) Noise causes fatigue and anxiety
      b. Decor
         (1) Pastel colors (yellow or pink) are soothing and relaxing
         (2) Harsh colors (red or black) overstimulate senses
         (3) Flowers and pictures enhance environment
      c. Odors
         (1) Foul or strong odors should be eliminated by means of room deodorizer or removal of causative agent
         (2) Mild, fragrant odors reduce antiseptic smell and patient embarrassment
      d. Privacy: curtains, screens, and proper draping should be used as indicated to reduce embarrassment and protect patient dignity
   3. Care of the environment: varies according to agency policy
      a. Responsibilities of housekeeping and ancillary services (central supply and maintenance)
         (1) Daily damp dusting and floor cleaning
         (2) Scrubbing, disinfecting, sterilizing, and storing of equipment after patient transfer, discharge, or death
         (3) Repairing or replacing defective equipment or furnishings
      b. Responsibilities of the nursing personnel
         (1) Place bedside table, call signal, phone, and personal articles within patient's reach

(2) Straighten and damp dust bedside unit (includes care of flowers)

(3) Care for patient belongings (clothing, valuables, glasses, dentures, and prostheses)

(4) Prevent cross-infection between patients

OTHER THERAPEUTIC NURSING MEASURES
Wound Care

A. Cleaning the wound
   1. Commonly used antiseptics
      a. 70% alcohol
      b. Povidone-iodine (Betadine)
   2. Hydrogen peroxide to remove dry and crusted secretions
   3. Always clean from innermost to outermost aspect of wound
B. Wound irrigation
   1. To remove secretions or excessive discharge from surfaces or body cavities or to apply moist heat
   2. May use clean or sterile technique depending on area to be irrigated
   3. Assemble equipment: may vary according to area to be irrigated (disposable kits are available)
      a. Container to hold irrigating solution
      b. Container for return flow of solution
      c. Irrigating solution
      d. Irrigator: usually bulb syringe or large plunger-type syringe
      e. Protection for patient and linens
      f. Gloves
      g. Replacement dressing if indicated
C. Dressing changes
   1. Dressing: material placed on a wound or incision to protect, absorb drainage, or promote healing
   2. Dressings are classified by method of application
      a. Clean
      b. Sterile
      c. Moist or dry
   3. Disposable kits or hospital-assembled kits
   4. Types of dressing material
      a. Gauze
      b. Petrolatum gauze
      c. Telfa
   5. Material for securing dressings
      a. Tape: in various widths
         (1) Adhesive
         (2) Paper
         (3) Nonallergic
      b. Montgomery straps
      c. Bandages and binders
   6. Nurse may be responsible for changing dressing or assisting physician in changing dressing
   7. Initial change of postoperative dressing is done by physician unless an order specifies otherwise
   8. Dressings that are not to be changed should be reinforced with additional material if drainage seeps through
D. Care of patient with wound infection
   1. Infection may be local (confined to wound) or systemic (generalized throughout body), often depending on the causative organism
   2. Signs of local infection result from increased circulation and accumulation of waste in the area
      a. Redness, heat, pain, and swelling
      b. Purulent drainage
      c. Loss of function
      d. Changes in vital signs
   3. Signs of systemic infection
      a. Increase in temperature, pulse, and respirations (TPR); possible decrease in blood pressure
      b. Nausea and vomiting
      c. General malaise
      d. Loss of appetite
   4. Basic principles of treatment
      a. Physical and mental rest
      b. Elevation and rest of infected part
      c. Application of heat or cold
   5. Special treatment may include
      a. Chemotherapy (sulfonamides and antibiotics)
      b. Incision and drainage of wound
      c. Debridement: removal of foreign, infected, or necrotic tissue
   6. Infection control committee investigates and follows up infections occurring in an agency

Bandages

A. Applied to give support, immobilize a part, apply pressure, or hold dressings
B. Types of bandages
   1. Strips or rolls of gauze, cotton flannel, or elastic material
   2. Many widths, depending on purpose and part to be bandaged
C. Types of basic turns in bandaging
   1. Circular
   2. Spiral
   3. Spiral reverse
   4. Recurrent
   5. Figure-of-eight
D. Safety factors
   1. Apply in direction from distal to proximal
   2. Apply tight enough to serve purpose but loose enough to permit circulation (presence of pulse)
   3. Do not fasten over bony prominence, area of pressure, or a wound
   4. Part being bandaged should remain in functional position

Binders

A. Purposes
   1. Support: abdomen or chest
   2. Hold dressings in place
   3. Apply pressure
B. Types
   1. Straight
   2. Tailed: T-binder, four-tailed, or scultetus (many-tailed)

Antiembolism Stockings

A. Purposes
   1. To help maintain circulation
   2. To prevent thrombi or phlebitis formation

B. Application and maintenance
1. Exact size is obtained by measuring calf or leg length and circumference
2. Be sure legs are clean and dry before applying
3. Apply with patient lying down
4. Periodically check foot and leg for redness, irritation, swelling, and presence of pulse
5. Occasional laundering is necessary

Application of Heat and Cold

A. Physiologic principles
1. Cold applications (by constricting blood vessels) prevent or reduce swelling, stop bleeding, decrease suppuration, and reduce pain
2. Heat applications (by dilating blood vessels) increase supply of oxygen and nutrients to body cells and increase amount of toxins and excess fluids carried away

B. Types of cold applications
1. Dry: ice bag, ice cap, ice collar, and hypothermic devices
2. Moist: cold packs and compresses

C. Nursing observations
1. White, mottled skin
2. Frostbite
3. Numbness
4. Lowered body temperature

D. Guidelines
1. Caps and bags are two-thirds filled and air is removed
2. Containers are closed securely
3. Caps and bags are always covered
4. Application is removed every half hour for 1 hour
5. Ice is replaced frequently

6. These treatments are contraindicated or used only with great care in patients with poor circulation or impaired sensation
7. Physician's order is always required

E. Types of heat
1. Dry: hot water bottle, sunlight, heating pad, and incandescent, ultraviolet, and infrared lights
2. Moist: warm compresses, hot soaks, hot packs, and K pad units

F. Nursing observations
1. Redness
2. Swelling
3. Pain
4. Change in vital signs
5. Loss of function in part

G. Guidelines
1. Always requires physician's order
2. Carefully observe body parts that are very sensitive and burn easily (eyes, neck, and inner aspect of arm)
3. Bottles and pads are always covered
4. Never allow patient to lie on heating device
5. Check for faulty electric wiring
6. Never use safety pins with electric devices
7. Check body temperature frequently
8. Check distance of heating bulbs from body area; should be at least 18 inches (45 cm) away
9. Wring out compresses well to prevent burn; if area is infected, use compresses only once and discard
10. Agency policy may require application of a thin layer of petrolatum to area receiving heat

H. Special baths
1. Hot (sitz) or cold (Fig. 2-14)
2. Medicated

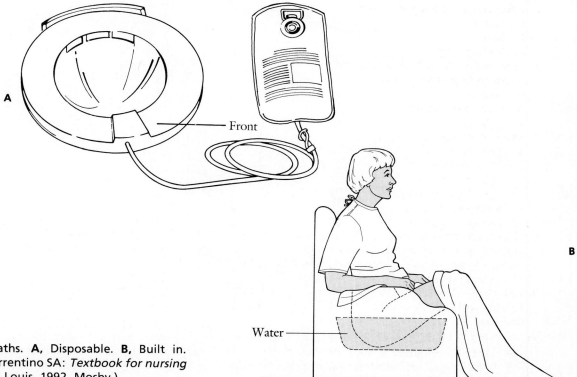

FIG. 2-14. Sitz baths. **A,** Disposable. **B,** Built in. (Adapted from Sorrentino SA: *Textbook for nursing assistants,* ed 3, St Louis, 1992, Mosby.)

Front

Water

MEASURES FOR EYE, EAR, AND THROAT DISORDERS
Eye Treatments

A. Hot compresses
1. Assemble equipment: sterile basin of solution as ordered, gauze pad, heating device, paper bag, and protective gloves
2. Put on protective gloves
3. Apply thin layer of petrolatum over lid
4. Wring out gauze pad with hands if clean technique or with two pairs of forceps if sterile technique and allow pad to stop steaming; apply compress slowly until patient is accustomed to heat, or allow patient to apply compress if able
5. Try to keep compress on eyelid only; if lid is inflamed, compress may be placed on lid and cheek; if eyeball is inflamed, compress may be placed on lid and brow
6. Change compresses every 30 to 60 seconds for 15 to 20 minutes as ordered
7. If discharge is present, use clean pad each time compress is applied
8. Use two sets of equipment if both eyes are involved

B. Irrigation
1. Assemble equipment: basin of sterile solution as ordered at 95° to 100° F, medicine dropper or ear syringe, basin for return flow, cotton balls to protect uninvolved eye and to dry treated eye, and face towel to protect bed; separate irrigating tip is needed for each eye
2. Direct flow of solution into conjunctival sac from inner angle to outer angle of eye; position patient toward affected side (Fig. 2-15)

Ear Treatment: Irrigation

A. Assemble equipment: sterile ear syringe, solution as ordered at 105° to 108° F, basin for return flow, and towel to protect bed
B. Position patient: patient may lie down, but sitting position is preferred, with head tilted slightly so affected ear is downward; patient may hold basin for return flow, if able
C. Retract pinna, in direction according to age, to expose orifice of external canal; direct flow gently against side of canal; interrupt irrigation if pain or dizziness occurs and notify physician

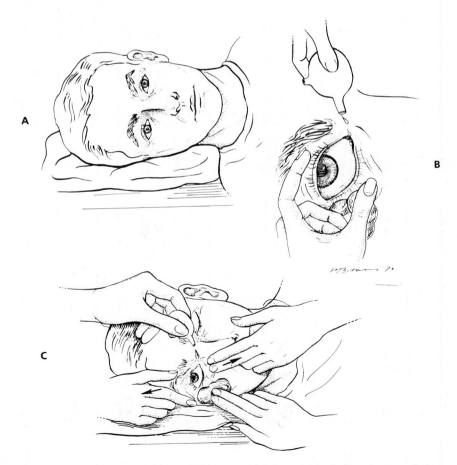

FIG. 2-15. Irrigation of the eye. **A,** The nurse turns the patient's head toward the eye that is to be irrigated. **B,** Solution flows from the inner canthus to the outer canthus of the eye. The irrigator is held less than 4 inches (10 cm) away from the eye. **C,** The patient may assist by retracting the lower eyelid and collecting irrigating solution with absorbent material. (From Dison N: *Clinical nursing techniques,* ed 4, St Louis, 1975, Mosby.)

Throat Treatments

A. Throat swab
  1. Assemble equipment: sterile applicators, tongue blade, medication as ordered, tissue wipes, flashlight, and paper bag
  2. When swabbing throat, avoid stimulating gag reflex by not touching uvula
B. Throat culture
  1. Assemble equipment: sterile culture tube, applicator, and tissue wipes
  2. After touching sides and back of throat with applicator, put applicator in culture tube without contaminating inside of tube by breaking off top of applicator that was touched by fingers
C. Throat irrigation
  1. Assemble equipment: irrigating container, solution as ordered at 110° F, tubing with rubber tip on end, tissue wipes, basin for return flow, towel to protect patient; protective gloves
  2. Put on protective gloves
  3. Have patient tilt head forward over basin and breathe through nose; discourage deep breathing
  4. Have patient do treatment if able
  5. Hold container slightly above patient's mouth; direct flow toward affected area
     a. Irrigation may be interrupted for patient's comfort
     b. Flow should not be directed toward uvula or base of tongue
  6. Tilt patient's head to one side and then the other to facilitate results

MEASURES FOR GASTROINTESTINAL DISORDERS
Gastric Intubation

A. Purposes
  1. To administer gavage feedings
  2. To obtain specimens (gastric analysis and cytology)
  3. To irrigate or cleanse (lavage)
  4. For decompression (suction)
B. Tube locations
  1. Nose to stomach: nasogastric
  2. Mouth to stomach: orogastric
  3. Artificial opening into stomach: gastrostomy
C. Insertion of tube
  1. Is not always a licensed practical/vocational nurse (LP/VN) responsibility: refer to your agency's policy
  2. Assemble equipment: flashlight, tongue blade, stethoscope, cup of water, irrigating syringe, water-soluble lubricant, 12- to 18-gauge French tube, gloves, and towel to protect patient's clothing
  3. If rubber tube is used, it should be chilled first
  4. Place patient in semi-Fowler's position with towel protecting clothing
  5. Approximate distance of tube insertion is the length from tip of nose to ear lobe to xiphoid process
  6. Apply water-soluble lubricant to tip of tube; if intubation is for cytology study, tube is lubricated with water or saline solution
  7. With gloved hands hold tube 3 inches (7.5 cm) from tip, place into nostril or mouth, and advance
  8. Have patient flex neck and take repeated shallow breaths when tube passes into pharynx (about 3 inches [7.5 cm])
  9. Have patient swallow while advancing tube
D. Checking placement of tube
  1. Check back of throat with tongue blade and flashlight to see if coiling has occurred
  2. Aspirate stomach contents; may need to advance tube if no stomach contents are obtained
  3. While injecting 5 ml of air, use stethoscope to listen for air entering stomach
  4. Observe patient's respirations and note ability to speak; respirations may be labored or patient will be unable to speak if tube is in trachea or lungs
E. Securing tube (Fig. 2-16)
  1. Anchor with strip of tape and secure to nose and cheek if nasogastric
  2. Anchor with strip of tape and secure to chin and cheek if orogastric
F. Removal of tube
  1. Clamp tube
  2. Remove anchoring tape
  3. Put on protective gloves
  4. Draw tube through towel so it is wiped of secretions
  5. Have patient inhale and exhale slowly
  6. Pull tube with one continuous, rapid motion
  7. Have basin ready if patient vomits

Suction and Irrigation

A. Nasogastric or GI tubes (Levin, Cantor, Miller-Abbott, or Salem sump) may be connected to mechanical suction apparatus
B. Suction
  1. Rate is ordered by physician or according to agency policy
  2. May be intermittent or continuous
  3. Collection container is emptied and rinsed; amount of drainage is measured and recorded at end of shift and when container becomes nearly filled
C. Irrigation
  1. Check orders for frequency, solution type, amount, and method of aspiration (force or gravity)
  2. Assemble equipment: solution as ordered, container for solution, basin for return flow, irrigating syringe (bulb or plunger type), and protective pad
  3. Fill syringe and free it of air
  4. Instill solution into tube slowly and gently
  5. Allow solution to return by aspirating or by gravity
  6. Remove syringe and reconnect to suction if ordered
D. Patients with indwelling tubes should be given frequent mouth and nose care
E. Accurate measurement of intake and output (subtracting irrigating solution) is essential

MEASURES FOR VAGINAL CARE
Perineal Care

A. Assemble equipment: solution as ordered, cotton balls for cleansing and drying, gloves, perineal pad with belt, and bedpan
B. With gloved hands put patient on bedpan; pour solution over vulva, clean with cotton balls; dry vulva; make patient comfortable
C. If using bottle method, fill bottle with warm water and squeeze solution over vulva; dry, wiping from urinary meatus toward anus and wiping only once with each cotton ball

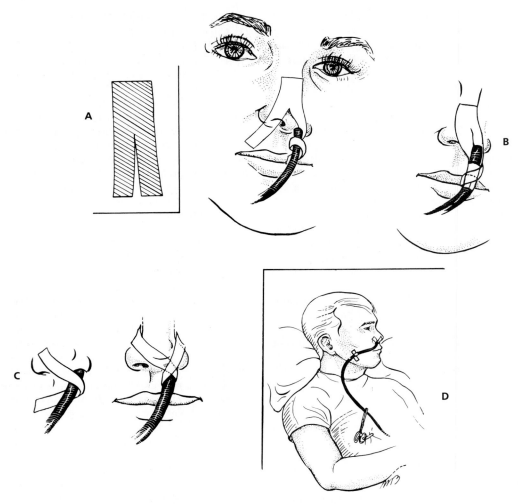

FIG. 2-16. Securing the nasogastric tube. **A,** A length of adhesive tape is split for use in anchoring the tube to the nostril. **B,** The unsplit portion is affixed to the nose: one of the split portions is wrapped around the tube, and then the other portion is wrapped around the tube. **C,** A narrow strip of tape may be used to secure the tube. **D,** The tube is taped to the nostril and cheek and clamped or connected to suction. (From Dison N: *Clinical nursing techniques,* ed 4, St Louis, 1975, Mosby.)

Vaginal Irrigation (Douche)

A. Assemble equipment: irrigating container with solution as ordered, tubing with douche tip, clamp, cotton balls for drying, gloves, perineal pad with belt, bedpan, and bed protection
B. Have patient void; place on bedpan, or patient may administer to self in bathroom if able
C. Insert tip down and back into vagina
D. Give irrigation under low pressure; have solution flowing before inserting douche tip; rotate douche tip until prescribed amount is used
E. If patient is on bedpan, raise head of bed slightly to allow fluid to drain into bedpan

MEASURES FOR PATIENTS UNDERGOING SURGERY
Preoperative Preparation

A. Psychosocial aspects
  1. Nurse assesses patient's knowledge and expected results of surgery
  2. Anxiety may interfere with learning
  3. Extremely frightened patients may respond poorly to surgery
  4. Planned, individualized, simple explanations will enhance patient cooperation and reduce anxiety
  5. Nurse assesses and responds to patient's religious needs
  6. Common preoperative fears
    a. Fear of mutilation
    b. Fear of death
    c. Fear of change in family role
    d. Fear of pain
  7. Family or significant others must understand measures taken to prepare patient
  8. Family or significant others should participate in explanations and encouragement
B. Physical preparation
  1. Explain preoperative tests (CBC, ECG, urinalysis, x-ray examinations)
  2. Explain, demonstrate, and have patient practice any special postoperative exercises that will need to be

done (turning, deep breathing, and pumping feet)
3. Follow preoperative orders as prescribed by physician (enema, diet, and medications)
4. Prepare appropriate skin area (see agency procedure manual)
5. Care for valuables
6. Follow and complete preoperative checklist
    a. Informed consents for surgery and anesthesia signed and witnessed
    b. Nail polish, prostheses, jewelry, and makeup removed
    c. Patient dressed in hospital gown only
    d. Hygienic measures performed (bath with mouth care and voiding or catheterization)
    e. Vital signs checked and recorded and abnormalities reported
    f. Identification and allergy bracelets in place
C. Observations and procedures recorded
D. After patient leaves for operative procedure, prepare postoperative bed and unit

Postoperative Care

A. Immediate care
    1. Ensure and maintain patent airway
    2. Maintain adequate circulation
    3. Observe for complications at operative site and in general (hemorrhage, shock, swelling, and severe pain)
    4. Assess and secure dressing, drainage, and IV tubings
    5. Assess mental status (orientation)
    6. Position patient properly; keep patient warm
    7. Assess vital signs as often as ordered or more frequently as condition warrants
    8. Follow physician's orders
    9. Report signs of restlessness, excessive drainage, or abnormal reactions
    10. Support patient and family by briefly answering questions and offering explanations
B. Routine care
    1. Follow physician's orders
    2. Assess and record vital signs frequently during first 24 hours; report changes immediately
    3. Assess dressing or surgical site frequently
    4. Give oral hygiene as needed
    5. Have patient turn, deep breathe, and, unless contraindicated, cough and exercise legs at least q2h
    6. Assess and record intake and output (patient may need order for catheterization if he or she does not void within 6 to 8 hours after surgery)
    7. Help patient with passive or active exercises unless contraindicated
    8. Encourage and assist patient to ambulate as much as orders permit
    9. Perform daily assessment
        a. Lungs: breath sounds and cough
        b. Circulation: pain in legs or chest and IV site
        c. GI tract: nausea, vomiting, distention, bowel sounds, and passage of flatus
        d. Urine: amount, color, odor, and frequency
        e. Mental status: withdrawal, confusion, anxiety, or restlessness
    10. Offer pain medication

MEASURES RELATED TO RADIATION THERAPY

A. Radiation
    1. Radiate: to send out rays (light, heat, or roentgen)
    2. Radiation is used in diagnosis and therapeutic treatment of various conditions (especially for malignancies)
    3. Types of radiation
        a. Alpha rays: harmless; do not travel far
        b. Beta rays: more penetrating; stop at person's body surface
        c. Gamma rays: very penetrating
B. Types of therapy
    1. Infrared lamp
    2. Ultraviolet
    3. Diatherapy
    4. Roentgen ray (x-ray: low voltage, external)
    5. Betatron, cobalt, cesium (high voltage, external)
    6. Internal radiation
        a. Implants (skin surface, intratumor, intracavitary)
        b. Liquid forms of radioisotopes
        c. Injection (intracavitary, systemic)
C. Radiation therapy and the nurse
    1. Internal implant
        a. Explain procedure and precautions to patient and family or significant others
            (1) Patient needs to know that he or she will be in isolation and how many days isolation is likely to last
            (2) Patient should know that nursing personnel and visitors will be spending a minimal amount of time at the bedside and yet will be available when needed
        b. Ensure good fluid intake
        c. Have patient move about as little as possible
        d. Assess for signs of radiation reactions (nausea, vomiting, or skin irritation)
        e. Communicate frequently with patient from doorway without entering room
        f. Use precautions at all times
    2. Radiation precautions with implant
        a. RADIATION IN USE sign with directions posted on patient's door
        b. No staff member or visitor spends more than 1 hour per day with patient; care must be well organized
        c. Pregnant women and children should not enter the patient's room
        d. Check placement of implant q4h
        e. Wear gown and gloves while handling excreta, secretions, and utensils
        f. Wash contaminated gloves with soap and water before removing
        g. Wash hands with soap and water
        h. If implant becomes dislodged, call radiologist immediately—do not touch implant
    3. Nursing care for specific situations
        a. Therapy involving mouth
            (1) Oral hygiene with brushing teeth (or dentures) should be done 3 times a day (tid)
            (2) Smoking should be discouraged
            (3) Teeth should be assessed for change in condition; if changes observed, notify physician

(4) Male patient should not shave if jaw is being treated

b. Uterine therapy
  (1) Bed rest is maintained to prevent displacement of implant
  (2) Bedpan is inspected for loss of implant before contents are discarded
  (3) Foley catheter with continuous irrigation may be ordered to reduce bladder irritation
  (4) Vaginal irrigation may be ordered after removal of implant

c. Radioactive gold administered intraperitoneally
  (1) Leakage on dressings appears bright red and may be confused with blood
  (2) Dressings should be wrapped in newspaper and disposed of in special container

4. External radiotherapy
  a. Explain procedure to patient and family or significant others
  b. Never remove skin markings
  c. Avoid washing the marked area
  d. Do not apply ointments, creams, or powders to marked area
  e. Encourage good fluid intake and nutrition
  f. Observe for radiation reactions

MEASURES CONCERNING PATIENT'S DEPARTURE

A. Transferring patient
  1. Patient may be transferred from one service to another, from one floor to another, or from one agency to another
  2. Physician's order is required
  3. Transfer patient ambulatory, by wheelchair, or on stretcher; follow agency's policy
  4. Explain transfer to patient; be sure all personal belongings are transferred with patient
  5. Avoid transferring during mealtime or change of shift to reduce confusion
  6. Make proper charting notations; notify significant others

B. Discharging patient
  1. Written order by physician is required
  2. Nurse's responsibilities
    a. Gather and check with patient all personal belongings
    b. Make sure patient understands all instructions regarding diet, medications, treatments, and follow-up appointments
    c. Notify family as necessary
    d. Accompany patient to exit
    e. Make proper charting notations
  3. Discharge planning
    a. Begins after initial nursing assessment and is included on care plan
    b. Nursing interventions are directed toward eventual discharge of patient
    c. Planning consists of teaching patient and family or significant other
      (1) Cause of illness
      (2) Drugs, treatments, and diet
      (3) Health care follow-up
      (4) Functions within limitations

CARING FOR THE DYING

A. Signs of approaching death
  1. Patient is pale with pinched expression of anxiety
  2. Eyes are glazed and dull; pupils do not react to light
  3. Mouth remains partially open unless patient attempts to speak; speech is mumbled and often confused
  4. Muscle tone becomes flaccid
  5. Skin is cool and clammy and may be mottled; this is caused by diminished circulation; body temperature is often elevated
  6. Respirations are rapid and shallow, often progressing to Cheyne-Stokes
  7. Pulse becomes weak and thready
  8. Patient may be diaphoretic, thirsty, and incontinent of urine and feces

B. Five stages in the process of reaction to a terminal illness or to dying: refer to Chapter 7 for more detailed information relative to death and dying
  1. Denial
  2. Anger
  3. Bargaining
  4. Grief/depression
  5. Acceptance

C. Nursing care of dying patient
  1. Give symptomatic nursing care
  2. Give good personal hygiene
  3. Turn patient frequently
  4. Give treatments and medications as long as possible or until discontinued
  5. Carry out desires of patient, family, or significant others as far as possible
  6. Be available to provide emotional support and privacy to patient, family, or significant other
  7. Remember that hearing may be the last sense to fail

D. Spiritual needs of patient
  1. Fulfill needs as requested by patient, family, or significant other
  2. Continue to adhere to patient's individual religious beliefs

E. Care of body after death (postmortem care)
  1. Lower head of bed
  2. Leave one pillow under head to prevent congestion of blood in vessels of face
  3. Close eyes
  4. Place dentures in mouth immediately and close mouth
  5. Clean body; follow agency's policy for removal of drains, IV needle and tubing, dressings, and tubes
  6. Straighten body and place in natural position
  7. Allow viewing of body by family or significant other if they desire
  8. Wrap in shroud and label with tags according to agency policy
  9. Gather, pack, label, and care for patient's personal belongings
  10. Record observations, procedures, disposition of valuables, and time of death; complete records

Suggested Reading List

Anderson K, Anderson L: *Mosby's pocket dictionary of medicine, nursing, and allied health,* St Louis, 1990, Mosby.

Bryant RA: Saving the skin from tape injury, *Am J Nurs* 88(2):189-191, 1988.

Carroll P: Safe suctioning, *Nurs 89* 19:48, 1989.

Clark A: The good wound guide, *Nurs Time* 84(2):63-65, 1988.

Cole G, editor: *Basic nursing skills and concepts,* St Louis, 1991, Mosby.

Cooper KM: Measuring blood pressure the right way, *Nurs 92* 4:75, 1992.

Dickerson M: Protecting yourself from AIDS: infection control measures, *Crit Care Nurs* 9(10):26, 1989.

Dowd SB: Radiation safety and the nurse, *J Pract Nurs* (12):31-33, 1990.

Ebersole P, Hess P: *Toward healthy aging,* ed 4, St Louis, 1990, Mosby.

Holder C, Alexander J: A new and improved guide to IV therapy, *Am J Nurs* 90:43, 1990.

Jaffe MS, Melson KA: Laboratory and diagnostic cards: clinical implications and teaching, St Louis, 1988, Mosby.

Kuehl PG: Immunizations for special situations, *J Pract Nurs* (3):52-61, 1992.

Larson E: Handwashing: it's essential even when you use gloves, *Am J Nurs* 89:934, 1989.

Potter PA, Perry AG: *Basic nursing theory and practice,* ed 2, St Louis, 1991, Mosby.

Skidmore-Roth L: *Mosby's 1993 nursing drug reference,* ed 6, St Louis, 1992, Mosby.

Weinberger B: Discharge planning, the sooner, the better, *Nurs 89* 2:75-76, 1989.

Basic Nursing Concepts and the Nursing Process Review Questions

Answers and rationales start on p. 419.

Situation: Ralph Jones, a 72-year-old widower, is admitted to your unit with pneumonia. He lives alone, and his two sons live out of state.

1. Because of Mr. Jones' age, you can assume his:
   ① Ability to remain independent will be lost after this hospitalization
   ② Eyesight is poor
   ③ Level of functioning must be carefully assessed
   ④ Short-term memory is limited

2. Assessment of Mr. Jones' cultural background may help the nurse understand his:
   ① Body defense mechanisms
   ② Immune response
   ③ Reactions to hospitalization
   ④ Socioeconomic level

3. While caring for Mr. Jones, you have become totally exasperated at his refusal to bathe, to cooperate with treatments, and to comply with the physician's orders. Your next action should be:
   ① Call the patient advocate
   ② Call the physician
   ③ Consult with the nursing staff
   ④ Request a psychiatric consult

4. Mr. Jones tells you he does not like to bathe in the morning; he prefers an evening shower. Your response should be:
   ① Bathing in the morning makes a patient feel more refreshed
   ② Hospital routine requires nurses to provide for bathing in the morning
   ③ The staff is too busy for patients to bathe in the evening
   ④ The staff will do its best to provide for an evening shower

5. Mr. Jones is receiving oxygen via nasal cannula and asks why it is attached to a container of water. Your response includes that:
   ① A water source is required to prevent friction formation
   ② Oxygen does not flow properly without a water source
   ③ Oxygen is more combustable without a source of water
   ④ Water provides humidity

6. In the middle of the night Mr. Jones becomes confused and tries to climb over the side rails. You consider applying a restraint knowing that:
   ① A physician's order is required
   ② Restraints provide patients with a sense of security
   ③ The restraint is tied to side rails to allow faster removal in an emergency
   ④ The restraint is applied loosely on the elderly to prevent skin abrasion

Situation: Mrs. Jackson is 69 years old and has uncontrolled hypertension.

7. Mrs. Jackson has an IV. Which of the following assessed data might indicate fluid excess?
   ① Poor skin turgor
   ② Thick, tenacious sputum
   ③ Wedding ring too tight to remove
   ④ Weight loss of 5 pounds

8. On Mrs. Jackson's physician's order sheet you read, "Start oxygen." Your next action is:
   ① Assess Mrs. Jackson's vital signs
   ② Obtain a complete oxygen order
   ③ Obtain the necessary equipment
   ④ Write a nurse's note indicating oxygen therapy will be started

9. As Mrs. Jackson's visitors leave, they tell you she is crying and won't talk to them. Your approach to Mrs. Jackson should include:
   ① Asking her if she would like to talk about what is bothering her
   ② Asking if she has ever seen a psychiatrist
   ③ Posting a NO VISITORS sign
   ④ Reminding her of how much her visitors care about her

10. Mrs. Jackson has developed a reddened area on her sacrum. The best method of treating the area is:
    ① Alternating pressure mattress
    ② Place a sheepskin on the bed
    ③ Range-of-motion exercises q2h
    ④ Turn and position q2h

11. Mrs. Jackson has become increasingly lethargic and requires nasopharyngeal suctioning. While performing this procedure you remember:
    ① The catheter is inserted with a rotating motion
    ② Each episode of suctioning lasts no more than 30 seconds
    ③ Only medical asepsis is required
    ④ Suction is only applied while the catheter is being withdrawn.

12. You and another nurse are moving Mrs. Jackson up in bed. Which of the following indicate use of good body mechanics?
    ① Back is straight, knees are flexed
    ② Feet are close together
    ③ Knees are straight, back is flexed
    ④ Nurses stand one step back from bed

Situation: Mrs. Fletcher is 92 years old and lives in a nursing home. Although she enjoys participating in all activities, she is weak and needs assistance with ambulation and with activities of daily living.

13. You observe that Mrs. Fletcher's skin is dry and that she has been itching. A priority in planning her care would be to:
    ① Apply a medicated lotion
    ② Avoid bathing
    ③ Avoid the use of soap
    ④ Call the physician

14. Mrs. Fletcher tells the nurse that she feels bad today. The nurse replies, "You're fine. You'll feel much better after the bingo game." This type of response:
    ① Demonstrates a therapeutic relationship
    ② Discourages communication
    ③ Encourages further communication
    ④ Enhances continuing assessment

15. Mrs. Fletcher has begun to seep liquid fecal material. You recognize that this may be an indication of:
    ① Diarrhea
    ② Flatulence
    ③ Impaction
    ④ Incontinence

16. A stool for hemocult has been ordered. Hemocult is a test for:
    ① Blood
    ② Cancer
    ③ Ova
    ④ Parasites

17. Which of the following is an objective symptom?
    ① Burning
    ② Nausea
    ③ Numbness
    ④ Redness

18. Mrs. Fletcher is to receive passive range-of-motion exercises bid (twice a day). The purpose of these exercises is to:
    ① Enhance muscle tone
    ② Prevent joint contractures
    ③ Prevent muscle atrophy
    ④ Strengthen bones

19. Trochanter rolls would be used to help maintain Mrs. Fletcher's alignment when she is in which position?
    ① Dorsal recumbent
    ② Lithotomy
    ③ Sims'
    ④ Supine

20. When performing a capillary puncture, the next step after swabbing the site with alcohol is to:
    ① Apply warmth to the site
    ② Explain the procedure to the patient
    ③ "Milk" the site
    ④ Puncture the site

21. You find Mrs. Fletcher crying in the dayroom. Your first intervention would be to:
    ① Ask her what is wrong
    ② Ask the other patients what happened
    ③ Return her to her room
    ④ Sit next to her

22. Mrs. Fletcher falls in the bathroom, resulting in a large bruised area on her right hip. This type of wound is a(n):
    ① Abrasion
    ② Concussion
    ③ Contusion
    ④ Laceration

23. A physician has determined that Mrs. Fletcher has fractured her hip and will have surgical repair in the morning. Preoperative teaching should include:
    ① How to cough and deep breathe postoperatively
    ② The length of the suture line
    ③ The method used to repair the bones
    ④ The type of sutures to be used

24. Makeup and nail polish are removed preoperatively to:
    1. Assess the patient's normal preoperative appearance
    2. Assess oxygenation and circulation during and after surgery
    3. Avoid smearing or marring them during surgery
    4. Prevent contamination of the surgical site

25. When transported to the operating room, the patient should be dressed:
    1. As ordered by the physician
    2. In a hospital gown only
    3. In a hospital gown and warm underwear
    4. With a warm robe over a hospital gown

26. When the patient is returned to bed from the recovery room, the priority nursing action is to assess the:
    1. Airway
    2. Dressing
    3. IV infusion
    4. Vital signs

27. During the early postoperative period, which of the following requires further assessment?
    1. Respiratory rate of 12 respirations per minute
    2. Response to verbal commands
    3. Restlessness
    4. Urine output of 30 ml/hr

28. After the patient's return from the recovery room, assessment of the dressing reveals a nickle-sized area of bright red blood. The nurse:
    1. Changes the dressing
    2. Notifies the physician
    3. Reinforces the dressing
    4. Removes the dressing to observe the wound

29. Postoperative catheterization may be necessary unless the patient voids within:
    1. 3 to 5 hours
    2. 6 to 8 hours
    3. 9 to 11 hours
    4. 12 hours

30. An indication that bowel function is returning after surgery is:
    1. Burping
    2. Gas pain
    3. Increased appetite
    4. Passing of flatus

31. Promoting the return of peristalsis postoperatively is best accomplished by:
    1. Administering an enema
    2. Encouraging coughing and deep breathing
    3. Inserting a nasogastric tube
    4. Providing for ambulation and exercise

32. One of the first signs of hypovolemic shock as a result of postoperative hemorrhage is:
    1. Flushed face
    2. Slow, deep respirations
    3. Warm skin
    4. Weak, rapid pulse

Situation: This morning you are assigned to 89-year-old Mr. McGinnis, who was admitted last evening with right-sided weakness.

33. You notice that Mr. McGinnis has a reddened skin discoloration over his coccyx area. The probable cause of this problem is:
    1. Body lice that have embedded in the skin
    2. Frequent moving up and down in the bed
    3. Inadequate nutrients in his regular diet
    4. Pressure over a bony prominence

34. While bathing Mr. McGinnis' legs, you would be careful *not* to:
    1. Bend the knee while bathing the posterior aspect of the leg
    2. Change the bath water when it becomes soapy
    3. Massage the lower legs
    4. Wash the bottom of his feet since he is ticklish

35. During the bath, assessment of the skin would include:
    1. Color, warmth, bruising
    2. Distribution and color of the hair
    3. Markings made by wrinkles in the sheets or crumbs
    4. Temperature, integrity, and condition

36. Measures that can help to make Mr. McGinnis less susceptible to infectious disease include:
    1. Assessing his vital signs (VS) on a regular basis
    2. Bathing him with soap and water bid
    3. Dressing him in street clothes each day (qd)
    4. Ensuring that he gets adequate rest and sleep

37. Using good body mechanics to help Mr. McGinnis from a sitting to a standing position, the nurse would:
    1. Stand about 2 ft (60 cm) out from his weak side while lifting him under his weak arm
    2. Stand close to his strong side while lifting him under his strong arm
    3. Stand in front of him keeping arms and legs straight to serve as levers while lifting under both arms
    4. Stand in front of him starting with knees bent, straightening them as he rises

38. Mr. McGinnis is embarrassed because he is incontinent of feces. To prevent further emotional stress and soiling of bed linen, you can:
    1. Administer an antidiarrheal drug
    2. Allow Mr. McGinnis to keep a pan of water near his bed to keep himself clean
    3. Offer Mr. McGinnis the bedpan at frequent intervals
    4. Use an absorbent diaper on him

39. Before having a member of the clergy visit Mr. McGinnis, the nurse would:
    1. Ask a family member if such a visit would be desired
    2. Find out if Mr. McGinnis wanted communion
    3. Find out if Mr. McGinnis wanted such a visit
    4. Wait until Mr. McGinnis seemed gravely ill

40. Which of the following religions, in addition to Judaism, observe the Sabbath from sundown Friday to sundown Saturday?
    1. Baptist
    2. Jehovah's Witnesses
    3. Mormon
    4. Seventh Day Adventist

41. In determining the distance to insert a nasogastric tube, the nurse measures the distance from:
    1. Bridge of nose to xiphoid process
    2. Mouth to earlobe to xiphoid process
    3. Tip of nose to earlobe to xiphoid process
    4. Tip of nose to navel

42. During a gavage feeding the patient is placed in which of the following positions?
    1. Fowler's
    2. Lithotomy
    3. Prone
    4. Supine

43. As you begin Mr. McGinnis' gavage feeding he becomes pale and starts to cough. The reason for this is probably that the feeding solution is:
    1. Being introduced too quickly
    2. Entering his trachea
    3. Too cold
    4. Too thick

44. When the patient receiving gastric gavage develops diarrhea, it may be due to:
    1. Air entering the stomach
    2. The feeding being administered too rapidly
    3. Too much water given after the feeding
    4. The tube being inserted too far into the stomach

45. Mr. McGinnis is to have a lumbar puncture this afternoon. An important nursing action after a lumbar puncture is to:
    1. Have the patient lie flat
    2. Keep the patient in the Trendelenburg position
    3. Measure intake and output for 24 hours
    4. Take vital signs qh

46. Mr. McGinnis has just had a glass of cold water. How many minutes must you wait before taking his oral temperature?
    1. 4 minutes
    2. 6 minutes
    3. 8 minutes
    4. 10 minutes

47. You have just taken Mr. McGinnis' pulse and found it to be 56 beats/min—much lower than his normal range. Which of the following should you do first?
    1. Ask another nurse to take the pulse
    2. Count his pulse again
    3. Notify the charge nurse
    4. Notify the physician

Situation: Mrs. Simpson is a 72-year-old woman admitted to the hospital with vaginal bleeding.

48. Therapeutic communication between the nurse and the patient provides communication that is:
    1. Easily understood and meets basic communication needs
    2. Beneficial to the nursing staff in determining attitudes
    3. Purposeful and directed toward goals that benefit the patient
    4. Representative of the type of communication to which the patient is accustomed

49. To prepare Mrs. Simpson for a vaginal examination by the physician, you would assist her into a:
    1. Knee-chest position
    2. Lithotomy position
    3. Prone position
    4. Sims' position

50. While cleaning Mrs. Simpson's dentures, you would be careful to:
    1. Hold dentures over a towel or basin of water
    2. Hold dentures with tissue paper under running water
    3. Soak in cool water before brushing dentures
    4. Soak in very hot water before brushing dentures

51. While seeing about another patient, you leave Mrs. Simpson alone. When you return to her room she screams, "I'm too sick to be left alone." Your best reply would be:
    1. "Don't worry, you're okay."
    2. "I'm sorry I had to leave you. How can I help you now?"
    3. "We nurses understand, but we're very busy."
    4. "Why don't you lie down and rest for awhile?"

52. As you consider Mrs. Simpson's statement, your assessment would be that she is:
    1. Anxious about the source of her illness
    2. A demanding woman
    3. Disrespectful to those trying to help her
    4. Used to a great deal of attention

53. Having written Mrs. Simpson's nurse's note, you realize you wrote it in Mr. Stinson's chart. To correct this error you:
    1. Completely cover the note with a black felt tip marker, write *error* below it and sign your name
    2. Draw a line through the note, write *error—wrong chart* followed by your signature
    3. Erase the note from Mr. Stinson's chart
    4. Remove the page from Mr. Stinson's chart and rewrite the entire page leaving out Mrs. Simpson's note

54. Mrs. Simpson states that although she is having a great deal of pain, she does not want to take her pain medication yet. Reluctance to take pain medication is most often influenced by a patient's:
    1. Cultural background
    2. Genetic background
    3. Economic status
    4. Social status

55. Besides medications, measures helpful in reducing patient's pain include:
    1. Giving a cool sponge bath
    2. Giving a relaxing backrub or changing their position
    3. Having them speak to their physician
    4. Performing range-of-motion exercises

56. The most effective means by which the nurse can protect other patients and self from infections is:
    1. Discarding linen in hamper and not dropping it on the floor
    2. Maintaining enteric isolation
    3. Washing hands between patients and before and after performing care or procedures
    4. Wear a mask around patients with productive coughs

57. To prevent the nurse from physical fatigue during the work day, the nurse must:
   ① Wear a girdle and not lift heavy objects
   ② Maintain good posture and use good body mechanics
   ③ Use back muscles when moving or lifting patients
   ④ Make beds one side at a time

58. In planning care for Mrs. Simpson, you want to increase her fluid intake to 2500 ml/24 hr. Which of the following is the best way to state the goal for Mrs. Simpson?
   ① Patient will be encouraged to drink as much as possible during day and evening shifts
   ② Patient will be given a glass of fluid q2h from 7 AM to 10 PM
   ③ Patient will drink 150 ml fluid qh from 7 AM to 10 PM in addition to drinking all fluids on meal trays
   ④ Patient will drink plenty of fluids during her waking hours

59. In the evening, before Mrs. Simpson goes to sleep, you can help her relax by:
   ① Adjusting the television so she can see the picture without straining
   ② Offering her oral hygiene, reading her the newspaper, and dimming the lights
   ③ Reading her a story or a magazine
   ④ Tightening bed covers and replacing soiled linen

Situation: Mrs. Rabb, an 89-year-old woman, is admitted to your unit. She is pale, weak, and frightened and has ankle edema. BP is 98/52. Temperature is 99°F, pulse is 64 beats per minute and regular, and respirations are 28 per minute. She is diagnosed as having congestive heart failure.

60. If Mrs. Rabb has an irregular pulse, it would be necessary to:
   ① Apply less pressure on the artery
   ② Count it for 1 full minute
   ③ Take an apical-radial pulse
   ④ Take it at the carotid artery

61. Assessment of Mrs. Rabb's IV infusion includes observation of the needle insertion site, tubing, fluid container, and:
   ① Peripheral venous pressure
   ② Rate of flow
   ③ Both of these
   ④ Neither of these

62. An independent nursing action that should be included in Mrs. Rabb's plan of care is:
   ① Range-of-motion exercises
   ② Having the dietician send up high-calorie meals
   ③ Application of elastic stockings to lower leg
   ④ Administration of multivitamins

63. Mrs. Rabb's fluids are restricted to 1200 ml/24 hr. Which of the following would be measured as intake?
   ① Pureed vegetables
   ② Pureed fruit
   ③ Custard
   ④ Beef stew

64. Mrs. Rabb asks why she is being weighed qd. The best explanation is that:
   ① The doctor wants to know her weight qd so that he can change medication dosages if necessary
   ② It is necessary to see that her low-calorie diet is working and that she is not cheating
   ③ Every patient gets weighed daily
   ④ Comparison of daily weights is a good indication of whether she is losing excess fluids

65. Mrs. Rabb is so weak that she needs to be fed. During the meal when she attempts to hold a slice of bread you should:
   ① Encourage her to do so
   ② Place the bread back on the tray so she does not drop it
   ③ Tell her she should not exert herself so much
   ④ Tell her that eating will be much easier if you do the work

66. A retention catheter is ordered for Mrs. Rabb. As part of the procedure, sterile gloves are donned after:
   ① Arranging the sterile drapes
   ② Cleansing the meatus
   ③ Explaining the procedure
   ④ Opening the sterile package

67. You know that the catheter needs to be inserted:
   ① 1 to 2 inches (2.5 to 5 cm)
   ② 3 to 4 inches (7.5 to 10 cm)
   ③ 5 to 6 inches (12.5 to 15 cm)
   ④ 6 to 8 inches (15 to 20 cm)

68. Your neighbor is surprised that after exposure to rubella, her six-week-old son did not get the disease. You explain to her that the baby has:
   ① Active acquired immunity
   ② Active natural immunity
   ③ Passive acquired immunity
   ④ Passive natural immunity

69. While obtaining a throat culture, you should *avoid* touching the swab to the following structure:
   ① Nasal turbinate
   ② Posterior pharynx
   ③ Tonsils
   ④ Uvula

70. You and another team member have just taken an apical-radial pulse. The results were apical—76 beats/ min, radial—82 beats/min. Your next action should be:
   ① Have the patient lie flat in bed
   ② Repeat the procedure
   ③ Report results to the charge nurse
   ④ Report results to the physician

71. While assessing your patient's ankle edema, in addition to inspection, which other technique would you use?
   ① Auscultation
   ② Evaluation
   ③ Palpation
   ④ Percussion

72. To obtain a urine culture and sensitivity from an indwelling catheter, you:
    ① Attach a sterile drainage bag and obtain the specimen from the outlet spout
    ② Protect the end of the drainage tubing while letting urine drip from the catheter into a sterile specimen tube
    ③ Use a needle and syringe, inserting the needle directly into the catheter
    ④ Use a needle and syringe, inserting the needle into the port

73. Your patient's care plan indicates he has orthopnea. Your nursing interventions will include:
    ① Keeping the bed in high-Fowler's position
    ② Maintaining oxygen at 40% by Venturi mask
    ③ Taking vital signs q2h
    ④ Using log-rolling technique to turn him to his side

74. Chickenpox has just been diagnosed in your 17-year-old patient. You should place your patient in which category-specific isolation?
    ① Drainage/secretion
    ② Respiratory
    ③ Strict
    ④ Universal blood and body fluid

75. The practical nurse observes a co-worker using the following techniques in caring for a patient on respiratory isolation. Which technique is in error?
    ① Leaving the patient's glass thermometer in his room
    ② Washing hands before entering the patient's room
    ③ Wearing a mask while applying TED stockings
    ④ Wearing a gown while obtaining a sputum specimen

CHAPTER 3

Anatomy and Physiology

Anatomy and physiology describe and explain how the body is structured and how it functions. The nurse must be familiar with the normal functions of the body to understand the abnormal conditions and the disease processes. Without this knowledge the physical and psychosocial needs of the patient cannot be met.

A. Anatomy: the study of the structure of the body, its many parts, and their relationship to one another
B. Physiology: the study of how the body and its many parts function
C. Homeostasis: a state of constancy or equilibrium within the body
D. Anatomic terminology
   1. Anatomic position: the body is erect, with arms at sides and palms turned forward
   2. Anterior: toward the front of the body
   3. Posterior: toward the back of the body
   4. Cranial: near the head
   5. Superior: toward the head
   6. Inferior: toward the lower aspect
   7. Medial: toward the midline
   8. Lateral: toward the side
   9. Proximal: nearest the origin of a structure
   10. Distal: farthest from the origin of a structure
E. Body cavities
   1. Dorsal: pertaining to the back; has two subdivisions that are continuous with each other
      a. Cranial: the space inside the skull; contains the brain
      b. Spinal: extends from the cranial cavity nearly to the end of the vertebral column; contains the spinal cord
   2. Ventral: pertaining to the front; contains structures of the chest and abdomen; has two subdivisions
      a. Thoracic: chest cavity; contains the heart, lungs and large blood vessels; separated from the lower cavity by the diaphragm
      b. Abdominopelvic: one large cavity with no separation
         (1) Abdominal: upper portion; contains stomach, liver, gallbladder, pancreas, spleen, kidneys, and most of the intestines
         (2) Pelvic: lower portion; contains urinary bladder, lower part of intestines and internal reproductive organs

STRUCTURAL UNITS
Cell

A. Definition: the basic unit oof structure and function of all living things; made of protoplasm (meaning "original substance"), which is composed of carbon, oxygen, hydrogen, sulfur, nitrogen, and phosphorus; vary in size and shape
B. Structures and functions
   1. Structural parts
      a. Cytoplasmic membrane: keeps cell whole and intact; allows certain substances to pass through and prevents others from entering
      b. Cytoplasm: area where most cellular activity occurs; the working and storage area
      c. Nucleus: the control center; directs cell activity and is necessary for reproduction; the site of the genetic material DNA
   2. Characteristics of cells
      a. Irritability: responds to stimuli
      b. Growth and reproduction: gets larger in size and continues species
      c. Metabolism: chemical reaction consisting of:
         (1) Anabolism: forming new substances to build new cell material
         (2) Catabolism: breaking down of substances into simpler substances and disposing of waste
      d. Contractability: the ability to shorten
      e. Conductivity: ability to transfer an electrical charge
   3. Functions
      a. Movement of substances through cell membranes
         (1) Diffusion: movement of particles and water molecules through a fluid or membrane; dissolved particles become evenly distributed throughout fluid
         (2) Osmosis: movement of water and particles through a semipermeable membrane

(3) Filtration: movement of water and particles through a membrane because of a greater pushing force on one side of the membrane

b. Reproduction mitosis: process of cell division; distributes identical chromosomes (DNA molecules) to each cell formed; enables cells to reproduce their own kind

Tissues

A. Definition: groups of similar cells having like functions
B. Classifications and functions
   1. Epithelial: cells are packed close together; contain no blood vessels; three main types
      a. Simple squamous: single layer of cells that substances can pass through; function is absorption; lines air sacs of lungs, lines blood vessels, and covers membranes that line body cavity
      b. Stratified squamous: several layers of closely packed cells; protect the body against invasion of microorganisms; outer layer of skin, epidermis
      c. Simple columnar: single layer of cells; lines the stomach, intestines, and respiratory tract; specializes in secreting mucus and in absorption
   2. Connective: cells are separated by intercellular material; located in all parts of the body; various types include areolar, adipose, bone, and cartilage; function is to support and protect
   3. Muscle: three types of muscle tissue
      a. Skeletal or striated (voluntary): cells have striations; attach to bones; contractions are controlled voluntarily; cause movement
      b. Cardiac or striated (involuntary): cells have cross striations; contractions cannot be controlled; compose heart muscle; cause movement
      c. Visceral or nonstriated (smooth involuntary): cells appear smooth; help form walls of blood vessels and intestines; contractions cannot be controlled; cause movement
   4. Nerve: composed of cells called neurons; all neurons receive and conduct electrochemical impulses; important in control of the entire body

Membranes

A. Definition: thin, soft sheets of tissue that cover, line, lubricate, and anchor body parts
B. Classification and functions
   1. Epithelial: lubricate and protect the body against infection; two types
      a. Mucous: line body cavities that open to the exterior (mouth, nose, intestinal tract, and urinary tract); secrete mucus, which protects against bacterial invasion
      b. Serous: line cavities that do not open to the exterior; cover the lungs, stomach, and heart; secrete thin fluid that prevents friction
   2. Connective: cover bone or hold body parts in place
      a. Skeletal: cover bones and cartilage; support the bony structure
      b. Synovial: line joint cavities and secrete synovial fluid, which lubricates
      c. Fascial or fibrous: hold organs in place; superficial, connects the skin to underlying structures; deep, supports the internal organs (the viscera)

Organs

Structures composed of several tissues grouped together; they perform a more complex function than a single tissue; their composition and structure are dependent on function

Systems

A. Definition: groups of organs that contribute to the function of the whole; they perform a more complex function than a single organ; no system can function independently of another system
B. Body systems and functions
   1. Integumentary (skin): covers and protects the body
   2. Musculoskeletal: supports and allows movement; body's framework
   3. Circulatory: transports food, water, oxygen, and waste
   4. Digestive: processes food and eliminates waste
   5. Respiratory: supplies oxygen and eliminates carbon dioxide
   6. Urinary: excretes waste
   7. Nervous: controls and coordinates body activities
   8. Endocrine: regulates body activities
   9. Reproductive: reproduction

INTEGUMENTARY SYSTEM

A. Structure of skin: includes epithelial, connective, and nerve tissue; consists of sweat and oil glands; is soft and has elasticity
   1. Epidermis: outermost layer; cells are flat and tough; no blood supply
      a. Cells undergo constant cellular change by mitosis
      b. Contains pigment (melanin); amount of pigment varies among races and individuals
   2. Dermis: "true skin"; the inner layer, composed of living cells
      a. Connective tissue framework
      b. Contains blood vessels, nerves, hair roots, and oil and sweat glands
      c. The ridges and grooves form the pattern for fingerprints, unique to each individual
      d. Nerve endings provide sensation
   3. Subcutaneous tissue: lies under dermis
      a. Contains fat cells, which give the skin its smooth appearance
      b. Serves as a shock absorber and insulates deeper tissues
   4. Glands
      a. Sebaceous (oil glands)
         (1) Excrete oily substance (sebum)
         (2) Keep skin soft and moist
      b. Sudoriferous (sweat glands)
         (1) Secrete perspiration
         (2) Part of the body's heating and regulating equipment
   5. Appendages
      a. Hair: covers the skin except on the palms of the hands and the soles of the feet; composed of dead keratinized cells
         (1) Shaft: the hair above the skin
         (2) Follicle: a tiny sac from which the hair root grows

b. Nails: tightly packed cells of scaly epidermis
  (1) Roots are living cells; visible ends are dead cells
  (2) They protect the tips of the fingers and toes
  (3) The pink coloring comes from the blood supply in the nail bed

B. Functions
  1. Protection: protects deeper tissues from pathogenic organisms and harmful chemicals
  2. Excretion: limited to water and urea; only a small amount of waste products are eliminated
  3. Regulation: helps regulate body temperature and fluid content
  4. Sensory: contains millions of nerve endings that provide sensory reception to pressure, touch, pain, and temperature

SKELETAL SYSTEM (Fig. 3-1)

A. Functions
  1. Support: forms framework for body structures and provides shape
  2. Protection: protects the internal organs
  3. Movement: serves as levers that are activated by the contraction of an attached muscle
  4. Mineral storage: stores calcium and minerals used by the body when needed
  5. Produces blood cells: forms erythrocytes and thrombocytes and red marrow of bone

B. Bone composition
  1. Bone composed of 33% organic material and 67% inorganic mineral salts
  2. Collagen: organic part derived from a protein; fibrous material with a jellylike substance between the fibers; gives bone flexibility
  3. Inorganic substance consists of large amount of mineral salts, calcium phosphate, calcium carbonate, calcium fluoride, magnesium phosphate, sodium oxide, and sodium chloride; these minerals give bone its hardness and durability

C. Classification of bones
  1. Long bone: consists of diaphysis, epiphysis, and medullary cavity (e.g., femur)
  2. Short bone: contains more spongy bone than compact; generally cube shaped (e.g., wrist bone)
  3. Flat bone: thin and flat; has two thin layers of compact bone with a spongy bone between them; red blood cells are manufactured here (e.g., sternum)
  4. Irregular: do not fall into preceding categories; are not symmetrical (e.g., vertebrae)

D. Structure of long bones
  1. Similar to other bones in the body as to structure, development, and function
  2. Longer than wide; have a shaft with heads at both ends; bones of extremities are long bones
  3. Diaphysis or shaft: hollow cylinder of hard compact bone; contains medullary canal, which is filled with yellow bone marrow; in the adult it is primarily a storage area for adipose fat
  4. Epiphysis: the ends of the diaphysis composed of spongy bone covered by a thin layer of compact bone; contains red marrow where some red blood cells are manufactured during childhood and adolescence; erythropoietic activity in the adult mainly occurs in flat bones and vertebrae
  5. Periosteum: strong fibrous membrane that covers the bone; contains blood vessels, lymph vessels, nerves, and bone cells necessary for growth, repair, and nutrition
  6. Epiphyseal disk (flat plate of hyaline cartilage): allows for lengthwise growth of long bones; at puberty when growth stops, it calcifies and becomes the epiphyseal line
  7. Haversian canals: run lengthwise through bone matrix, carrying blood vessels and nerves to all areas of the bone; nourish the osteocytes or bone cell

E. Processes: bony prominences that serve as landmarks
  1. Acromion: highest point of the shoulder
  2. Olecranon: the upper end of the ulna, forms the point of the elbow
  3. Iliac crest: curved rim along the upper border of the ilium
  4. Ischial spine: lies at the back of the pelvic outlet
  5. Acetabulum: the deep socket in the hip bone
  6. Greater trochanter: the large protuberance located at the top of the shaft of the femur

F. Factors that affect bone growth and maintenance
  1. Heredity: each person has a genetic potential for height with genes inherited from both parents
  2. Nutrition: nutrients such as calcium, phosphorus, and proteins are raw materials of which bones are made of; without nutrients bones cannot grow properly
  3. Hormones: produced by endocrine glands; help regulate cell division, protein synthesis, calcium metabolism, and energy production
  4. Exercise: bearing weight, such as walking; without exercise bones become thin and fragile

G. Joints: point where bones meet; classification is determined by extent of movement
  1. Synarthroses: fibrous connective tissue holds joining bones close together; no movement (e.g., sutures in skull)
  2. Amphiathroses: slight movement (e.g., joints between the vertebrae)
  3. Diathroses: free movement; all have a joint capsule, a joint cavity, and a layer of cartilage
    a. Ball-and-socket joint: ball-shaped head of one bone fits into a concave socket of another bone (e.g., hip joint)
    b. Hinge joint: allows movement in only two directions, flexion and extension (e.g., knee)
    c. Pivot joint: small projection of one bone pivots in an arch of another bone (e.g., vertebrae of the neck)
    d. Saddle joint: exists only between the metacarpal bone and a carpal bone of the wrist (e.g., thumb and wrist)
    e. Gliding joint: bone surfaces slide over one another (e.g., wrist/ankle)

H. Ligaments: connective tissue bands that hold bones together

I. Tendons: connective tissue bands that attach bones to muscles

J. Bursa: a sac or cavity filled with fluid that reduces friction

SKELETON

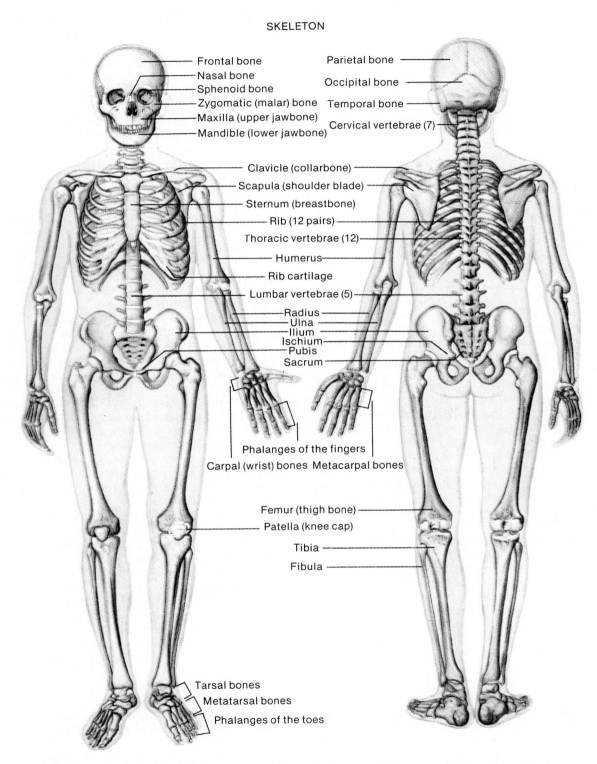

FIG. 3-1. The skeletal system. (From Milliken ME, Campbell G: *Essential competencies for patient care,* St Louis, 1985, Mosby.)

MUSCULAR SYSTEM (Fig. 3-2)

A. Functions
  1. Produces movement by contraction (Table 3-1)
  2. Maintains posture
  3. Produces heat and energy
B. Structure and types
  1. Striated: skeletal, voluntary muscle; attached to bones and accounts for body movement; controlled consciously
  2. Smooth: visceral, nonstriated, involuntary muscle; found in the walls of internal organs and blood vessels; works automatically
  3. Cardiac: found only in the heart; striated, branched, and involuntary
C. Characteristics
  1. Excitability: capacity to respond to stimulus
  2. Contractility: ability to shorten and tighten

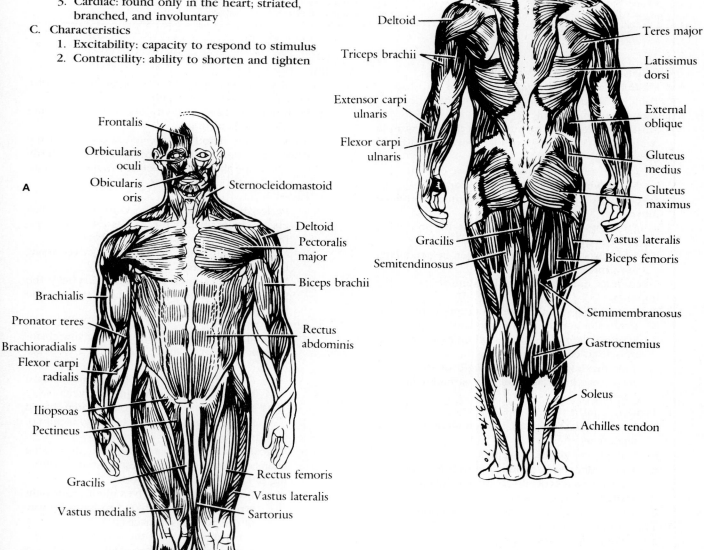

FIG. 3-2. Muscles of the body. **A,** Anterior view. **B,** Posterior view. (From Austrin M: *Young's learning medical terminology step by step,* ed 6, St Louis, 1986, Mosby.)

Table 3-1. The skeletal muscles

Muscle	Location	Function
Sternocleidomastoid	Neck	Flexion and rotation of head
Trapezius	Upper back	Helps hold head erect; also assists in moving the head sideways
Latissimus dorsi	Lower back	Extension and adduction of upper arm
Pectoralis major	Chest	Flexion and adduction of upper arm
Deltoid	Shoulder	Abduction of upper arm
Biceps brachii	Anterior upper arm	Flexion of arm and forearm
Triceps brachii	Posterior upper arm	Extension of arm and forearm
Gluteus maximus	Fleshy part of hips and buttocks	Extension of thigh
Gluteus medius	Lateral part of hips and buttocks	Abduction of thigh when limb is extended
Hamstring group	Posterior thigh	Flexion of lower leg and extension of thigh
Quadriceps femoris	Anterior thigh	Flexion of thigh and extension of lower leg
Gastrocnemius	Calf of leg	Helps in extension of foot and flexion of leg

3. Extensibility: ability to stretch
4. Elasticity: ability to regain original size and shape
5. Tonicity: ability to maintain steady contraction

D. Contraction and movement
  1. Muscles move bones by pulling on them; as muscle contracts, it pulls insertion bone toward its original bone
    a. Origin: attached to fixed structure of bone
    b. Insertion: attached to movable part
  2. Several muscles contract at the same time to produce movement
    a. Prime mover: mainly responsible for producing movement
    b. Synergists: aid the prime mover in producing movement
  3. To contract, muscle must first be stimulated by nerve impulses
    a. Subminimal stimulus: does not cause contraction
    b. Minimal stimulus: does cause contraction
    c. Maximal stimulus: causes all muscle fibers in muscle to contract
    d. Supramaximal stimulus: strength of stimulus is above maximal; no effect on strength of contraction
  4. Types of contraction
    a. Isometric: increases the tension without causing movement
    b. Isotonic: produces movement
    c. Tonic: does not produce movement but increases firmness of muscles that maintain posture
    d. Twitch: a quick, jerky contraction
    e. Tetanic (tetanus): sustained contraction
  5. Types of movement
    a. Flexion: makes angle at joint smaller
    b. Extension: makes angle at joint larger
    c. Abduction: moves part away from midline
    d. Adduction: moves part toward midline

CIRCULATORY SYSTEM

A. Functions
  1. Major function: transports oxygen, carbon dioxide, cell wastes, nutrients, enzymes, and antibodies throughout the body
  2. Secondary function: contributes to the body's metabolic functions and maintenance of homeostasis

B. Heart (Fig. 3-3)
  1. Hollow, cone-shaped muscular organ the size of a man's fist; functions as pump
  2. Positioned in thoracic cavity between the sternum and thoracic vertebrae
  3. Apex extends slightly to the left and rests on the diaphragm, approximately at the level of the fifth rib; a stethoscope should be placed at the apex to count an apical pulse
  4. Layers
    a. Pericardium: outer covering; consists of two layers of serous membrane that is lubricated and prevents friction when the heart beats
    b. Myocardium: dense fibrous connective tissue; the wall of the heart
    c. Endocardium: a thin, serous lining that helps the blood flow smoothly through the heart; lines the heart chamber
  5. Chambers
    a. Atria: upper chambers: primarily receiving chambers; not important in the pumping action of the heart
      (1) Right atrium: receives deoxygenated blood from the superior and inferior vena cava
      (2) Left atrium: receives oxygenated blood from the lungs by way of the four pulmonary veins
    b. Ventricles: lower chambers; the dispensing chambers; have the major responsibility of forcing blood out into large arteries
      (1) Right ventricle: receives blood from right atrium and pumps blood to lungs by way of the pulmonary artery
      (2) Left ventricle: does the major work of the heart; has the thickest wall; pumps blood to all parts of the body by way of the aorta
      (3) Interventricular or interatrial septum: divides the heart longitudinally
  6. Valves: permit flow of blood in only one direction
    a. Tricuspid: allows blood to flow from right atrium into right ventricle
    b. Mitral or bicuspid: allows blood to flow from left atrium to left ventricle
    c. Pulmonary semilunar: allows blood to flow out of right ventricle into pulmonary artery

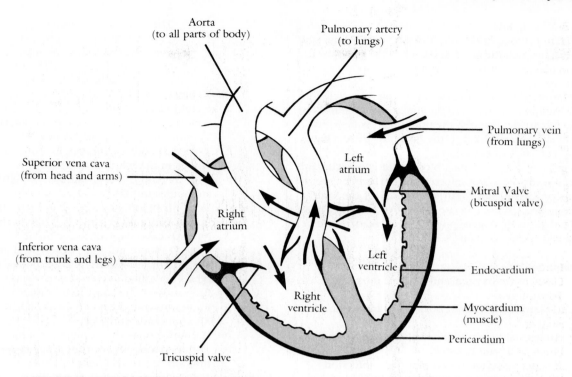

Aorta
(to all parts of body)

Pulmonary artery
(to lungs)

Pulmonary vein
(from lungs)

Superior vena cava
(from head and arms)

Left
atrium

Mitral Valve
(bicuspid valve)

Right
atrium

Left
ventricle

Endocardium

Inferior vena cava
(from trunk and legs)

Myocardium
(muscle)

Right
ventricle

Pericardium

Tricuspid valve

FIG. 3-3. Structures of the heart. (From Sorrentino SA: *Mosby's textbook for nursing assistants,* ed 2, St Louis, 1987, Mosby.)

d. Aortic semilunar: allows blood to flow out of left ventricle into aorta
7. Physiology
  a. Cardiac cycle: refers to one complete heartbeat, consisting of contraction or systole and relaxation or diastole of the atria and ventricles
  b. Auscultatory sounds: heard through a stethoscope; the first sound, systolic, is longer and louder because of the closure of the cuspid valves; the second sound, diastole, is shorter and softer because of the closure of the semilunar valves
  c. Conduction system
    (1) Functions: initiates heartbeat; conducts electrical impulses around heart; coordinates heartbeat
    (2) Components
      (a) Sinoatrial (SA) node: the pacemaker of the heart, sets and regulates the beat by sending electrical impulses to the atria and the AV node
      (b) Atrioventricular (AV) node: receives impulses from SA node; transmits electrical impulses by way of bundle of His to the ventricles
      (c) Bundle of His: fibers that begin at AV node and follow the interventricular septum; divides into Purkinje's fibers
      (d) Purkinje's fibers: conducting fibers; stimulate the ventricles to contract
  d. Heart rates: controlled by internal and external factors

    (1) Bradycardia: slower than normal rate, less than 60 beats/min
    (2) Tachycardia: faster than normal rate, more than 100 beats/min
    (3) Extrasystole: premature beat
    (4) Sinus arrhythmia: a regular variation in heart rate resulting from changes in the rate and depth of breathing
C. Blood vessels
  1. Arteries: elastic, muscular-conducting tubes; carry blood away from the heart and to the capillaries; all arteries (except pulmonary) carry oxygenated blood
    a. Aorta: the largest artery, from which all other arteries branch out and become smaller and smaller
    b. Arterioles: extremely small arteries; branch into the capillaries
  2. Veins: thin-walled tubes that have one-way valves to prevent backflow of blood; transport blood back to the heart; all veins (except pulmonary) carry deoxygenated blood
    a. Venae cavae: largest veins; enter the right atrium
      (1) Superior vena cava: returns blood from the head, arms, and thoracic region
      (2) Inferior vena cava: returns blood from body regions below the diaphragm
    b. Venules: extremely small veins; collect blood from the capillaries
  3. Capillaries: microscopic vessels; carry blood from arterioles to venules; exchange of nutrients and waste products occurs in capillaries

D. Types of circulation
 1. Systemic: blood flows from the left ventricle into the aorta, through the body, and back to the right atrium; provides oxygen-rich, nutrient-laden blood to body organs
 2. Pulmonary: blood flows from the right ventricle into the pulmonary artery, to the lungs, and then back to the left atrium through the pulmonary vein; its function is to carry blood to the lungs for gas exchange and return it to the heart
 3. Portal: detour of venous blood from stomach, pancreas, intestines, and spleen through the liver, where it is processed, and returned by way of the inferior vena cava; excess glucose is removed and stored in the liver as glycogen; poisonous substances are removed and detoxified
E. Blood
 1. Functions
  a. Transports oxygen and carbon dioxide to and from lungs
  b. Transports nutrients, hormones, and waste products
  c. Helps maintain acid-base balance, electrolyte balance, and fluid balance
  d. Carries substances that help fight infection
  e. Acts to maintain homeostasis
 2. Composition
  a. Plasma: liquid, straw-colored portion of blood
   (1) Approximately 90% water
   (2) Contains blood proteins (fibrinogen, prothrombin, albumin, gamma globulin)
   (3) Contains mineral salts (electrolytes), hormones, nutrients, oxygen, carbon dioxide, and waste products (urea, lactic acid, and uric acid)
  b. Formed elements
   (1) Erythrocytes: red blood cells (RBCs)
    (a) Contain hemoglobin, which carries oxygen to cells and carbon dioxide from cells
    (b) Originate in red bone marrow
    (c) Life span is 100 to 120 days
    (d) Destroyed by the spleen, liver, and bone marrow
    (e) Normal range: male, 4.5 to 6.2 million per cubic millimeter; female, 4 to 5.5 million per cubic millimeter
   (2) Leukocytes: white blood cells (WBCs)
    (a) Principal function is to fight infection
    (b) Able to multiply rapidly
    (c) Classified according to whether they contain visible granules in their cytoplasm
     ■ Granulocytes: include neutrophils, eosinophils, and basophils
     ■ Agranulocytes: include lymphocytes and monocytes
    (d) Formation is in red bone marrow and by lymphatic tissue in lymph nodes, thymus, and spleen
    (e) Normal range: 5000 to 10,000 per cubic millimeter

   (3) Thrombocytes: platelets
    (a) Aid in clotting process
    (b) Originate in bone marrow
    (c) Normal range: 200,000 to 400,000 per cubic millimeter
 3. Blood types
  a. Every person belongs to one of the four groups: type A, type B, type AB, or type O; and is classified as either Rh positive or Rh negative
  b. Type A blood: A antigens in RBCs, anti-B antibodies in plasma
  c. Type B blood: type B antigens in RBCs, anti-A antibodies in plasma
  d. Type AB blood: has type A and type B antigens in RBCs; no anti-A or anti-B antibodies in plasma; type AB called universal recipient
  e. Type O blood; no type A or type B antigens in RBCs; both anti-A and anti-B antibodies in plasma; type O is called universal donor blood
  f. Rh-positive blood: Rh-factor antigen in RBCs
  g. Rh-negative blood: no Rh factor in RBCs; no anti-Rh antibodies in plasma
  h. Harmful effects can result from a blood transfusion if donor's RBCs become agglutinated by antibodies in the recipient's plasma
F. Lymphatic system: represents an accessory route for return of fluid from interstitial spaces to cardiovascular system; consists of lymphatic vessels, lymph nodes or glands, and spleen
 1. Lymph: transparent fluid in surrounding spaces between tissue cells; made of water and end products of cell metabolism; referred to as intercellular or interstitial fluid
 2. Function of system
  a. Lymphatic vessels: return fluid and proteins to blood
  b. Lymph nodes: filter injurious particles such as microorganisms and cancer cells
  c. Tonsils: filter and remove bacteria or pathogens entering the throat
  d. Thymus: most active during early life; relates immune reaction through puberty; atrophies at adulthood
 3. Spleen: consists of lymphoid tissue
  a. Forms lymphocytes and monocytes
  b. Destroys old RBCs
  c. Stores blood until needed and then releases it into circulation
G. Immunity: the body's defense system against diseases and substances interpreted as nonself; mediated by T- and B-lymphocytes of the circulatory system; the functions of lymphocytes in immunity by cell type are
 1. T-lymphocytes: originate from stem cells in thymus; responsible for cellular immunity (a slow response) to an antigen; act against most bacteria, viruses, tumor cells, and foreign organs or grafts; clone into types of regulatory cells—helper and suppressors
  a. Helper T-cells: interact directly with B-cells by stimulating activity of B-cells on killer T-cells
  b. Killer T-cells: directly attack virus-infected cells, promote lysis
  c. Suppressor T-cells: terminate normal immune response

2. B-lymphocytes: originate mainly in fetal liver and lymphoid tissue during first few months of life; responsible for humoral immunity (a rapid response) to an antigen
    a. Clone antibody-producing plasma cells
    b. Protect against toxin
3. Naturally acquired immunity
    a. Active: acquired through contact with disease
    b. Passive: acquired from antibodies obtained through placenta and mother's milk
4. Artificially acquired immunity
    a. Active: immunization with vaccines
    b. Passive: administration of immune serum

NERVOUS SYSTEM

The nervous system functions as a coordinated unit both structurally and functionally

A. Functions
    1. Regulates system
    2. Controls communication among body parts
    3. Coordinates activities of body system
B. Divisions
    1. Central nervous system (CNS): brain and spinal cord; interprets incoming sensory information and sends out instruction based on past experiences
    2. Peripheral nervous system (PNS): cranial and spinal nerves extending out from brain and spinal cord; carry impulses to and from brain and spinal cord
    3. Autonomic nervous system: function classification of the PNS; regulates involuntary activities
    4. Somatic nervous system: functional classification of the PNS; allows conscious or voluntary control of skeletal muscles
C. Structure and physiology
    1. Neurons or nerve cells: respond to a stimulus, connect it into a nerve impulse (irritability), and transmit the impulse to neurons, muscle, or glands (conductivity); consists of three main parts
        a. Cell body: contains nucleus and one or more fibers or processes extending from cell body
        b. Dendrites: conduct impulses toward cell body; neuron has many dendrites
        c. Axons: conduct impulses away from cell body; neuron has one axon
    2. Types of neurons
        a. Motor (efferent): conduct impulses from CNS to muscle and glands
        b. Sensory (afferent): conduct impulses toward CNS
        c. Connecting (interneuron): conduct impulses from sensory to motor neurons
    3. Synapse: chemical transmission of impulses from axon to dendrites
    4. Myelin sheath: protects and insulates the axon fibers; increases the rate of transmission of nerve impulses
    5. Neurilemma: sheath covering the myelin; found in PNS; function is regeneration of nerve fiber
    6. Neuroglia: connective or supporting tissue, important in reaction of nervous system to injury or infection
    7. Ganglia: clusters of nerve cells outside CNS
    8. White matter: bundles of myelinated nerve fibers; conducts impulses along fibers
    9. Gray matter: clusters of neuron cell bodies; fibers not covered with myelin; distributes impulses across selected synapses
D. Central nervous system
    1. Brain (Fig. 3-4)
        a. Cerebrum: largest part of brain; outer layer called cerebral cortex; cortex composed of dendrites and cell bodies; controls mental processes; highest level of functioning
        b. Cerebellum: controls muscle tone coordination and maintains equilibrium

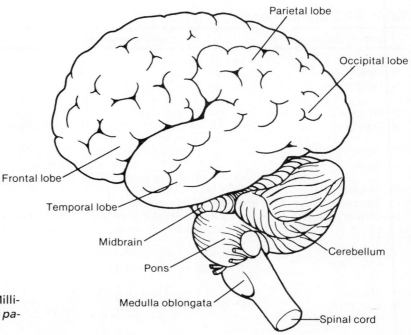

FIG. 3-4. Lateral view of the cerebrum. (From Milliken ME, Campbell G: *Essential competencies for patient care,* St Louis, 1985, Mosby.)

c. Diencephalon: consists of two major structures located between cerebrum and midbrain
  (1) Hypothalamus: regulates the autonomic nervous system, controls blood pressure, helps maintain normal body temperature and appetite and controls water balance and sleep
  (2) Thalamus acts as a relay station for incoming and outgoing nerve impulses; produces emotions of pleasantness and unpleasantness associated with sensations
d. Brainstem: connects the cerebrum with the spinal cord
  (1) Midbrain: relay center for eye and ear reflexes
  (2) Pons: connecting link between cerebellum and rest of nervous system
  (3) Medulla oblongata: contains center for respiration, heart rate, and vasomotor activity
2. Spinal cord
  a. Inner column composed of gray matter, shaped like an H, made up of dendrites and cell bodies; outer part composed of white matter, made up of bundles of axons called tracts
  b. Function: sensory tract conducts impulses to brain; motor tract conducts impulses from brain; center for all spinal cord reflexes
3. Protection for CNS
  a. Bone: vertebrae surround cord; skull surrounds brain
  b. Meninges: three connective tissue membranes that cover brain and spinal cord
    (1) Dura mater: white fibrous tissue; outer layer
    (2) Arachnoid: delicate membrane, middle layer; contains subarachnoid fluid
    (3) Pia mater: inner layer, contains blood vessels

c. Spaces
  (1) Epidural: between dura mater and the vertebrae
  (2) Subdural space: between dura mater and arachnoid
  (3) Subarachnoid space: between arachnoid and pia mater, contains cerebrospinal fluid
d. Cerebrospinal fluid: acts as a shock absorber; aids in exchange of nutrients and waste materials
E. Peripheral nervous system
  1. Carries voluntary and involuntary impulses
  2. Cranial nerves: (Table 3-2)
  3. Spinal nerves: 31 pairs; conduct impulses necessary for sensation and voluntary movement; each group named for the corresponding part of the spinal column
F. Autonomic nervous system
  1. Part of PNS; controls smooth muscle, cardiac muscle, and glands
  2. Two divisions
    a. Sympathetic: "fight or flight" response; increases heart rate and blood pressure; dilates pupils
    b. Parasympathetic: dominates control under normal conditions; maintains homeostasis

RESPIRATORY SYSTEM

A. Respiration: the taking in of oxygen, its use in the tissues, and the giving off of carbon dioxide; has two stages
  1. External: exchange of oxygen and carbon dioxide between body and outside environment; consists of inhalation and exhalation
  2. Internal: exchange of carbon dioxide and oxygen between the cells and the interstitial fluid surrounding the cells
B. Organs (Fig. 3-5)
  1. Nose:
    a. Divides into two cavities separated by nasal septum

Table 3-2. Cranial nerves

Cranial nerves	Conducts impulses	Function
I Olfactory	From nose to brain	Sense of smell
II Optic	From eye to brain	Vision
III Oculomotor	From brain to eye and eye muscles	Contraction of upper eyelid; maintain position of eyelid; pupillary reflexes
IV Trochlear	From brain to external eye muscles	Eye movements
V Trigeminal	From skin and mucous membranes of head and teeth to chewing muscles	Sensations of head and teeth; muscles of chewing
VI Abducens	From brain to external eye muscles	Eye movements
VII Facial	From taste buds of tongue and facial muscles to muscles of facial expression	Taste; facial expression
VIII Acoustic	From organ of Corti to brain	Hearing
Vestibular branch	From semicircular canals to brain	Balance
IX Glossopharyngeal	From pharynx and posterior third of tongue to brain; also from brain to throat muscles and salivary glands	Sensations of tastes, sensations of pharynx; swallowing; secretion of saliva
X Vagus	From throat and organs in thoracic and abdominal cavities to brain; to muscles of throat and abdominal cavities	Important in swallowing, speaking, peristalsis, and production of gastric juices
XI Accessory	From brain to shoulder and neck muscles	Rotation of head and raising shoulders
XII Hypoglossal	From brain to muscles of tongue	Movement of tongue

FIG. 3-5. Organs of the respiratory system. (From Anthony CP, Kolthoff NJ: *Textbook of anatomy and physiology,* ed 9, St Louis, 1975, Mosby.)

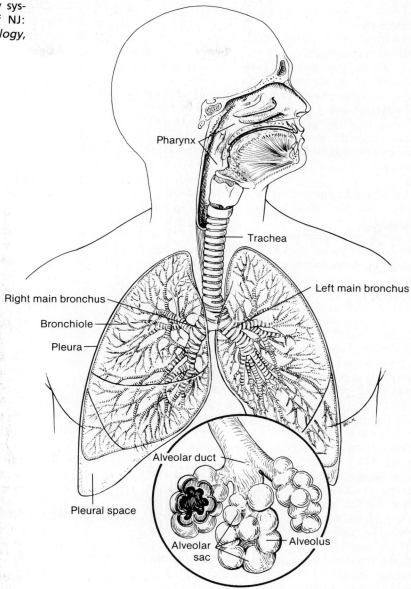

Pharynx

Trachea

Right main bronchus

Left main bronchus

Bronchiole

Pleura

Alveolar duct

Pleural space

Alveolar sac

Alveolus

b. Ciliated mucosa lines the cavities and traps inhaled foreign particles

c. Filters, warms, and moistens air

d. Serves as organ of smell

e. Paranasal sinuses: lighten skull, act as resonance chamber in speech

2. Pharynx: passageway for food and air; divided into three parts

   a. Nasopharynx (behind nose): contains adenoids; eustachian tube, which drains the middle ear, opens into the nasopharynx

   b. Oropharynx (mouth): contains tonsils, which are lymphatic tissue

   c. Laryngopharynx: opens into larynx toward front and into esophagus toward back

3. Larynx (voice box)

   a. Formed by nine cartilages in boxlike formation

b. Thyroid cartilage forms the Adam's apple

c. Epiglottis: flap of elastic cartilage that closes off the larynx when swallowing food

d. Produces sound; vocal cords vibrate with expelled air

e. Passageway for air to the trachea

4. Trachea (windpipe): tube reinforced by C-shaped rings; open ends of rings face posteriorly toward the esophagus and allow esophagus to expand when swallowing food; solid portion keeps the trachea open for the passage of air

5. Bronchi

   a. Formed by the division of the trachea into two branches; distribute air to the lungs' interior; called bronchial tree

   b. Right main bronchus is larger and more vertical; aspiration is more common by this route

c. Bronchi divide into smaller branches called bronchioles

d. Bronchioles divide into smaller tubes and terminate in the alveoli

e. Alveoli: microscopic air sacs that resemble bunches of grapes; composed of a single, thin layer of squamous epithelium; external surface surrounded with spider-webbed pulmonary capillaries; here the gas exchanges occur, oxygen passes from the alveoli into the capillary blood, and carbon dioxide leaves the blood to enter the alveoli

6. Lungs

a. Cone shaped; upper part is the apex; broad lower part is the base; base is concave and rests on diaphragm

b. Tissue is porous and spongy

c. Pleura: thin, moist, slippery membrane covering lungs; prevents friction during breathing movement

C. Physiology

1. Two phases of breathing: inspiration and expiration

2. Respiration controlled by respiratory center in medulla oblongata

3. Carbon dioxide stimulates respiration

4. Muscles of respiration

a. Diaphragm: dome shaped; separates thoracic and abdominal cavities; contracts and relaxes

b. Intercostals: between the ribs; elevate the ribs and enlarge the thorax during inspiration

5. Mechanism of inspiration

a. Contraction of diaphragm causes thorax to expand

b. The lungs cling to the thoracic wall as a result of the attachment of the pleural membranes

c. Intrathoracic pressure decreases

d. The volume within the lungs (intrapulmonary) increases, and gases in the lungs spread out to fill the space

e. Result is a decrease in gas pressure, and a partial vacuum sucks air into the lungs; air continues to move into the lungs until intrapulmonic pressure equals atmospheric pressure

6. Mechanism of expiration

a. Respiratory muscles relax and thorax decreases in size

b. Intrathoracic and intrapulmonary volumes decrease

c. As volume decreases, gases are forced closer together, and intrapulmonary pressure rises higher than atmospheric pressure

d. Gases flow out of lungs and equalize pressure inside and outside the lung

7. Volumes of air exchanges

a. Total lung capacity (TLC): total volume of air present in the lungs after maximum inspiration

b. Vital capacity (VC): volume of air that can be expelled after maximum inspiration

c. Tidal volume (TV): volume of air exhaled after normal inspiration

d. Residual volume (RV): amount of air remaining in lung after maximum expiration

DIGESTIVE SYSTEM

A. Organs (Fig. 3-6)

1. Mouth (buccal cavity)

a. Receives food; aids in digestion; aids in speaking

b. Consists of hard and soft palate, teeth, tongue, and salivary glands

(1) Teeth:

(a) Deciduous: baby teeth

(b) Permanent: appear at approximately 6 years of age

(c) Incisors: cut food

(d) Canines: tear food

(e) Molar: grind food

(2) Salivary glands: parotid, submandibular, submaxillary; manufacture saliva, which contains ptyalin to begin the chemical breakdown of food

c. Functions

(1) Ingestion of food

(2) Mastication of food

(3) Lubrication of food

(4) Digestion of starch with salivary amylase

2. Pharynx: transports food

3. Esophagus: muscular tube; conducts food from pharynx to stomach

4. Stomach:

a. J-shaped pouch; varies in size depending on contents; stores food and changes it into chyme

b. Three divisions

(1) Fundus: upper portion; the cardiac sphincter between the esophagus and fundus; controls the entrance of food

(2) Body: the largest, central portion

(3) Pylorus: lower portion above the small intestine; the pyloric sphincter controls the passage of food into the duodenum

c. Glands: secrete gastric juices and enzymes (including hydrochloric acid): the chemical breakdown of protein begins in the stomach

(1) Pepsin: begins digestion of protein

(2) Lipase: acts on emulsified fat

(3) Renin: acts on casein (a protein) in milk

(4) Gastrin (hormone): related to the control of gastric secretions; not an enzyme

(5) Hydrochloric acid: makes stomach content acid and activates enzymes

d. Chyme: the semiliquid contents of the stomach, consisting of partially digested food and gastric enzymes

e. Functions

(1) Storage of food

(2) Breakdown of food by churning

(3) Liquefying of food with hydrochloric acid

(4) Digestion of protein with enzyme, pepsin

5. Small intestine: extends from the pyloric sphincter to the ileocecal valve, which prevents backflow of material and regulates forward flow

a. Size: approximately 20 ft (600 cm) long and 1 inch (2.5 cm) in diameter

b. Three major divisions

(1) Duodenum: approximately 10 inches (25 cm) long; curves around head of the pan-

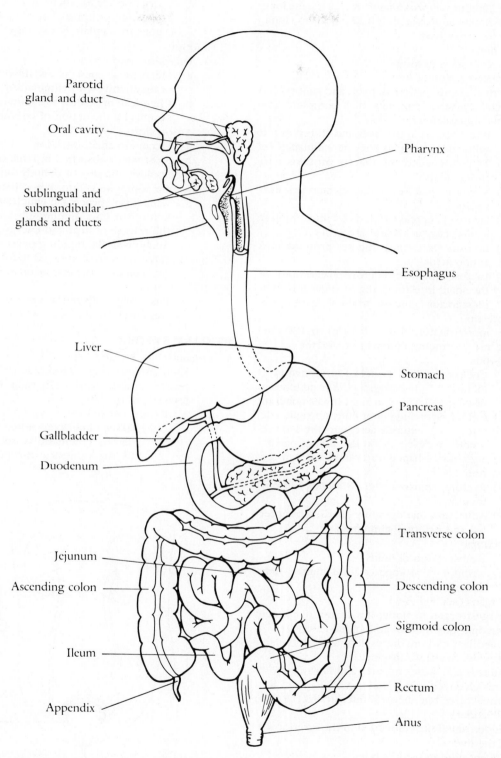

FIG. 3-6. Digestive system. (From Sorrentino, SA: *Mosby's textbook for nursing assistants,* ed 2, St Louis, 1987, Mosby.)

creas; pancreatic and common bile duct enter below pyloric sphincter
   (2) Jejunum: approximately 8 ft (240 cm) long
   (3) Ileum: approximately 12 ft (360 cm) long; terminal part
  c. Functions
    (1) Digestion of food
    (2) Absorption of food
  d. Intestinal glands, pancreas, liver, and gallbladder secrete digestive enzymes that complete the chemical breakdown of food
    (1) Bile (formed in the liver and stored in the gallbladder): not an enzyme; emulsifies fat
    (2) Trypsin (pancreas): digests proteins into amino acids
    (3) Amylase (pancreas): digests starches into sugars
    (4) Lipase (pancreas): digests fat into simplest forms (fatty acids and glycerol)
    (5) Erepsin (intestine): digests proteins into amino acids
    (6) Lactose, maltose, sucrose (secretions of the small intestine): digest sugar into simplest forms (glucose, fructose, galactose)
 6. Large intestine
  a. Size: approximately 5 to 6 ft (150 to 180 cm) long and 2½ inches (6 cm) in diameter
  b. Divisions
    (1) Cecum: a blind pouch approximately 3 inches (7.5 cm) long; appendix attaches to distal end; located in right lower quadrant
    (2) Colon: ascending, continues up right side; transverse, extends across to the left; descending, descends on left side of pelvis
    (3) Sigmoid: S-shaped portion; extends to rectum
    (4) Rectum: approximately 8 inches (20 cm) long
    (5) Anus: terminal opening: guarded by internal and external sphincters
  c. Functions
    (1) Reabsorption of fluids
    (2) Temporary storage of fecal matter; defecation

B. Accessory organs (see Fig. 3-6)
 1. Liver: largest organ in body; lies below diaphragm in upper right quadrant of abdominal cavity
  a. Metabolizes carbohydrates, fats, and proteins
  b. Detoxifies harmful substances
  c. Produces and stores heparin and fibrinogen
  d. Stores glycogen and vitamins A, B, B_{12}, and K
  e. Manufactures bile; hepatic duct drains bile into gallbladder
 2. Gallbladder: small sac embedded in the interior surface of the liver
  a. Concentrates and stores bile
  b. Releases bile through the common bile duct into the duodenum when fat enters the small intestine
 3. Pancreas: long, triangular gland; lies behind the stomach; produces enzymes that break down food particles; secretes enzymes into the duodenum; has two functions

  a. Exocrine gland: secretes digestive enzymes that neutralize chyme
  b. Endocrine gland: islets of Langerhans; secretes insulin for utilization of glucose; secretes glucagons to regulate blood sugar level

C. Functions
 1. Digestion: two process
  a. Mechanical: chewing, swallowing, and peristalsis of food; ends with elimination
  b. Chemical: breakdown of food into simpler compounds by the action of enzymes on food
 2. Absorption
  a. Occurs in small intestine
  b. Most water absorbed in large intestine
 3. Metabolism: the sum of all body functions to convert simple compounds into living tissue
  a. Catabolism: process in which substances are broken down into simpler substances, resulting in the release of heat and energy
  b. Anabolism: the building phase in which simpler substances are combined to form more complex substances (conversion of food into living tissues)
  c. Basal metabolism: the amount of energy (calories) used by the body when at rest

URINARY SYSTEM

A. Organs (Figs. 3-7 and 3-8)
 1. Kidneys: bean shaped and reddish brown; lie against posterior abdominal wall; right kidney is slightly lower than the left
  a. External structure
    (1) Hilus: concave notch; blood vessels, nerves, lymphatic vessels, and ureters enter the kidneys at this point

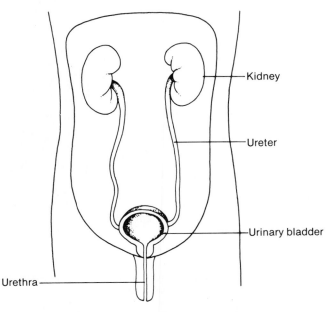

FIG. 3-7. Organs of the urinary system. (From Milliken ME, Campbell G: *Essential competencies for patient care,* St Louis, 1985, Mosby.)

(2) Renal capsule; protective fibrous tissue surrounding kidneys
  b. Internal structure
    (1) Cortex: outer portion; the greater portion of the nephron is located here
    (2) Medulla: inner portion; consists of 12 cone-shaped structures (pyramids); tip of pyramid points toward renal pelvis and drains waste and excess water into pelvis
    (3) Pelvis: funnel shaped; forms upper end of ureter and receives waste and water
  c. Nephron: basic unit of function; microscopic structure composed of capillaries; approximately 1 million per kidney; control the processes of filtration, reabsorption, and secretion
    (1) Glomerulus: filtering unit; process of urine formation begins
    (2) Renal tubules: reabsorption occurs in the proximal convoluted tubules, through Henle's loops, and the distal convoluted tubules; then the collecting tubules pass the final urine product into the pelvis
  2. Ureters: two long, narrow tubes; transport urine from kidney to bladder by peristalsis
  3. Bladder: elastic, muscular organ, capable of expansion; stores urine; assists in voiding (micturition: the release of urine or voiding)
  4. Urethra: narrow, short tube from bladder to exterior; exterior opening called the meatus
    a. Female: approximately 1¼ to 2 inches (3 to 5 cm) long; transports urine
    b. Male: approximately 8 inches (20 cm) long; transports urine and is a passageway for semen
B. Functions
  1. Excretion: nitrogen-containing waste (urea, uric acid, and creatinine) is excreted; normal daily output is 1200 to 1500 ml
  2. Maintenance of water balance: absorbs more or less water depending on intake; normally, intake is approximately equal to output
  3. Regulates acid balance; reabsorbs or actively secretes excess acids and bases produced by cell metabolism
C. Urine composition
  1. Clear, yellowish, slightly aromatic, and slightly acid
  2. Contains 95% water and 5% solids, which includes urea, uric acid, creatinine, ammonia, sodium, and potassium; specific gravity (sp gr) indicates amount of the dissolved solids; normal range: 1.05 to 1.03 sp gr
  3. Abnormal substances: glucose, blood protein, RBCs, bile, and bacteria

ENDOCRINE SYSTEM

A. Classification and secretions
  1. Exocrine glands: have ducts (tubes); secretions carried to an external or internal surface of the body by ducts (e.g., lacrimal gland)
  2. Endocrine glands: ductless; secretions by glands (hormones) carried to body tissue by blood and lymph
B. Endocrine glands and hormones (Fig. 3-9 and Table 3-3)

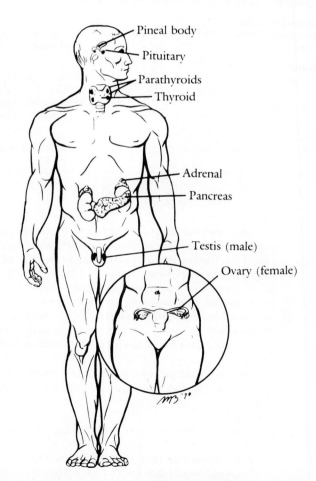

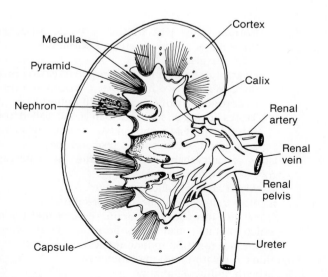

FIG. 3-8. Structure of the kidney. (From Milliken ME, Campbell G, *Essential competencies for patient care*, St Louis, 1985, Mosby.)

FIG. 3-9. Endocrine system. (From Austin M, *Young's learning medical terminology step by step*, ed 6, St Louis, 1986, Mosby.)

Table 3-3. Endocrine glands, hormones and actions

Endocrine glands and hormones	Actions of hormones
Anterior pituitary	
Corticotropin (adrenocorticotropic hormone [ACTH])	Stimulates the adrenal cortex to produce and secrete glucocorticoid hormones
Somatotropic hormone (STH)	Stimulates growth of body cells
Thyroid-stimulating hormone (TSH)	Stimulates the thyroid gland to produce and release thyroid hormone
Gonadotropic hormones (GTH)	Affect growth, maturity, and function of primary and secondary sex organs
Luteinizing hormone (LH)	
Follicle-stimulating hormone (FSH)	
Lactogenic hormone (prolactin)	
Posterior pituitary	
Antidiuretic hormone (ADH)	Promotes sodium and water retention in the kidney; increases blood pressure
Oxytocin	Initiates and maintains labor; influences the breasts to release milk
Thyroid	
Thyroxine	Regulates the metabolic rate of all body cells
Pancreas	
Insulin	Promotes glucose use by the cell and decreases blood sugar level
Glucagon	Promotes glucose release from the liver and increases blood sugar level
Adrenal cortex	
Glucocorticoids (includes cortisol and cortisone)	Assist the body to respond to stress; concerned with carbohydrate, fat, and protein metabolism; reduces inflammation
Mineralcorticoids (includes aldosterone)	Promote sodium and water retention in the kidney and potassium excretion
Sex hormones (androgens, estrogen, and progesterone)	Mainly affect development of secondary sex characteristics
Adrenal medulla	
Epinephrine (adrenaline) and norepinephrine (noradrenaline)	Constrict blood vessels and channel the blood to vital internal organs to prepare the body for emergency situations
Ovaries	
Estrogen	Promotes development of female sex characteristics, growth of female sex organs, and development of the uterine wall for implantation of the fertilized ovum; regulates menstruation
Progesterone	Prepares the uterine wall for implantation of the fertilized ovum; maintains the placenta and pregnancy; regulates menstruation
Testes	
Androgens (includes testosterone)	Stimulates development of the secondary male sex characteristics; essential for normal functioning of male sex organs

1. Pituitary: located at base of the brain in a saddle-like depression of the sphenoid bone at the base of brain; called the master gland, approximately the size of a grape; composed of two parts
   a. Anterior lobe: secretes many hormones
   b. Posterior lobe: secretes two hormones
2. Thyroid: located in the neck inferior to the Adam's apple; easily palpated; the largest of the endocrine glands; consists of two lobes joined by a narrow band (isthmus)
3. Parathyroid (four glands): located on posterior surface of the thyroid; regulates calcium level in the blood
4. Adrenal
   a. Two small glands; curve over the top of the kidneys
   b. Each gland has two separate parts: inner area (medulla) and outer area (cortex); produces different hormones
   c. Medulla: mimics the action of the sympathetic nervous system
   d. Cortex: outer part of the adrenals: produces three major groups of steroid hormones
5. Gonads (sex glands)
   a. Ovaries in female: located in pelvic cavity; produce ova and two hormones, estrogen and progesterone; do not function until puberty
   b. Testes in male: suspended in a sac called the scrotum outside the pelvic cavity; produce sperm and sex hormone, testosterone
6. Islets of Langerhans: located within the pancreas; consist of alpha and beta cells
   a. Alpha cells: produce glucagon
   b. Beta cells: secrete hormone insulin
7. Pineal: lies just above midbrain; secretes melatonin, which inhibits gonadotropic hormone (GTH) secretion; exact function in man unclear
C. Functions: regulators of body functions
   1. Growth and development
   2. Reproduction
   3. Metabolism
   4. Fluid and electrolyte balance

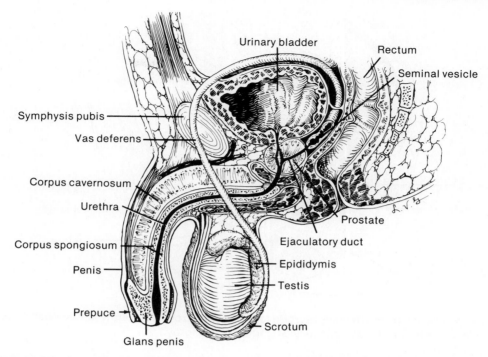

FIG. 3-10. Organs of the male reproductive system. (From Milliken ME, Campbell G: *Essential competencies for patient care,* St Louis, 1985, Mosby.)

REPRODUCTIVE SYSTEM
Male Reproductive System (Fig. 3-10)
A. External genitals
1. Scrotum: skin-covered pouch; lies outside of pelvic cavity; contains testes, epididymis, and lower part of vas deferens; lower body temperature here is necessary for reproduction
2. Penis: erectile tissue; organ of coitus (sexual intercourse); serves as passageway for urine and semen
B. Testes: small oval glands in scrotum; produce spermatozoa; secrete testosterone
C. Ducts
1. Seminiferous tubules: formation of sperm
2. Epididymis: narrow, tightly coiled tubes; provides temporary storage space for immature sperm
3. Vas deferens: continuation of the epididymis; lies near surface of scrotum; called the spermatic cord
4. Ejaculatory: pass through prostate; ejaculate semen into urethra
D. Accessory glands
1. Seminal vesicles: located on each side of the prostate; empty secretion into the prostatic ampulla
2. Prostate: encircles the upper area of the urethra; secretes alkaline fluid; increases sperm motility
3. Cowper's gland: located below prostate; produces an alkaline secretion that is primarily a lubricant during sexual intercourse
E. Semen: alkaline fluid (pH 7.5); the major bulk (60%) is secreted by the seminal vesicles; the remaining 40% is secreted by other accessory organs
F. Function
1. Reproduction
2. Production of testosterone

Female Reproductive System (Fig. 3-11)
A. External genitals
1. Vulva
   a. Labia majora: two long folds of skin on each side of the vaginal orifice outside of the labia minora
   b. Labia minora: two flat, thin, delicate folds of skin that are highly sensitive to manipulation and trauma; enclose the region called the vestibule, which contains the clitoris, the urethral orifice, and the vaginal orifice
   c. Clitoris: very sensitive erectile tissue; becomes swollen with blood during sexual excitement
   d. Vaginal orifice: opening into vagina; hymen, fold of mucosa, partially closes orifice and generally is ruptured during first sexual intercourse
   e. Bartholin's glands: located on each side of vaginal orifice; secrete lubrication fluid
2. Perineum: between vaginal orifice and anus; forms pelvic floor
B. Internal organs
1. Ovaries: main sex glands
   a. Located on either side in pelvic cavity
   b. Produce ova, which form in the graafian follicles
   c. Graafian follicle produces estrogen
   d. Rupture of a follicle releases an ovum (ovulation)
   e. Ruptured follicles becomes glandular mass called corpus luteum
   f. Corpus luteum secretes estrogen, but mainly progesterone
2. Fallopian tubes
   a. Extend from point near ovaries to uterus; no direct connection between ovaries and tubes

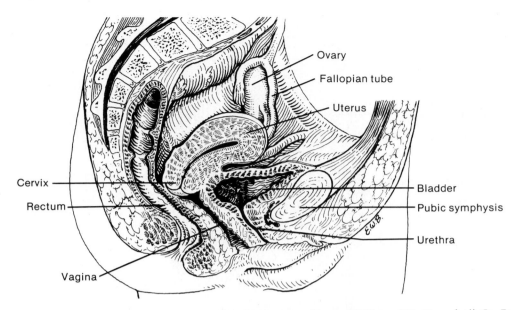

FIG. 3-11. Organs of the female reproductive system. (From Milliken ME, Campbell G: *Essential competencies for patient care*, St Louis, 1985, Mosby.)

b. Fimbriae: fingerlike extensions on tubes; pick up ova and transport into fallopian tubes
c. Fertilization occurs in outer one third of the fallopian tubes

3. Uterus
  a. Upper portion rests on upper surface of bladder; the lower portion is embedded in pelvic floor between the bladder and the rectum
  b. Pear-shaped, hollow organ that expands tremendously to accommodate a fetus
  c. Divisions
    (1) Body: upper main part
    (2) Fundus: bulging upper surface of the body
    (3) Cervix: neck of the uterus
  d. Endometrium: uterine lining; sloughs off during menstruation
  e. Functions
    (1) Menstruation
    (2) Pregnancy
    (3) Labor

4. Vagina
  a. Located between rectum and urethra
  b. Structure: wrinkled mucous membrane (rugae); capable of great distention
  c. Functions
    (1) Lower part of birth canal
    (2) Receives semen from male
    (3) Passageway for menstrual flow

C. Breasts (mammary glands)
  1. Located over pectoral muscles
  2. Size depends on adipose tissue rather than glandular tissue
  3. Consists of lobes, lobules, and milk-secreting cells (acini)

4. Ducts lead to the opening called the nipple
5. Areola: pigmented area surrounding the nipple

D. Function
  1. Reproduction
  2. Production of estrogen and progesterone

E. Menstrual Cycle
  1. Phases: regulated primarily by the hormonal control of pituitary gland, ovaries, and uterus
    a. One ovum discharged each month from an ovary; ripens in the graafian follicle; follicle-stimulating hormone (FSH) from anterior lobe of pituitary stimulates the formation of the follicle
    b. Estrogen produced by the follicle builds up the endometrium in expectation of a fertilized ovum
    c. Ovum is discharged into the fallopian tube by luteinizing hormone (LH) from the anterior lobe pituitary; follicle is converted into the corpus luteum
    d. Postovulation: corpus luteum secretes progesterone and estrogen for final preparation of the endometrium
    e. Premenstrual: the gradual drop in progesterone and estrogen leads to menses
  2. Length of cycle: usually 28 days; highly variable; ovulation occurs midway
  3. Menopause (climacteric): the gradual cessation of menstrual cycle; the ability to bear children ends; occurs at approximately 45 years of age
    a. Ovaries lose their ability to respond to hormones
    b. Decrease in levels of estrogen and progesterone
      (1) Failure to ovulate
      (2) Monthly flow is less, irregular, and gradually ceases
      (3) Reproductive organs atrophy

FIG. 3-12. Structure of the eye: lateral view: (From Milliken ME, Campbell G: *Essential competencies for patient care,* St Louis, 1985, Mosby.)

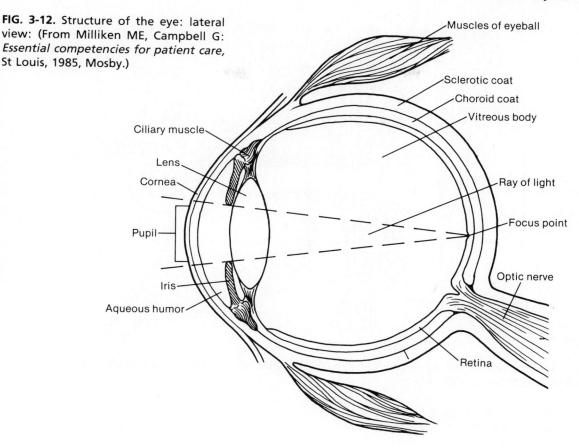

Ciliary muscle
Lens
Cornea
Pupil
Iris
Aqueous humor

Muscles of eyeball
Sclerotic coat
Choroid coat
Vitreous body
Ray of light
Focus point
Optic nerve
Retina

SENSORY SYSTEM
Eye (Fig. 3-12)

A. Lies in a protective bony orbit in the skull
B. Eyebrows, eyelids, and lashes also protect the eye
C. Sphere consists of three layers of tissue
   1. Sclera: thick, white fibrous tissue (white of eye); a transparent section over the front of the eyeball, the cornea, permits light rays to enter
   2. Choroid: the middle vascular area: brings oxygen and nutrients to the eye: choroid extends to ciliary body (two smooth muscle structures), which helps control shape of the lens; the front is a pigmented section (iris), which gives the eye color; in the center of the iris lies the pupil, the "window of the eye" (allows light to pass to lens and retina)
   3. Retina: inner layer; physiology of vision takes place; contains receptors of optic nerve; neurons are shaped like rods and cones; cones permit perception of color, rods permit perception of light and shade
D. Chambers
   1. Anterior: contains aqueous humor; maintains slight forward curve in cornea
   2. Posterior: contains vitreous humor: maintains spherical shape of eyeball
E. Conjunctiva: mucous membrane that covers eyeball and eyelid; keeps eyeball moist

F. Lens: transparent structure behind iris; focuses light rays on retina
G. Lacrimal apparatus: gland located in upper, outer part of eye; produces tears to lubricate and cleanse; nasolacrimal duct is located in nasal corner, tears drain into nose
H. Function: vision

Ear (Fig. 3-13)

A. External ear (pinna or auricle): outer, visible portion, shaped like a funnel; gathers sound and sends it into the auditory canal, which is lined with tiny hairs and secretes cerumen, a waxy substance; canal extends to the eardrum, also called the tympanic membrane
B. Middle ear: small, flattened space; contains three small bones called ossicles: malleus (hammer), incus (anvil), and stapes (stirrup); bones are mobile and vibrate; conduct sound waves, the eustachian tube extends into nasopharynx and equalizes the pressure in the middle ear to that of atmospheric pressure
C. Internal ear (labyrinth): vestibule; cochlea, snail-shaped bony tube, contains organ of Corti (organ of hearing); semicircular canals are the receptors for equilibrium and head movements
D. Function
   1. Transmission of sound waves; result is hearing
   2. Maintenance of equilibrium

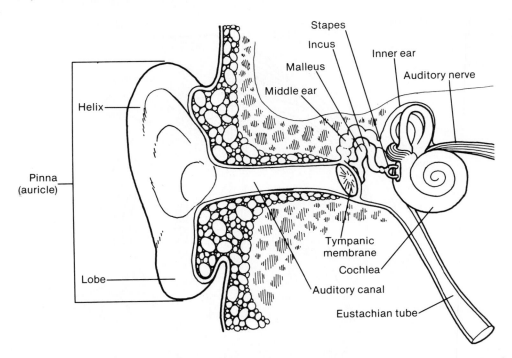

FIG. 3-13. Structure of the ear. (From Milliken ME, Campbell G: *Essential competencies for patient care,* St Louis, 1985, Mosby.)

Special Sense Organs

A. Taste
1. Receptors (taste buds, located in tongue): stimulated only if substance is in solution
2. Four kinds: sweet (tip of tongue); sour (side of tongue); salty (tip of tongue); bitter (back part of tongue)
3. Stimulates appetite and flow of digestive juices

B. Smell
1. Receptors located in olfactory epithelium of upper part of nasal cavity
2. Stimulates appetite and flow of digestive juices
3. Senses of smell and taste work together to give flavor to food

C. Touch
1. Receptors: small, round bodies (tactile corpuscles)
2. Located in dermis; numerous in tips of fingers, toes, and tongue
3. Allows perception of heat, cold, and pain

Suggested Reading List

Anthony CP, Thibodeau GA: *Basic concepts in anatomy and physiology,* ed 8, St. Louis, 1988, Mosby.

Hole JW Jr: *Essentials of human anatomy and physiology,* Dubuque, Iowa, 1986, William C Brown.

Marieb E: *Human anatomy and physiology,* laboratory manual, Reading, Mass, 1988, Addison-Wesley.

Memmler RL, Wood DL: *Structure and function of the human body,* ed 5, Philadelphia, 1992, JB Lippincott.

Physicians' desk reference, Montvale, NJ, Medical Economics (published annually).

Scanlon V, Sanders T: *Essentials of anatomy and physiology,* Philadelphia, 1991, FA Davis.

Tortora GJ, Anagnostakos NP: *Principles of anatomy and physiology,* ed 5, New York, 1989, Harper & Row.

Anatomy and Physiology Review Questions

Answers and rationales begin on p. 423.

1. Formed elements in the blood that aid in blood clotting are called:
   ① Antibodies
   ② Leukocytes
   ③ Erythrocytes
   ④ Platelets

2. The body's continual response to changes in the external and internal environment is called:
   ① Homeostasis
   ② Diffusion
   ③ Osmosis
   ④ Filtration

3. The ability of a cell to reproduce is called:
   ① Osmosis
   ② Crenation
   ③ Lyse
   ④ Mitosis

4. The immunity that occurs when a person is given a substance containing antibodies or antitoxins is called:
   ① Active
   ② Autoimmune
   ③ Passive
   ④ Permanent

5. The part of the cell necessary for reproduction is the:
   ① Cytoplasm
   ② Nucleus
   ③ Protoplasm
   ④ Cytoplasmic membrane

6. The hormone that regulates the metabolic rate of body cells is:
   ① Oxytocin
   ② Aldosterone
   ③ Thyroxin
   ④ Cortisone

7. The ovaries produce the hormones:
   ① Estrogen and testosterone
   ② Progesterone and testosterone
   ③ Estrogen and progesterone
   ④ Progesterone and prolactin

8. A greater amount of body heat is lost when surface blood vessels:
   ① Contract
   ② Dilate
   ③ Increase the production of sweat
   ④ Help the skeletal muscles relax

9. The pigmented area surrounding the nipple is the:
   ① Areola
   ② Bartholin's gland
   ③ Cowper's gland
   ④ Urochrome

10. The hormone produced by the testes is:
    ① Progesterone
    ② Estrogen
    ③ Testosterone
    ④ Aldosterone

11. Connective tissue that attaches muscles to bones is called:
    ① Tendons
    ② Ligaments
    ③ Cartilage
    ④ Osseous

12. The lymphatic system is a collection of vessels and tissues that:
    ① Destroys enzymes
    ② Manufactures erythrocytes
    ③ Localizes infections and filters foreign cells
    ④ Filters and aids in blood clotting

13. A patient with a low hemoglobin level would be deficient in which of the following essential minerals:
    ① Copper
    ② Magnesium
    ③ Calcium
    ④ Iron

14. Bile is important in the digestive process because it:
    ① Dissolves meat fibers and makes them easier to digest
    ② Breaks down fat globulars so they can be more easily digested
    ③ Digests simple fats and sugars
    ④ Changes complex sugars to glucose

15. The tissue that forms a protective covering for the body and lines the intestinal and respiratory tract is called:
    ① Periosteum
    ② Pericardium
    ③ Epithelial
    ④ Connective

16. Regurgitation of food is prevented by the:
    ① Cardiac sphincter
    ② Rugae
    ③ Chyme
    ④ Pyloric sphincter

17. Nutrients that the body uses are absorbed primarily in the:
    ① Liver
    ② Stomach
    ③ Small intestine
    ④ Large intestine

18. Muscles whose functions are to close off body openings are:
    ① Abductors
    ② Sphincters
    ③ Extensors
    ④ Flexors

19. Tears drain into the nose through the:
    ① Ciliary body
    ② Lacrimal gland
    ③ Eustachian tube
    ④ Nasolacrimal duct

20. The first eight deciduous teeth to appear through the gums of a baby are:
    ① Eye teeth
    ② Molars
    ③ Incisors
    ④ Canines

21. Respiration and heart rate are controlled by the:
    ① Cerebellum
    ② Cerebrum
    ③ Medulla
    ④ Pons

22. The main function of the large intestine is to:
    ① Absorb digested food
    ② Absorb water from waste material
    ③ Produce digestive enzymes
    ④ Secrete digestive enzymes

23. The movement that propels food down the digestive tract is called:
    ① Pylorospasm
    ② Rugae
    ③ Mastication
    ④ Peristalsis

24. The end product of protein metabolism is:
    ① Amino acids
    ② Ptyalin
    ③ Hydrochloric acid
    ④ Glucose

25. The completion of digestion occurs in the:
    ① Large intestine
    ② Stomach
    ③ Small intestine
    ④ Sigmoid

26. The function of the liver includes the following *except*:
    ① Production of digestive enzymes
    ② Detoxification of harmful substances
    ③ Manufacture of bile
    ④ Production of heparin and fibrinogen

27. To function adequately, the thyroid gland must have a sufficient supply of:
    ① Calcium
    ② Phosphorus
    ③ Iron
    ④ Iodine

28. The exchange of nutrients and waste products occurs in the:
    ① Capillaries
    ② Veins
    ③ Arterioles
    ④ Venules

29. The chamber of the heart that receives venous blood from body tissues is:
    ① Right atrium
    ② Left atrium
    ③ Right ventricle
    ④ Left ventricle

30. The hormone released by the medulla at times of an emergency is called:
    ① Insulin
    ② Aldosterone
    ③ Epinephrine
    ④ Testosterone

31. The reabsorption of water from the kidney tubules is promoted by:
    ① Oxytocin
    ② Calcitonin
    ③ Antidiuretic hormone (ADH)
    ④ Prolactin (PRL)

32. The exchange of oxygen and carbon dioxide in the lungs occurs in the:
    ① Bronchi
    ② Alveoli
    ③ Bronchioles
    ④ Venules

33. The pacemaker of the heart is the:
    ① AV node
    ② Bundle of His
    ③ Purkinje fibers
    ④ SA node

34. All arteries carry oxygenated blood with the exception of the:
    ① Pulmonary
    ② Aorta
    ③ Coronary
    ④ Carotid

35. Immunity occurring in the early months of an infant's life results from the functioning of which gland?
    ① Thyroid
    ② Thymus
    ③ Pineal
    ④ Pituitary

36. The large, rounded portion at the upper and lateral portion of the femur most often involved in hip fractures is the:
    ① Acetabulum
    ② Acromion
    ③ Greater trochanter
    ④ Olecranon process

37. The major function of the periosteum is to:
    ① Produce RBCs
    ② Produce yellow bone marrow
    ③ Provide a structure for blood, lymph, and nerves
    ④ Provide storage for adipose fat

38. The muscular structure that forms the floor of the pelvis is the:
    ① Peritoneum
    ② Perineum
    ③ Mons pubis
    ④ Rectus abdominis

39. Assessment of a patient's integumentary system includes checking:
    ① Blood pressure and pulse
    ② Blood sugar levels
    ③ Rashes, bruises, and decubitus
    ④ Rashes, bruises and blood sugar levels

40. Observing that a teenager has many blackheads, you know one cause would be blockage of the:
    ① Ceruminous gland
    ② Lacrimal gland
    ③ Sebaceous gland
    ④ Sudoriferous gland

41. Normal urine has the following characteristics *except*:
    ① Clear, amber liquid
    ② Nitrogenous waste products
    ③ Slightly aromatic
    ④ High specific gravity

42. Grooves and ridges that make up fingerprints are located in the:
    ① Elastic skin tissue
    ② Subcutaneous layer of tissue
    ③ Upper surface of the dermis
    ④ Upper surface of the epidermis

43. The hormone that regulates blood composition and blood volume by acting on the kidney is:
    1. Antidiuretic (ADH)
    2. Aldosterone
    3. Parathormone
    4. Oxytocin
44. Muscles obtain energy from:
    1. Glycogen and acetylcholine
    2. Carbohydrates and lactic acid
    3. Oxygen and acetylcholine
    4. Oxygen and glycogen
45. An injury to the left motor area of the cerebrum would cause paralysis of:
    1. The right side of the body
    2. The left side of the body
    3. Both arms and legs
    4. Both arms
46. The large, flat, dome-shaped muscle that assists in breathing is the:
    1. Latissimus dorsi
    2. Sternocleidomastoid
    3. Diaphragm
    4. Gastrocnemius
47. The part of the nervous system that directs the digestion of food and the circulation of blood is the:
    1. Sensory
    2. Interneurons
    3. Sympathetic
    4. Parasympathetic
48. Regulation of body temperature is a function of the:
    1. Medulla
    2. Hypothalamus
    3. Cerebral cortex
    4. Cerebellum
49. The organ of hearing is the:
    1. Tympanic membrane
    2. Organ of Corti
    3. Semicircular canal
    4. Malleus
50. The equalizing of pressure in the middle ear with atmospheric pressure is the function of the:
    1. Eustachian tube
    2. Labyrinth
    3. Oval window
    4. Ossicles
51. Electrolyte balance is maintained chiefly by the action of the:
    1. Bladder
    2. Kidney
    3. Islets of Langerhans
    4. Gonads
52. Insulin is produced in the:
    1. Pineal gland
    2. Duodenum
    3. Islets of Langerhans
    4. Liver
53. A muscle commonly used as a location for intramuscular injections is the:
    1. Gluteus maximus
    2. Gluteus medius
    3. Iliopsoas
    4. Sartorius
54. Which statement best describes the T-cells in the immunity response
    1. Responsible for humeral immunity
    2. Act against bacteria, viruses, tumor cells, and foreign organs
    3. Clone into helpers and suppressors
    4. Clone antibody-producing plasma cells
54. Moving a body part away from the midline is called:
    1. Abduction
    2. Adduction
    3. Flexion
    4. Pronation
55. The primary function of the fluid within the eyeball is to:
    1. Dilate the pupil
    2. Produce tears
    3. Regulate the thickness of the lens
    4. Give and maintain shape of the eyeball

CHAPTER 4

Pharmacology

This chapter encompasses two major areas: (1) administration of medications and (2) pharmacologic aspects of nursing care. The nursing process as it applies to drugs and drug administration is explained and integrated throughout the text.

Calculation of dosage and intravenous infusion rate, principles of medication administration, procedures and sites for medication administration, blood transfusion administration, and pediatric drug administration are reviewed.

The major classifications of drugs are presented as to their action, adverse effects, and nursing process application. Commonly used clinical drugs are listed with generic name and brand name.

The role of the licensed practical/vocational nurse (LP/VN) in the administration of medications is determined by the state nurse practice acts and agency policy. However, knowledge of drugs has a significant impact on the quality of nursing care provided each patient by the LP/VN.

PHARMACOLOGY AND THE NURSING PROCESS

A. Assessment: systematic collection and interpretation of data
B. Management
  1. Planning: defining objectives, setting priorities, selecting the best approach
  2. Implementation: plan is carried out
C. Evaluation: determination of effectiveness of the plan and making necessary modification

Nursing Assessment

A. Assessing the patient
  1. Variables
    a. Age
    b. Body build
    c. Pathologic conditions
    d. Diet and fluid intake
    e. Concurrent drug use
    f. Allergies
    g. Health-illness values
    h. Understanding of disease and drugs
    i. Cognitive function
    j. Physical abilities and disabilities
  2. Medication history
    a. Prescription and nonprescription drugs
    b. Caffeine-containing products
    c. Alcohol
    d. Tobacco
    e. Street drugs
B. Assessing the drug
  1. Medication order
    a. Accuracy
    b. Legibility
    c. Need for clarification

  2. Types of medication orders
    a. Routine or standard
    b. Prn order: given on a "when necessary" basis
    c. Single order: to be given only once
    d. Stat order: to be given only once and immediately
    e. Standing order: established for all patients with a specific condition

Nursing Management

A. Planning
  1. Goal setting: statement of expected outcomes of actions taken in relation to the problem
  2. Establishing priorities: weighing the importance of one problem against the others
  3. Selecting the best approach: identifying the approach most likely to succeed with minimal risk and high acceptability to the patient
B. Implementation
  1. Proper administration technique
  2. Measures to support the therapeutic effect
  3. Observation for desired therapeutic response
  4. Observation for adverse effects
  5. Teaching patients
  6. Accurate recording
C. Institutional level management: drug distribution systems
  1. Floor stock
  2. Individual patient medication system: a supply of medication is dispensed and labeled for a particular patient
  3. Unit dose: individual doses of each medication ordered are dispensed
D. Individual patient care management
  1. Approach to patient
    a. "Therapeutic use of self" attitude of nurse

b. Consistency of approach

c. Informed consent for patient

d. Compliance and right to refuse

2. Patient teaching: explain drug dose, side effects, food-drug interactions, and so forth

   a. Identify need for teaching

   b. Establish realistic teaching goals

   c. Select teaching methods

   d. Implement teaching

   e. Evaluate effect of teaching

3. Patient observation: establish observational parameters—vital signs, laboratory studies, etc.—to evaluate effects of drugs

4. Supportive therapy: nursing actions can complement drug therapy or minimize unpleasant, adverse reactions

5. Documentation of medications (form is set by agency policy)

   a. Information must be complete and accurate

   b. Legal implications: if drug administration is not documented, it is assumed not to have been administered

   c. Data should include

      (1) Observations relevant to therapeutic effects

      (2) Actions taken to prevent or treat adverse reactions

      (3) Time when a drug is discontinued

      (4) Reason(s) for discontinuation of drug

E. Dosage form and route

1. Factors influencing route of administration

   a. Specific chemical and physical properties of the drug

   b. Pathologic condition of the patient

   c. Adequacy of medication compliance

2. Dose: amount of the drug to be given at one time

3. Dosage: regulation of the frequency, size, and number of doses

4. Dosage form: final product administered to the patient

   a. Tablet: solid dosage form made by compression of a powdered drug

      (1) Enteric-coated tablet: tablet coated with material to prevent dissolution in stomach; disintegrates in small intestine to prevent stomach irritation

      (2) Press-coated or layered tablet: tablet with a second layer of material pressed on or around it, which allows incompatible ingredients to be separated and to dissolve at different rates

      (3) Sublingual tablet: dissolves under the tongue

      (4) Buccal tablet: dissolves between the cheek and gum

      (5) Troche or lozenge: Dissolves in mouth over a long period of time

   b. Capsule: gelatin shell containing a drug; it dissolves quickly in stomach or small intestine

   c. Caplet: coated tablet in the shape of a capsule

   d. Timed release or sustained action: slow, continuous dissolution for an extended time, allowing larger doses to be given fewer times

   e. Solution: a liquid, usually water, in which one or more compounds are dissolved

      (1) Oral solutions: may contain flavoring

      (2) Intravenous solutions: must be sterile and particle free

      (3) Other injectable solutions: need only be sterile

      (4) Solutions for external use

   f. Syrup: medication dissolved in a concentrated solution of a sugar to which flavors may have been added

   g. Elixir: clear fluid that serves as a vehicle for drugs; contains primarily water, alcohol, glycerine, and a sweetener

   h. Tincture: alcohol or water-alcohol solutions of a drug

   i. Suppository: solid dosage form that dissolves after insertion into a body cavity such as rectum, vagina, or urethra

   j. Suspension: a liquid in which fine drug particles are suspended; shake vigorously before use; not for intravenous use

      (1) Emulsion: an aqueous medium in which microscopic oil particles are dispersed

      (2) Lotion: a suspension for external application

   k. Ointment: semisolid mixture of a drug, which is rubbed onto the skin

   l. Cream: semisolid mixture of a drug in a thick emulsion, which is rubbed into the skin

5. Dosage route: means of access to the site of action or systemic circulation

   a. Oral: drug is ingested and absorbed from stomach or small intestine; convenient, economical; can irritate stomach; may be destroyed by digestive juices

   b. Sublingual: drug dissolved under tongue and absorbed through mucous membrane of mouth; can irritate oral mucosa

   c. Buccal: drug dissolved between cheek and gum and absorbed through mucous membrane of the mouth

   d. Rectal: drug inserted into rectum and absorbed through rectal mucous membrane; may be used in unconscious or vomiting patient

   e. Lung: drug inhaled as a gas or aerosol; useful for drugs intended to act directly on the lung

   f. Subcutaneous: drug injected under the skin into subcutaneous fascia; sterile procedure

   g. Intramuscular: drug injected into muscle mass; relatively rapid absorption due to good blood supply; sterile procedure

   h. Intravenous: drug injected into vein for immediate effect; permits direct control of blood drug concentrations; sterile procedure

   i. Intradermal: drug injected directly under skin; sterile procedure

   j. Vaginal: drug inserted into the vagina and absorbed through the mucous membrane

   k. Intraarterial: drug injected directly into an artery

   l. Intraarticular: drug injected directly into a joint

   m. Intraspinal (intrathecal): drug injected directly into spinal canal

n. Ophthalmic: drug applied to the eye in form of drops or ointments; must be sterile

o. Otic or aural: drugs applied in the ear

p. Nasal: drugs applied to the nasal cavity by dropper or atomizer

Nursing Evaluation

A. Therapeutic goals: evaluate therapeutic effectiveness of drugs

B. Diagnostic goals: observation for potential adverse reactions

C. Teaching goals: verifying patient's knowledge of drug or ability to perform a skill necessary for administration of the drug

D. Patient compliance: evaluate adherence by the patient to a prescribed plan of treatment

SOURCES OF DRUGS

A. Animals

B. Plants

C. Microorganisms

D. Synthetic chemical substances

E. Food substances

DRUG LEGISLATION

A. Food, Drug, and Cosmetic Act: 1938 (amended 1952, 1962)
   1. Contains detailed regulations to ensure that drugs meet standards of safety and effectiveness
   2. Requires physician's prescription for legal drug purchase

B. Controlled Substances Act: 1970
   1. Defines drug dependency and drug addiction
   2. Classifies drugs according to potential abuse and medical usefulness
   3. Establishes methods for regulating manufacture, distribution, and sale of controlled substances
   4. Establishes education and treatment programs for drug abuse

C. Controlled substances schedule

Schedule I: Drugs that have a high potential for abuse and are not approved for medical use in the United States (e.g., cocaine)

Schedule II: Drugs that have a high potential for abuse but have a currently accepted medical use in the United States; abuse may lead to severe psychologic or physical dependence (e.g., morphine sulfate)

Schedule III: Drugs that have a lower potential for abuse than those in schedules I and II; abuse may lead to high psychologic or low-to-moderate physical dependence (e.g., aspirin [Empirin] with codeine)

Schedule IV: Drugs that have some potential for abuse; abuse may lead to limited psychologic or physical dependence (e.g., diazepam [Valium])

Schedule V: Drugs that have the lowest potential for abuse; products that contain moderate amounts of controlled substances that may be dispensed by the pharmacist without a physician's prescription but with some restrictions such as amount, record keeping, and other safeguards (e.g., Robitussin A-C)

PRINCIPLES OF DRUG ACTION
Mechanisms of Drug Therapy

A. Dissolution: disintegration of dosage form; dissolution of an active substance

B. Absorption: the process that occurs between the time a substance enters the body and the time it enters the bloodstream

C. Distribution: the transport of drug molecules within the body

D. Metabolism: biotransformation—the way in which drugs are inactivated by the body

E. Excretion: elimination of a drug from the body

Variables That Affect Drug Action

A. Dosage

B. Route of administration

C. Drug-diet interactions: food slows absorption of drugs; some foods containing certain substances react with certain drugs

D. Drug-drug interactions
   1. Additive effect: occurs when two drugs with similar actions are taken together
   2. Synergism (potentiation): a total effect of two similar drugs that is greater than the sum of the effects if each is taken separately
   3. Interference: occurs when one drug interferes with the metabolism or elimination of a second drug, resulting in intensification of the second drug
   4. Displacement: occurs when one drug is displaced from a plasma protein-binding site by a second, causing an increased effect of the displaced drug
   5. Antagonism: a decrease in the effects of drugs caused by the action of one on the other

E. Age
   1. Fetus: metabolism and elimination mechanisms immature
   2. Newborn: organ systems not fully developed
   3. Children: depends on age and developmental stage
   4. Elderly adults: physiologic changes may alter a drug's actions in the body

F. Body weight: affects drug action mainly in relation to dosage

G. Pregnancy: influence on drug interactions can be pronounced

H. Pathologic conditions: disease processes are capable of altering drug mechanisms (e.g., patients with kidney disease have increased risk of drug toxicity)

I. Psychologic considerations: attitudes and expectations influence patient response (e.g., anxiety can decrease effect of analgesics)

Adverse Reactions to Drugs

A. Idiosyncratic reaction: unusual, unexpected reaction usually the first time a drug is taken

B. Allergic reactions: stimulate antibody reactions from the immune system of body
   1. Urticaria (hives)
   2. Anaphylaxis: severe allergic reaction involving cardiovascular and respiratory systems; may be life threatening

C. Gastrointestinal effects
   1. Anorexia
   2. Nausea, vomiting

3. Constipation
4. Diarrhea
5. Abdominal distention
D. Hematologic effects
1. Blood dyscrasia
2. Bone marrow depression
3. Blood coagulation disorders
E. Hepatotoxicity
1. Hepatitis
2. Biliary tract obstruction or spasms
F. Nephrotoxicity: renal insufficiency or failure; kidney stones
G. Drug dependence
1. Physiologic: physical need to relieve shaking; pain
2. Psychologic: need to relieve feeling of anxiety; stress
H. Teratogenicity: ability of a drug to cause abnormal fetal development

Tolerance and Cross Tolerance

A. Tolerance: acclimation of the body to a drug over a period of time so that larger doses must be given to achieve the same effect
B. Cross tolerance: tolerance to pharmacologically related drugs

Sources of Drug Information

A. Resource people
1. Pharmacists
2. Physicians
3. Registered nurses
B. Poison control centers
C. Published sources of information
1. *United States Pharmacopeia (USP)* and *National Formulary (NF)*
a. Official reference books
b. Establish legally binding standards to which drugs must conform
c. Revised every 5 years with periodic supplements
2. Package insert: Food and Drug Administration (FDA)–approved label for drug products in the United States
3. *Physicians' Desk Reference (PDR)*
a. Published annually with interim supplements
b. Contains information supplied by manufacturers
c. Is most useful for finding drugs according to brand name
4. American Hospital Formulary Service
a. Contains data on almost every drug available in the United States
b. Kept current by periodic supplements
5. Pharmacology textbooks; drug reference books/cards
6. Nursing journals

Nursing Process

A. Nursing assessment: obtain data on patient regarding problems related to
1. Route of administration
2. Elimination or metabolism
B. Nursing management
1. Proper timing of dosage
2. Ways to improve effectiveness of the drug
3. Instruction of patient concerning drugs

C. Nursing evaluation: if therapy is ineffective, examine possible causes such as drug interactions

ADMINISTERING MEDICATIONS
Calculation of Dosage

A. Practical nurse responsibility
1. Abide by the guidelines of the health care agency
2. Check for accuracy in dosage calculation before preparing and administering drug
3. Check calculations with another knowledgeable person
4. Measure doses exactly as prescribed by physician
B. Systems of measurement
1. Household system: measurements commonly used in the home; not as accurate as other systems; following are examples:
a. 1 teaspoon (tsp or t) = 60 drops (gtt)
b. 3 or 4 tsp = 1 tablespoon (tbsp or T)
2. Apothecary system: an older system but one that continues to be used in dosage calculations
a. Common units of measurement
(1) Weight: grain (gr)
(2) Volume
(a) 60 minims (m) = 1 dram (dr or ℨ)
(b) 8 dr = 1 ounce (oz or ℥)
b. Notations in this system use lowercase Roman numerals; quantities less than 1 are expressed as common factors; exception: one half is written as $\overline{ss}$
3. Metric system: international decimal system
a. Common units of measurement
(1) Weight: unit is expressed in terms of the gram (g)
(a) Prefix kilo indicates 1000
(b) Prefix milli indicates $\frac{1}{1000}$
(c) 1 g = 1000 milligrams (mg)
(2) Volume: unit is expressed in terms of the liter (L)
(a) Prefix milli indicates $\frac{1}{1000}$
(b) 1 L = 1000 milliliters (ml)
b. Notations in this system use Arabic numbers; fractions are expressed as decimals
4. Equivalents between systems: a given quantity considered to be of equal value to a quantity expressed in a different system; some common approximate equivalents are
a. 1 kilogram (kg) = 2.2 pounds (lb)
b. 1 g = 15 gr
c. 60 mg = 1 gr
d. 1 cubic centimeter (cc) = 1 ml
e. 1000 ml = 1 quart (qt)
f. 30 ml = 1 oz
g. 1 ml = 15 or 16 m
h. 1 tsp = 4 or 5 ml
i. 1 ml = 15 or 16 gtt
C. Mathematics of conversion within and between systems; ratio and proportion method:
1. Household

EXAMPLE: 3 tsp = _____ gtt
teaspoons : drops :: teaspoons : drops
$1 : 60 :: 3 : x$
$x = 180$
Answer: 3 tsp = 180 gtt

2. Apothecary system

EXAMPLE: 3 oz = _____ dr
ounces : drams :: ounces : drams
1 : 8 :: 3 : x
$x = 24$
Answer: 3 oz = 24 dr

3. Metric system

EXAMPLE: 250 mg = _____ g
milligram : gram :: milligram : gram
1000 : 1 :: 250 : x
1000 $x = 250$
$x = 0.25$
Answer: 250 mg = <u>0.25 g</u>

4. Conversion between systems

EXAMPLE: gr $\frac{1}{6}$ = _____ mg
grains : milligrams :: grains : milligrams
1 : 60 :: $\frac{1}{6}$: x
$1x = 60 \times \frac{1}{6}$
$x = 10$
Answer: gr $\frac{1}{6}$ = <u>10 mg</u>

D. Dosage calculations: The dose for oral tablets, capsules, and liquids or solutions for injections can be calculated by using the following formula:

$$\frac{\text{Desired dose (D)}}{\text{Dose on hand (H)}} \times \text{Quantity (Q)} = \text{Amount to be given}$$

EXAMPLE: Give 500 mg of tetracycline (Achromycin) using capsules containing 250 mg
$$\frac{D}{H} \times Q = \frac{500 \text{ mg}}{250 \text{ mg}} \times 1 \text{ capsule} =$$
Answer: 2 capsules

EXAMPLE: Physician orders digoxin 0.125 mg to be given orally; stock bottle is labeled "Digoxin 0.25 mg" scored tablets
$$\frac{D}{H} \times Q = \frac{0.125 \text{ mg}}{0.25 \text{ mg}} \times 1 \text{ tablet} =$$
Answer: 0.5 tablet or $\frac{1}{2}$ tablet

EXAMPLE: Erythromycin suspension 750 mg is ordered orally. The bottle is labeled 250 mg/5 ml
$$\frac{D}{H} \times Q = \frac{750 \text{ mg}}{250 \text{ mg}} \times 5 \text{ ml} =$$
Answer: 15 ml

EXAMPLE: Morphine sulfate gr $\frac{1}{4}$ is to be given by subcutaneous injection; the vial is labeled "Morphine Sulfate gr $\frac{1}{2}$/ml"
$$\frac{D}{H} \times Q = \frac{\text{gr } \frac{1}{4}}{\text{gr } \frac{1}{2}} \times 1 \text{ ml} =$$
Answer: 0.5 ml

EXAMPLE: Penicillin 600,000 units is to be given by intramuscular injection; the vial is labeled "Penicillin 300,000 units per ml"
$$\frac{D}{H} = Q = \frac{600,000 \text{ units}}{300,000 \text{ units}} \times 1 \text{ ml} =$$
Answer: 2 ml

NOTE: This formula can be used with any system of measurement. When two systems are involved, it is necessary to convert to the system of measurement of the dose on hand.

EXAMPLE: Codeine sulfate gr $\overline{ss}$ is ordered by mouth; on hand are codeine sulfate tablets labeled 30 mg

STEP 1: conversion between systems
grain : milligram :: grain : milligram
1 : 60 :: $\frac{1}{2}$: x
$x = 60 \times \frac{1}{2}$
$x = 30$
Answer: codeine gr $\overline{ss}$ = 30 mg
STEP 2: Formula
$$\frac{D}{H} \times Q = \frac{30 \text{ mg}}{30 \text{ mg}} \times 1 \text{ tablet}$$
Answer: 1 tablet

Calculation of Drip Rate for Intravenous Infusion

A. Information that must be known
   1. Volume of solution to be infused
   2. Length of time over which this volume is to be infused
   3. Number of drops per milliliter delivered by the administration set being used
B. The drip rate may be calculated as follows:
   1. Find the volume of fluid to be administered per hour

   $$\frac{\text{Milliliters of fluid to be infused}}{\text{Number of hours for infusion}}$$
   = Milliliters of fluid per hour

   2. Find the volume of fluid to be administered per minute

   $$\frac{\text{Milliliters of fluid per hour}}{60 \text{ min/hr}}$$
   = Milliliters to run per minute

   3. Multiply the milliliters of fluid to run per minute by the number of drops per milliliter delivered by the infusion set; this gives the number of drops that should fall in the drip chamber per minute

   Milliliters per minute $\times$ Drops per milliliter
   = Drops per minute

   EXAMPLE: Administer 1000 ml of dextrose 5% in water (D5W) over 8 hours using an infusion set that delivers 10 gtt per minute
   $$\frac{1000 \text{ ml}}{8 \text{ hr}} = 125 \text{ ml/hr}$$
   $$\frac{125 \text{ ml/hr}}{60 \text{ min/hr}} = 2.1 \text{ ml/min}$$
   2.1 ml/min $\times$ 10 gtt/ml =
   Answer: 21 gtt/min

C. If the administration rate has been ordered as milliliters per hour, step 1 above is omitted
D. Alternate formula to calculate drip rate

   $$\frac{\text{Milliliters to administer} \times \text{Drops per milliliter}}{\text{Hours to run} \times 60 \text{ min/hr}}$$
   = Drops per minute

   EXAMPLE: Administer 1000 ml of D5W over 8 hours using an infusion set that delivers 10 gtt/min
   $$\frac{1000 \text{ ml} \times 10 \text{ gtt/ml}}{8 \text{ hr} \times 60 \text{ min/hr}} =$$
   Answer: 21 gtt/min

E. Adjust the flow rate to the number of drops per minute as calculated; assess the fluid volume at hourly intervals to see that the fluid is being administered at the desired rate; the calculated drip rate is an approximation of the actual flow rate; the type of solution, additives, position of the patient or infusion tubing, height of the reservoir, and volume of fluid in the container can influence the actual drip rate; the practical nurse should verify computations with another knowledgeable person before readjusting the drip rate to ensure volume delivery for the prescribed time

Methods of Administering Medications

A. Nurse's responsibilities
  1. Knowledge of drug
    a. Its actions
    b. Ranges of dosage
    c. Methods of administration
    d. Common use
    e. Adverse reactions
    f. Contraindications
    g. Patient education
  2. Assess patient regarding history of allergies or sensitivities to drugs
  3. Be aware of and follow agency's policy regarding procedure by which the medication order is checked
  4. Know agency's system of medication distribution
    a. Cards
    b. Kardex/Medex
    c. Computer printout sheet
  5. Know occasions when drugs may be withheld
    a. Fasting for diagnostic tests or surgery; illness
    b. Required laboratory blood work before medication administration
    c. Specific guidelines for certain drugs, for example, apical pulse rate before cardiotonics or blood pressure (BP) readings before antihypertensive agents
  6. Position the patient to properly administer medications; assist as needed
  7. Observe the "five rights" of medication administration
    a. *Right patient*
    b. *Right drug*
    c. *Right dose*
    d. *Right route*
    e. *Right time*
  8. Inform patient of any anticipated change in normal body functions such as drowsiness, nausea, or change in color of urine
  9. Report patient noncompliance or adverse reactions to other responsible person, that is, registered nurse or physician
  10. Be aware of and follow procedure for controlled substances
  11. Never leave medications at patient's bedside unless specifically ordered
  12. Ensure accuracy in drug calculation; when in doubt, verify with other responsible person, that is, registered nurse or pharmacist
  13. Check expiration date on all medication labels and orders
  14. Accurately document medications given and, if omitted, inclusion of explanation for omission
  15. Document effectiveness of medication
  16. Be aware of and follow agency procedure in event of medication error

B. Safety measures in preparing medications
  1. Environment
    a. Quiet
    b. Free from distractions
    c. Good lighting
  2. Do not leave prepared medications unattended; keep in a locked area
  3. Read each label three times
    a. When reaching for the container
    b. Immediately before pouring the medication
    c. When replacing or discarding the container
  4. Transport drugs for administration by using trays or carts that allow the identifying information and the medication container to be kept together safely
  5. Do not allow tray or cart to be left out of sight during administration
  6. Make positive identification of patient before administering the medication, preferably by checking the patient's identification bracelet; having patient state his or her name; having second person identify patient
  7. Remain with the patient until patient takes the medication
  8. Document necessary supplemental information according to agency policy, for example, pulse rate, blood pressure, site of application or injection

C. Oral administration of medications
  1. General information
    a. Simplest and most convenient route
    b. Liquid preparations
      (1) Pour into a container placed on a flat surface
      (2) Read at eye level
      (3) Measure amount by using the bottom of meniscus
    c. Irritating drugs should be dissolved or diluted and given with food or immediately after a meal
    d. Distasteful oral medications can be disguised, for example, by having patient suck on a piece of ice for a few minutes to numb taste buds, by storing oily medications in a refrigerator, by having patient use a straw, or by mixing medication with a small amount of fruit juice, milk, applesauce, or gelatin; always inform patient that a food vehicle contains the medication
    e. For patients who have difficulty taking liquid medications from a cup a medication extractor resembling a syringe or a syringe with the needle removed may be used; this allows for accurate measurement of certain liquids in amounts measured in minims, since the syringe or extractor is calibrated in cubic centimeters and minims; device can be placed directly in patient's mouth; must be done carefully and administered slowly to avoid choking or aspiration
    f. For patients who have difficulty swallowing tablets, some tablets may be crushed to facilitate swallowing; be aware of contraindications for crushing of certain medications, for example, enteric coated tablets, or of opening capsules containing timed-release medications

Table 4-1. Administration of oral medications

Suggested action	Rationale
Check the order and read label three times while preparing the drug	Frequent checking prevents errors and ensures accuracy
Observe practices of medical asepsis while preparing and administering medications	Careful handwashing and separate medication cups prevent cross-contamination between nurse and patients
Pour tablets and capsules into the cap of a stock container and then transfer proper amount into medication cup	Pouring medications into the nurse's hand contaminates the tablet or capsule
Pour liquids from the side of the bottle opposite the label	Liquid that may spill onto the label makes reading the label difficult
Transport medications to patient's bedside carefully	Prevent accidental or deliberate disarrangement of medications
Keep medications in sight at all times	
Identify patient carefully	Illness and different environment can often cause confusion
Assist patient to an upright position as necessary	Proper positioning facilitates swallowing
Offer sufficient water or other permitted fluids	Liquids allow for ease in swallowing and help to dissolve solid drugs
Remain with patient until each medication is swallowed	Patient may discard unwanted medications or may accumulate them with intent to harm himself or herself
Document each medication administered, promptly and according to agency's policy; report/document medications not taken	The patient's chart is a legal record; prompt documentation avoids the possibility of repeating administration of the same drug
If patient's intake is being measured, record the amount of fluid taken with the medication	All fluids taken are to be recorded for determining total intake

Table 4-2. Selection of syringe and needle

Type of injection	Syringe size	Needle size
Intradermal	1 ml calibrated in tenths or hundredths of a milliliter or in minims	26 or 27 gauge, ½ or ¾ inch
Subcutaneous	2, 2½, or 3 ml calibrated in 0.1 ml	25 gauge, ½ or ⅝ inch
Intramuscular	2-5 ml calibrated in 0.2 ml	20 or 22 gauge, 1½ inch
Insulin (subcutaneous)	1-2 ml calibrated in units	25, 26, or 27 gauge, ½ or ⅝ inch

    g. Liquid medications that are harmful to teeth, for example, liquid iron preparations, should be administered with a straw

  2. Specific procedure is described in Table 4-1

D. Parenteral administration of medications: administration by a route other than through the enterol or gastrointestinal (GI) tract, such as intradermal, subcutaneous, intramuscular, or intravenous routes

  1. General information: maintain surgical aseptic technique in preparation and administration; it is preferable to use prepackaged, disposable sterile needles and syringes

  2. Selection of syringe and needle: thick or oily solutions require a large lumen; short needles are used for children and adults with little adipose tissue; obese individuals may require longer needles to ensure delivery of medications to proper tissue level (Table 4-2)

  3. Putting the drugs into the syringe

    a. Manufacturer prefilled syringes or cartridges: contain the name and dose of the drug and the intended parenteral route; should not be given by any route other than the one specified

    b. Rubber-capped vials: single or multidose container; solution or powder form; dry form of drug dissolved according to label instructions; to remove the drug

      (1) Remove the soft metal cover on top of the vial

      (2) Using friction; wipe the rubber cap with a pledget soaked with antiseptic solution

      (3) Fill syringe with air equal to amount of solution to be withdrawn in order to increase pressure within the vial and to facilitate withdrawal of solution

      (4) Insert needle into the rubber cap while holding the needle in a slightly lateral position to prevent a piece of the stopper from entering the vial

      (5) Inject the air and remove prescribed amount of solution while holding the syringe in a vertical position

    c. Glass ampules: prescored or unscored tops; constricted neck ampules require that solution be in base of ampule

      (1) Quickly snap finger on the stem to move the solution into the base of the ampule

      (2) Use a saw-toothed file for unscored ampules to scratch the glass on opposite sides of the stem, where it will be broken

      (3) Hold the ampule in one hand

      (4) Protecting the fingers of the other hand with a sterile, dry gauze pledget, break off the stem of the ampule; check solution for fragments of glass

      (5) Insert needle into the opened ampule, avoiding needle contamination by not touching the rim of the ampule with the needle

      (6) Keep needle under solution and withdraw the prescribed amount of the solution

  4. Skin preparation

    a. Heavily soiled skin in area of intended injection site should be washed with soap and water

    b. Antiseptic-soaked gauze or pledget is then used to disinfect injection site and thus prevent injection of harmful organism into body tissue

      (1) Wipe in a circular motion, starting at point

of injection and moving outward to carry debris away from injection site

    (2) Use firm pressure and friction when wiping to help remove soil

5. Reduce discomfort
   a. Use sharp needle
   b. Use appropriate gauge
   c. Select site free of irritation or nodules from previous injections
   d. Numb skin receptors: cold compresses or ice cube over injection site
   e. Hold tissue taut or compress tissue to form a pad, depending on type of injection
   f. Be sure there is no solution on the needle
   g. Help patient to relax
   h. Insert needle without hesitation
   i. Aspirate when appropriate
   j. Inject solution slowly
   k. Remove needle quickly
   l. Massage area after injection unless contraindicated with certain medications
6. Care of equipment after injections: use needle disposal unit; follow agency policy
7. Injection sites
   a. Intradermal injection: solutions injected directly under the epidermis into the dermis, (10- to 15-degree angle)
      (1) Absorption occurs slowly through the capillaries
      (2) Common site: inner aspect of the forearm
   b. Subcutaneous injection: solutions injected into the subcutaneous layer of the skin (45- to 90-degree angle)
      (1) Common sites
         (a) Outer aspect of upper arm
         (b) Thigh
         (c) Lower abdomen
         (d) Upper back
      (2) Suggested procedure for subcutaneous injection is described in Table 4-3
   c. Intramuscular injection: solutions injected into the muscular layer of tissue (90-degree angle)
      (1) Common sites
         (a) Dorsogluteal site
         (b) Ventrogluteal site
         (c) Vastus lateralis muscle
         (d) Deltoid muscle
         (e) Posterior triceps muscle
         (f) Rectus femoris muscle
      (2) Suggested procedure for intramuscular injection is described in Table 4-4
   d. Z-track injection: technique used to prevent damage to and staining of the skin and subcutaneous tissues; common site is the upper outer quadrant of the gluteal region
   e. Intravenous infusion: administration of a large amount of fluid into a vein
      (1) Purposes
         (a) To restore or maintain electrolyte balance
         (b) To supply drugs for immediate effect
         (c) To replace nutrients and vitamins
         (d) To replace blood loss

Table 4-3. Administration of subcutaneous injection

Suggested action	Rationale
Verify physician's order and read medication label three times; check expiration date	Ensures accuracy and prevents errors
Obtain and assemble equipment maintaining sterile technique	Prevents contamination
Draw the drug into syringe and protect needle with sterile needle cover	Exposure to air or contact with moist surface contaminates needle
Identify patient by identification bracelet and by having patient state name, if possible	Prevents potential medication error
Select appropriate injection site and cleanse area with antiseptic pledget, using firm, circular motion moving outward from injection site	Friction helps to clean skin and decreases possibility of introducing bacteria into body tissue
Grasp the tissue surrouding the injection site and hold it to form a cushion pad	Ensures placement of medication into subcutaneous tissue and helps prevent deposition of medication into muscle tissue
Inject the needle quickly at an angle of 45 to 90 degrees, depending on the quality and amount of tissue and length of needle	Ensures placement of medication into subcutaneous tissue
After needle is in proper tissue level, release grasp of the tissue	Reduces discomfort of injeciton
Aspirate to determine whether needle is in a blood vessel	Prevents discomfort and possible serious reaction if medication is injected into vein
If there is no blood return, inject solution slowly	Reduces discomfort by reducing pressure in subcutaneous tissue
Withdraw needle quickly	Reduces discomfort
Massage area gently, unless contraindicated with certain medications	Helps to distribute the solution and hasten absorption of the medication

    (2) Nurse practice acts and agency policy dictate who may administer intravenous infusions

    (3) Nurse's responsibilities for intravenous infusion
        (a) Verifying physician's order
        (b) Calculating rate of flow
        (c) Monitoring rate of flow
        (d) Assessing patient for adverse reactions
            ■ Infiltration
            ■ Circulatory overload
            ■ Thrombophlebitis

   f. Hyperalimentation: total parenteral nutrition (TPN), that is, an intravenous infusion containing sufficient nutrients to sustain life; provides amino acids, glucose, vitamins, and electrolytes for those patients unable to ingest nutrients normally for extended periods and for whom standard infusions are inadequate

   g. Hypodermoclysis: administration of relatively large amounts of fluid into subcutaneous tissue

Table 4-4. Administration of intramuscular injection

Suggested action	Rationale
Verify physician's order and read medication label three times; check expiration date	Ensures accuracy and prevents errors
Obtain and assemble equipment, maintaining sterile technique	Prevents contamination
Draw the drug into syringe; create small air bubble in the syringe; protect needle with sterile needle cover	Air bubble forces medication out of needle shaft when injected; Exposure to air or contact with most surfaces contaminates needle
Identify patient by identification bracelet and by having patient state name, if possible	Prevents potential medication error
Have the patient assume appropriate position according to site selected	Helps to relax muscles and eases discomfort
Select appropriate injection site and cleanse area with antiseptic pledget, using firm, circular motion moving outward from injection site	Friction helps to clean the skin, thus decreasing possibility of introducing bacteria into body tissue
Press down and hold tissue taut over the injection site	Ensures needle reaches muscle layer
Hold syringe at 90-degree angle and quickly thrust needle into the tissue	Minimizes discomfort
Aspirate to determine whether needle is in a blood vessel	Prevents discomfort and possible serious reaction if medication injected into vein
If there is no blood return, inject medication slowly, followed by the air bubble	Reduces discomfort and allows medication to disperse into the tissue; air bubble clears medication from needle
Withdraw needle quickly	Reduces discomfort
Massage area gently, unless contraindicated with certain medications	Helps to distribute the solution and hasten absorption of the medication

  h. Blood transfusion: infusion of whole blood from a healthy person into a recipient's vein
    (1) Blood is typed and cross matched before administration to determine compatibility
    (2) Nurse's responsibility for blood transfusion
      (a) Check and double-check
        ■ The labels
        ■ The numbers
        ■ The Rh factor
        ■ Compatibility
      (b) Stay with patient for at least the first 5 minutes after transfusion is started
      (c) Monitor rate of transfusion
      (d) Assess patient for signs of adverse reactions
        ■ Hemolytic reaction: stop transfusion immediately, keep vein open with slow drip normal saline solution, and notify physician; indications include
          □ Headache
          □ Sensations of tingling
          □ Difficulty in breathing
          □ Pain in lumbar region or legs
        ■ Allergic reactions: stop transfusion immediately and notify physician; indications include
          □ Pruritus
          □ Hives (urticaria)
          □ Difficulty in breathing
        ■ Febrile reactions resulting from contaminant in the blood: usually occurs late in the transfusion or after it is completed; indications include
          □ Flushed skin
          □ Elevated temperature
          □ General malaise
          □ Signs of systemic infection
        ■ Circulatory overload can lead to pulmonary edema; indications include
          □ Increased pulse rate
          □ Dyspnea
          □ Respiratory distress
          □ Moist coughing
          □ Expectoration of blood-tinged mucus
        ■ Anticoagulant reaction: indications include
          □ Tingling in the fingers
          □ Muscular cramping
          □ Convulsions
  i. Blood extracts: specific components of whole blood that meet specific needs of the patient
    (1) Packed red blood cells (RBCs)
    (2) Plasma
    (3) Human albumin
    (4) Fibrinogen
    (5) Gamma globulin
E. Percutaneous administration
  1. Description: application of medication for absorption through mucous membrane or skin
  2. Common sites
    a. Instilling solution into the ear, eye, nose, mouth or vagina
    b. Applying topical creams, powders, ointments, or lotions onto the skin
    c. Using aerosolized liquids/gases to medicate nasal passages, sinuses, or lungs

PEDIATRIC DRUG ADMINISTRATION
General Rules

A. Pediatric drug therapy should be guided by the child's age, weight, and level of growth and development
B. The nurse's approach to the child should convey the impression that he or she expects the child to take the medication
C. Explanation regarding the medication should be based on the child's level of understanding
D. The nurse must be honest with the child regarding the procedure
E. It may be necessary to mix distasteful medication or crushed tablets with a small amount of honey, applesauce, or gelatin

F. Never threaten a child with an injection if he refuses an oral medication
G. All medications should be kept out of the reach of children, and medications should never be referred to as candy

Calculating the Pediatric Dose

Safe dosage ranges of drugs are less well defined for children than for adults. Not all drug dosage ranges for children are listed in the literature. It is not the nurse's responsibility to determine the dose of a drug for the infant or child, but at times it may be necessary to verify or calculate a dose as a fraction of the adult dose. The following methods may be used:

A. Body surface area: considered most accurate; requires a nomogram—a device for rapid estimation of body surface area

$$\text{Child's dose} = \frac{\text{Body surface area (in square meters)}}{1.73 \text{ sq m}^2} \times \text{Adult dose}$$

B. Clark's rule: based on weight and used for children at least 2 years old

$$\text{Child's dose} = \frac{\text{Weight (in pounds)}}{150} \times \text{Adult dose}$$

C. Young's rule: based on age and used for children at least 2 years old

$$\text{Child's dose} = \frac{\text{Age (in years)}}{\text{Age (in years)} + 12} \times \text{Adult dose}$$

D. Fried's rule: used for children less than 2 years old

$$\text{Child's dose} = \frac{\text{Age (in months)}}{150} \times \text{Adult dose}$$

Identifying the Patient

A. Check the child's identification bracelet
B. Ask the older child his name

Oral Medication

Verify, calculate, and document all medications

A. Infants
1. Draw up liquid medication in a dropper or a syringe without the needle
2. Elevate infant's head and shoulders; hold infant in a feeding position
3. Depress the chin with the thumb to open infant's mouth
4. Using the dropper or syringe, direct the medication toward the inner aspect of the infant's cheek and release the flow of medication slowly
5. Release the thumb and allow the infant to swallow
6. Liquid medication can also be measured into a nipple and the infant allowed to suck the medication through the nipple
7. Crushed tablets can be mixed with a small amount of honey or applesauce and fed slowly with a teaspoon

B. Toddlers
1. Draw up medication in a syringe or measure into a medication cup
2. Elevate the child's head and shoulders

3. Place the syringe in the child's mouth and slowly release the medication, directing it toward the inner aspect of the cheek, or allow the child to hold the medicine cup and drink it at own pace; offer praise

C. School-age children
1. When the child is old enough to take medicine in tablet or capsule form, direct him or her to place the medicine near the back of the tongue and to immediately swallow fluid such as water or juice
2. Offer the child praise after he or she has taken medication

Intramuscular Injection

A. Infants
1. Common site: largest muscle group is the quadriceps femoris, located in the anterolateral thigh; largest muscle of this group is the vastus lateralis, situated on the anterior surface of the midlateral thigh
   a. Place infant in supine position
   b. Compress muscle tissue at upper aspect of thigh, pointing the nurse's fingers toward the infant's feet
   c. Needle is inserted at a 90-degree angle; maximum length of needle for an infant is 1 inch (2.5 cm)
2. Alternate site: rectus femoris muscle, located on the anterolateral surface of the upper thigh; needle is inserted at a 45-degree angle and is directed toward the knee

B. Toddlers and school-age children: common sites are
1. Dorsogluteal muscle: upper outer quadrant; gluteal muscle does not develop until child begins to walk; should be used for injections only after the child has been walking for a year or more
2. Ventrogluteal muscle: a dense muscle mass; the disadvantage is that the site is visible to the child
3. Deltoid muscle may be used for older, larger children
4. Lateral and anterior aspect of thigh: upper outer quadrant of thigh

Administration of Injections

A. Infants
1. Place infant in a secure position to avoid movement of the extremity
2. Usually, have a second person to secure the infant
3. Hold, cuddle, and comfort the infant after the injection

B. Toddlers and school-age children
1. Have syringe and needle completely prepared before contact with the child
2. Keep needle outside of child's visual field
3. Explain according to the child's developmental age, the reason for an injection and where it will be given; do not say "it won't hurt"
4. Inspect injection site before injection for tenderness or undue firmness
5. Have a second person available to help secure the child and offer comfort during the procedure
6. Allow the child to express fears
7. Perform the procedure quickly and gently
8. Praise the child for his or her behavior after the injection

CENTRAL NERVOUS SYSTEM
Depressants

A. Characteristics of drug-induced central nervous system (CNS) depression
  1. Mild: disinterest in surroundings, inability to focus on a topic or to initiate talking or movement, slowed pulse and respirations
  2. Moderate or progressive: drowsiness or sleep, decreased muscle tone and ability to move, diminished acuity of all sensations—touch, vision, hearing, heat, cold, or pain
  3. Severe: unconsciousness or coma, loss of reflexes, respiratory failure, death

B. Analgesics: drugs used to relieve pain (Table 4-5)
  1. Narcotic analgesics (opioids: morphine, prototype)
    a. Actions
      (1) Raises pain perception threshold
      (2) Reduces fear and anxiety
      (3) Induces sleep
      (4) Depresses respiratory and cough centers in medulla
      (5) Inhibits gastric, biliary, and pancreatic secretions; depressing gastrointestinal tract
      (6) Stimulates release of antidiuretic hormone, resulting in decreased urine volume
      (7) Induces hypotension
      (8) Slows heart rate
      (9) Causes pupillary constriction
    b. Agents

Examples	Comments
Alphaprodine hydro-chloride (Nisentil)	Not given orally; schedule II drug
Anileridine hydrochlo-ride (Leritine)	Schedule II drug
Butorphanol tartrate (Stadol)	Currently not classified as a controlled drug
Codeine sulfate	Schedule II drug
Codeine phosphate	
Hydromorphone hydro-chloride (Dilaudid)	Schedule II drug
Levorphanol tartrate (Levo-Dromoran)	Schedule II drug
Meperidine hydrochlo-ride (Demerol)	Schedule II drug
Methadone hydrochlo-ride (Dolophine, Methadose)	Also used as a replacement drug for opiate dependence or to ease withdrawal; schedule II drug
Morphine sulfate	Poor oral absorption; schedule II drug
Nalbuphine hydrochlo-ride (Nubain)	Currently not classified as a controlled drug
Oxycodone hydrochlo-ride (Percodan)	Schedule II drug
Oxymorphone hydro-chloride (Numorphan)	Schedule II drug
Pentazocine hydrochlo-ride (Talwin)	Schedule IV drug; oral preparation
Pentazocine (Talwin) lactate	Schedule IV drug; parenteral preparation
Propoxyphene hydro-chloride (Darvon)	Schedule IV drug
Propoxyphene napsylate (Darvon-N)	Schedule IV drug

  c. Adverse reactions and contraindications
    (1) Nausea and vomiting
    (2) Constipation
    (3) Urinary retention
    (4) Pruritus
    (5) Hypotension
    (6) Morphine can cause respiratory depression, so is used cautiously for patients with impaired respiratory function; it is not used for patients with head injury as it will obscure CNS evaluation
  d. Dependency: develops rapidly
    (1) There is a distinct physical reaction when the drug is suddenly stopped and the body readjusts to functioning in the absence of the drug (abstinence syndrome); symptoms include
      (a) Runny nose
      (b) Goose flesh
      (c) Tearing
      (d) Yawning
      (e) Muscle twitching and abdominal cramping
      (f) Insomnia
      (g) Nausea and vomiting
      (h) Diarrhea
    (2) Methadone hydrochloride is used for detoxification and maintenance
  e. Acute toxicity: usual cause of death is respiratory depression; treated with support to respiration and with a narcotic antagonist such as levallorphan tartrate (Lorfan), nalorphine hydrochloride (Nalline), or naloxone hydrochloride (Narcan)
  2. Nonnarcotic analgesics/antiinflammatory analgesics
    a. Action: sensitization of peripheral pain receptor
    b. Agents
      (1) Acetylsalicylic acid (aspirin): effective in management of low-intensity pain
        (a) Adverse reactions
          ■ Gastric irritation
          ■ Ulceration and gastric bleeding
          ■ Intoxication (salicylism): tinnitus, reversible hearing loss, hyperventilation, fever, metabolic acidosis, vomiting, hypokalemia, convulsions, coma, and death
        (b) Drug interactions with aspirin
          ■ Anticoagulants: increase likelihood of bleeding
          ■ Alcohol: increases likelihood of gastrointestinal irritation and bleeding
      (2) Acetaminophen (Datril, Tylenol): effective in management of low-intensity pain; does not produce gastric irritation or alter platelet function and bleeding times as does aspirin; does not interact with oral anticoagulants; prolonged use or frequent high doses can cause liver and kidney damage
      (3) Nonsteroidal antiinflammatory drugs (NSAIDs): effective in treatment of osteoarthritis, degenerative joint disease, rheumatic diseases

Table 4-5. Composition of oral narcotic preparations

Name	Narcotic	Other components
Empirin compound no. 1	Codeine phosphate 8 mg	Aspirin
2	Codeine phosphate 16 mg	Phenacetin
3	Codeine phosphate 32 mg	Caffeine
4	Codeine phosphate 65 mg	
Fiorinal with codeine no. 1	Codeine phosphate 7.5 mg	Aspirin
2	Codeine phosphate 15 mg	Phenacetin
3	Codeine phosphate 30 mg	Caffeine
4	Codeine phosphate 60 mg	Butalbital
Percodan	Oxycodone hydrochloride	Aspirin
		Phenacetin
		Caffeine
Darvon compound	Propoxyphene hydrochloride	Aspirin
Darvon compound-65		Phenacetin
		Caffeine
Darvon with ASA	Propoxyphene hydrochloride	Aspirin
Darvon-N with ASA	Propoxyphene napsylate	Aspirin
Darvocet-N	Propoxyphene napsylate	Acetaminophin
Percobarb	Oxycodone hydrochloride	Aspirin
		Phenacetin
		Caffeine
		Hexobarbital
Percocet	Oxycodone hydrochloride	Acetaminophen
Phenaphen with codeine no. 1	Codeine phosphate 8 mg	Aspirin
2	Codeine phosphate 16 mg	Phenacetin
3	Codeine phosphate 32 mg	Phenobarbital
4	Codeine phosphate 65 mg	Hyoscamine sulfate
Tylenol with codeine no. 1	Codeine phosphate 7.5 mg	Acetaminophen
2	Codeine phosphate 15 mg	Acetaminophen
3	Codeine phosphate 30 mg	Acetaminophen
4	Codeine phosphate 60 mg	Acetaminophen

(a) Adverse reactions
- Heartburn/indigestion
- Nausea/vomiting
- Constipation or diarrhea
- Fluid retention
- Hypertension
- Dizziness
- Blurred vision
- Skin rash

(b) Drug interactions vary because of the chemical makeup of the various NSAIDs

(c) Agents: the following are examples

Ibuprofen (Motrin, Nuprin, Advil)
Indomethacin (Indocin)
Meclofenemate sodium (Meclomen)
Phenylbutazone (Azolid)
Piroxicam (Feldene)

3. Nursing assessment: determine character, location, onset, contributing factors, duration of pain, time of last dose

4. Nursing management
 a. Determine the most effective way to manage the pain: drug versus nondrug measure (i.e., positioning, turning)
 b. Obtain vital signs
  (1) Be alert to hypotension/hypertension
  (2) Analyze rate and character of respiration
  (3) Withhold drug and notify physician in presence of respiratory depression: respiratory rate of 10 or less respirations per minute or a decrease of 8 or more respirations per minute from baseline data
 c. Caution patient to remain quiet after drug administration to decrease possible nausea and vomiting
 d. Implement safety measures: use side rails and advise patient to remain in bed if there are changes in mental status: alterations in judgment or unsteadiness
 e. Initiate intake and output records to determine effectiveness of bladder function
 f. Determine efficacy of bowel activity
 g. Patient instruction concerning
  (1) How to take drug
  (2) Safe storage in the home
  (3) Avoidance of driving
  (4) Danger of simultaneous administration of alcohol or other CNS depressant with narcotics

5. Nursing evaluation
 a. Subjective interviewing: ask if patient is comfortable
 b. Objective observations
  (1) Decreased restlessness and anxiety
  (2) Ability of the patient to function

C. Anesthetics: provide a pain-free experience during an operative procedure along with a relaxed state of mind and sense of security
   1. General anesthetics: provide loss of pain sensation, loss of consciousness, loss of memory, and loss of voluntary and some involuntary muscle activity
      a. Inhalation agents: the following are examples

Cyclopropane	Methoxyflurane
Ether	(Penthrane)
Halothane	Nitrous oxide

      b. Intravenous agents: the following are examples

Droperidol	Methohexital (Brevital)
(Inapsine)	sodium
Droperidol–Fentanyl	Thiamylal sodium
citrate (Innovar)	(Surital)
Ketamine hydrochlo-	Thiopental (Pentothal)
ride	sodium

   2. Regional anesthetics: provide loss of sensation and motor activity in localized areas of the body
      a. Types
         (1) Topical
         (2) Infiltration
         (3) Peripheral nerve blocks
         (4) Spinal
         (5) Epidural
         (6) Caudal
      b. Agents: the following are examples

Carbocaine	Pontocaine
Novocain	Xylocaine
Nupercaine	

   3. Nursing assessment
      a. Preoperative: obtain health history including allergies, psychologic status, physiologic baseline data
      b. Intraoperative: implement safety measures in presence of explosive or flammable agents
      c. Postoperative: determine vital signs and respiratory function
   4. Nursing management
      a. Preoperative: prepare patient physically and psychologically; initiate measures to prevent complications: deep breathing and bed exercises; administer preoperative medications; initiate safety measures and provide quiet environment
      b. Intraoperative: maintain quiet during stage 2 anesthesia; position patient properly and pad pressure points adequately; transfer patient from operating table in a smooth, coordinated manner to avoid severe hypotension
      c. Postoperative: preserve quiet atmosphere; maintain airway, control pain using careful nursing judgment; prevent complications by encouraging deep breathing, coughing
   5. Nursing evaluation
      a. Preoperative: effects of preoperative medication
      b. Intraoperative: ongoing evaluation of patient's status, usually the responsibility of the anesthesiologist
      c. Postoperative: concerned with pulmonary complications, thrombophlebitis, infection, or other complications

D. Anticonvulsants: drugs used to control seizures
   1. Action: not completely understood; thought to depress neuron excitability and to modify the ability of brain tissue to respond to stimuli that initiate seizure activity
   2. Agents

	Examples	Adverse reactions
a.	Long-acting barbiturates Mephobarbital (Mebaral) Phenobarbital (Luminal) Primidone (Mysoline)	Sedation, drowsiness, tolerance, nystagmus, ataxia, anemia, congenital malformations in fetus; sudden withdrawal can induce convulsions
b.	Hydantoins Ethotoin (Peganone) Mephenytoin (Mesantoin) Phenytoin (Dilantin)	Nystagmus, ataxia, slurred speech, tremors, nervousness, drowsiness, fatigue, overgrowth of the gums (gingival hyperplasia), occasional folic acid or vitamin D deficiency; congenital malformations in fetus
c.	Succinimides Ethosuximide (Zarontin) Methsuximide (Celontin) Phensuximide (Milontin)	Gastrointestinal irritation, dizziness, drowsiness, headache, fatigue
d.	Oxazolidinediones Trimethadione (Tridione)	Serious allergic dermatitis, kidney and liver damage, vertigo, photophobia, spontaneous abortion, congenital malformations
e.	Benzodiazepines Clonazepam (Clonopin) Diazepam (Valium)	Drowsiness, ataxia, personality changes
f.	Miscellaneous Acetazolamide (Diamox)	Loss of appetite, drowsiness, confusion
	Carbamazepine (Tegretol)	Drowsiness, dizziness, ataxia, double vision, gastrointestinal upset
	Lidocaine (Xylocaine) hydrochloride	Depressed heart action
	Paraldehyde	Bronchopulmonary irritation, thrombophlebitis at intravenous injection site
	Valproic acid (Depakene)	Gastrointestinal distress, sedation

   3. Nursing assessment: observe course of the seizure; assist in case finding; assess baseline data with concentration on areas known to be affected by the drug, e.g., phenytoin (Dilantin): assess mouth, teeth, and gums for development of gingival hyperplasia
   4. Nursing management: instruct patient concerning
      a. Drug characteristics
      b. Importance of taking medication even when patient is seizure free; awareness that reaching a therapeutic level may take time

c. Wearing or carrying identification indicating seizure activity and drugs and dosages being taken

d. Reducing gastric irritation by taking drug with meals

e. Good gum massage

5. Nursing evaluation: continued medical follow-up; blood level tests

E. Skeletal muscle relaxants: drugs used to treat muscle spasticity

1. Action: thought to restore some inhibitory tone in neural pathways from the brain or spinal cord or by acting within the muscle itself by interfering with the intracellular release of calcium necessary to initiate contraction

2. Agents

Examples	Adverse reactions
a. Drugs to treat spasticity	
Baclofen (Lioresal)	Drowsiness, incoordination, gastrointestinal upset
Dantrolene sodium (Dantrium)	Liver damage
Diazepam (Valium)	Drowsiness, incoordination
b. Drugs to treat muscle spasm	Drowsiness, dizziness
Carisoprodol (Rela, Soma)	
Chlorphenesin carbamate (Maolate)	
Chlorzoxazone (Paraflex)	
Cyclobenzaprine hydrochloride (Flexeril)	
Dantrolene (Dantrium)	
Diazepam (Valium)	
Methocarbamol (Delaxin, Robaxin)	
Meprobamate (Miltown, Equanil)	
Orphenadrine citrate (Flexon, Norflex)	

3. Nursing assessment: obtain baseline data, focusing on spasticity, including degree, aggravating factors, associated pain, and interference with activities of daily living (ADL); observe baseline liver function studies

4. Nursing management: monitor for drug effectiveness and side effects; institute safety measures if drowsiness occurs

5. Nursing evaluation: at regular intervals, assess the continuing degree of spasticity

F. Antiparkinsonian drugs: drugs used in the management of Parkinson's disease

1. Action: restores action of the neurotransmitter dopamine to the basal ganglia of the brain or blocks the effects of excessive action of acetylcholine

2. Agents

Examples	Adverse reactions
a. Anticholinergics	Dry mouth, constipation, urinary retention, blurred vision; impairment of recent memory, confusion, insomnia, and restlessness
Benztropine mesylate (Cogentin)	
Biperiden (Akineton)	
Cycrimine hydrochloride (Pagitane hydrochloride)	
Ethopropazine hydrochloride (Parsidol)	

Examples	Adverse reactions
Procyclidine hydrochloride (Kemadrin)	
Trihexyphenidyl hydrochloride (Artane, Pipanol, Tremin)	
b. Antihistamines	Sedation
Chlorphenoxamine hydrochloride (Phenoxene)	
Diphenhydramine hydrochloride (Benadryl)	
Orphenadrine citrate (Disipal)	
c. Other drugs	
Amantadine hydrochloride (Symmetrel)	Dry mouth, constipation, urinary retention, blurred vision
Levodopa (Dopar, Larodopa)	Nausea, vomiting, anorexia, orthostatic hypotension, GI bleeding, cough, hoarseness, dyspnea, blurred vision, increased sex drive
Carbidopa-levodopa (Sinemet)	Same as levodopa

G. Sedatives, hypnotics, antianxiety drugs

1. Sedatives: small dose to calm an anxious patient

2. Hypnotics: larger dose to induce sleep

3. Antianxiety drugs (minor tranquilizers): drugs used to treat anxiety

4. Barbiturates: classified according to duration of action: ultra short acting, short acting, intermediate acting, and long acting

a. Action: produce CNS depression ranging from sedation to anesthesia

b. Adverse reactions

(1) Mild withdrawal symptoms: rebound REM sleep, nightmares, daytime agitation, and a "shaky" feeling

(2) Acute overdose: depression of medullary centers regulating respiration and cardiovascular system—tachycardia, hypotension, loss of reflexes, marked depression of respiration

c. Agents: the following are examples

Amobarbital (Amytal, Tuinal)	Pentobarbital (Nembutal)
Butabarbital sodium (Butalan, Butisol Sodium)	Phenobarbital (Luminal)
	Secobarbital (Seconal)

5. Benzodiazepines

a. Action: produce CNS depression

b. Adverse reactions: daytime sedation, motor incoordination, dizziness, headaches; schedule IV substances

c. Agents: the following are examples

Chlordiazepoxide hydrochloride (Librium)	Lorazepam (Ativan)
Clorazepate dipotassium (Tranxene)	Oxazepam (Serax)
Diazepam (Valium)	Prazepam (Verstran, Centrax)
Flurazepam hydrochloride (Dalmane)	

6. Miscellaneous
   a. Action: produce CNS depression; generally short acting
   b. Agents

Examples	Adverse reactions
Chloral betaine (Beta-Chlor)	Gastric irritation; schedule IV substance
Chloral hydrate (Noctec)	Gastric irritation; schedule IV substance
Ethchlorvynol (Placidyl)	Muscular weakness; schedule IV substance
Glutethimide (Doriden)	Dilated pupils, dry mouth; schedule III substance
Hydroxyzine hydrochloride (Vistaril)	Dry mouth, hypotension, blurred vision, urinary retention
Meprobamate (Equanil, Miltown)	Schedule IV substance
Methaqualone (Quaalude, Sopor, Parest)	Paresthesia, peripheral neuropathy; schedule II substance
Methyprylon (Noludar)	Schedule II substance

7. Nursing assessment: give special attention to vital signs, level of consciousness, sleep patterns
8. Nursing management: observe for signs of CNS depression; identify nondrug solutions to sleep problems; monitor safety aspects of patient care
9. Nursing evaluation: review purpose for which drug is given and observe effectiveness; instruct patient concerning self-medication, medical follow-up, and drug-dependence potential

H. Alcohol
1. Action: produces CNS depression: sedation, disinhibition, sleep, anesthesia; vasodilation; gastric irritation
2. Effects of an acute overdose: death, accidents, hangover: upset stomach, thirst, fatigue, headache, depression, anxiety; chronic toxicity can lead to liver, esophagastrointestinal and cardiovascular disorders
3. Withdrawal symptoms after chronic use: tremors, anxiety, tachycardia, increased blood pressure, diaphoresis, anorexia, nausea, vomiting, insomnia, hallucinations, seizures, delirium tremens
4. Treatment of withdrawal: one of the benzodiazepines; restoration of normal metabolic functions, and vitamin B_1, B_{12}, and folic acid
5. Aversion therapy: disulfiram (Antabuse) given to detoxified patient who wishes to avoid drinking again; produces unpleasant reaction in presence of alcohol: flushing, throbbing in head and neck, respiratory difficulty, nausea, copious vomiting, diaphoresis, fainting, dizziness, blurred vision, confusion

Psychotherapeutic Agents

A. Antidepressants: Characteristic of drug-induced prevention or relief of depression
1. Tricyclic antidepressants
   a. Action: primarily used to relieve symptoms of endogenous depression; also used to treat mild exogenous depression
   b. Agents: the following are examples

Amitriptyline hydrochloride (Elavil)	Imipramine hydrochloride (Tofranil)
Clomipramine hydrochloride (Anafranil)	Nortriptyline hydrochloride (Aventyl Hydrochloride, Pamelor)
Doxepin hydrochloride (Adapin, Sinequan)	

2. Monoamine oxidase (MAO) inhibitors
   a. Action: relieve symptoms of severe reactive or endogenous depression that has not responded to tricyclic antidepressant therapy, electroconvulsive therapy, or other modes of psychotherapy
   b. Agents: the following are examples

Isocarboxazid (Marplan)
Phenelzine sulfate (Nardil)
Tranylcypromine sulfate (Parnate)

3. Nursing assessment: obtain complete health history, history of insomnia, fatigue, or loss of motivation; observe motor movements, facial expression and posture; assess for any feelings of suicide
4. Nursing management: administer medication with food to avoid gastric distress
5. Nursing evaluation: observe for adverse effects such as drowsiness
6. Patient teaching: stress compliance of taking medication as ordered; instruct patient to avoid using alcohol with sleeping pills and hay fever or cold medications because doing so increases the effects of these medications

B. Antipsychotic drugs
1. Phenothiazines/thioxanthenes
   a. Action: primarily to reduce or relieve symptoms of acute and chronic psychoses, including schizophrenia, schizoaffective disorders, and involutional psychoses
   b. Agents: the following are examples

Chlorpromazine (Thorazine)	Trifluoperazine hydrochloride (Stelazine)
Promazine hydrochloride (Sparine)	Triflupromazine hydrochloride (Vesprin)
Thioridazine hydrochloride (Mellaril)	

2. Nursing assessment: obtain complete health history, current use of medications, and possibility of pregnancy; obtain history of emotional unrest, agitation, paranoid ideation, delusions, and inability to cope with reality
3. Nursing management: administer medication with food or milk to avoid or reduce gastric distress
4. Nursing evaluation: observe for adverse effects such as urinary retention, change in vision, sore throat with fever, muscle spasms, trembling or shaking of

hands, skin rash, yellow tinge to skin or eyes, uncontrollable movements of the tongue

C. Antimanic drugs: used to treat manic-depressive psychoses in the acute manic phase; also used to prevent recurrent episodes of mania in the manic-depressive patient
   1. Agent: Lithium carbonate (Lithane, Carbolith)
   2. Nursing assessment: obtain complete health history, possibility of pregnancy, and medications currently being taken; observe for restlessness, hyperactivity, aggressiveness
   3. Nursing management: ensure adequate fluid and electrolyte balance
   4. Nursing evaluation: monitor serum lithium levels to avoid drug toxicity and reduce side effects
   5. Patient teaching: stress compliance of taking medication as ordered; instruct patient to wear medical identification tag

Stimulants

Stimulants are medically accepted only for treatment of narcolepsy, hyperkinetic behavior in children, and obesity. Occasionally they are used for depression in the elderly and to reverse respiratory depression from CNS depressants.

A. Amphetamines
   1. Action: increase the release and effectiveness of catecholamine neurotransmitters in the brain and peripheral nerves and create increased alertness and sensitivity to stimuli
   2. Adverse reactions
      a. Gastrointestinal system: vomiting, diarrhea, abdominal cramps, dry mouth, anorexia
      b. Central nervous system: restless behavior, tremor, irritability, talkativeness, insomnia, mood changes, excessive aggressiveness, confusion, panic, increased libido
      c. Autonomic nervous system: headache, chilliness, palpitation, pallor or facial flushing
      d. Children: growth retardation
   3. Agents: the following are examples

Amphetamine sulfate	Methylphenidate (Ritalin)
Dextroamphetamine sulfate (Dexedrine, Ferndex)	Pemoline (Cylert)
Methamphetamine hydrochloride (Desoxyn)	

   4. Nursing assessment: obtain thorough history of patient's presenting problem; obtain vital signs, weight, and height in children
   5. Nursing management: monitor height, weight, and vital signs; inquire about relief of subjective symptoms such as insomnia, agitation, headache, and irritability; begin preparation of patient and family for long-term management
   6. Nursing evaluation: success of goals of therapy evaluated
      a. Hyperkinesis: less hyperactivity and a more normal attention span
      b. Narcolepsy: ability to remain awake and alert during specified appropriate time periods

B. Appetite suppressants: used to help control obesity
   1. Action: exert an anorectic effect on the appetite-control center in the brain
   2. Agents

Examples	Adverse reactions/comments
Amphetamine sulfate (Benzedrine)	See Amphetamines
Benzphetamine (Didrex)	See Amphetamines
Caffeine	Nervousness, jitteriness, gastrointestinal bleeding, nausea, vomiting, excessive CNS stimulation, and convulsions
Caffeine sodium benzoate injection	Same as caffeine
Dextroamphetamine sulfate (Dexedrine)	See Amphetamines
Diethylpropion hydrochloride (Propion, Tenuate)	Dry mouth, constipation; schedule IV drug
Doxapram hydrochloride (Dopram)	Dizziness, apprehension, disorientation
Fenfluramine hydrochloride (Pondimin)	Sedation and depression; schedule IV drug
Mazindol (Sanorex)	Insomnia, dizziness, agitation; schedule III drug
Methamphetamine hydrochloride (Desoxyn, Obedrin-LA)	See Amphetamines
Nikethamide (Coramine)	Hypertension, tachycardia, tremors, flushing, increased body temperature, convulsion
Phendimetrazine tartrate (Bacarate)	Gastrointestinal distress; schedule III drug
Phenmetrazine hydrochloride (Preludin)	Schedule II drug; see Amphetamines
Phentermine hydrochloride (Adipex-P, Fastin, Tora)	Insomnia; schedule IV drug
Phenylpropanolamine hydrochloride (Acutrim, Control, Diadax, Dexatrim)	Blood pressure increases
Theophylline	Increased heart rate, nervousness, jitteriness, nausea, vomiting, excessive CNS stimulation, and convulsions

   3. Nursing assessment: obtain vital signs and weight; discuss usual eating habits and establish reasonable goals for losing weight
   4. Nursing management: promote weight reduction; monitor for adverse reactions; offer support
   5. Nursing evaluation: instruct patient concerning medication and its potential for drug abuse; assess achievement of goal—weight loss

C. Respiratory stimulants (analeptics): used to stimulate respiration when it has been depressed by drugs, asphyxiation, or electric shock
  1. Action: stimulates central nervous system medullary centers controlling respiration, vasomotor tone, and vagal tone
  2. Agents: see Amphetamines
  3. Nursing assessments: check respiratory rate and depth of respirations; may measure vital capacity and arterial blood gas levels
  4. Nursing management: monitor vital signs with focus on respirations; keep suction machine at bedside
  5. Nursing evaluation: observe whether patient is breathing at a rate and depth nearing normal and whether short-term hospitalization is necessary

AUTONOMIC NERVOUS SYSTEM
Cholinesterase Inhibitors (Cholinergic Agents)

A. Description: drugs that produce a physiologic response similar to that of acetylcholine released on nerve stimulation
B. Action
  1. Direct-acting cholinergic stimulants: mimic the action of acetylcholine
  2. Indirect-acting cholinergic stimulants: inhibit the enzyme cholinesterase, which acts to limit acetylcholine action
C. Effects
  1. Vasodilation
  2. Lowered blood pressure
  3. Slowing of heart rate
  4. Salivation
  5. Perspiring
  6. Increased tone and movement in the gastrointestinal and genitourinary systems
  7. Increased tone and contractility in striated muscles
D. Adverse reactions: heart block, arrhythmias, hypotension, hypertension, nausea, vomiting, cramps, diarrhea, heartburn, muscle weakness, increase in intraocular pressure
E. Agents: the following are examples

Ambenonium chloride (Mytelase Chloride, Mysuran)
Demecarium bromide (Humorsol)
Echothiophate iodide (Phospholine iodide)
Edrophonium chloride (Tensilon)
Isoflurophate (Floropryl)
Neostigmine bromide (Prostigmin)
Pyridostigmine bromide (Mestinon)

F. Nursing assessment: history of lung disease, hyperthyroidism
G. Nursing management: monitor vital signs; insert rectal tube to relieve flatus
H. Nursing evaluation: observe for adverse reactions, bowel activity, intake and output records

Parasympathetic Blocking Agents (Parasympatholytic or Cholinergic Blocking Agents)

A. Action: prevent acetylcholine released by nerve stimulation from exerting its effects

B. Effects:
  1. Gastrointestinal: slows peristalsis
  2. Heart: increases rate
  3. Secretions: depresses all body secretions including perspiration and respiratory, salivary, pancreatic, and gastric secretions
  4. Eye: dilates pupils (mydriasis); paralyzes ciliary muscles; increases intraocular pressure
C. Adverse reactions: dry skin, delirium, convulsions, tachycardia, convulsions, mydriasis, hypertension, dry mouth, urinary retention
D. Agents

Examples	Clinical uses
Atropine sulfate	Adjunct to anesthesia, antispasmodic, cardiac stimulant
Cyclopentolate hydrochloride (Cyclogyl)	Mydriatic, cycloplegic
Homatropine hydrobromide	Mydriatic, cycloplegic
Scopolamine hydrobromide (Hyoscine)	Sedative-hypnotic, adjunct to anesthesia, antiemetic, mydriatic, cycloplegic
Isopropamide iodide (Darbid)	Antispasmodic
Methantheline bromide (Banthine)	Antispasmodic
Propantheline bromide (Pro-Banthine)	Antispasmodic
Benztropine mesylate (Cogentin)	Antiparkinsonian agent
Procyclidine hydrochloride (Kemadrin)	Antiparkinsonian agent
Trihexyphenidyl hydrochloride (Artane)	Antiparkinsonian agent

E. Nursing assessment: monitor vital signs; tachycardia; bowel functions; stimulation or depression of central nervous system; elevation in temperature; respiratory status; history of urinary difficulty, familial history of glaucoma
F. Nursing management: maintain oral hygiene for dry mouth; initiate methods to prevent abdominal distention, and constipation and safety measures in presence of blurred vision
G. Nursing evaluation: establish intake and output records when these drugs are given to elderly males; observe for effectiveness of drug

Neuromuscular Blocking Agents

A. Action: act at the striated neuromuscular junction to produce paralysis of the voluntary muscles
B. Effects
  1. Produce muscular relaxation for insertion of endotracheal tubes during surgical interventions
  2. Protect against violent thrashing that occurs with electroconvulsive therapy
  3. Alleviate spasms that accompany tetanus
C. Adverse reactions: paralysis of respiration, which may be reversed with neostigmine or Tensilon
D. Agents: the following are examples

Decamethonium bromide (Syncurine)
Pancuronium bromide (Pavulon)
Succinylcholine chloride (Anectine)
Tubocurarine chloride (Tubarine)

E. Nursing assessment: elicit medical history: asthma, myasthenia gravis remission; potassium blood levels

F. Nursing management: cardiopulmonary resuscitation skills—have resuscitative equipment available; monitor vital signs

G. Nursing evaluation: observe for early signs of flaccid paralysis in muscles of face, neck, eyes

Sympathomimetic Drugs: Adrenergic Stimulants

A. Actions
   1. Act directly on adrenergic receptors to produce either excitation or inhibition of a particular effector organ
   2. Act indirectly by releasing the stored catecholamines norepinephrine and epinephrine

B. Major effects
   1. Excitation of the heart, both its rate and force of contraction
   2. Excitation and constriction of smooth muscle in blood vessels
   3. Inhibition and relaxation of smooth muscles in bronchi, gastrointestinal tract, and skeletal muscle blood vessels
   4. Metabolism: release of fatty acids from adipose tissue and increased gluconeogenesis in muscle and liver
   5. Excitation of functions controlled by central nervous system, for example, respiration
   6. Suppression of appetite
   7. Lessening of fatigue

C. Adverse reactions: anxiety, apprehension, headache, arrhythmias, cerebral hemorrhage, heart failure, pulmonary edema

D. Agents

Examples	Clinical indications
Dopamine hydrochloride (Intropin)	Hypotension
Ephedrine hydrochloride (Bronkotabs)	Bronchospasms, nasal decongestion, allergy
Epinephrine bitartrate (Medihaler-Epi)	Acute or chronic bronchial asthma, allergic disorders, acute hypersensitivity to drugs
Epinephrine hydrochloride (Adrenalin Chloride)	Cardiac arrest, heart block, acute asthma, adjunct to local anesthesia, acute hypersensitivity to drugs
	Ophthalmic use: control hemorrhage, decrease intraocular pressure
Isoproterenol (Isuprel) hydrochloride	Bronchodilation, cardiac stimulant
Isoproterenol sulfate (Medihaler-Iso)	Bronchodilation
Mephentermine (Wyamine) sulfate	Maintain blood pressure during anesthesia
Metaraminol bitartrate (Aramine)	Hypotension
Naphazoline (Privine) hydrochloride	Nasal decongestion
Norepinephrine (Levophed, Noradrenalin) bitartrate	Shock, cardiac arrest
Nylidrin hydrochloride (Arlidin)	Peripheral vascular disease

E. Nursing assessment: obtain history of hyperthyroidism, diabetes, hypertension, emotional lability, heart disease

F. Nursing management: monitor vital signs; check infusion rate often; observe for infusion infiltration; record bowel and urinary activity

G. Nursing evaluation: monitor effect on blood pressure, pulse rate, and regularity of heart rate; observe for therapeutic and adverse effects

Adrenergic Receptor Blockers and Neuron Blockers

A. Action: interfere with peripheral adrenergic activity by blocking alpha and beta receptors, by depleting peripheral neural stores of norepinephrine, and by inhibiting peripheral sympathetic activity through an action on the central nervous system

B. Adverse reactions: postural hypotension, miosis, inhibition of ejaculation, headache, intense vasoconstriction, diarrhea, nausea, disturbances of vision, insomnia, depression

C. Agents

Examples	Clinical indications
Clonidine (Catapres-TTS)	Chronic hypertension
Ergoloid mesylate (Hydergine)	Mental and emotional complaints of the elderly
Guanethidine monosulfate (Ismelin)	Hypertension
Methyldopa (Aldomet)	Hypertension
Metoprolol tartrate (Lopressor)	Chronic hypertension, angina prophylaxis
Nadolol (Corgard)	Chronic hypertension, angina prophylaxis
Phenoxybenzamine hydrochloride (Dibenzyline)	Peripheral vascular disease
Phentolamine mesylate (Regitine)	Hypertension secondary to pheochromocytoma, adrenal tumor surgery
Prazosin hydrochloride (Minipress)	Chronic hypertension
Propranolol hydrochloride (Inderal)	Chronic hypertension, angina prophylaxis, cardiac dysrhythmias, migraine headaches
Reserpine (Serpasil)	Chronic hypertension
Timolol maleate (Timoptic)	Glaucoma
Tolazoline (Priscoline) hydrochloride	Peripheral vascular disease

D. Nursing assessment: ascertain if patient has history of ulcer disease, diabetes, ulcerative colitis, emotional depression, renal problems, coronary heart disease, predisposition to asthma, or congestive heart failure

E. Nursing management: aim instruction toward patient compliance; administer medications with meals or milk; maintain safety measures in presence of postural hypotension; monitor vital signs

F. Nursing evaluation: observe for therapeutic and adverse reactions; observe for changes in sleep patterns and appetite and depression or suicidal tendencies

Ganglionic Agents

A. Action: reduces sympathetic tone, particularly in the cardiovascular system
B. Adverse reactions: postural hypotension, pupillary dilation, blurring vision, dry mouth, constipation
C. Agents

Examples	Clinical indications
Mecamylamine hydrochloride (Inversine)	Hypertensive crisis, chronic hypertension
Pentolinium (Ansolysen) tartrate	Hypertensive crisis, chronic hypertension
Trimethaphan camsylate (Arfonad)	Hypertensive crisis

D. Nursing assessment: obtain baseline vital signs; assess factors contributing to hypertension such as diet, weight, exercise, and life-style
E. Nursing management: instruction aimed at patient compliance
F. Nursing evaluation: observe for therapeutic effects and adverse reactions

RESPIRATORY SYSTEM
Antihistamines

A. Action: blocks histamine effects at the receptor site
B. Adverse reactions: sedation, drowsiness, dry mouth, blurred vision, urinary retention, constipation; can also stimulate the nervous system, especially in children, causing insomnia, irritability, and nervousness
C. Agents

Examples	Clinical indications
Brompheniramine maleate (Dimetane)	Colds, allergies
Carbinoxamine maleate (Clistin)	Colds, allergies
Chlorpheniramine maleate (Chlor-Trimeton, Teldrin, Chlortab)	Colds, allergies
Cyproheptadine hydrochloride (Periactin)	Pruritus
Dexchlorpheniramine maleate (Polaramine)	Colds, allergies
Dimethindene (Forhistal) maleate	Colds, allergies
Diphenhydramine hydrochloride (Benadryl)	Allergic reactions, motion sickness, mild parkinsonism
Meclizine hydrochloride (Bonine)	Motion sickness
Methdilazine (Tacaryl) hydrochloride	Pruritus
Promethazine hydrochloride (Phenergan, Promine, Remsed, Zipan)	Sedation, pruritus, motion sickness, nausea, vomiting
Trimeprazine tartrate (Temaril)	Pruritus
Tripelennamine (Pyribenzamine) hydrochloride	Colds, allergies

D. Nursing assessment: obtain vital signs; assess respiratory and cardiovascular status; ascertain if patient has history of allergy and extent and type of rash if present
E. Nursing management: Monitor respiratory response, vital signs, urinary and bowel function
F. Nursing evaluation: observe for therapeutic effects and adverse reaction; instruct patient on dangers of operating machinery and to wear medical identification tag in presence of allergies

Nasal Decongestants

A. Action: sympathomimetic agents (see the Autonomic Nervous System) when applied to nasal mucosa or taken orally constrict the smooth muscle of arterioles in the nasal mucosa and thus reduce blood flow and edema
B. Adverse reactions: rebound nasal congestion if used too frequently; nervousness, irritability
C. Agents: the following are a few examples of the numerous preparations available

Allerest	Neo-Synephrine
Afrin	Privine
Contac	Sine-Off
Coricidin	Sinutab
Dristan	Sudafed

D. Nursing assessment: obtain history of irritants or environmental conditions contributing to symptoms and such objective data as respiratory rate and vital signs
E. Nursing management: instruct patient regarding medication use
F. Nursing evaluation: monitor for therapeutic effects and adverse reactions

Expectorants, Antitussives, Mucolytic Drugs

A. Definitions
   1. Expectorant: increases output of respiratory tract fluid that coats the bronchi and trachea
   2. Antitussive: suppresses cough
   3. Mucolytic: breaks up viscous mucus to allow for ease in expectoration of drainage
B. Adverse reactions
   1. Expectorants: nausea, drowsiness; iodide base drugs: skin rash, metallic taste, fever, skin eruptions, mucous membrane ulcerations, salivary gland swelling
   2. Antitussives: nausea, dizziness, constipation
   3. Mucolytics: gastrointestinal upset
C. Agents: the following are examples
   1. Expectorants: Robitussin, iodinated glycerol (Organidin), potassium iodide, SSKI
   2. Antitussives: codeine, hydrocodone bitartrate, dextromethorphan hydrobromide (Romilar), Benylin, benzonatate (Tessalon)
   3. Mucolytics: acetylcysteine (Mucomyst), Alevaire
D. Nursing assessment: obtain history relevant to cough, vital signs, and such objective data as character and quantity of secretions
E. Nursing management: monitor symptoms, vital signs, and amount of secretions with mucolytics
F. Nursing evaluation: instruct patient regarding drugs, how/when to take them and when they should be discontinued; encourage patients with persistent coughs to seek follow-up treatment

Bronchodilators

A. Action: act on bronchial cells to dilate the bronchioles
B. Adverse reactions: CNS stimulation, increased heart rate, muscle tremors, headache, nausea, epigastric pain, bronchospasms
C. Agents: the following are examples

Aminophylline
Dyphylline
  (Dilin, Protophylline)
Ephedrine sulfate
  (Slo-Fedrin)
Epinephrine
  (Sus-Phrine)
Epinephrine bitartrate
  (AsthmaHaler,
    Medihaler-Epi,
    Primatene Mist)
Epinephrine hydrochloride
  (Adrenalin Chloride)
Isoetharine hydrochloride
  (Bronkosol)

Isoetharine mesylate
  (Bronkometer)
Isoproterenol hydrochloride
  (Iprenol, Isuprel
    Hydrochloride)
Metaproterenol sulfate
  (Alupent, Metaprel)
Oxtriphylline
  (Choledyl)
Terbutaline sulfate
  (Brethine, Bricanyl)
Theophylline
  (many preparations)

D. Nursing assessment: obtain relevant history and vital signs; note amount and characteristics of secretions
E. Nursing management: monitor vital signs and closely monitor intravenous drugs
F. Nursing evaluation: observe for therapeutic effects; instruct patient regarding drug knowledge and usage

CARDIOVASCULAR SYSTEM
Drugs to Improve Circulation

A. Action: vasoconstriction (direct- and indirect-acting sympathomimetic amines cause release of norepinephrine, which stimulates alpha receptors and thus produces vasoconstriction)
B. Adverse reactions: headache, anxiety, palpitation, nausea, vomiting, insomnia, tremors
C. Agents: the following are examples

Dobutamine hydrochloride
  (Dobutrex)
Dopamine hydrochloride
  (Intropin)
Epinephrine hydrochloride
  (Adrenalin Chloride)
Isoproterenol
  hydrochloride
  (Isuprel Hydrochloride)
Mephentermine
  (Wyamine) sulfate

Metaraminol bitartrate
  (Aramine)
Methoxamine
  hydrochloride
  (Vasoxyl)
Norepinephrine bitartrate
  (Levarterenol bitartrate;
    Levophed)
Phenylephrine
  hydrochloride
  (Neo-Synephrine
    Hydrochloride,
    Isophrin)

D. Principal clinical use: treatment of cardiogenic and anaphylactic shock; to maintain blood pressure in life-threatening situations and during anesthesia
E. Nursing assessment: obtain pulse, respirations, and blood pressure; note level of consciousness
F. Nursing management: use infusion-control device to monitor intravenous administration; monitor vital signs frequently
G. Nursing evaluation: observe for therapeutic effects

Vasodilator Drugs (Antianginal Drugs)

A. Action: dilate arterioles and veins to lower blood pressure, which reduces work load on the heart and decreases the heart's oxygen demand; increases circulation to cardiac muscle
B. Adverse reactions: flushing, headache, dizziness
C. Agents: the following are examples

Amyl nitrite (Vaporole)
Erythrityl tetranitrate
  (Cardilate)
Isosorbide dinitrate
  (Iso-Bid, Isordil,
    Sorbide, Sorbitrate)
Mannitol hexanitrate
  (Nitranitol)

Nitroglycerin (Nitro-Bid)
Nitroglycerine lingual aerosol
  (Nitrolingual Spray)
Nitroglycerin ointment, 2%
  (Nitrol)
Pentaerythritol tetranitrate
  (Peritrate)
Trolnitrate phosphate
  (Metamine)

D. Nursing assessment: obtain vital signs and history relevant to onset and duration of pain
E. Nursing management: observe and monitor for additional angina attacks; instruct patient about prescribed drugs
F. Nursing evaluation: observe for therapeutic effects

Vasodilator Drugs for Peripheral Vascular Disease

A. Action: work directly on vascular smooth muscle to cause relaxation or stimulate beta receptors in blood vessels to produce vasodilation
B. Adverse reactions: gastrointestinal upset, flushing, hypotension, dizziness, increased heart rate, headache
C. Agents: the following are examples

Cyclandelate
  (Cyclospasmol)
Ergoloid mesylates
  (dihydrogenated
    ergot alkaloids;
    Hydergine)
Isoxsuprine
  hydrochloride
  (Vasodilan)

Nylidrin hydrochloride
  (Arlidin, Rolidrin)
Papaverine hydrochloride
  (many trade names)
Tolazoline (Priscoline)
  hydrochloride

D. Nursing assessment: obtain history of onset and course of vascular disease; assess blood pressure, pulses, including peripheral pulses, mental status, and color of affected extremities
E. Nursing evaluation: observe for therapeutic and adverse effects
F. Nursing management: monitor presenting signs and symptoms; instruct patient regarding medications

Antihypertensives

There are several subgroups of drugs that can lower blood pressure

A. Action
  1. Adrenergic drugs
    a. Beta-1 adrenergic receptor antagonists (beta-blockers): reduce cardiac output; reduce renin release from kidney (blocks response to sympathetic impulses)
    b. Alpha-1 adrenergic receptor antagonists: prevent norepinephrine from constricting blood vessels to increase resistance to blood flow
  2. Centrally acting antihypertensive drugs that inhibit

the activity of the sympathetic nervous system: decrease sympathetic tone and activate alpha receptors in the medulla that decrease heart rate and cardiac output

3. Vasodilators: relax arteriolar smooth muscle
4. Vasodilators in hypertensive emergencies: rapidly relax smooth muscle

B. Adverse reactions: bradycardia, hypotension, nasal congestion, reflex tachycardia, dry mouth, fluid retention, arthralgia, depression, drowsiness

C. Agents: the following are examples

1. Beta adrenergic receptor antagonists
   Metoprolol tartrate (Lopressor)
   Nadolol (Corgard)
   Propranolol hydrochloride (Inderal)

2. Alpha adrenergic receptor antagonists
   Phenoxybenzamine hydrochloride (Dibenzyline)
   Phentolamine mesylate (Regitine)
   Prazosin hydrochloride (Minipress)

3. Drugs interfering with norepinephrine
   Deserpidine (Harmonyl)
   Guanethidine monosulfate (Ismelin)
   Rauwolfia serpentina (Raudixin)
   Reserpine (Serpasil, Sandril)

4. Centrally acting antihypertensive drugs
   Clonidine hydrochloride (Catapres)
   Methyldopa (Aldomet)

5. Vasodilators
   Hydralazine (Apresoline) hydrochloride
   Minoxidil (Loniten)

6. Vasodilators: hypertensive emergencies
   Diazoxide (Hyperstat)
   Sodium nitroprusside (Nipride)
   Trimethaphan camsylate (Arfonad)

D. Nursing assessment: obtain vital signs and additional baseline data, such as weight, diet, and blood studies
E. Nursing management: monitor vital signs, intake and output, weight, blood studies; instruct patient regarding drugs
F. Nursing evaluation: observe for therapeutic effects and adverse reactions
G. Patient teaching: stress the importance of knowing acceptable ranges of blood pressure and pulse; taking medication as ordered; preventing orthostatic hypotension; and reporting asthmalike signs and symptoms

Diuretics

A. Action: increase the excretion of sodium ion and thus increase urine flow
B. Agents

Examples	Adverse reactions
Ethacrynic acid (Edecrin)	Dehydration, thrombosis, emboli, electrolyte imbalance
Furosemide (Lasix)	Acute dehydration, sodium and potassium depletion, calcium loss, dermatitis, blood dyscrasias

Examples	Adverse reactions
1. Thiazide diuretics Bendroflumethiazide (Naturetin) Benzthiazide (Aquatag, Urazide) Chlorothiazide (Diuril) Chlorthalidone (Hygroton) Cyclothiazide (Anhydron) Hydrochlorothiazide (Esidrix, HydroDiuril) Hydroflumethiazide (Saluron) Methyclothiazide (Enduron) Metolazone (Zaroxolyn) Polythiazide (Renese) Trichlormethiazide (Diurese, Naqua)	Fluid and electrolyte imbalance, increased calcium serum levels, gastrointestinal irritation, dizziness, headache, paresthesias, blood dyscrasias, allergy, hypotension
2. Carbonic anhydrase inhibitors Acetazolamide (Diamox) Ethoxzolamide (Cardrase, Ethamide)	
3. Organomercurials Mercaptomerin sodium (Thiomerin) Merethoxylline (Dicurin) procaine	Electrolyte imbalance, skin irritation, bone marrow toxicity, kidney toxicity
4. Potassium-sparing diuretics Spironolactone (Aldactone) Triamterene (Dyrenium)	Hyperkalemia, fatal cardiac dysrhythmias, endocrine alterations, blood dyscrasias

C. Nursing assessment: perform total patient assessment with emphasis on presenting signs and symptoms, vital signs, and laboratory blood studies
D. Nursing management: to foster drug therapy such as by restrictions of fluid and diet; monitor weight, intake and output, and vital signs
E. Nursing evaluation: observe for therapeutic effects and adverse reactions; instruct patient regarding drugs and diet

Cardiotonic Drugs (Cardiac Glycosides)

A. Action: act directly on myocardial cells to increase contractility and thus cardiac output; slows heart rate
B. Adverse reactions: anorexia, nausea, vomiting, bradycardia, weakness, fatigue, visual dimming, double vision, altered color vision, mood alterations, hallucinations, dysrhythmias
C. Agents: the following are examples

Digitoxin (Crystodigin)　　Digoxin (Lanoxin)

D. Nursing assessment: obtain baseline data, weight, vital signs, electrocardiogram (ECG) results

E. Nursing management: monitor vital signs, weight, fluid intake and output, serum electrolyte level, especially potassium; instruct patient regarding drugs

F. Nursing evaluation: observation for therapeutic effects and adverse reactions

Drugs to Control Dysrhythmias

A. Action: slow conduction through atrioventricular (AV) node; block effects of vagal nerve stimulation; block beta adrenergic stimulation; suppress automaticity; increase electrical threshold for stimulation

B. Agents

Examples	Adverse reactions
Atropine	Dry mouth, cycloplegia, mydriasis, fever, urinary retention
Bretylium tosylate (Bretylol)	Anginal attacks, bradycardia, hypotension
Deslanoside (Cedilanid-D) Digitoxin (Crystodigin, Purodigin) Digoxin (Lanoxin)	Bradycardia, premature ventricular beats, atrioventricular tachycardia, anorexia, nausea, vomiting
Disopyramide phosphate (Norpace)	Dry mouth, constipation, urinary retention, blurred vision
Lidocaine (Xylocaine without epinephrine)	Muscle twitching, respiratory depression, convulsions, coma
Phenytoin (Dilantin)	Bradycardia, cardiac arrest, nausea, dizziness, drowsiness
Procainamide hydrochloride (Pronestyl)	Hypotension, decreased cardiac output, gastrointestinal distress
Propranolol hydrochloride (Inderal)	Bradycardia, lowered cardiac output, bronchospasm
Quinidine sulfate (Cin-Quin, Quinora) Quinidine gluconate (Duraquin) Quinidine polygalacturonate (Cardioquin)	Peripheral vasodilation, hypotension, gastrointestinal distress

C. Nursing assessment: obtain baseline data, history of subjective and objective symptoms, vital signs

D. Nursing management: monitor vital signs; instruct patient regarding drugs

E. Nursing evaluation: observe for therapeutic effects and adverse reactions

Anticoagulants

A. Action: inhibit the aggregation of platelets; interfere with any of the steps leading to the formation of fibrin

B. Adverse reactions: hemorrhage, hematuria, melena, rashes, depression of bone marrow

C. Agents: the following are examples

1. Antiplatelet drugs
   Aspirin
   Dipyridamole (Persantine)
   Sulfinpyrazone (Anturane)

2. Heparin sodium (Liquaemin Sodium, Panheprin, Lipo-Hepin)

3. Coumarins
   Dicumarol
   Phenprocoumon (Liquamar)
   Warfarin sodium (Coumadin, Panwarfin)

4. Indanediones
   Anisinodione (Miradon)
   Phenindione (Hedulin)

D. Nursing assessment: obtain baseline data relevant to general condition of the patient, history of problems with clots, and blood coagulation studies: prothrombin time (PT), partial thromboplastin time (PTT), platelet count, and clotting times

E. Nursing management: monitor blood coagulation studies carefully; use infusion monitoring device for constant infusions of heparin; have drug antidotes readily available

F. Nursing evaluation: observe for therapeutic effects and adverse reactions

G. Patient teaching: stress home safety factors to prevent tissue trauma and bleeding; advise to avoid foods high in vitamin K; instruct patient to observe excreta for signs of bleeding

H. Drug interactions
   1. Drugs potentiating response: clofibrate (Atromid S), disulfiram (Antabuse), neomycin sulfate, phenylbutazone (Butazolidin), salicylates, sulfisoxazole (Gantrisin)
   2. Drugs diminishing response: barbiturates, cholestyramine (Questran), ethchlorvynol (Placidyl), glutethimide (Doriden), griseofulvin (Grifulvin-V)

I. Antidotes
   1. Heparin: protamine sulfate
   2. Coumarins: vitamin K

Thrombolytic Drugs

A. Action: promote the digestion of fibrin to dissolve the clot

B. Agents: enzymes urokinase and streptokinase

C. Adverse reaction: hemorrhage

D. Special considerations: reserved for use in acute pulmonary embolism, deep vein thrombosis, or peripheral arterial occlusion; posttreatment: treated with heparin

E. Nursing assessment: obtain baseline data relevant to size, location, and symptoms of clot

F. Nursing management: used only in acute care setting; monitor laboratory blood studies and for signs of clot dissolution

G. Nursing evaluation: observe for therapeutic effects and adverse reactions

Hemostatic Agents

A. Action: inhibit the dissolution of blood clots

B. Adverse reactions: nausea, cramps, dizziness, tinnitus, thrombophlebitis, flushing, vascular collapse

C. Agents

Examples	Clinical indications
1. Systemic agents Aminocaproic acid (Amicar)	Used in special surgical situations
Menadiol sodium diphosphate (Synkayvite) Menadione sodium bisulfite (Hykinone)	Correction of secondary hypoprothrombinemia, correction of severe vitamin K deficiency

Examples	Clinical indications
Phytonadione; vitamin K (AquaMEPHYTON, Konakion, Mephyton)	Oral anticoagulant overdose emergency
2. Local hemostatic agents	
Absorbable gelatin sponge (Gelfoam)	Control bleeding in wound or at operative site
Microfibrillar collagen hemostat (Avitene)	Control bleeding in wound or at operative site
Oxidized cellulose (Oxycel)	Control hemorrhage and absorb blood
Thrombin	Control bleeding in wound or at operative site

D. Nursing assessment: obtain baseline data relevant to type, location, and amount of bleeding, appropriate laboratory blood studies, and general condition of patient
E. Nursing management: monitor appropriate laboratory blood studies
F. Nursing evaluation: observe for therapeutic effects and adverse reactions

Drugs That Lower Blood Lipid Levels

A. Action: in general these drugs lower blood lipid concentrations
   NOTE: no present proof that lowering blood lipid concentrations will reverse or halt atherosclerosis
B. Adverse reactions: bloating, nausea, constipation, muscle cramps, impotence, flushing, weight loss, insomnia, water retention
C. Agents: the following are examples

Aluminum nicotinate (Nicalex)	Colestipol hydrochloride (Colestid)
Beta sitosterol (Cytellin)	Dextrothyroxine (Choloxin)
Cholestyramine resin (Questran)	Niacin; nicotinic acid (Nicobid, Niac, Nicolar)
Clofibrate (Atromid S)	Probucol (Lorelco)

D. Nursing assessment: obtain baseline data relevant to weight, serum cholesterol and triglyceride levels, blood pressure, and dietary history
E. Nursing management: observe for any new symptoms; instruct patient regarding drugs
F. Nursing evaluation: observe for adverse effects; monitor blood levels for therapeutic effects

Drugs That Treat Nutritional Anemias

A. Action: supplement or replace essential vitamins and minerals
B. Agents

Examples	Clinical indications
1. Iron salts	Acute toxicity: acute nausea and vomiting, metabolic acidosis, extensive liver and kidney damage
Ferrous sulfate (Feosol, Fer-In-Sol, Fero-Gradumet, Mol-Iron)	
Ferrous gluconate (Fergon, Ferralet Plus, Entron)	Chronic toxicity: bronze coloration of skin, development of diabetes mellitus, heart failure
Ferrocholinate (Chel-Iron, Kelex)	

Examples	Clinical indications
Ferrous fumarate (Ferranol, Feostat)	
Iron dextran injection (Imferon)	
2. Antidote for iron toxicity	
Deferoxamine mesylate (Desferal)	
3. Vitamin B_{12}	Virtually free of adverse reactions
Cyanocobalamin (Betalin 12 Crystalline, Redisol, Rubramin PC, Sytobex)	
Hydroxocobalamin (alphaRedisol)	
4. Folic acid for anemia	Nontoxic
Folic acid (Folvite)	
Leucovorin calcium	

C. Nursing assessment: obtain baseline data for vital signs, weight, dietary history, blood studies, and presence of neurologic symptoms
D. Nursing management: monitor blood studies, vital signs
E. Nursing evaluation: observe for therapeutic effects and adverse reactions; instruct patient regarding medications
F. Patient teaching: expect dark or black stools and the possibility of gastrointestinal distress

GASTROINTESTINAL SYSTEM
Drugs That Increase Tone and Motility

A. Action: cholinomimetic action to stimulate or restore intestinal tone or urinary bladder tone
B. Adverse reactions: salivation, skin flushing, sweating, diarrhea, abdominal cramps
C. Agents: bethanechol chloride (Urecholine); neostigmine methylsulfate (Prostigmin)
D. Nursing assessment: obtain baseline data regarding vital signs, bowel sounds, fluid intake and output, bowel activity
E. Nursing management: stay with patient at least 15 minutes after administration to observe for adverse reactions; monitor vital signs, fluid intake and output, bowel activity
F. Nursing evaluation: observe for therapeutic effects and adverse reactions

Drugs That Decrease Tone and Motility (Anticholinergics)

A. Action: inhibit gastric secretion and depress gastrointestinal motility
B. Adverse reactions: dry mouth, mydriasis, blurred vision, tachycardia, constipation, and acute urinary retention
C. Agents: the following are examples

Anisotropine methylbromide (Valpin 50)	Hyoscyamine hydrobromide Hyoscyamine sulfate (Anaspaz, Levsin)
Atropine sulfate	Mepenzolate bromide (Cantil)
Belladonna extract	Methantheline bromide (Banthine)
Belladonna tincture	Methixene hydrochloride (Trest)
Dicyclomine hydrochloride (Bentyl, Di-Spaz)	Methscopolamine bromide (Pamine)

Diphemanil methylsulfate (Prantal)	Oxyphencyclimine hydrochloride (Daricon)
Glycopyrrolate (Robinul)	Propantheline bromide (Pro-Banthine)
Homatropine methylbromide (Homapin)	Thiphenamil hydrochloride (Trocinate)
	Tridihexethyl chloride (Pathilon)

D. Nursing assessment: obtain baseline data for vital signs, frequency and character of stools, and presence of occult blood in stools

E. Nursing management: monitor vital signs

F. Nursing evaluation: observe for therapeutic effects and adverse reactions; instruct patient regarding medication

Drugs to Treat Ulcers

A. Action
1. Antacids: neutralize gastric hydrochloric acid
2. Anticholinergic drugs: see drugs under the Autonomic Nervous System
3. Antihistamines: block the histamines' receptors and decrease gastric acid production

B. Adverse reactions: constipation, diarrhea; can interfere with absorption of some drugs: tetracycline, digoxin, quinidine

C. Agents (antacids): the following are examples

Aluminum hydroxide (Amphojel)	Aluminum hydroxide ⎫
Calcium carbonate (Dicarbosil, Tums)	Magnesium hydroxide ⎬ (Maalox)
Dihydroxyaluminum aminoacetate (Robalate)	Aluminum hydroxide ⎫
Dihydroxyaluminum sodium carbonate (Rolaids)	Magnesium trisilicate ⎬ (Trisogel)
Magnesium hydroxide (Milk of Magnesia)	Aluminum hydroxide gel ⎫ (Maalox Plus, Mylanta, Gelusil)
Aluminum hydroxide ⎫	Magnesium hydroxide ⎬
Calcium carbonate ⎬ (Camalox)	Simethicone
Magnesium hydroxide ⎭	Aluminum phosphate gel (Phosphaljel)
	Magaldrate (Riopan)

D. Agents (Histamine H_2-receptor antagonists): the following are examples

Cimetidine (Tagamet)	Ranitidine hydrochloride (Zantac)
Famotidine (Pepcid)	

E. Nursing assessment: obtain baseline data relevant to vital signs, level of consciousness, character and quality of emesis and stool, appropriate laboratory blood studies

F. Nursing management: monitor vital signs, fluid intake and output, level of consciousness, and character of stools and vomitus

G. Nursing evaluation: observe for therapeutic effects and adverse reactions

Antiemetics

A. Action: control nausea and vomiting by reducing stimulation of labyrinthine receptors; dopamine antagonists, which act on the chemoreceptor trigger zone in the medulla

B. Adverse reactions: drowsiness, blurred vision, dilated pupils, dry mouth, extrapyramidal symptoms

C. Agents: the following are examples

1. Anticholinergics
   Scopolamine hydrobromide
2. Antihistamines
   Dimenhydrinate (Dramamine)
   Diphenhydramine hydrochloride (Benadryl)
   Hydroxyzine pamoate (Vistaril)
   Meclizine hydrochloride (Antivert, Bonine)
   Promethazine hydrochloride (Phenergan)
3. Miscellaneous drugs
   Benzquinamide hydrochloride (Emete-con)
   Diphenidol hydrochloride (Vontrol)
   Trimethobenzamide hydrochloride (Tigan)
4. Dopamine antagonists
   Chlorpromazine hydrochloride (Thorazine)
   Fluphenazine hydrochloride (Prolixin)
   Haloperidol (Haldol)
   Perphenazine (Trilafon)
   Prochlorperazine (Compazine)
   Promazine hydrochloride (Sparine)
   Triflupromazine hydrochloride (Vesprin)

D. Nursing assessment: obtain baseline data regarding vital signs, character and quantity of any emesis, presence of bowel sounds, fluid intake and output

E. Nursing management: monitor vital signs and fluid intake and output

F. Nursing evaluation: observe for therapeutic effects and adverse reactions

Antidiarrhetic Agents

A. Action: decrease tone of small and large bowel; depress smooth muscle contraction; decrease release of acetylcholine; absorb toxins

B. Adverse reactions: respiratory depression, constipation, impaction

C. Agents: the following are examples

Bismuth subsalicylate (Pepto-Bismol)	Loperamide hydrochloride (Imodium)
Codeine phosphate	
Codeine sulfate	
Diphenoxylate hydrochloride with atropine sulfate (Diphenatol, Lomotil, Lofene)	

D. Nursing assessment: obtain baseline data relevant to vital signs, fluid and solid intake and output, nature and character of stools

E. Nursing management: monitor vital signs, intake and output, frequency and character of stools

F. Nursing evaluation: observe for therapeutic effects and adverse reactions

Laxatives

A. Action: retain water to keep stools large and soft; stimulate motility in large intestine; inhibit reabsorption of water; attract water by osmosis; soften feces

B. Adverse reactions: loss of bowel tone, dehydration, hypokalemia, hyponatremia, malabsorption of fat-soluble vitamins

C. Agents: the following are examples

1. Bulk-forming agents
   Gum karaya
   Plantago seed
     (psyllium)
   Psyllium
     hydrocolloid
     (Effersyllium)
   Psyllium hydrophilic
     mucilloid
     (Metamucil)
2. Stimulant cathartics
     (irritants)
   Bisacodyl (Bisco-Lax,
     Dulcolax)
   Cascara sagrada
   Castor oil
   Glycerin
     suppositories
   Phenolphthalein (Ex-
     Lax,
     Feen-A-Mint,
     Phenolax)
   Senna concentrate
     (Senokot)
   Senna pod
3. Saline cathartics
   Magnesium hydroxide
     (Milk of Magnesia)
   Magnesium sulfate (Epsom
     salt)
   Monosodium phosphate
     (Sal Hepatica)
   Sodium phosphate with
     sodium biphosphate
     (Phospho-Soda)
4. Lubricants
   Mineral oil (Agoral Plain,
     Petrogalar Plain)
5. Fecal softeners
   Docusate calcium (dioctyl
     calcium sulfosuccinate;
     Surfak)
   Docusate sodium (dioctyl
     sodium sulfosuccinate;
     Colace, Comfolax, D-S-S)

D. Nursing assessment: obtain baseline data relevant to vital signs, intake and output, presence of bowel sounds, bowel habits, dietary history, medications

E. Nursing management: monitor diet and fluid intake; instruct patient regarding drugs

F. Nursing evaluation: observe for therapeutic effects and adverse reactions

ENDOCRINE SYSTEM
Drugs Affecting Pituitary Gland

A. Action
1. Antidiuretic hormone (ADH): increases renal tubule's permeability and thus its ability to reabsorb water
2. Oxytocin: promotes uterine contractions during last stages of labor when cervix is fully dilated
3. Growth hormone: anabolic agent that increases cell size and cell numbers
4. Gonadotropic hormone (GTH): regulates maturation and function of male and female sexual organs
5. Adrenocorticotropic hormone (ACTH): stimulates adrenal cortex to release its hormone

B. Adverse reactions: hyponatremia, water retention, glycosuria, vasoconstriction, nausea

C. Agents

Examples	Clinical indications
Desmopressin actate (DDAVP)	Diabetes insipidus
Lypressin (Diapid)	Diabetes insipidus
Posterior pituitary extract (Pituitrin)	Smooth muscle contraction
Vasopressin (Pitressin)	Short-term maintenance of unconscious patient

D. Nursing assessment: obtain baseline data relative to excesses or deficiencies of specific hormone

E. Nursing management: monitor fluid intake and output, laboratory values; instruct patient regarding medications

F. Nursing evaluation: observe for therapeutic effects and adverse reactions

Drugs Affecting Adrenal Glands

A. Action: replace the body's normal amount of hormones; block inflammatory responses; antineoplastic; antagonize autoimmune responses

B. Adverse reactions: impaired glucose tolerance or hyperglycemia; fat deposition; muscle weakness or wasting; peptic ulcer; growth inhibition; mood changes or psychosis; osteoporosis; sodium retention; potassium loss

C. Agents: dosage is individualized to patient and diagnosis; the following are examples

Betamethasone valerate (Valisone)
Cortisone (Cortone) acetate
Desoxycorticosterone (Doca, Percorten) acetate
Dexamethasone (Decadron, Hexadrol)
Fludrocortisone (Florinef) acetate
Hydrocortisone (cortisol; Cortef, Cortril, Hydrocortone)
Hydrocortisone (Cortef) acetate

Methylprednisolone (Medrol, Wyacort)
Methylprednisolone acetate (Depo-Medrol)
Methylprednisolone sodium succinate (Solu-Medrol)
Prednisolone (Delta-Cortef, Paracortol)
Prednisolone sodium phosphate (Hydeltrasol)
Prednisone (Meticorten, Delta-Dome)
Triamcinolone (Aristocort, Kenacort)
Triamcinolone acetonide (Kenalog)
Triamcinolone hexacetonide (Aristospan)

D. Nursing assessment: obtain baseline data relevant to vital signs, weight, glycosuria

E. Nursing management: monitor vital signs, weight, serum electrolyte levels, sugar concentrations in blood and urine, signs of masked infection; instruct patient regarding medications

F. Nursing evaluations: observe for therapeutic effects and adverse reactions

Drugs Affecting Thyroid Gland

A. Action
1. Hypothyroidism: replace the body's normal amount of hormone
2. Hyperthyroidism
   a. Control the symptoms of hyperthyroidism
   b. Inhibit the synthesis of thyroid hormones
   c. Inhibit iodine uptake by thyroid gland
   d. Inhibit thyroid hormone release and symptoms
   e. Suppress continued uptake of iodine
   f. Destroy surrounding tissue by emission of low-energy radiation

B. Adverse reactions to drugs for hyperthyroidism: agranulocytosis, skin rash, nausea, vomiting, twitching muscles, bronchospasm, iodism, symptoms of hyperthyroidism

C. Adverse reactions to drugs for hypothyroidism: dysrhythmias, hypertension, headache, insomnia, irritability, vomiting, weight loss

D. Agents: the following are examples

1. Hypothyroidism
   a. Natural thyroid hormones
      Thyroglobulin (Proloid)
      Thyroid (Delcoid, Thyrar, Thyrocrine)
   b. Synthetic thyroid hormones
      Levothyroxine sodium (Eltroxin, Levoid, Synthroid)
      Liothyronine sodium (Cytomel)
      Liotrix (Euthroid, Thyrolar)
   c. Adenohypophyseal hormone
      Thyroid-stimulating hormone (TSH) (thyrotropin; Thytropar)
      Protirelin (Thypinone)

2. Hyperthyroidism
   a. Thioamides
      Methimazole (Tapazole)
      Propylthiouracil
   b. Beta adrenergic blocker
      Propranolol hydrochloride (Inderal)
   c. Iodine
      Potassium or sodium iodide (Lugol's solution)
   d. Radioactive iodine (^{131}I)

E. Nursing assessment: obtain baseline data relevant to vital signs, weight, level of energy, and symptoms of hypofunctioning or hyperfunctioning of gland

F. Nursing management: monitor vital signs, weight; instruct patient regarding medications

G. Nursing evaluation: observe for therapeutic effects and adverse reactions

Drugs Affecting Parathyroid Gland

A. Action: maintain blood calcium levels in the blood

B. Adverse reactions: nausea, local irritation at injection sites, drowsiness; gastrointestinal complaints, hypertension

C. Agents: the following are examples

Calcitonin (Calcimar)
Calcitriol (Rocaltrol)
Parathyroid hormone

D. Nursing assessment: obtain baseline data relevant to vital signs and blood calcium levels

E. Nursing management: monitor vital signs, blood calcium levels

F. Nursing evaluation: observe for therapeutic effects (i.e., decreased muscle cramping) and adverse reactions; instruct patient regarding medications

FEMALE REPRODUCTIVE SYSTEM
Estrogens

A. Action: replace or supplement natural body hormones; alter cell environment in neoplastic processes

B. Adverse reactions: breast tenderness, increased risk of endometrial cancer, nausea, vomiting, anorexia, malaise, depression, salt and water retention

C. Agents: the following are examples

Chlorotrianisene (TACE)
Diethylstilbestrol (DES) (Stilbestrol)
Ethinyl estradiol (Estinyl)
Estradiol (Estrace)
Estrone (Theelin, Femogen)
Estrogen, conjugated (Premarin)

Progestins

A. Action: suppress endometrial bleeding; withdrawal of drug induces tissue sloughing

B. Adverse reactions: edema, breast tenderness, depression, midcycle bleeding

C. Agents: the following are examples

Dydrogesterone (Gynorest)
Hydroxyprogesterone caproate (Delalutin, Gesterol LA)
Medroxyprogesterone acetate (Depo-Provera, Provera)
Megestrol acetate (Megace)
Norethindrone (Norlutin)
Porgesterone (Gesterol-50, Lipo-Lutin)

Fertility Drugs

A. Action: stimulate ovulation by pituitary or ovarian mechanisms

B. Adverse reactions: relatively rare

C. Agents: the following are examples

Clomiphene citrate (Clomid)
Menotropins (Perganol)
Human chorionic gonadotropin (HCG) (Antuitrin S, Follutein)

Contraceptive Drugs

A. Action: suppress ovulation; induce changes in cervical mucus, making uterine entry by sperm difficult; produce changes in endometrium, making implantation difficult

B. Adverse reactions: thromboembolitic diseases, stroke, hypertension

C. Agents: the following examples contain varying amounts of progesterone and estrogen

Brevicon
Enovid
Norlestrin
Ortho-Novum
Ovrette
Ovulen

Oxytocic Drugs

A. Action: induce contraction of the myometrium

B. Adverse reactions: fetal or maternal cardiac dysrhythmias, acute hypertension, nausea, water intoxication, uterine hypertonicity with fetal or maternal injury

C. Agents: the following are examples

Dinoprost tromethamine (Prostin F2 Alpha)
Dinoprostone (Prostin E2)
Ergonovine (Ergotrate) maleate
Methylergonovine maleate (Methergine)
Oxytocin (Pitocin, Syntocinon)

Uterine Relaxants

A. Action: stimulation of beta-2 adrenergic receptors produces relaxation of uterine muscle
B. Adverse reactions: heart palpitations, nausea, vomiting, trembling, flushing, and headache
C. Agents: Ritodrine

Nursing Process

A. Assessment: obtain baseline data relevant to vital signs, weight, current problem; elicit history of previous pregnancies and deliveries, fetal heart tones
B. Management: inform of possible side effects and benefits; monitor vital signs, weight; with oxytocics: maternal and fetal monitoring; infusion monitoring device
C. Evaluation: observe for therapeutic effects and adverse reactions; instruct patient regarding medications

MALE HORMONES
Androgens

A. Action: replace or supplement normal body hormone; relieve postpartum breast engorgement; alter cell environment in neoplastic disease in females
B. Adverse reactions: female masculinization; premature closure of epiphyses in children; nausea, vomiting, diarrhea
C. Agents: the following are examples

Fluoxymesterone (Halotestin)	Testosterone (Testaqua, Oreton)
Methyltestosterone (Android)	

Anabolic Steroids

A. Action: increase nitrogen retention and protein formation; stimulate red blood cell formation and increase bone deposition
B. Adverse reactions: increased libido; priapism (continuous erection), female masculinization, precocious sexual development in children, premature epiphyseal fusion
C. Agents: the following are examples

Ethylestrenol (Maxibolin)	Nondrolone phenpropionate (Durabolin)
Methandrostenolone (Dianabol)	Oxandrolone (Anavar)
Methandriol	Stanozolol (Winstrol)
Nonrolone decanoate (Deca-Durabolin)	

Nursing Process

A. Assessment: obtain baseline data relevant to vital signs, weight, height (children), current problem
B. Management: monitor vital signs, weight, height (children); review possible side effects with patient
C. Evaluation: observe for therapeutic effects and adverse reactions; instruct patient regarding medications

THE EYE
Anticholinergic Drugs

A. Action: cause mydriasis (dilated pupils) and cycloplegia (blurred vision)
B. Adverse reaction: dry mouth and skin, fever, thirst, confusion, hyperactivity

C. Agents: the following are examples

Atropine sulfate (Atropisol, Isopto Atropine)	Scopolamine hydrobromide (hyoscine hydrobromide; Isopto Hyoscine)
Cyclopentolate hydrochloride (Cyclogyl)	
Homatropine hydrobromide (Isopto Homatropine, Homatrocel)	Tropicamide (Mydriacyl)

Adrenergic Drugs

A. Action: cause mydriasis
B. Adverse reactions: rare
C. Agents: the following are examples

Hydroxyamphetamine hydrobromide (Paredrine)	Phenylephrine hydrochloride (Alconefrin, Mydfrin, Neo-Synephrine Hydrochloride)

Drugs Used to Treat Glaucoma

A. Action: cause miosis (pupil constriction); reduce resistance to outflow of aqueous humor; decrease production of aqueous humor
B. Adverse reactions: blood vessel congestion causing increased intraocular pressure, ocular pain, headache, tachycardia or bradycardia, hypertension, diaphoresis, anorexia, gastrointestinal upset, lethargy, depression, diuresis, dehydration
C. Agents: the following are examples

Acetazolamide (Diamox)	Epinephryl borate (Epinal, Eppy/N)
Carbachol (Isopto Carbachol)	Epinephrine hydrochloride (Epifrin, Glaucon)
Demecarium bromide (Humorsol)	Ethoxzolamide (Cardrase, Ethamide)
Dichlorphenamide (Daranide, Oratrol)	Glycerin (Glyrol, Osmoglyn)
	Isoflurophate (Floropryl)
Echothiophate iodide (Phospholine Iodide)	Isosorbide (Ismotic)
	Mannitol (Osmitrol)
	Methazolamide (Neptazane)
Epinephrine bitartrate (Epitrate, Primatene Mist Suspension)	Physostigmine (Eserine) sulfate
	Pilocarpine hydrochloride (Isopto Carpine, Pilocar)
	Timolol maleate (Timoptic)
	Urea (Ureaphil, Urevert)

Nursing Process

A. Nursing assessment: obtain history of eye-related symptoms, such as difficulty in driving or ambulating; examine eyes for signs of infection, exudate, tearing, or drying
B. Nursing management: advise patient about effects of drugs such as blurred vision and photophobia; instruct patient regarding drugs (i.e., do not skip doses)
C. Nursing evaluation: observe for therapeutic effects and adverse reactions

DRUGS USED TO CONTROL MUSCLE TONE
Acetylcholinesterase Inhibitors (Anticholinergic Agents)

A. Action: allow the accumulation of acetylcholine at neuromuscular junctions and thus ensure muscle contractility; drugs are not used during pregnancy or with patients that have hyperexcitability of muscular symptoms
B. Adverse reactions: muscle cramps, fasciculations (rapid,

small contractions), weakness; excessive salivation, perspiration, nausea, vomiting

C. Agents: the following are examples

Ambenonium chloride (Mytelase)

Neostigmine bromide (Prostigmin)

Edrophonium chloride (Tensilon)

Pyridostigmine bromide (Mestinon, Regonol)

D. Nursing assessment: obtain baseline data relevant to vital signs, ability to swallow, muscle strength, and eyelid ptosis

E. Nursing management: monitor disease symptoms and vital signs; have suction and intubation equipment at bedside

F. Nursing evaluation: observe for therapeutic effects and adverse reactions

Neuromuscular Blocking Agents

A. Action: produce muscle paralysis

B. Adverse reactions: hypotension, bronchospasm, tachycardia, bradycardia, cardiac dysrhythmias, respiratory distress

C. Agents: the following are examples

Decamethonium bromide (Syncurine)

Succinylcholine chloride (Anectine Quelicin, Sucostrin)

Gallamine triethiodide (Flaxedil)

Tubocurarine chloride (Tubarine)

Pancuronium bromide (Pavulon)

D. Nursing assessment: obtain baseline data relevant to pulse, respiration, and blood pressure

E. Nursing management: monitor vital signs; observe rate, quality, and depth of respiration

F. Nursing evaluation: observe for therapeutic effects: sufficient muscle relaxation to allow procedure to be done; observe for adverse reactions: cough and inability to breathe unassisted and to handle secretions

DIABETES MELLITUS
Insulin

A. Action: restores the cell's ability to use glucose and to correct the metabolic changes that occur with diabetes mellitus

B. Adverse reactions: Table 4-6; allergic reactions, insulin resistance, injection-site lipoatrophy

C. Agents: Table 4-7 lists insulin preparations

Table 4-7. Insulin preparations

	Onset of action	Peak action	Duration of action
Rapid acting			
Insulin injection (Regular Insulin)	Within 1 hr	2-4 hr	6-8 hr
Prompt insulin zinc suspension (Semilente Iletin, Semilente Insulin)	1.5-2 hr	4-7 hr	12-16 hr
Intermediate acting			
Globin zinc insulin injection	2-4 hr	10-14 hr	14-22 hr
Isophane insulin suspension (NPH Iletin, NPH Insulin)	1-2 hr	10-16 hr	18-30 hr
Insulin zinc suspension (Lente Iletin, Lente Insulin)	1-2 hr	10-16 hr	18-30 hr
Long acting			
Protamine zinc insulin suspension (Protamine Zinc Iletin, Protamine Zinc Insulin, PZI)	6-8 hr	14-24 hr	24-36 hr or longer
Extended insulin zinc suspension (Ultralente Iletin, Ultralente Insulin)	5-8 hr	16-18 hr	24-36 hr or longer

Table 4-6. Hyperglycemic and hypoglycemic reactions

	Hyperglycemia: ketoacidosis, diabetic coma, too little insulin	Hypoglycemia: Insulin reaction, too much insulin
Onset	Gradual—Days	Minutes to hours
Causes	Neglect of therapy, untreated diabetes, intercurrent disease or infection, increase in emotional or psychologic stress	Insulin overdose, omission or delay of meals, excessive exercise before meals
Signs and symptoms	Thirst, headache, excessive urination, nausea, vomiting, abdominal pain, dim vision, coma, flushed face, Kussmaul breathing—rapid, deep—air hunger, dehydration, acetone breath, soft eyeballs, normal or absent reflexes	Nervousness, hunger, weakness, cold clammy sweat, nausea, dizziness, double or blurred vision, behavioral changes, stupor, convulsions, pallor, shallow respirations, normal eyeballs, Babinski's reflex may be present
Urine glucose	Positive	Negative or low
Urine acetone	Positive	Negative
Blood glucose	High (above 250 mg)	Low (below 60 mg)
Blood CO_2	Low	Usually normal
Treatment	Insulin, fluid replacement, electrolyte replacement, close observation	Glucose, glucagon, close observation
Response to treatment	Slow	Rapid

Oral Hypoglycemic Agents

A. Action: stimulate release of insulin from pancreas
B. Adverse reactions: gastrointestinal distress, muscle weakness, paresthesias, skin reactions, hypoglycemia
C. Agents

Examples	Duration of action
Tolbutamide (Orinase)	6 to 12 hours
Acetohexamide (Dymelor)	12 to 24 hours
Tolazamide (Tolinase)	12 to 24 hours
Glyburide (Micronase)	up to 24 hours
Chlorpropamide (Diabinese)	up to 72 hours

Nursing Process

A. Nursing assessment: obtain baseline data relevant to vital signs, weight, blood and urine glucose levels, and other signs and symptoms of the disease
B. Nursing management: monitor vital signs, blood and urine glucose levels, and other appropriate laboratory results; instruct patient regarding medications and administration
C. Nursing evaluation: observe for therapeutic effects and adverse reactions

PREVENTION AND TREATMENT OF INFECTIONS (ANTIMICROBIALS/ANTIINFECTIVES)
Penicillins and Cephalosporins

A. Action: bacteriocidal by interfering with the synthesis of the bacterial cell wall
B. Adverse reactions: allergies—rash, anaphylaxis; convulsions with high parenteral doses; gastrointestinal distress—nausea, vomiting, and diarrhea
C. Agents: the following are examples

1. Penicillins
   Amoxicillin
      (Amoxil, Larotid,
      Polymox,
      Trimox)
   Ampicillin
      (Amcill, Omnipen,
      Polycillin,
      Principen)
   Carbenicillin disodium
      (Geopen)
   Cloxacillin sodium
      (Cloxapen,
      Tegopen)
   Dicloxacillin sodium
      (Dycill, Dynapen)
   Methicillin sodium
      (Celbenin,
      Staphcillin)
   Nafcillin sodium
      (Nafcil, Unipen)
   Oxacillin sodium
      (Bactocill,
      Prostaphlin)
   Penicillin G potassium
      (Pentids, Pfizerpen)
   Penicillin G benzathine (Bicillin)

Penicillin G procaine
   (Crysticillin,
   Duracillin, Wycillin)
Penicillin V
   (Pen·Vee K,
   V-Cillin, Veetids)
2. Cephalosporins
Cefaclor
   (Ceclor)
Cefamandole nafate
   (Mandol)
Cefazolin sodium
   (Ancef, Kefzol)
Cefoxitin
   (Mefoxin)
Cephalexin
   (Keflex)
Cephaloridine
   (Loridine)
Cephalothin sodium
   (Keflin)
Cephapirin sodium
   (Cefadyl)
Cephradrine
   (Anspor, Velosef)

D. Clinical indications
   1. Wound and skin infections
   2. Respiratory infections
   3. Prophylaxis for patients with rheumatic fever or congenital heart disease
   4. Gram-positive infections caused by streptococci and some staphylococci
   5. Gram-negative infections caused by *Haemophilus influenza, Escherichia coli,* and *Neisseria gonorrhoeae*

Erythromycin, Clindamycin (Penicillin Substitutes)

A. Action: bacteriostatic or bacteriocidal (dosage related) by inhibiting protein synthesis
B. Adverse reactions: abdominal discomfort, cramping, nausea, vomiting, diarrhea, urticaria, anaphylaxis, colitis, liver dysfunction, deafness (vancomycin), permanent kidney damage (systemic bacitracin)
C. Agents: the following are examples

1. Erythromycins
   Erthromycin
      (E-Mycin,
      Ilotycin,
      Robimycin,
      RP-Mycin)
   Erythromycin
      estolate (Ilosone)
   Erythromycin
      ethylsuccinate
      (E.E.S.)
   Erythromycin
      (Erythrocin)
      stearate
2. Clindamycins/Lincomycins
   Clindamycin
      (Cleocin)
   Lincomycin hydrochloride
      (Lincocin)
3. Penicillin substitutes
   Bacitracin
   Novobiocin sodium
      (Albamycin)
   Spectinomycin
      hydrochloride (Trobicin)
   Vancomycin (Vancocin)
      hydrochloride

D. Clinical indications
   1. See clinical indications for penicillins
   2. Used for patients allergic to penicillin

Tetracyclines and Chloramphenicol

A. Action: bacteriostatic by preventing the start of protein synthesis (tetracyclines) or inhibiting protein synthesis (chloramphenicol)
B. Adverse reactions
   1. Tetracyclines: nausea, vomiting, stomach pain, diarrhea, superimposed infections, impaired kidney functions, jaundice, delayed blood coagulation, brown discoloration of teeth in children under 8 years of age
   2. Chloramphenicol: bone marrow toxicity, aplastic anemia, allergies, gastrointestinal irritation, headache, mental confusion, depression
C. Agents: the following are examples

Chloramphenicol
   (Chloromycetin)
Chlortetracycline
   hydrochloride
   (Aureomycin)
Demeclocycline
   hydrochloride
   (Declomycin)
Doxycycline hyclate
   (Vibramycin,
   Doxychel)

Methacycline hydrochloride
   (Rondomycin)
Minocycline hydrochloride
   (Minocin, Vectrin)
Oxytetracycline
   hydrochloride
   (Terramycin, Oxlopar)
Tetracycline hydrochloride
   (Achromycin, Panmycin
   Hydrochloride, Sumycin,
   Tetracyn)

D. Clinical indications
1. Gram-negative and gram-positive infections
2. Severe acne vulgaris
3. Used for patients allergic to penicillin

Aminoglycosides and Polymyxins

A. Action
1. Aminoglycosides: inhibit early stages of protein synthesis
2. Polymyxins: alter bacterial cell membrane permeability
B. Adverse reactions: eighth cranial nerve damage, renal damage, respiratory paralysis
C. Agents: the following are examples

1. Aminoglycosides
   Amikacin sulfate
     (Amikin)
   Gentamicin sulfate
     (Garamycin)
   Kanamycin sulfate
     (Kantrex)
   Neomycin sulfate
     (Mycifradin,
     Neobiotic)

   Streptomycin
   Tobramycin sulfate
     (Nebcin)
2. Polymyxins
   Colistimethate sodium
     (Coly-Mycin M)
   Colistin sulfate
     (Coly-Mycin S)
   Polymyxin B sulfate
     (Aerosporin)

D. Clinical indications
Drugs are potentially dangerous and are used only in cases of severe infections, such as gram-negative bone and joint infections and septicemia

Sulfonamides, Trimethoprim, Nitrofurantoins, Nalidixic Acid

A. Action: block bacterial synthesis of folic acid; inhibit bacterial enzymes required for proper metabolism of sugar; interfere directly with DNA synthesis
B. Adverse reactions
1. Sulfonamides, trimethoprim, nitrofurantoins: allergies, nausea, vomiting, diarrhea, stomatitis, blood dyscrasias, renal calculi, and hematuria
2. Nalidixic acid: convulsions, mental instability, headache, dizziness, visual disturbances, photosensitivity
C. Agents: the following are examples

1. Sulfonamides
   Sulfadiazine
   Sulfameter
     (Sulla)
   Sulfamethizole
     (Microsul,
     Thiosulfil, Forte)
   Sulfamethoxazole
     (Gantanol)
   Sulfamethoxazole-
     phenazopyridine
     (Azo Gantanol)
   Sulfamethoxazole-
     trimethoprim
     (Bactrim, Septra)
   Sulfamethoxypyridazine
     (Midicel) acetyl
   Sulfasalazine
     (Azulfidine,
     Salazopyrin)
   Sulfisoxazole
     (Gantrisin,
     Rosoxol, Sulfalar)

   Sulfisoxazole–
     phenazopyridine
     hydrochloride
     (Azo Gantrisin,
     SK-Soxazole, Azosul)
2. Sulfonamides: topical
   agents
   Mafenide
     (Sulfamylon)
   Nitrofurantoin
     (Furadantin, Furalan,
     Nephronex)
   Nitrofurantoin macro-
     crystals (Macrodantin)
   Nalidixic acid
     (NegGram)
   Silver sulfadiazine
     (Silvadene)
   Sulfacetamide
     (Sulamyd) sodium
   Sulfisoxazole diolamine
     (Gantrisin Ophthalmic)
   Trimethoprim
     (Proloprim, Trimpex)

D. Clinical indications
1. Used to treat acute and chronic urinary tract infections
2. Other uses include trachoma, chancroid, toxoplasmosis, acute otitis media, and prophylactic therapy in cases of recurrent rheumatic fever
3. Treatment of ulcerative colitis
4. Prophylaxis for patients scheduled for bowel surgery

Drugs Used to Treat Tuberculosis and Leprosy

A. Action: alter several metabolic processes in mycobacteria
B. Adverse reactions: peripheral neuropathies, visual disturbances, gastrointestinal distress, ototoxicity, headache
C. Agents: the following are examples

1. First-line antitubercular
   drugs
   Ethambutol
     hydrochloride
     (Myambutol)
   Isoniazid
     (Isotamine, Niconyl,
     Nydrazid)
   Para-aminosalicylic
     acid (PAS)
     (aminosalicylic acid,
     Teebacin acid)
   Rifampin
     (Rifadin, Rimactane)
   Streptomycin
2. Second-line
   antitubercular drugs
   Capreomycin (Capastat)
   Cycloserine
     (Seromycin)
   Ethionamide
     (Trecator S.C.)
   Pyrazinamide
3. Antileprosy agents
   Clofazimine
     (Lamprene)
   Dapsone
     (Avlosulfon)
   Rifampin
     (Rifadin, Rimactane)
   Sulfoxone
     (Diasone) sodium

D. Patient teaching: stress importance of long-term compliance and follow-up visits with the physician; report any adverse reactions promptly; refrain from using alcohol; refrain from taking other medications without the knowledge and permission of the physician; wear a medical identification tag indicating medication being taken

Antifungal Drugs

A. Action: selectively damages the membranes of fungi
B. Adverse reactions: renal damage, anemia, nausea, diarrhea
C. Agents: the following are examples

1. Systemic agents
   Amphotericin B
     (Fungizone)
   Flucytosine
     (Ancobon)
   Hydroxystilbamidine
     isethionate
   Miconazole
     (Monistat-IV)
2. Topical agents
   Acrisorcin
     (Akrinol)
   Amphotericin B
     (Fungizone)
   Candicidin
     (Vanobid)
   Clioquinol
     (Vioform)

   Clotrimazole
     (Gyne-Lotrimin, Lotrimin)
   Griseofulvin
     (Fulvicin-P/G, Grifulvin V,
     Grisactin)
   Haloprogin
     (Halotex)
   Miconazole nitrate
     (Micatin, Monistat)
   Nystatin
     (Mycostatin, Nilstat)
   Tolnaftate
     (Aftate, Tinactin)
   Undecylenic acid–zinc
     undecylenate
     (Desenex, Ting, Cruex)

Drugs Used to Treat Viral Diseases

A. Action: selective toxicity in various processes of virus reproduction
B. Adverse reactions: ataxia, slurred speech, lethargy, local irritation, anorexia, nausea, vomiting, diarrhea
C. Agents: the following are examples

Acyclovir (Zovirax)
Amantadine (Symmetrel)
Idoxuridine (Dendrid, Herplex Liquifilm, Stoxil)
Methisazone
Vidarabine (Vira-A)
Zidovudine* (AZT, Retrovir)

Antiprotozoal and Anthelmintic Agents

A. Action: destroy the protozoa and helminths at various stages of development
B. Adverse reactions: gastrointestinal distress, flatulence, vision changes, irritability, hemolysis, skin eruptions, blood dyscrasias
C. Agents: the following are examples

1. Amebic infestations
   Chloroquine (Aralen) phosphate
   Diloxanide (Furamide)
   Emetine hydrochloride
   Iodoquinol (Yodoxin)
   Metronidazole (Flagyl)
2. Malaria
   Amodiaquine (Camoquin) hydrochloride
   Chloroquine (Aralen) hydrochloride
   Primaquine phosphate
   Quinine
3. Others
   Povidone-iodine (Betadine, Proviodine)
   Quinacrine hydrochloride
4. Anthelmintics
   Mebendazole (Vermox)
   Niclosamide (Yomesan)
   Piperazine citrate (Antepar)
   Pyrantel pamoate (Antiminth)
   Pyrvinium pamoate (Povan)

Nursing Process

A. Nursing assessment: obtain history of allergies; evaluate baseline data relevant to signs and symptoms of infection, vital signs, pertinent laboratory tests, appearance of wounds, incisions, or lesions, amount and description of drainage, swelling, erythema, subjective symptoms of pain or pressure
B. Nursing management: obtain culture for specimens before starting antibiotics; maintain supportive measures such as rest, comfort, nutrition, fluids and electrolyte balance; maintain proper administration regarding route, time, and dosage; monitor vital signs and laboratory results
C. Nursing evaluation: observe for therapeutic effects and adverse reactions; instruct patient regarding medications to ensure compliance

---

*Used in treatment of AIDS; prevents replication of HIV virus, thus delaying disease progression.

NEOPLASTIC DISEASES
Specific Antineoplastic Agents

A. Action: selective toxicity during various stages of the cell cycle
B. Agents

Examples	Adverse reactions
Asparaginase (Elspar)	Central nervous system depression
Bleomycin sulfate (Blenoxane)	Pulmonary toxicity, skin reactions
Busulfan (Myleran)	Bone marrow and kidney toxicity
Calusterone (Methosarb)	Mild virilism, edema, hypercalcemia, nausea, vomiting
Carmustine (BiCNU)	Bone marrow suppression, nausea
Chlorambucil (Leukeran)	Bone marrow suppression
Cisplatin (Platinol)	Renal damage, nausea and vomiting, ototoxicity, neurotoxicity, and anaphylactic reactions
Cyclophosphamide (Cytoxan)	Hemorrhagic cystitis, bladder fibrosis
Cytarabine (Cytosar-U)	Bone marrow suppression
Dacarbazine (DTIC-Dome)	Bone marrow suppression
Dactinomycin (Cosmegen)	Bone marrow suppression, gastrointestinal irritation, skin reactions
Diethylstilbestrol diphosphate (Stilphostrol)	Risk of thromboembolic disease, edema, mood changes
Doxorubicin hydrochloride (Adriamycin)	Bone marrow suppression, gastrointestinal distress, alopecia
Dromostanolone propionate (Drolban)	Mild virilism, edema, hypercalcemia
Estradiol (Progynon)	Risk of thromboembolic disease, edema, mood changes
Etoposide	Bone marrow suppression
Floxuridine (FUDR)	Gastrointestinal and hematologic toxicity
Fluorouracil (5-FU, Adrucil)	Gastrointestinal and hematologic toxicity
Hydroxyurea (Hydrea)	Bone marrow suppression
Lomustine (CeeNU)	Myelosuppression, nausea
Mechlorethamine hydrochloride or nitrogen mustard (Mustargen)	Bone marrow suppression
Medroxyprogesterone (Depo-Provera)	Menstrual irregularities, rashes, and thrombolic diseases
Megestrol acetate (Megace)	Thromboembolic disease
Melphalan (Alkeran)	Leukopenia, anemia, menstrual irregularities
Mercaptopurine (Purinethol)	Hematologic toxicity, immunosuppression
Methotrexate	Gastrointestinal toxicity, bone marrow suppression, immunosuppression
Mitomycin (Mutamycin)	Bone marrow suppression, gastrointestinal irritation, alopecia, renal toxicity

Examples	Adverse reactions
Mitotane (Lysodren)	Gastrointestinal disturbances, skin reactions
Plicamycin (mithramycin; Mithracin)	Gastrointestinal, skin, liver, and kidney toxicity
Polyestradiol phosphate (Estradurin)	Risk of thromboembolic disease, edema, mood changes
Prednisone (Deltasone, Panasol, Meticorten)	Cushing's syndrome
Procarbazine hydrochloride (Matulane)	Bone marrow suppression, gastrointestinal disturbances
Tamoxifen citrate (Nolvadex)	Hot flashes, nausea, vomiting
Teniposide	Bone marrow suppression
Testolactone (Teslac)	Pain and irritation at injection site, hypercalemia
Thioguanine	Hematologic toxicity
Thiotepa	Bone marrow toxicity
Vinblastine sulfate (Velban)	Peripheral neuropathy and bone marrow suppression
Vincristine sulfate (Oncovin)	Alopecia, abdominal pain, peripheral neuropathy

C. Nursing assessment: obtain baseline data regarding possible adverse reactions of drugs; evaluate condition of hair, skin, nails, weight, vital signs and necessary blood laboratory studies (especially WBC and RBC count)

D. Nursing management: monitor weight, vital signs, and laboratory studies; institute regular inspection of mouth; maintain good medical asepsis; use infusion monitoring device for IV administration; provide patient/family teaching and psychologic support

E. Nursing evaluation: observe for therapeutic effects and adverse reactions

NUTRIENTS, FLUIDS, AND ELECTROLYTES

Substances required for human nutrition include water, carbohydrates, proteins, fats, vitamins, and minerals; necessary to maintain health, prevent illness, and promote recovery from illness.

Nutritional Products: Oral and Tube Feedings

A. Nutritionally complete formulas
1. Action
   a. Provide United States Recommended Daily Allowance for protein, minerals, and vitamins
   b. Provide 1 calorie per milliliter (Sustagen: 1.84 cal/ml)
2. Agents: the following are examples

Compleat-B	Osmolite
Ensure	Sustacal
Isocal	Sustagen
Meritene	

B. Nutritional agents for limited use
1. Vital H.N.: contains easily digested forms of protein, carbohydrate, and fat; used for critically ill patients
2. Lofenalac: a low-phenylalanine preparation used for infants and children with phenylketonuria (PKU)
3. MBF (Meat Base Formula): hypoallergenic infant formula for those who are allergic to milk or have galactosemia
4. Neo-Mull-Soy, Pro Sobee, Isomil: soybean products used as hypoallergenic, milk-free formulas
5. Pregestimil: infant formula containing easily digested protein, fat, and carbohydrate; used in infants with diarrhea or malabsorption syndromes
6. Vivonex: nutritionally complete diet containing amino acids as its protein

C. Nutritionally incomplete supplements
1. Amin-Aid: source of protein for patients with renal insufficiency
2. Casec: carbohydrate calories supplement
3. Lipomul: unsaturated fat supplement
4. Liprotein: high caloric and protein oral supplement for use in burn or debilitated patients
5. Lonalac: milk substitute for sodium-restricted diets
6. Probana: iron-free, high-protein formula for infants and children with diarrhea or malabsorption syndromes

D. Complete infant formulas
1. May be used alone for bottle-fed babies or to supplement breast-fed babies, similar to human breast milk; iron deficient
2. Preparations: Enfamil and Similac are examples

Intravenous Fluids

A. Dextrose injection: contains 2.5%, 5%, 10%, 20%, 40%, 50%, 60%, and 70% dextrose; the 20% to 50% solutions are used for calories in total parenteral nutrition (TPN) and administered through a central or subclavian catheter

B. Dextrose and sodium chloride injection: most commonly used concentrations are 5% dextrose in 0.25% or 0.45% sodium chloride

C. Amino acid solution (Aminosyn): contains essential and nonessential amino acids; most often used with dextrose in TPN

D. Liposyn, Intralipid: concentrated calories and essential fatty acids; most often used as part of TPN

Vitamins

A. General information
1. Group of substances that act as coenzymes to help in the conversion of carbohydrate and fat into energy and to form bones and tissues; necessary for metabolism of fat, carbohydrate, and protein; normally obtained from foods
2. Subclassified as
   a. Fat soluble: A, D, E, K
   b. Water soluble: B complex, C

B. Agents
1. Fat-soluble vitamins: the following are examples

Vitamin A (Alphalin, Aquasol A)	Vitamin K Menadiol sodium diphosphate (Synkayvite)
Vitamin E (Tocopherol, Aquasol E)	Phytonadione (Mephyton, AquaMEPHYTON)

2. Water-soluble vitamins: the following are examples
   a. B-complex

Calcium	Niacin
pantothenate	Pyridoxine hydrochloride
(B_5)	(B_6)
(Pantholin)	(Hexa-Betalin)
Cyanocobalamin	Riboflavin
(B_{12})	(Riobin-50, B_2)
(Rubramin PC,	Thiamine hydrochloride (B_1)
Betalin 12)	(Betalin S)
Folic acid	
(Folvite)	

   b. Vitamin C: ascorbic acid

Minerals and Electrolytes

A. General information: basic constituents of living tissues and components of many enzymes; function to maintain fluid, electrolyte, and acid-base balance; maintain muscle and nerve function; assist in transfer of materials across cell membranes and contribute to the growth process
B. Agents: the following are examples

Ammonium chloride	Potassium chloride
Deferoxamine mesylate	(Kay Ciel, K-Lor)
(Desferal)	Potassium gluconate
Ferrous gluconate	(Kaon)
(Fergon)	Sodium bicarbonate
Ferrous sulfate (Feosol)	Sodium polystyrene sulfonate
Iron dextran injection	(Kayexalate)
(Imferon)	Tromethamine
Magnesium sulfate	(THAM)
Potassium bicarbonate—	
potassium citrate	
(K-Lyte)	

Multiple mineral-electrolyte preparations

Normosol-R	Plasma-Lyte 148
Pedialyte (oral)	Polysal M
Plasma-Lyte 56	Ringer's lactate

Nursing Process

A. Nursing assessment: obtain baseline data with emphasis on presenting signs and symptoms, vital signs, and laboratory blood studies
B. Nursing management: perform nursing actions to foster drug therapy; monitor diet and laboratory blood studies
C. Nursing evaluation: observe for therapeutic effects specific to type of nutrient supplement; instruct patient regarding medications and diet

Suggested Reading List

Asperheim M, Eisenhauer L: *The pharmacological basis of patient care,* ed 5, Philadelphia, 1986, WB Saunders.

Brown M, Mulholland JL: *Drug calculations: process and problems for clinical practice,* ed 4, St Louis, 1992, Mosby.

Clark JF, Queener SF, Karb VB: *Pharmacologic basis of nursing practice,* ed 4, St Louis, 1992, Mosby.

Clayton BD: *Mosby's handbook of pharmacology in nursing,* ed 4, St Louis, 1989, Mosby.

Clayton BD, Stocks YN, Squire JE: *Squire's basic pharmacology for nurses,* ed 9, St Louis, 1989, Mosby.

Dison N: *Simplified drugs and solutions for nurses,* ed 10, St Louis, 1991, Mosby.

Gahart BL: *Intravenous medications,* ed 8, St Louis, 1992, Mosby.

Loebl S, Spratto G: *The nurse's drug handbook,* ed 4, New York, 1988, John Wiley & Sons.

McKenry LM, Salerno E: *Mosby's pharmacology in nursing,* ed 18, St Louis, 1992, Mosby.

Pagliaro LA, Pagliaro AM: *Pharmacologic aspects of nursing,* St Louis, 1986, Mosby.

Physicians' desk reference, Montvale, NJ, Medical Economics (published annually).

Scherer JC: *Introductory clinical pharmacology,* ed 3, Philadelphia, 1987, JB Lippincott.

Skidmore L: Medication cards for clinical use, rev ed, Bowie, Md, 1984, Brady Communications.

Skidmore-Roth L: *Mosby's nursing drug reference,* St Louis, Mosby (published annually).

Pharmacology Review Questions

Answers and rationales begin on p. 426.

1. When preparing narcotics and other controlled substances for administration the nurse must:
   1. Confirm the dosage with another nurse
   2. Sign for the drugs on separate record forms
   3. Be sure the order sheet has been signed by two physicians
   4. Have a witness during preparation

2. The law that regulates the manufacture, distribution, advertisement, and labeling of drugs to ensure safety and effectiveness is the:
   1. Harrison Narcotic Act
   2. Consumer Protection Act
   3. Controlled Substances Act
   4. Federal Food, Drug, and Cosmetic Act

3. The study of drugs is called:
   1. Pharmacokinetics
   2. Pharmacology
   3. Pharmacy
   4. Pharmacodynamics

4. The name given to a drug that is designated and patented by the manufacturer is the:
   1. Official name
   2. Generic name
   3. Chemical name
   4. Brand name

5. When assessing a patient's medication history, the nurse should:
   1. Only be interested in prescribed medication taken
   2. Know the names of all medications kept in the patient's home
   3. Record all nonprescription and prescription medication being taken
   4. Only be interested in nonprescription medication being taken

6. Preparations coated to dissolve in the intestines and not in the stomach are referred to as:
   1. Sustained-action
   2. Enteric coated
   3. Lozenges
   4. A tablet within a tablet

7. When the appearance, odor, or color of a medication changes, the nurse should:
   1. Disregard this and give the medication as ordered
   2. Have the registered nurse give the medication
   3. Withhold the medication and consult the pharmacist
   4. Understand that this is a normal occurrence when dealing with chemicals

8. The parenteral route of medication administration that allows for the fastest absorption is the:
   1. Intradermal route
   2. Subcutaneous route
   3. Intramuscular route
   4. Intrastitial route

9. Morphine affects respiration by:
   1. Depressing the rate and depth
   2. Accelerating the rate and depth
   3. Depressing the rate and accelerating the depth
   4. Accelerating the rate and depressing the depth

10. For accurate drug administration the nurse should read the drug label:
    1. Two times
    2. Three times
    3. Four times
    4. Five times

11. When a medication is being administered, the most accurate way to verify a patient's identification is to:
    1. Call the patient by the name on the drug card or Kardex
    2. Ask the patient to state his or her name
    3. Ask another nurse to identify the patient
    4. Check the patient's identification bracelet

12. When the nurse is administering medications, the patient informs the nurse that the tablet usually received is a different color. The nurse should:
    1. Insist that the patient take the tablet she poured
    2. Have the patient take the tablet and then recheck the order
    3. Leave the medication at the bedside and recheck the order
    4. Recheck the order before giving the drug

13. To instill ear drops in the adult patient, the ear canal is opened by pulling the ear:
    1. Up and back
    2. Down and back
    3. Up and forward
    4. Back and forward

14. The physician's order reads to administer 3L of IV fluid 5%D/0.45% normal saline over 24 hours. The drop factor is 60 gtt/ml. The nurse regulates the IV at:
    1. 25 gtt/min
    2. 100 gtt/min
    3. 125 gtt/min
    4. 150 gtt/min

15. If the nurse is unable to read the physician's order or if the order seems erroneous, the nurse must:
    1. Administer what seems to be the correct dose
    2. Ignore the order, since it is not clear
    3. Question the order before she gives the drug
    4. Verify the order with another nurse

16. The position of choice for instilling nose drops for the adult patient is:
    1. Lying on the right side
    2. Lying down or sitting with the neck hyperextended
    3. Lying down or sitting with the neck flexed
    4. Lying on the left side

17. The patient is to receive an IV of Ringer's lactate at 75 ml/hr. The drop factor is 20 gtt/ml. The nurse runs the IV at:
    1. 5 gtt/min
    2. 15 gtt/min
    3. 25 gtt/min
    4. 35 gtt/min

18. The patient suffering from salicylate (aspirin) toxicity is most likely to complain that:
    1. "My head hurts all the time."
    2. "My stools are hard and tarry."
    3. "I'm beginning to have diarrhea."
    4. "I hear ringing in my ears."

19. A poisonous effect of a drug, either from a regular dose or an overdose of a drug, is referred to as a/an:
① Side effect
② Untoward effect
③ Toxic action
④ Idiosyncratic action

20. The physician orders administration of 1 g of Kefzol in 100 ml of D5W in 20 minutes q6h. The drop factor is 15 gtt/ml. The nurse regulates the IV at:
① 25 gtt/min
② 50 gtt/min
③ 75 gtt/min
④ 100 gtt/min

21. The action of a drug in the body other than the main effect for which the drug was given is called:
① Side effect
② Idiosyncratic action
③ Synergistic action
④ Antagonistic action

22. In relation to drugs, the term *blood level* refers to the:
① Metabolism of the drug
② Excretion of the drug
③ Amount of the drug in the circulating fluids
④ Effect of the drug on red blood cells (RBCs)

23. The patient is to receive an IV of 5%D/0.33% normal saline at 1000 ml/8 hr. The drop factor is 10 gtt/ml. The nurse is to run the IV at:
① 7 gtt/min
② 14 gtt/min
③ 20 gtt/min
④ 28 gtt/min

24. The drug of choice in the treatment of AIDs is:
① Acetylsalicylic acid (ASA) (aspirin)
② Azidothymidine (AZT)
③ Pralidoxime chloride (PAM)
④ Phencyclidine hydrochloride (PCP)

25. When treating the pain associated with angina pectoris, sublingual nitroglycerin:
① Dilates blood vessels and increases circulation
② Inhibits the pain sensors in the brainstem
③ Increases respirations and causes drowsiness
④ Dulls nerve endings in the myocardium

26. The process by which drugs are inactivated by the body is:
① Absorption
② Distribution
③ Metabolism
④ Excretion

27. The process that occurs from the time a drug is taken into the body and the time it enters the circulatory or lymphatic system is called:
① Absorption
② Distribution
③ Metabolism
④ Excretion

28. The usual hypnotic dose for secobarbitol (Seconal) is 100 mg. The apothecary equivalent for this dose is:
① gr v
② gr $\overline{\text{iss}}$
③ gr iii
④ gr $\frac{1}{150}$

29. 7.5 L is equivalent to:
① 75 ml
② 0.075 ml
③ 750 ml
④ 7500 ml

30. 125 ml is equivalent to:
① 0.125 L
② 1.25 L
③ 12.5 L
④ 1250 L

31. 8 dr is equivalent to:
① ½ oz
② 1 oz
③ 1½ oz
④ 2 oz

32. 500 mg is equivalent to:
① 500 g
② 0.5 g
③ 0.05 g
④ 0.005 g

33. Which of the following is the correct needle gauge and length to use for a subcutaneous injection?
① 19 gauge; 1½ inch
② 24 gauge; 1 inch
③ 22 gauge; 1 inch
④ 25 gauge; ⅝ inch

34. The patient is to receive 50 mg of Demerol with 25 mg of Vistaril at 7:30 PM. The charge nurse states that she drew up the medication for you and hands you the syringe. Which of the following actions is the most appropriate?
① Place the syringe in the medication drawer for the patient
② Recheck the physician's order before administering
③ Check drug compatibility chart for drug interactions
④ Refuse to give the injection

35. Digitalis preparations must not be given without the specific direction of the physician whenever:
① The systolic blood pressure is above 100
② The rectal temperature is subnormal
③ The pulse rate is 60 beats/min or below
④ A patient is flushed and perspiring

36. Toxicity to digitalis occurs more rapidly when the body stores of what ion are depleted?
① Sodium
② Potassium
③ Calcium
④ Chloride

37. Intramuscular injection sites are selected to avoid:
① Injecting into subcutaneous tissue
② Injuring nerves and blood vessels
③ Injecting into a blood vessel
④ Injuring organs

38. Drugs absorbed into the bloodstream and circulated to various parts of the body are said to have a:
① Systemic effect
② Local effect
③ Palliative effect
④ Curative effect

39. Early signs of digoxin toxicity are:
① A sustained pulse rate above 60 beats/min
② Nausea and vomiting
③ Diarrhea and rectal bleeding
④ Elevated respiration and blood pressure

40. An important nursing consideration in the administration of diuretics is to:
① Limit the patient's intake of fluids
② Withhold the diuretic if pulse rate is below 80 beats/min
③ Give in the early morning if ordered daily
④ Delay the administration if BP is below 110/80

41. Foods to avoid when patients are receiving an MAO-inhibitor drug include:
① Aged cheeses, coffee, chocolate
② Poultry, bananas, eggs
③ Green, leafy vegetables, raisins, milk
④ Pork, pickles, whole wheat bread

42. Which of the following is effective in the treatment of status epilepticus?
① Diazepam
② Hydroxyzine
③ Meprobamate
④ Chlordiazepoxide

43. The major action of amitriptyline hydrochloride (Elavil) is to decrease:
① Euphoria
② Depression
③ Confusion
④ Hallucinations

44. The nursing implication for digoxin toxicity would be to:
① Give the drug if the apical pulse rate is above 60 beats/min and report to the physician
② Omit the drug, take an apical pulse rate, and report to the physician
③ Administer an antacid with the digoxin
④ Administer O₂ by nasal cannula with the digoxin

45. The major adverse reaction associated with the use of sedative-hypnotics is:
① Hypertension
② Hypotension
③ Respiratory depression
④ Hypothermia

46. Objective evidence of the therapeutic effects of antianxiety drug therapy would be:
① Crying, facial grimaces, rigid posture
② Anger, aggressive behavior
③ Decreased blood pressure, pulse, respiration
④ Verbal statements of worry, feeling ill, resting poorly

47. An important nursing action to institute when administering a sedative to a geriatric patient is to:
① Apply a posey jacket restraint
② Leave on the overhead light in the room
③ Raise the side rails on the bed and tell patient not to get out of bed unassisted
④ Check the patient every half hour to determine effectiveness of the medication

48. Sodium pentobarbital (Nembutal Sodium) acts to:
① Depress the coughing center in the brain
② Relieve moderate-to-severe pain
③ Allay apprehension and induce sleep
④ Increase blood pressure and decrease respirations

49. The brand name for meperidine hydrochloride is:
① Dilaudid
② Demerol
③ Dilantin
④ Dicumerol

50. A drug used as a substitute for morphine or heroin in the management of addiction is:
① Meperidine
② Nalline
③ Methadone
④ Talwin

51. The major adverse reactions with the use of meperidine hydrochloride (Demerol) are:
① Increased perspiration, euphoria, nausea
② Increased blood pressure and decreased respirations
③ Diarrhea and decreased blood pressure
④ Dysphagia and urinary retention

52. The therapeutic effectiveness of the bronchodilating drugs can be assessed by observing for:
① Cardiac dysrhythmias
② Nausea and vomiting
③ Insomnia, restlessness
④ Decreased dyspnea and wheezing

53. An example of a rapid-acting insulin is:
① Insulin injection (Regular Insulin)
② Isophane insulin suspension (NPH Insulin)
③ Insulin zinc suspension (Lente Insulin)
④ Protamine zinc insulin suspension

54. The primary purpose for instilling silver nitrate or erythromycin in the eyes of a newborn is to:
① Protect against bacteria encountered during the birthing process
② Protect against ophthalmia neonatorum
③ Protect against blindness caused by syphilis
④ Establish antibodies for the first 6 months of life

55. The most serious adverse reaction to anticoagulant therapy is:
① A rapid fall in blood pressure
② Formation of thrombi in major blood vessels
③ Hemorrhage
④ Infection

56. Doses of warfarin sodium (Coumadin) are ordered on the basis of measurement of the patient's:
① Clotting time
② Prothrombin time (PT)
③ Bleeding time
④ Capillary fragility testing

57. Common adverse reactions to corticosteroid therapy include:
① Tachycardia, insomnia
② Bradycardia, mental dullness
③ "Moon face," obese trunk
④ Anorexia, polyuria

58. Oral corticosteroid drugs should be given:
① Before meals
② With or after meals
③ At bedtime
④ With orange juice

59. The pharmacologic effect of IV administration of oxytocin solution is to:
    1. Produce rhythmic contractions of uterine muscle fibers
    2. Relax smooth muscle fibers of the cervix
    3. Initiate vigorous sustained contractions of the abdominal muscles
    4. Produce relaxation of vaginal walls and perineal muscles

60. When administering insulin, the nurse should:
    1. Give medication intramuscularly
    2. Use a 1½-inch needle to administer
    3. Rotate injection sites
    4. Massage insulin into tissues

61. An example of an intermediate-acting insulin is:
    1. Insulin injection (Regular Insulin)
    2. Prompt insulin zinc suspension
    3. Insulin zinc suspension (Lente Insulin)
    4. Extended insulin zinc suspension (Ultralente Insulin)

62. After taking a nitroglycerin tablet sublingually, the patient may expect pain relief in approximately:
    1. 2 to 3 seconds
    2. 20 to 30 seconds
    3. 1 to 3 minutes
    4. 20 to 30 minutes

63. An example of a long-acting insulin is:
    1. Prompt insulin zinc suspension
    2. Isophane insulin suspension (NPH Insulin)
    3. Insulin zinc suspension (Lente Insulin)
    4. Protamine zinc insulin suspension

64. When injecting the patient on blood and body fluid precautions, the Centers for Disease Control (CDC) recommends that the nurse:
    1. Wear two pairs of gloves
    2. Wear a gown
    3. Wear a mask
    4. Wash the injection site with povidine-iodine (Betadine)

65. Emergency treatment of hyperinsulinism consists of administering:
    1. Glucose intravenously
    2. Insulin hypodermically
    3. Epinephrine (Adrenalin) intramuscularly
    4. High-calorie liquids by gavage feeding

66. Which of the following symptoms suggest that a patient had received an overdose of insulin?
    1. Flushed skin, nausea, and vomiting
    2. Pallor, fatigability, dyspnea
    3. Nervousness, anxiety, sweating
    4. Hyperpnea, drowsiness, fever

67. Bulk-forming laxatives, such as psyllium husk (Metamucil), should be administered:
    1. At bedtime
    2. With meals
    3. With a full glass of fluid
    4. With an antacid

68. The effectiveness of placebos is generally credited to:
    1. The production of endorphins in the brain
    2. The nurturing attitude of the nurse
    3. The action of the active drug in the placebo
    4. The patient's ability to metabolize the placebo

69. Phenobarbital may be ordered for a patient with hyperthyroidism to achieve which of the following effects?
    1. Sedative
    2. Anticonvulsant
    3. Spasmolytic
    4. Vasodilation

70. Thyroid drugs should be administered:
    1. In a single dose, usually before breakfast
    2. In divided doses, before meals
    3. In divided doses, after meals
    4. As the patient's energy level decreases

71. Cimetidine (Tagamet) should be administered:
    1. With a liquid antacid preparation
    2. After meals and at bedtime
    3. With meals and at bedtime
    4. Only when the patient has gastric distress

72. To assess the therapeutic effectiveness of a parkinsonian drug, the nurse would observe the patient's:
    1. Increased sleep patterns
    2. Increased ability to ambulate and speak
    3. Decreased emotional stability
    4. Decreased caloric and nutritional intake

73. The correct method for instilling eye drops is to drop the medication on:
    1. The eyeball itself
    2. The inner canthus of the eye
    3. The lower conjunctival sac
    4. The outermost point of the eye

74. Drug levels are routinely monitored for which of the following medications?
    1. Cephalothin sodium; clindamycin
    2. Cephalexin (Keflex); aspirin
    3. Gentamicin sulfate; theophylline
    4. Meperidine hydrochloride (Demerol); morphine sulfate

75. A major adverse reaction with the use of antineoplastic drugs is:
    1. Bone marrow depression
    2. Oliguria
    3. Lethargy
    4. Photosensitivity

76. Your patient is to receive antitubercular medications at home. Which of the following instructions is essential for the patient to understand before discharge?
    1. Eat foods high in calcium to improve the absorption of the drug
    2. Continue the drug therapy regime as ordered by the physician
    3. Perform postural drainage each morning before taking the medication
    4. Have those with whom you work take the medication also

77. Daily assessment of the integrity of the oral mucous membranes is important when the patient is receiving:
    1. Antibiotics
    2. Cancer drugs
    3. Antiparkinsonian drugs
    4. Vitamins

78. Body functions decline with age, thus making an individual prone to which of the following reactions to medication?
    ① Developing a tolerance to medications
    ② Metabolizing medications more rapidly
    ③ Developing more frequent adverse effects
    ④ Experiencing more cumulative effects

79. When a mydriatic eye medication has been administered, the nurse should observe for:
    ① Decreased drainage
    ② Constriction of the pupil
    ③ Dilation of the pupil
    ④ Decreased intraocular pressure

80. When asked about medications to be taken after the signs and symptoms have disappeared, the nurse appropriately tells the patient to:
    ① Discard what is left
    ② Finish what is left
    ③ Save what is left
    ④ Call the physician

81. Drugs that relieve pain are classified as:
    ① Sedatives
    ② Hypnotics
    ③ Analgesics
    ④ Antipyretics

82. When a medication is ordered for "swish and swallow," the nurse tells the patient to:
    ① Thoroughly rinse the mouth and then swallow
    ② Swallow immediately followed by 60 ml of water
    ③ Thoroughly rinse the mouth and spit out the remains
    ④ Gargle deep in the throat and then swallow

83. Adverse reactions associated with the use of acetylsalicylic acid (aspirin) include:
    ① Vomiting, petechiae, tinnitus
    ② Constipation, polyphagia, hematuria
    ③ Hypertension, anaphylactic shock, tachycardia
    ④ Bradycardia, hypotension, dermatitis

84. Antipyretic medication ordered for the patient experiencing nausea and vomiting should be given:
    ① Orally
    ② Rectally
    ③ Sublingually
    ④ Topically

85. Patients receiving antihypertensive drugs should be cautioned to avoid sudden changes in position, especially from a supine to an upright position, because:
    ① A thrombus may become dislodged
    ② Severe nausea may result
    ③ Postural hypotension may occur
    ④ Increased diuresis occurs

86. A side effect of a cholinergic drug may be:
    ① Increased peristalsis
    ② Decreased peristalsis
    ③ Increased urine output
    ④ Decreased urine output

87. Anticholinergic drugs are usually contraindicated in:
    ① Hypertension
    ② Diabetes mellitus
    ③ Cardiac failure
    ④ Glaucoma

88. An adverse reaction to atropine sulfate that may be serious for patients with underlying heart disease is:
    ① Delirium
    ② Tachycardia
    ③ Constipation
    ④ Dry mouth

89. Patients who receive atropine sulfate as a preoperative medication should not be allowed out of bed after the drug is given because:
    ① There is depression of the central nervous system
    ② Vertigo may occur because of dilation of the pupils
    ③ One effect of the drug is the development of postural hypotension
    ④ Diaphoresis may predispose to a chill

90. A patient is to receive temazepam (Restoril) 0.015 g by mouth (PO), at bedtime (HS) for insomnia. The label indicates 15-mg tablets. How many tablets would you give?
    ① 1
    ② 1.5
    ③ 2
    ④ 2.5

91. Iron preparations should be administered:
    ① At bedtime
    ② Before breakfast
    ③ With meals
    ④ Between meals

92. The patient with glaucoma should not receive:
    ① Atropine sulfate
    ② Morphine sulfate
    ③ Meperidine hydrochloride (Demerol)
    ④ Hydroxyzine hydrochloride (Vistaril)

93. A patient with emphysema is receiving aminophylline. As his nurse, you know this medication will act to:
    ① Relax the diaphragm and intercostals to increase chest expansion
    ② Decrease contraction of the smooth muscles of the bronchi
    ③ Increase the contraction of the bronchi and alveoli
    ④ Decrease the amount of mucous secretion from the bronchi

94. A life-threatening blood alcohol concentration in the average person exceeds:
    ① 0.5%
    ② 5.0%
    ③ 0.25%
    ④ 2.5%

95. When chest pain is not relieved by nitroglycerin, the dose should be repeated in:
    ① 1 minute
    ② 5 minutes
    ③ 10 minutes
    ④ 30 minutes

96. Before administering medication through a nasogastric tube, the nurse must make sure:
    ① The tube is in the esophagus
    ② The tube is in the stomach
    ③ The pill will dissolve
    ④ The pill is enteric coated

97. A patient receiving meperidine hydrochloride (Demerol) 100 mg, q4h prn for relief of pain should be monitored for which of the following:
    ① Decreased blood pressure
    ② Increased respirations
    ③ Increased heart rate
    ④ Decreased respirations

98. Some adrenergic drugs can be used in stopping bleeding and relieving nasal and ocular congestion by causing:
    ① Constriction of blood vessels
    ② Vasodilation of blood vessels
    ③ Astringent action on mucous membranes
    ④ A rise in arterial blood pressure

99. A nursing measure requiring the use of the anticholinesterase agent neostigmine bromide (Prostigmin) is:
    ① Inserting a Foley catheter
    ② Inserting a rectal tube
    ③ Encouraging oral fluids
    ④ Assisting the patient to ambulate

100. A patient has just returned from the postoperative recovery room and is complaining of pain. The most appropriate nursing action would be to first:
    ① Call the physician
    ② Administer the pain medication as ordered
    ③ Ask the patient to describe pain and location
    ④ Check when the medication was given last

CHAPTER 5

Nutrition

Nutrition is the combination of processes by which the body uses food for growth, energy, and maintenance. Nutrition is also the study of food and its relation to health and disease. The nurse plays an especially important role in the nutritional aspects of patient care. Because of close and continual contact with the patient, the nurse is able to evaluate and monitor the patient's nutritional status and inform the dietitian about the patient's nutritional needs and acceptance of the nutritional plan of care. Good nutrition is essential to good health throughout the life cycle, and the nurse is in an excellent position to encourage sound nutritional practices for each patient.

PRINCIPLES OF NUTRITION

A. Functions of food
1. Provides energy
2. Builds and repairs body tissues
3. Regulates and controls the body's chemical processes, which are essential for providing energy and building tissues
B. Evidence of good nutrition (Table 5-1)
C. Primary causes of nutritional deficiency
1. Dietary lack of specific essential nutrients caused by
a. Anorexia (resulting from a variety of causes)
b. Alcoholism (and the resulting lack of proper nutrition)
c. Poor food habits or eating nutritionally deficient foods
2. Inability of the body to use a specific nutrient properly as a result of
a. Diseases of the digestive tract such as ulcerative colitis
b. Faulty absorption in digestive tract (such as the way in which the excessive use of mineral oil impedes the absorption of fat-soluble vitamins)
c. Metabolic disorders such as diabetes
d. Drug interactions and/or toxicity
D. Classification of nutrients
1. Nutrients are chemical substances that are present in food and needed by the body to function
2. Six prime nutrients
a. Carbohydrates
b. Fats
c. Proteins
d. Vitamins
e. Minerals
f. Water

ASSIMILATION OF NUTRIENTS
Digestion and Absorption

A. Digestion: the process of changing foods to be absorbed and used by cells; mechanical digestion and chemical digestion occur simultaneously
1. Mechanical digestion (chewing, swallowing, peristalsis) breaks food into small pieces, mixes it with digestive juices, and moves it along the digestive tract
2. Chemical digestion occurs through the action of enzymes, which break large food molecules into smaller molecules
a. Carbohydrate digestion begins in the mouth and occurs primarily in the small intestine; carbohydrates are reduced to simple sugars (monosaccharides), such as glucose, for absorption
b. Protein digestion begins in the stomach and is completed in the small intestine; proteins are broken down into amino acids for absorption
c. Fat digestion begins in the stomach but occurs primarily in the small intestine; fats are reduced to fatty acids and glycerol for absorption
B. Absorption: the process by which end products of digestion (fatty acids, glycerol, amino acids, and glucose) are absorbed from the small intestine into circulation (blood and lymph) to be distributed to the cells

Metabolism

A. Use of food by the body cells for producing energy and for building complex chemical compounds
B. Consists of two processes
1. Catabolism: the breakdown of food molecules into carbon dioxide and water, which releases energy; carbohydrates are primarily catabolized for energy

Table 5-1. Clinical signs of nutritional status

Features	Good	Poor
General appearance	Alert, responsive	Listless, apathetic; cachexia
Hair	Shiny, lustrous; healthy scalp	Stringy, dull, brittle, dry, depigmented
Neck glands	No enlargement	Thyroid enlarged
Skin, face, and neck	Smooth, slightly moist, good color, reddish pink mucous membranes	Greasy, discolored, scaly
Eyes	Bright, clear; no fatigue circles	Dryness, signs of infection, increased vascularity, glassiness, thickened conjunctivae
Lips	Good color, moist	Dry, scaly, swollen, angular lesions (stomatitis)
Tongue	Good pink color; surface papillae present; no lesions	Papillary atrophy, smooth appearance; swollen, red, beefy (glossitis)
Gums	Good pink color; no swelling or bleeding; firm	Marginal redness or swelling; receding, spongy
Teeth	Straight, no crowding; well-shaped jaw; clean, no discoloration	Unfilled cavities, absent teeth, worn surfaces; mottled, malpositioned
Skin, general	Smooth, slightly moist; good color	Rough, dry, scaly, pale, pigmented, irritated; petechiae, bruises
Abdomen	Flat	Swollen
Legs, feet	No tenderness, weakness, swelling; good color	Edema, tender calf; tingling, weakness
Skeleton	No malformations	Bowlegs, knock-knees, chest deformity at diaphragm, beaded ribs, prominent scapulae
Weight	Normal for height, age, body build	Overweight or underweight
Posture	Erect, arms and legs straight, abdomen in, chest out	Sagging shoulders, sunken chest, humped back
Muscles	Well developed, firm	Flaccid, poor tone; undeveloped, tender
Nervous control	Good attention span for age; does not cry easily; not irritable or restless	Inattentive, irritable
Gastrointestinal function	Good appetite and digestion; normal, regular elimination	Anorexia, indigestion, constipation or diarrhea
General vitality	Endurance; energetic; sleeps well at night; vigorous	Easily fatigued; no energy; falls asleep in school; looks tired, apathetic

From Williams SR: *Basic nutrition and diet therapy*, ed 9, St Louis, 1992, Mosby.

2. Anabolism: the process by which food molecules are built up into more complex chemical compounds; proteins are primarily anabolized (used for building)

Energy

A. Energy is required for the metabolic processes of catabolism and anabolism; energy needs of the body are based on three factors
   1. Physical activity: the type of activity and how long it is performed
   2. Basal metabolism: the energy required for the body to sustain life while in a resting state (1 calorie per kilogram of body weight per hour)
   3. Thermic effects of food: energy required for the digestion, absorption, and metabolism of foods
B. Measurement of energy
   1. The calorie (or kilocalorie) is the unit used to measure the energy value of food
   2. Fuel values of basic nutrients
      a. Carbohydrate: 4 calories per gram
      b. Fat: 9 calories per gram
      c. Protein: 4 calories per gram
   3. Total number of calories needed per day
      a. Moderately active man: 20.5 calories per pound (0.45 kg) of ideal weight
      b. Moderately active woman: 18 calories per pound (0.45 kg) of ideal weight

Drugs and Nutrition

Drugs affect taste, appetite, intestinal motility, absorption, metabolism, and excretion of nutrients; many of these interactions may compromise nutritional status and health

NUTRIENTS
Carbohydrates

A. Classification
   1. Monosaccharides: single sugars, which require no digestion and are easily absorbed into the bloodstream (e.g., glucose, fructose, and galactose)
   2. Disaccharides: double sugars, which must be broken down before absorption (e.g., sucrose [table sugar], lactose, and maltose)
   3. Polysaccharides: complex carbohydrates composed of many sugar units (e.g., starches, glycogen, and dietary fiber)
B. Functions
   1. Provide energy (the only source of energy for the brain)
   2. Protein-sparing effect allows protein to be used for tissue building rather than energy
   3. Essential for complete metabolism of fats (incomplete fat metabolism leads to buildup of ketones and acidosis)
C. Sources
   1. Bread, cereal, grain, and macaroni products

2. Fruits such as bananas, pears, and apples
3. Vegetables such as peas, corn, and potatoes
4. Sugars such as honey, molasses, and candy

D. Metabolism
1. Carbohydrates must be broken down into monosaccharides before being absorbed
2. Monosaccharides are carried to the liver, where glucose is released to the cells
3. Excess glucose is stored as glycogen to be used when needed or converted to fat and stored as fat tissue
4. Insulin regulates the use of glucose for use by the cells, thereby lowering blood sugar
5. The hormone glucagon regulates the conversion of glycogen back to glucose, causing an increase in blood glucose

E. Excess carbohydrates in diet may lead to
1. Obesity
2. Tooth decay and gum disease
3. Malnutrition (if empty calorie foods such as candy and soft drinks are eaten extensively)

F. Dietary considerations
1. Approximately 50% to 60% of total caloric intake may come from carbohydrates (mainly starches)
2. Encourage the intake of whole grain bread and cereal products; if refined cereal products are used, they should be enriched
3. Reduce the dietary intake of simple sugars (which provide empty calories) and substitute starches as sources of carbohydrates

Protein

A. Composed of amino acids
1. Essential amino acids: amino acids the body cannot manufacture and therefore must be supplied in the diet; there are eight essential amino acids
2. Nonessential amino acids: those the body can manufacture and therefore are not needed in the diet

B. Functions
1. Build and repair body tissue (primary function)
2. Furnish energy if there is insufficient carbohydrate or fat for this purpose
3. Maintain normal circulation of tissue and blood vessel fluids through the action of plasma protein
4. Aid metabolic functions by combining with iron to form hemoglobin; used to manufacture enzymes and hormones
5. Aid body defenses by manufacturing lymphocytes and antibodies

C. Metabolism
1. Protein must be broken down into amino acids to be absorbed and distributed to the cells
2. End products of protein metabolism are hydrogen, oxygen, nitrogen, water, uric acid, and urea

D. Types and sources
1. Complete proteins: foods that contain all eight essential amino acids in amounts capable of meeting human requirements (e.g., mainly animal sources, such as meats, fish, poultry, eggs, milk, and cheese)
2. Incomplete proteins: foods that lack one or more of the essential amino acids (e.g., mainly plant sources, such as cereal grains, nuts, legumes, and lentils)
3. Complementary proteins: foods that, when eaten together, supply the amino acid that is missing or in short supply in the other food (e.g., peanut butter with bread, beans with rice, and baked beans with brown bread)

E. Dietary considerations
1. The recommended daily protein intake for adults is 0.8 g/kg of body weight (15% of total caloric intake)
2. Protein is not stored in the body; good quality protein (either complete animal protein or carefully selected combinations of complementary plant proteins) should be eaten at each meal
3. Increased protein is necessary during periods of growth, illness, or injury; after surgery; and when bed rest is prescribed (especially for the elderly)
4. Kwashiorkor, a protein deficiency disease, is seen in many underdeveloped countries
5. Marasmus is overt starvation caused by a deficiency of calories from any source

Fats (Lipids)

A. Functions
1. Supply energy for body activities; all body tissues except brain and nervous cells can use fat for energy; most concentrated form of energy yields 9 calories per gram
2. Act as insulation to maintain body temperature and protect organs from mechanical injury
3. Carry fat-soluble vitamins A, D, E, and K and aid in their absorption
4. Provide a feeling of fullness and satisfaction after eating because of their slow rate of digestion
5. Furnish the essential fatty acid, linoleic acid, which is found primarily in vegetable oils; called essential because it cannot be synthesized in the body and is vital to body functioning

B. Types
1. Saturated fats: those whose structure is completely filled with all the hydrogen it can hold; they are usually from animal sources and are usually solid at room temperature (e.g., fats in meat, dairy products, and eggs; coconut oil, palm oil, and chocolate are also highly saturated)
2. Unsaturated fats: those whose chemical structure has one or more places where hydrogen can be added; they are less dense, usually liquid at room temperature, and are chiefly from plant sources (e.g., vegetable oils such as cottonseed, soybean, corn oil)
   a. Monounsaturated fats have one place for hydrogen to be added
   b. Polyunsaturated fats have two or more places for hydrogen to be added
   c. Hydrogenation: the process of adding hydrogen to a liquid or polyunsaturated fat and changing it to a solid or semisolid state (however, hydrogenation reduces the polyunsaturated fat content and therefore possibly reduces its health value)

C. Digestion and metabolism
1. Digestion of fat begins in the stomach, where gastric lipase acts on emulsified fats
2. Major portions of fat digestion occur in the small intestine, where bile emulsifies fats (breaks it into small droplets); pancreatic lipase changes the emul-

sified fats into fatty acids and glycerol, the end products of fat digestion

3. Fats are carried as lipoproteins to body cells, where they are either broken down for use as energy or stored as adipose tissue

D. Sources
1. Visible fats: those readily seen (e.g., butter and oleo, salad oils, shortening, and fat in meats)
2. Invisible fats: those in which the fat is less obvious (e.g., milk, avocado, cheese, and lean meat)

E. Cholesterol: a complex fat-related compound
1. A normal component of blood and of all body cells, especially brain and nerve tissue
2. Necessary for normal body functioning as structural material in cells, in the production of vitamin D, and in the production of a number of hormones
3. Supplied by food (mainly animal sources); some synthesized within the body, mainly in the intestinal walls and liver, in response to need
4. Blood cholesterol levels are affected by a variety of factors including diet, heredity, emotional stress, and exercise; saturated fats tend to raise blood cholesterol, whereas polyunsaturated fats are recommended for lowering cholesterol levels
5. Cholesterol is carried to and from body cells by special carriers called *lipoproteins*
   a. High-density lipoprotein (HDL), or "good" cholesterol, carries cholesterol away from the arteries and back to the liver for removal from the body
   b. Low-density lipoprotein (LDL), or "bad" cholesterol, tends to circulate in the bloodstream and form plaque on the inner walls of arteries
6. Risk is classified according to total cholesterol level as follows
   a. Desirable—below 200 mg/dl
   b. Borderline high—200 to 239 mg/dl
   c. High—above 240 mg/dl
7. If the total cholesterol level is borderline high or high, then the levels of LDL and HDL should be evaluated
8. High cholesterol levels predispose individuals to atherosclerosis
9. Foods high in cholesterol: organ meats, animal fat, egg yolk, and shellfish

F. Dietary considerations
1. U.S. Dietary Goals suggest a decrease in total fat intake to no more than 30% of total caloric intake; decrease in saturated fats and cholesterol is also recommended
2. To decrease dietary fat
   a. Use leaner cuts of meat and more poultry; trim fats from all meats
   b. Use fewer eggs
   c. Use low-fat milk products
   d. Limit use of fat in cooking as much as possible

G. Effects of excess fat intake
1. Obesity
2. Predisposition to serious conditions such as heart disease and diabetes
3. Increased surgical risk

Vitamins

A. Definitions
1. Vitamins: organic compounds needed in small amounts for growth and maintenance of life
2. Precursor (or provitamin): substances that precede and can be changed into active vitamins (e.g., carotene is the precursor of vitamin A)
3. Hypervitaminosis: the excess of one or more vitamins
4. Synthetic: man-made vitamins
5. Enriched or fortified: the addition of nutrients to a food often in amounts larger than might be found naturally in that food
6. Restored: the replacement of nutrients in food lost during processing

B. Characteristics
1. Totally lacking in calories
2. Essential to life because they generally cannot be synthesized by the body and are necessary for cell metabolism
3. Functions include tissue building and regulation of body functions
4. Needed in minute amounts (milligrams [mg] or micrograms [μg]); the safety of taking megadoses is debatable
5. Well-balanced diet should provide adequate vitamins to fulfill body requirements

C. Classified on basis of solubility (Table 5-2)
1. Fat-soluble vitamins: A, D, E, and K
   a. Sufficient fats needed in diet to carry fat-soluble vitamins
   b. Stored in body, so deficiencies are slow to appear
   c. Absorbed in the same manner as fats so anything that interferes with absorption of fats interferes with absorption of fat-soluble vitamins (mineral oil, an undigestible substance, carries fat-soluble vitamins with it out of the body)
   d. Fairly stable in cooking and storage
2. Water-soluble vitamins: C and B complex (Table 5-2)
   a. Not stored in body
   b. Easily destroyed by air and in cooking

Minerals

A. Definition: Inorganic elements essential for growth and normal functioning (Table 5-3)

B. Types
1. Major minerals, or macrominerals, are found in the largest amounts in the body and are needed in large amounts (100 mg or more per day); they are calcium, phosphorus, potassium, sodium, chlorine, magnesium, and sulfur
2. Microminerals, or trace elements, are needed in small amounts (e.g, iron, zinc, copper, and iodine)

C. Characteristics
1. Found in all body tissues and fluids
2. Occur naturally in foods (especially unrefined foods)
3. Do not furnish energy but regulate body processes that furnish energy
4. Remain stable in food preparation

Table 5-2. Vitamins

Vitamin	Sources	Functions	Deficiency symptoms
Fat-soluble vitamins			
A (retinol) Precursor: carotene	Fish liver oils Liver Green, leafy vegetables Yellow vegetables (corn, carrots, and sweet potatoes) Yellow fruits (apricots and peaches) Egg yolk Whole milk	Regenerates visual purple (necessary for good vision) Formation of bones and teeth Maintains skin and mucous membranes	Night blindness Retardation of skeletal growth Dry, scaly skin Dry mucous membranes Susceptibility to epithelial infection Xerophthalmia (corneal cells become opaque, slough off, could lead to blindness)
D (calciferol)	Sunshine Fish liver oils Fortified milk	Regulates calcium and phosphorus absorption and metabolism Essential for normal formation of bones and teeth	Lowered levels of calcium and phosphorus in blood Soft bones Rickets Malformed teeth
E (tocopherol)	Wheat germ Vegetable oils Dark green, leafy vegetables	Inconclusive at present Preserves integrity of RBCs Antioxidant (protects materials that oxidize easily) Protects structure and function of muscle	Increased hemolysis (breakdown) of red blood cells (RBCs) Anemia Breakdown of vitamin A and essential fatty acids
K (menadione)	Synthesis by intestinal bacteria Green, leafy vegetables Pork liver	Formation of prothrombin (necessary in blood clotting)	Prolonged clotting time (bleeding tendencies) Hemorrhagic diseases
Water-soluble vitamins			
C (ascorbic acid)	Citrus fruits Tomatoes, broccoli, strawberries, green peppers, cantaloupes, potatoes	Formation and maintenance of capillary walls and collagen formation Aids in absorption of iron	Scurvy (deficiency disease) Sore gums Tendency to bruise easily Poor wound healing Anemia
B_1 (thiamine)	Wheat germ Whole or enriched grains Legumes Pork and organ meats	Maintains carbohydrate metabolism Maintains muscle and nerve functioning Maintains appetite	Beriberi (deficiency disease) Anorexia, fatigue, nerve disorders, irritability
B_2 (riboflavin)	Milk Organ meats Green leafy vegetables Enriched bread and cereals	Maintains healthy eyes Maintains color and structure of lips Metabolism of nutrients	Sensitivity to light, dim vision Inflammation of lips and tongue Loss of appetite and weight
B_6 (pyridoxine)	Red meats (especially organ meats) Whole grain cereals Pork, lamb, veal	Synthesis and metabolism of proteins Hemoglobin synthesis Maintenance of muscles and nerves	Nausea and vomiting, anorexia, anemia, irritability, CNS dysfunction, kidney stones, dermatitis
B_{12} (cobalamin)	Found only in animal products Organ and muscle meats Dairy products	Protein metabolism Production of RBCs Normal functioning of nervous system	Pernicious anemia (resulting from lack of intrinsic factor needed for B_{12} absorption)
Niacin (nicotinic acid) Precursor: tryptophan	Meats (especially organ meats) Poultry and fish Peanut butter	Essential for normal functioning of digestive and nervous systems Essential for growth and metabolism	Pellagra (deficiency disease) Nervous disorders Diarrhea and nausea Dermatitis
Folic acid (folacin)		Essential in formation of all body cells especially RBCs Protein metabolism	Anemia (macrocytic) Gastrointestinal disturbances Glossitis Stomatitis

Table 5-3. Major minerals and trace elements

Mineral	Sources	Functions	Deficiency symptoms
Calcium (Ca): absorption aided by vitamin D	Milk and milk products Cheese Some green, leafy vegetables (turnips, collards, kale, broccoli)	Bone and tooth formation Blood clotting Muscle (including heart muscle) contraction) Nerve transmission Cell wall permeability	Poor bone and tooth formation Rickets (deficiency disease) Stunted growth Osteoporosis Poor blood clotting Tetany
Phosphorus (P): absorption with Ca aided by vitamin D	Milk and cheese Meat Egg yolk Whole grains (Diet adequate in protein and Ca should be adequate in P)	Functions as calcium phosphate in the calcification of bones and teeth Energy metabolism Regulation of acid-base balance Cell structure and enzyme activity	Poor bone and tooth formation Retarded growth Rickets (deficiency disease) Weakness Anorexia
Sodium (Na)	Salt Baking powder and soda Dairy products Meat, fish, and poultry	Regulation of acid-base balance Fluid balance Nerve transmission and muscle contraction Glucose absorption	Nausea and vomiting Apathy Exhaustion Abdominal and muscle cramps
Potassium (K)	Meat, fish, and poultry Whole grain breads and cereals Fruits (oranges, bananas)	Regulates nerve conduction and muscle contraction Necessary for regular heart rhythm Fluid and acid-base balance Cell metabolism	Abnormal heart beat Muscle weakness Nausea and vomiting
Chlorine (Cl)	Table salt (NaCl)	Formation of hydrochloric acid and maintaining gastric acidity Maintenance of acid-base balance, osmotic pressure, and water balance	Deficiency results from fluid loss through vomiting, diarrhea, and heavy sweating
Magnesium (Mg)	Green, leafy vegetables Legumes Milk Whole grains	Component of bones and teeth Enzymes essential in general metabolism Conduction of nerve impulses Muscle contraction	Tremors leading to convulsive seizures
Sulfur (S)	Protein foods Meat Milk Eggs Cheese Nuts and legumes	Component of all body cells; important in building connective tissue Component in several B vitamins and several amino acids Energy metabolism	None documented
Iron (Fe): absorption enhanced by vitamin C	Organ meats (especially liver) Egg yolk Green, leafy vegetables Lean red meats Dried fruits (apricots, raisins)	Synthesis of hemoglobin General metabolic activities	Anemia
Iodine (I)	Iodized salt Saltwater fish	Normal functioning of thyroid gland	Goiter
Zinc (Zn)	Oysters Liver High-protein foods	Component of enzymes Assists in regulation of cell growth Protein synthesis	Impaired wound healing Poor taste sensitivity Retarded sexual and physical development
Copper (Cu)	Liver Cocoa Nuts Raisins	Aids in absorption of iron Component of hemoglobin Component of enzymes	Unknown at present, although secondary conditions may develop

D. Functions
1. Constitute bones and teeth (calcium and phosphorus)
2. Transmit nerve impulses and aid in muscle contraction
3. Control water balance (sodium and potassium)
4. Maintain acid-base balance
5. Synthesize essential body compounds (e.g., iodine for thyroxine)
6. Act as catalysts for tissue reactions (e.g., calcium needed for blood clotting)

Water

A. Definition: principal body constituent; most indispensable of all nutrients
1. Intracellular: within cells
2. Extracellular: outside the cells: in blood lymph, secretions, and fluid surrounding the cells (interstitial fluid)
B. Functions
1. Essential component of all tissues and fluids
2. Transportation of nutrients from the digestive tract to the bloodstream and from cell to cell; also removal of waste products from cells to outside the body
3. Lubrication of joints
4. Maintenance of stable body temperature (as temperature increases, sweating occurs, evaporates, and cools the body)
5. Solvent for all the body's chemical processes
C. Overall water balance in the body
1. Intake: under ordinary conditions, adults need 2 to 3 L of liquid per day—5 to 6 glasses of which should be water
   a. Ingested fluids such as water, soups, and beverages
   b. Water in foods that are eaten
   c. Water formed from cell oxidation (when nutrients are burned)
2. Output: averages 2600 ml daily
   a. Normal routes of excretion: primarily the kidney but also the skin, lungs, and feces
   b. Abnormal and extensive losses can occur from vomiting and diarrhea, open or draining wounds, fever, extensive burns, hemorrhage, and anything that causes excessive perspiration
D. Additional fluids are required
1. By infants
2. During fever or disease process
3. In warm weather
4. During heavy work or extensive physical activity

Cellulose

A. Definition: a polysaccharide that makes up the framework of plants; provides bulk (fiber or roughage) for the diet; cannot be broken down by the human digestive system and therefore is not absorbed
B. Function: to absorb water, provide bulk, and stimulate peristalsis
C. Found in the stalks and leaves of plants, in the skins of fruit and vegetables, and in the outer covering of seeds and cereals (refined cereals have most of the fiber removed and provide little bulk)

NUTRITIONAL GUIDELINES
Recommended Dietary Allowances (RDA)

A. Developed by the Food and Nutrition Board of the National Academy of Science
B. Suggested levels of essential nutrients (proteins, vitamins, and minerals) known from current research to be adequate to meet nutritional needs of most healthy individuals
C. Used as a guideline for most federal, state, and local feeding programs but not to be used as requirements for individuals with specific nutritional deficiencies

U.S. DIETARY GOALS OR DIETARY GUIDELINES

A. Developed by the U.S. Department of Agriculture, Department of Health and Human Services
B. Seven factors to discourage excesses in the diet
1. Eat a variety of foods (for a variety of nutrients)
2. Maintain ideal weight (obesity is linked to several chronic diseases such as hypertension and diabetes)
3. Avoid too much fat, saturated fat, and cholesterol (which contributes to increased risk of cardiovascular disease)
4. Eat foods with adequate starch and fiber (better sources of fuel than simple sugars; contain more essential nutrients and add more bulk to the diet)
5. Avoid excessive sugar
6. Avoid excessive sodium
7. If you drink alcoholic beverages, do so in moderation (alcohol is high in calories but low in nutrients; also heavy drinking contributes to many chronic liver and neurologic disorders)

Four Basic Food Groups

A. Developed by the U.S. Department of Agriculture as a guide for planning a well-balanced diet
B. Milk group
1. Milk, cheese, ice cream, and yogurt
2. Daily recommended servings vary with age
   a. Adults, two servings
   b. Children under 9 years of age, two to three servings
   c. Children 9 to 12 years of age, three or more servings
   d. Pregnant women, three or more servings
   e. Nursing mothers, four or more servings
3. Nutrients primarily supplied are calcium, protein, and riboflavin
C. Meat group
1. Beef, veal, lamb, pork, organ meats, poultry, fish, eggs, dry peas and beans, nuts, and peanut butter
2. Recommended servings, two or more per day
3. Nutrients primarily supplied are protein, iron, and B vitamins
D. Vegetable and fruit group
1. All fruits and vegetables except dry peas, beans, and lentils
2. Recommended servings, four or more per day including
   a. One source rich in vitamin C (or two fair sources)
   b. One dark green or deep yellow vegetable or fruit rich in vitamin A

3. Nutrients primarily supplied are vitamins A and C, carbohydrates (sugar), and most dietary fiber

E. Bread and cereal group
   1. All enriched and restored breads, cereals, pasta products, crackers, and other baked goods made with flour
   2. Recommended servings, four or more per day
   3. Nutrients primarily supplied are iron, B complex vitamins, and carbohydrates (starches); refined products contain fewer vitamins, whereas the enriched, fortified, or restored products contain many more vitamins

F. Food guide pyramid (Fig. 5-1)
   1. Emphasizes grains, fruits, and vegetables as the foundation of a balanced diet and downplays meats, dairy products, and fats; fats, oils, and sweets are recommended sparingly
   2. Specific guidelines
      a. Breads, cereals, rice, pasta: six to eleven servings daily (1 serving equals 1 slice of bread, 1 oz of ready-to-eat cereal, or ½ cup of cooked cereal, rice, or pasta)
      b. Fruits: two to four servings daily (1 serving equals 1 medium apple, banana, or orange or ½ cup of cooked, chopped, or canned fruit)
      c. Vegetables: three to five servings daily (1 serving equals 1 cup of raw, leafy vegetables or ½ cup of other vegetables cooked, chopped, or raw)
      d. Milk, yogurt, cheese: two to three servings daily (1 serving equals 1 cup of milk or yogurt or 1 ½ oz of natural cheese)
      e. Meat, poultry, fish, dry beans, eggs, and nuts: two to three servings daily (1 serving equals 2 to 3 oz of cooked lean meat, poultry, or fish; ½ cup of cooked dry beans, or 1 egg; 2 tbsp of peanut butter equals 1 oz of lean meat)

FOOD MANAGEMENT
Economic Considerations in Menu Planning

A. Plan menus in advance
   1. Take advantage of specials to prepare balanced meals
   2. Shop from a list to avoid impulse buying
B. Choose foods wisely
   1. Buy foods in season and in good supply
   2. Buy in quantity if adequate storage is available (larger quantities cost less per unit)
   3. Buy sale items only if they can be used
   4. Use unit pricing to find the best buys among brands
   5. Know grades and brands of foods; grading of canned goods has no bearing on nutritive value; generic labeling can save up to 25% of name brand items
   6. Purchase staples and canned goods when on sale
   7. Remember that cost per serving rather than per pound is important, especially in buying meat
   8. Compare labels for weights and ingredients
   9. Buy less expensive forms of food (margarine is less expensive than butter)
   10. Limit purchase of empty-calorie foods
   11. Decrease the cost of protein in the diet by using small amounts of meats, fish, and poultry and by using lower grades and less expensive cuts of meat; also legumes, peanut butter, eggs, and cheese are good sources of less expensive protein
   12. Try to avoid convenience foods (any food bought partially prepared and ready to eat with little home preparation); they are usually more expensive than those prepared entirely at home and are less nutritionally balanced, containing high proportions of fat, calories, and sodium
C. Care for foods after purchase
   1. Store foods properly to avoid spoilage and loss of nutrients
   2. Use leftover foods

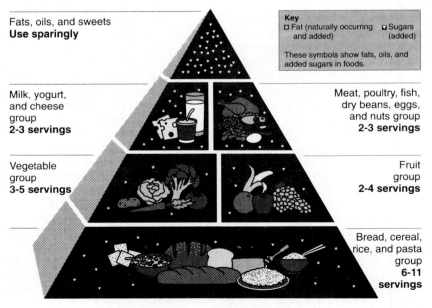

FIG. 5-1. Food guide pyramid: a guide to daily food choices. (Courtesy U.S. Department of Agriculture, Washington, DC, 1992.)

Storage and Preparation of Basic Foods

A. Milk
1. Store refrigerated in covered container; powdered milk: store in cool, dry place; refrigerate after re-constituting
2. Cook over low heat; avoid scorching

B. Cheese
1. Refrigerate well wrapped or in tight containers
2. Most palatable if served at room temperature; cook at low temperatures for a short time

C. Eggs
1. Refrigerate promptly; if cracked, use only in foods that will be well cooked
2. Cook at lower temperatures to prevent discoloration, curdling, or toughness

D. Cereals and breads
1. Store in cool, dry place; bread retains freshness best at room temperature, but molds faster; bread freezes well
2. Cook cereals according to directions; overcooking reduces vitamin content

E. Meat, fish, and poultry
1. Store in refrigerator for a short time or freeze for longer storage
2. Less expensive meats, although nutritionally equivalent to more expensive ones, require longer cooking at lower temperatures

F. Fruits and vegetables
1. Store ripe fruits and vegetables in the refrigerator (fruits ripen best at room temperature)
2. Cook only until tender, using as little water as possible (cooking liquids contain valuable nutrients and should be used if possible); raw fruits and vegetables are especially nutritious

Types of Milk

A. Skim: fat and vitamin A removed (may have vitamins A and D added); contains all other nutrients of whole milk
B. Homogenized: fat particles evenly dispersed so cream does not separate
C. Pasteurized: heated to a specific temperature to destroy pathogenic bacteria (but nutrients are not affected)
D. Condensed: water removed and sugar added so carbohydrate content is increased; low in calcium and vitamins and high in sugar compared with whole milk
E. Evaporated: heated above the boiling point so that more than half the water evaporates
F. Low fat: contains 0.5% to 2% fat; lower in calories than whole milk but comparable in nutrient value
G. Powdered or dry: water removed; least expensive form of milk on the market; when reconstituted, it has the same nutrient value as the milk from which it was made

NUTRITION THROUGHOUT THE LIFE CYCLE
Infant Nutrition

A. Infants require more protein and calories per pound of body weight than adults do because they have more body surface in proportion to weight and because of their growth and activity
B. Breast-feeding is the recommended method of feeding if possible; provides more vitamin C and more easily digested protein and sugar than cow's milk; also provides the infant with antibodies against disease and assists in establishing the mother-child bond
C. Bottle-feeding is an acceptable alternative if close mother-child contact is maintained; cow's milk is higher in protein, fat, and most minerals and lower in sugar than human milk; specialized products such as Isomil, a soy milk product, can be given in cases of allergies to milk products
D. Introduction of solid foods varies among pediatricians, most favoring a delay until the infant is at least 3 months of age and preferably 5 to 6 months of age
1. Infant cereal is usually given first (often with added iron to supplement a possible lack in the infant's diet; prenatal iron reserves last 5 to 6 months)
2. Fruits, vegetables, and egg yolk are frequently given next (because of possible allergic reactions, egg white is delayed until late in the first year)
3. Solid foods should be introduced one at a time and at 4- to 5-day intervals to observe for any allergic reactions
4. Adding sugar or salt to infant's food is undesirable
5. Infants can choke on small foods such as berries, corn, popcorn, or candy
6. Infants should not receive honey, because honey contains botulism spores, which could harm the infant (even though quantities are too low to harm older children and adults)

Preschool Children

A. Growth rate is slower and more erratic, and food intake will vary accordingly
B. A variety of foods should be offered
1. "Finger foods" such as carrot sticks are enjoyed
2. Serve small amounts because too large a serving can discourage a child from eating
3. Avoid refined sweets
4. Do not coax a child to eat; if a food is refused, offer it at a later date
5. Nutritious snacks are a viable alternative for a child who is a poor eater
C. Teach healthy eating habits; avoid rewarding good behavior with food

School Children (5 to 10 Years of Age)

A. Gradual increase in growth at this age (approximately equal for boys and girls)
B. Proper nutrition is important to proper mental and physical, development (adequate breakfast is important for alertness during class)
C. Children are usually good eaters at this age and should be encouraged by the examples set at home and at school; promote healthy eating

Adolescents

A. Tremendous growth spurt occurs at puberty (age of sexual maturity)
1. For girls, usually between 10 and 13 years of age
2. For boys, between 13 and 16 years of age
B. Diets are influenced by peers, with much empty-calorie foods being consumed
C. Boys gain mostly lean muscle tissue; they consume large amounts of food to meet energy requirements

D. Girls gain more fat tissue; their diets may be more influenced by a desire to remain thin; frequently require iron supplements to meet their needs; adequate nutrition during adolescence helps avoid complications during pregnancy; promote healthy eating along with exercise

Adults

A. Adequate nutrition throughout the life span is important in avoiding many serious illnesses
B. Proper nutrition is based on guidelines set by U.S. government agencies (such as the four basic food groups)
C. Persons who consume a balanced diet usually do not need vitamin supplements

Geriatrics

A. Physiologic changes affect nutrition of the elderly
   1. Aging slows the basal metabolic rate (BMR); combined with decreased activity the result is decreased energy requirements and decreased number of calories needed
   2. Taste may be adversely affected by gradual diminishment of the senses of smell, sight, and taste
   3. Loss of teeth may affect food intake or the enjoyment thereof
   4. Decreased body secretions make swallowing more difficult and digestion less efficient
   5. Decreased movement of wastes through intestines contributes to constipation
B. Economic and social considerations
   1. Decrease in income among the elderly, combined with an increase in the amount spent for medical care, leaves less for adequate nutrition; tendency is to eat less protein (which is expensive) and more carbohydrates (which are cheaper and easier to prepare)
   2. Loss of spouse, friends, or mobility results in isolation, depression, and often decreased will to obtain adequate nutrition
C. Planning diets
   1. Diet should be well balanced in protein, vitamins, and minerals (especially calcium and iron) to allow for diminished absorption
   2. Calories sufficient to maintain energy and activity (reduced from those previously required)
   3. Soft bulk in diet to prevent constipation (cooked fruits and vegetables)
   4. Increased fluid intake required to eliminate metabolic wastes
   5. Meals should be light and easily digested, that is, contain only a small amount of fats; frequent small meals may be easier to digest than three large meals
   6. Individual preferences should be respected and the diet built around them; make changes slowly
   7. Meals eaten with others are often more appetizing than those eaten alone

Pregnancy

A. A well-balanced diet with increased amounts of essential nutrients is important to the well-being of the mother and baby
   1. An increased intake of protein of 50% over the normal diet is recommended to allow for growth of the baby, placenta, maternal tissues, and increased circulating blood volume, amniotic fluid, and storage
   2. An increase in calories meets increased energy demands and allows protein to be used for tissue building
   3. Increased amounts of the following: calcium, phosphorus, and vitamin D are needed both for the mother and for the bones and teeth of the baby; iron for hemoglobin and prenatal storage for the baby; iodine for thyroxine for the mother's increased BMR; and vitamins A, B complex, and C
   4. Weight should not be severely restricted; a gain of 25 lb (11.25 kg) is considered healthy
   5. Severe restriction of salt is unfounded
B. Vomiting (morning sickness)
   1. Lower fat intake with more high-carbohydrate foods
   2. Fluids between instead of with meals
   3. Dry toast or crackers on awakening

Lactation

A. A baby requires 2 to 2 ½ oz (60 to 75 ml) of breast milk per pound (488 g) of body weight (1 oz [30 ml] = 20 calories); there is an increased need for all nutrients during lactation
B. Diet of a lactating mother should be high in protein and calories
C. Increased fluids are also required; at least 6 cups (1.5 L) of milk in some form is recommended

DIET THERAPY
Nursing Responsibilities

A. Prepare the patient for mealtime
B. See that each person receives the correct tray unless foods are being withheld
C. Serve and remove tray promptly
D. Teach patients the value of proper nutrition and urge compliance with the nutritional care plan

Purposes

A. To increase or decrease weight
B. To allow a particular organ or system to rest (e.g., a low-fat diet in gallbladder disease)
C. To regulate the diet to correspond with the body's ability to metabolize a specific nutrient (e.g., diabetes)
D. To correct conditions caused by deficiencies
E. To eliminate harmful substances from the diet (e.g., caffeine, cholesterol, and alcohol)

Diet Modifications

A. Calories may be increased or decreased
B. Nutrients may be adjusted (high or low protein)
C. Certain foods may be omitted
D. Modifications in texture (consistency—soft diet)
E. Frequency of meals: more than the standard three

Standard Hospital Diets (Modifications in Consistency)

A. Clear liquid (surgical liquid)
   1. Temporary diet of clear liquids, nonresidue, nonirritating, non-gas forming; inadequate in protein, vitamins, minerals, and calories
   2. Used postoperatively to replace fluids, before certain tests, and to lessen amount of fecal matter in colon

3. Includes water, coffee, tea, fat-free broth, pulp-free fruit juices (apple), gelatin, and ginger ale

B. Full liquid diet
1. Foods liquid at room or body temperatures; may be adequate if carefully planned, although frequently deficient in iron
2. Used postoperatively as a transition between clear and soft diet, in infections and acute gastritis; in febrile conditions; and for patients unable to chew or swallow or with an intolerance to food for other reasons
3. Includes all clear liquids, milk, creamed soups, ice creams, sherbets, plain puddings, and thin, strained cereal

C. Soft diet
1. Normal diet modified in consistency to have limited fiber; easily digested; nutritionally adequate
2. Used between full liquid and regular, for chewing difficulties, and in gastrointestinal disorders
3. Includes tender meats and tender, well-cooked vegetables (those with a great deal of fiber should be pureed or omitted); fruits (no fiber) and plain cakes are allowed; no spicy or coarse foods are allowed

D. Regular (general or house) diet
1. Adequate, well-balanced diet designed to appeal to most people
2. Used for those not requiring a modified or therapeutic diet
3. Includes all foods from the four basic food groups

Additional Modified (or Therapeutic) Diets

Table 5-4 lists diets; foods allowed and omitted; and when the diets are used.

DIETS FOR SPECIFIC DISEASE CONDITIONS
Diabetes Mellitus

A. Classification
1. Type I, or insulin dependent: onset is usually before the age of 20; difficult to manage and requires both dietary restrictions and insulin injections
2. Type II, or maturity onset: usually develops after age 35; frequently controlled by diet alone, and insulin or oral hypoglycemics or both may be needed

B. Diet is determined by age, sex, body build, weight, and activity; maintenance requirements are the same as for a nondiabetic patient
1. Calories: sufficient to maintain ideal body weight (approximately 30 cal/kg ideal weight)
2. Protein: 1 g/kg of body weight is the baseline (15% to 20% of total calories)
3. Carbohydrates: 50% to 60% of total calories (obtain greatest portion from complex carbohydrates such as starches and the least from simple sugars)
4. Fats: moderately controlled; 25% to 30% of total calories
5. High-fiber foods, which decrease postprandial blood glucose levels, are encouraged

C. Exchange system is used for planning the diabetic diet
1. Based on simple grouping of common foods according to equivalent nutritional values
2. Six basic food groups or food exchanges; each food within the group contains approximately the same food value as other foods within the same group
   a. Milk: equal to 1 cup (240 ml) whole milk
   b. Vegetables: variety of low-carbohydrate vegetables
   c. Fruit: fresh or canned without sugar
   d. Bread: starchy items (breads, cereals, and vegetables equal to 1 slice bread)
   e. Meat: protein food equal to 1 oz (28 g) lean meat
   f. Fat equal to 1 tsp (5 ml) margarine
3. Total exchanges per day is determined by individual nutritional needs based on nutritional standards (Table 5-5 shows a sample diet based on the exchange system)
4. Advantages of exchange system
   a. Is easy to understand
   b. Allows diabetic patients more freedom to choose foods they like
   c. Allows choice of foods that fit into their economic status
   d. Can be used for other types of diets
   e. Does not require dietetic or specialized diabetic foods

Surgery

A. Surgery increases the nutritional demands on the body
1. Protein: increased for tissue repair, to prevent tissue breakdown, and to help replace blood and fluid losses
2. Calories increased to meet body demands for energy and to spare protein for tissue building
3. Vitamins: especially important in wound healing; vitamin C cements cells, and builds connective tissue and capillaries

B. Types of feeding available postoperatively
1. Intravenous: immediately administered to supply essential water, electrolytes, and vitamins; intended only as short-term nutritional supplement
2. Parenteral hyperalimentation (total parenteral nutrition [TPN]): administered through a larger central vein to provide a higher percentage of glucose, amino acids, and electrolytes; requires surgical insertion, careful monitoring, and special care; may also be indicated preoperatively or for debilitated patients whose intake does not meet body requirements
3. Oral feedings: most patients should begin oral feedings as soon as bowel sounds return; provides nutrients essential to recovery; progress from clear liquid onward

Burns

A. Rate of tissue breakdown and loss of other body nutrients is greater with serious burns than with any other disease process

B. Increase of fluids and nutrients is required
1. Increased energy requires 3000 to 5000 calories
2. Protein increase of 50% above normal
3. Vitamin C requirements greatly increased for wound healing
4. B vitamins increased for higher metabolic rate
5. Increased fluids to replace lost body fluids and help eliminate waste products

Table 5-4. Modified or therapeutic diets

Diet	Condition	Foods allowed	Purpose of diet
High calorie	Underweight (10% or more) Anorexia nervosa Hyperthyroidism	Emphasis on increase in calories Easily digested foods (carbohydrates) recommended Full meals with high-calorie snacks	To meet the increased metabolic needs of the body or provide increased calories for weight gain
Low calorie	Overweight	Fruits and vegetables especially recommended	To reduce the caloric intake below what the body requires so weight loss will occur
High protein	Children who need additional protein for growth Following surgery Pregnancy and lactation Conditions that cause protein loss Extensive burns	Added amounts of poultry, meat, fish, milk, cheese, and eggs Nonfat dry milk added to soups and baked goods	To increase the intake of high-protein foods for maintaining and rebuilding tissues and correcting protein loss
Low protein	Liver diseases Kidney diseases leading to renal failure	Fruits and vegetables Severely limited in amounts of meats, fish, poultry, eggs, and dairy products	To limit the end products of protein metabolism to avoid disturbing the fluid, electrolyte, and acid-base balances
Bland	Gastric and duodenal ulcer Postoperative stomach surgery	Milk and protein foods Refined cereals Simple desserts Avoid Highly seasoned foods Raw foods Fried foods Alcohol and carbonated beverages Extremes in temperatures	To promote healing of the gastric mucosa by refraining from foods that are chemically or mechanically irritating To reduce peristalsis and excessive flow of gastric juices
High residue	Constipation (atonic) Diverticulitis (when inflammation has ceased)	Increased whole grain cereals Increased fruits and raw vegetables Fibrous meats	Mechanically stimulate the gastrointestinal tract
Low residue	Before and after bowel surgery Ulcerative colitis Diverticulitis (during inflammatory stage) Diarrhea	Soft cheeses Tender meats Refined cereals and breads Pureed fruits and vegetables Plain puddings	To soothe and be nonirritating to gastrointestinal tract
Low fat	Gall bladder disease Obesity Cardiovascular disease	Vegetables and fruits Skim milk Sherbet Increased carbohydrates and proteins	To lower fat content in diet (may be deficient in fat-soluble vitamins)
Low cholesterol	Cardiovascular disease	Lean meats and fish Poultry without the skin Liquid vegetable oils Skim milk	To decrease the blood cholesterol levels or maintain them at acceptable levels
High iron	Anemias	Regular diet with high-iron foods Liver and organ meats Red meats Dried fruits Egg yolks	To correct an iron deficiency
Sodium restricted	Kidney disease Cardiovascular disease Hypertension	Natural foods without salt Fruits and vegetables without salt Milk and meat in limited quantities	To control or correct the retention of sodium and water in the body by controlling sodium intake
High carbohydrate	Preparation for surgery Liver disease Kidney disease	Emphasis on carbohydrate foods Full meals with high carbohydrate snacks	To provide increased energy and spare protein for tissue building
Low carbohydrate	Dumping syndrome Hyperinsulinism Diabetes mellitus (although severe restriction of carbohydrates is currently considered unwarranted)	Proteins Only enough carbohydrate to maintain health and perform activities	To decrease the amounts of glucose in the bloodstream (increased blood glucose causes increased amounts of insulin to be produced by the body)
Lactose restricted	Lactose intolerance	Avoid Foods containing lactose such as milk, cheese, and ice cream	To eliminate or cut down on lactose—a substance certain individuals cannot metabolize

Table 5-5. 1800-calorie diet translated into food exchanges

Exchange group	Total exchanges for the day
Milk	2
Vegetables	2
Fruit	5
Bread	9
Meat	8
Fat	7

Sample diet	Food	Exchange list
Breakfast	Black coffee	Free
	2 eggs	2 meat
	2 pieces toast with butter	2 bread
		2 fat
	Cereal with milk	1 bread
		1 milk
	and plain blueberries	1 fruit
Lunch	Turkey sandwich (3 oz or 84 g)	2 breads
		3 meat
	with mayonnaise (2 tsp or 10 ml)	2 fat
	and tomatoes	1 vegetable
	Sponge cake	1 bread
	with strawberries	1 fruit
	and whipped cream	2 fat
Supper	Roast beef (3 oz or 84 g)	3 meat
	Mashed potatoes, butter	3 bread
		1 fat
	Carrots and butter	1 vegetable
		1 fat
	Applesauce	1 fruit
	1 small apple	1 fruit
Snack	Raspberries (1 cup or 224 g) in	1 fruit
	light cream (2 tbsp or 30 ml)	1 fat
	Milk (8 oz or 240 ml)	1 milk

C. Intravenous dextrose, electrolytes, and plasma are given initially; a high-protein, high-calorie diet is given when oral foods can be taken

D. Victims of extensive burns may require parenteral hyperalimentation to meet their extensive nutritional requirements

Cancer

A. The American Institute for Cancer Research developed the following guidelines to reduce the risk of cancer
  1. Reduce intake of dietary fat, both saturated and unsaturated, to 30% of total calories
  2. Increase intake of fruits, vegetables, and whole grain cereals
  3. Decrease intake of salt-cured, smoked, or charcoal-broiled foods
  4. Drink alcohol only in moderation

B. Diet for the patient with cancer must supply enough protein, fats, carbohydrates, vitamins, minerals, and fluids to meet increased energy demands, prevent weight loss, and rebuild body tissues during treatment; energy and protein needs may increase up to 20%; dietary supplements may be given to supply all necessary nutrients

Cardiovascular Disease

A. Cardiovascular diseases are the primary causes of death in the United States; research has shown that diet may be a risk factor in determining whether a person develops heart disease

B. Objectives in dietary treatment of heart disease
  1. Provide an adequate diet
  2. Prevent gas- and bulk-forming foods from distending stomach and exerting pressure against the heart
  3. Maintain patient's weight as near to ideal as possible to reduce work load of heart
  4. Prevent edema by lowering sodium intake
  5. Reduce the risk of atherosclerosis by reducing circulating blood lipids (low-saturated fat, low-cholesterol diet)

C. Sodium restriction
  1. Component of many diets used in cardiovascular diseases
  2. Helps reduce excess edema and is thought to reduce the risk of hypertension
  3. Sources of sodium
     a. Naturally present in foods, especially animal products such as meat, poultry, fish, milk, and eggs; fruits have little sodium
     b. Sodium added to foods in the form of table salt and preservatives in processed foods; most canned, packaged, and frozen foods have sodium added
     c. Water supplies may have a high-sodium content; water softeners add a significant amount of sodium to a diet
     d. Nonprescription medicines and home remedies such as baking soda, alkalizers for indigestion, cough medicines, and laxatives may contain large amounts of sodium
  4. Sodium-restricted diets limit the intake of sodium to a level prescribed by the physician
     a. Mild sodium-restricted diet (2 to 3 g) contains about half of the salt previously used; no additional salting of processed foods; no salty foods allowed
     b. 1000 mg sodium diet (moderate)
     c. 500 mg sodium diet (strict)
     d. 250 mg sodium diet (severe)

COMMON TYPES OF FOOD POISONING
Staphylococcal Food Poisoning

A. Caused by *Staphylococcus aureus* bacteria; quite resistant to heat

B. Involves foods such as custard, potato, macaroni, egg, chicken salad, cheese, ham, and salami

C. Exhibited by symptoms such as abdominal cramps, diarrhea, and vomiting; usually mild and attributed to other causes

D. Prevented by keeping foods above 140° F (60° C) or below 40° F (4° C); toxin is destroyed by boiling for several hours or heating in a pressure cooker at 240° F (138.5° C) for 30 minutes

Clostridial Food Poisoning

A. Perfringens
  1. Caused by *Clostridium perfringens,* spore-forming bacteria that grow in the absence of oxygen

2. Involves foods such as stews, soups, and gravies made from poultry and red meat
3. Exhibited by symptoms such as nausea without vomiting, diarrhea, and acute inflammation of the stomach and intestine
4. Prevented by storing foods properly and keeping foods above 140° F (60° C) or below 40° F (4° C)

B. Botulism
1. Caused by *Clostridium botulinum*, spore-forming bacteria that grow and produce toxins in absence of oxygen
2. Involves canned low-acid foods, especially home-canned foods such as meats, corn, peas, green beans, asparagus, and mushrooms
3. Exhibited by symptoms such as inability to swallow; double vision, and progressive respiratory paralysis; fatality rate is high
4. Prevented by pressure cooking canned foods for specified length of time; any can or jar with a bulging top should be discarded

Salmonellosis

A. Caused by *Salmonella*, bacteria widespread in nature and live in the intestinal tracts of humans and animals; transmitted by eating infected food or by contact with people who are infected or are carriers of the disease; also transmitted by insects or rodents
B. Involves poultry, red meats, dairy products, and eggs
C. Exhibited by symptoms such as severe headache, vomiting, diarrhea, abdominal cramps, and fever
D. Prevented by heating foods to 140° F (60° C) for 10 minutes or higher temperatures for less time

FOOD: FADS AND FACTS
Meat Eaters Versus Vegetarians

A. Problems exist when too large a portion of the diet consists of meat
1. Excess calories tend to be consumed; meat (and the fat therein) is high in calories, and because of the taste the tendency is to eat more than is required
2. When a large portion of the meal is meat, a smaller portion of fruits and vegetables is consumed; therefore less fiber and fewer of the nutrients in fruits and vegetables are consumed

B. Vegetarians also can have nutritional deficiencies
1. Calories may be insufficient despite large amounts of foods being consumed
2. Protein can be lacking; incomplete protein must be supplemented with complementary proteins

C. The ideal diet combines both types of diet with a variety of foods
1. Meat eaters should eat smaller servings of leaner meats with more fruits, vegetables, and cereals
2. Vegetarians should improve the quality of their diet by adding dairy products such as eggs and milk (if no dairy products are taken, complementary proteins should be carefully selected)

Vitamin C

A. Current research indicates that the effects of vitamin C on the common cold are minimal
B. Effects of vitamin C on cancer still require further study

Vitamin E

A. Claims list vitamin E as "cure-all," especially in prolonging virility in males, preventing miscarriages, and curing muscular weakness
B. Current research has not established the validity of these claims; however, the amounts usually taken in supplements have caused no damage

Suggested Reading List

Bodinski LH: *The nurse's guide to diet therapy*, New York, 1982, John Wiley & Sons.

Christian JL, Greger JL: *Nutrition for living*, Reading, Mass, 1985, Addison-Wesley.

Eschleman MM: *Introductory nutrition and diet therapy*, ed 2, Philadelphia, 1991, JB Lippincott.

Green ML et al: *Nutrition in contemporary nursing practice*, New York, 1987, John Wiley & Sons.

Guthrie H: *Introductory nutrition*, ed 7, St Louis, 1986, Mosby.

Lewis CM: *Nutrition and nutritional therapy in nursing*, 1986, Appleton & Lange.

Mahan LK, Rees JM: *Nutrition in adolescence*, St Louis, 1984, Mosby.

Physicians' desk reference, Montvale, NJ, Medical Economics (published annually).

Pipes PL, Trahms CM: *Nutrition in infancy and childhood*, ed 5, St Louis, 1993, Mosby.

Poleman CR: *Practical nurse nutrition education*, ed 5, Philadelphia, 1984, WB Saunders.

Poleman CR: *Nutrition: essentials and diet therapy*, ed 6, Philadelphia, 1991, WB Saunders.

Robinson C, Lawler M: *Normal and therapeutic nutrition*, New York, 1986, Macmillan.

Robinson CH, Weigley ES: *Basic nutrition and diet therapy*, New York, 1984, Macmillan.

Williams SR: *Basic nutrition and diet therapy*, ed 9, St Louis, 1992, Mosby.

Nutrition Review Questions

Answers and rationales begin on p. 429.

Situation: Helen Anderson is a 44-year-old, slightly overweight woman. She is married, the mother of three children, and an excellent cook who takes pride in her family and her homemaking skills. She has recently been experiencing right upper quadrant pain and is now hospitalized preoperatively for a cholecystectomy.

1. Preoperatively, which diet would be given to Mrs. Anderson to prevent further recurrence of her abdominal discomfort?
   ① Broiled fish, boiled potatoes, canned peaches, and skim milk
   ② Lamb, mashed potatoes, ice cream, and coffee
   ③ Hamburger, french fries, and milkshake
   ④ Avocado salad, cookies, and chocolate milk

2. Which of the following vegetables would supply a vitamin that might be lacking in a diet used in the treatment of gallbladder disease?
   ① Oranges and cantaloupe
   ② Sweet potatoes and carrots
   ③ Oranges and bananas
   ④ Raisins and prunes

3. Postoperatively, Mrs. Anderson will be on intravenous (IV) fluids for the first several days. What remark made by the patient indicates that she is probably ready to be started on oral feedings?
   ① "I can't wait to see some real food rather than this IV bottle!"
   ② "My stomach is feeling a little distended. Do you think it's because I haven't had anything in it for so long?"
   ③ "My stomach is really rumbling—I don't know why—there's nothing in it!"
   ④ "I'm so glad I don't have any more nausea—what a nuisance that was!"

4. Mrs. Anderson has progressed to a full liquid diet. Which of the following meals meets the specifications for a full liquid diet?
   ① Cottage cheese, custard, and coffee
   ② Pureed sweet potatoes, ground beef, and tea
   ③ Banana, baked squash, and custard
   ④ Cream of tomato soup, ice cream, and coffee with cream and sugar

5. In the days following surgery, Mrs. Anderson progressed satisfactorily and is now on a regular diet. Which of the following menus best meets her needs for a vitamin especially important in tissue healing?
   ① Baked chicken, white rice, and sliced peaches
   ② Liver, mashed potatoes, and carrots
   ③ Roast pork, egg noodles, and baked squash
   ④ Swiss steak in tomato sauce, mashed potatoes, and strawberries

Situation: You are working in the office of Dr. James Harrison, a busy general practitioner. As part of the daily routine, you receive many questions from patients regarding nutrition.

6. Faith Davenport, a patient of Dr. Harrison, stops you one day and states her confusion over what she hears about vitamin C. When discussing this vitamin with her, you should include:
   ① Vitamin C is fat soluble and readily stored in the body
   ② Vitamin C has been proven to reduce significantly the incidence and severity of colds
   ③ Deficiency symptoms include night blindness and dry, scaly skin
   ④ Improper storage and cooking can result in food losing its vitamin C

7. Alice Adams has had diverticulosis for 5 years. She seems confused about the type of diet to follow. You tell her that current evidence suggests the best diet for diverticulosis is a:
   ① High-fiber diet
   ② Bland diet
   ③ Low-fiber diet
   ④ Low-fat diet

8. Alex Sargent has come to Dr. Harrison's office with a complaint of irregular heartbeat. Following laboratory studies, hypokalemia was diagnosed and he was advised to increase his dietary intake of potassium. He asks you, "What foods are high in potassium?" Your answer would include:
   ① Apricots, oranges, and bananas
   ② Fish liver oils and fortified milk
   ③ Wheat germ and dark green, leafy vegetables
   ④ Dairy products

9. Alex Jackson, whose blood pressure has been elevated, tells you that Dr. Harrison has recommended that he reduce his intake of dietary sodium. You advise Mr. Jackson to:
   ① Increase canned and processed meats in his diet
   ② Increase dairy products in his diet
   ③ Limit fresh fruits and vegetables
   ④ Substitute spices, herbs, or lemon juice for salt in seasoning his food

10. Allison Armstrong has been told by Dr. Harrison that she has a lactose intolerance. In discussing dietary adjustments you advise Allison to avoid:
    ① Foods containing seeds and nuts
    ② Milk and milk products
    ③ Highly seasoned foods
    ④ Citrus fruits

Situation: Edward and Carolyn Turner have been married for 22 years. They have two children, Audra, aged 14 years, and Gerald, aged 16 years. Mrs. Turner's elderly mother, Dorothy Thompson, also resides with them. Mrs. Thompson has just been put on a bland diet. Refer to this family situation when considering the following six questions:

11. Which of the following should Mrs. Turner remember when cooking for her family?
    ① Raw fruit and vegetables contain more nutrients than cooked vegetables
    ② The more expensive the meat, the more nutrients it contains
    ③ The higher the grade on canned goods, the more nutritious the contents
    ④ Refined cereal products are more nutritious than fortified cereal products

12. Audra, the Turner's 14-year-old daughter, has just announced that she is going on a completely vegetarian diet, which includes no meat or dairy products of any kind. In what nutrient would Audra be particularly deficient if she continues on this diet?
    1. Iron
    2. B complex vitamins
    3. Protein
    4. Fat-soluble vitamins

13. The nutritional requirements of an elderly person such as Mrs. Thompson differ from those of younger people. In particular, Mrs. Thompson will require:
    1. Increased fats
    2. Fewer vitamins and minerals
    3. Decreased fluid intake
    4. Fewer calories

14. Mrs. Thompson has been taking a diuretic for the past 3 months. Of the following statements made by Mrs. Thompson, which would alert you to a possible dietary deficiency caused by the diuretic?
    1. "My eyes seem especially sensitive to that light."
    2. "I seem to bruise so easily these days."
    3. "Every once in awhile my heart feels like it's skipping beats!"
    4. "I feel so terribly nervous. Do you think I need a tranquilizer?"

15. Mrs. Turner tells you that she uses mineral oil as a base for her salad dressing. Your best response to this would be:
    1. "Why don't you try a vegetable oil instead. Mineral oil can hinder the absorption of some important vitamins."
    2. "That's a good idea! Mineral oil doesn't add any calories to your diet."
    3. "That's a good idea! It even fits into your mother's bland diet."
    4. "I would use another type of oil. Mineral oil is high in calories with very few vitamins."

16. Mrs. Thompson is on a bland diet. Her choice of which of the following menus would indicate a good understanding of what a bland diet contains?
    1. Roast beef, tomato salad, and coffee
    2. Hamburger, french fries, and coke
    3. Steak, baked potatoes, salad, and iced tea
    4. Baked filet of sole, baked potato, canned peaches, and milk

Situation: You have volunteered to teach a class on nutrition at the local community church. Your students range from mothers with young children to retired senior citizens. All are extremely interested in what constitutes good nutrition and pose a variety of questions to you on the subject.

17. Sheri Adams is the mother of 2-week-old Nicholas, and she is somewhat nervous about his feedings. Your advice to Ms. Adams would include:
    1. Begin infant cereal at 1 month of age
    2. Do not give honey to the baby until he is at least 1 year old
    3. Add sugar or salt to foods if he finds something unpalatable
    4. Delay giving egg yolk to the baby until he is 1 year old because this portion of the egg causes most instances of allergic reactions

18. Sally Davis, who has a history of family allergies, asks what foods she can feed her 4-month-old son Benjamin that would be least likely to cause an allergic reaction. You reply:
    1. Scrambled eggs
    2. Cow's milk
    3. Wheat cereal
    4. Rice cereal

19. Sandra Betheny, a young school teacher, has recently learned that she is pregnant. Her question concerns how she can eliminate the morning sickness that she has been experiencing. Your suggestions to her might include:
    1. Eat dry toast or crackers when you wake in the morning
    2. Drink liquids with your meals
    3. Increase fat products within your diet
    4. Decrease the carbohydrates within your meals

20. Lois Adelson has decided to decrease her intake of red meat, but she is concerned that she will also be decreasing her intake of iron. You suggest that she can increase her intake of iron by eating additional:
    1. Yellow vegetables, such as carrots and sweet potatoes
    2. Milk and dairy products
    3. Refined cereal products
    4. Dried fruits, such as raisins and apricots

21. The absorption of iron, especially nonmeat sources, can be enhanced significantly if iron is ingested with:
    1. Milk and dairy products
    2. Fish liver oils
    3. Citrus juices
    4. Green leafy vegetables

Situation: Miss Irma Van Houten is a 32-year-old librarian. She has lived a sedentary life and consequently is somewhat overweight. Following a series of unexplained physical complaints, a physical examination determined that she has diabetes. The physician placed her on a 1500-calorie diabetic diet and 30 units isophane insulin suspension (NPH Insulin) daily.

22. The diabetic diet is based on the exchange system. In using this system the patient should be instructed to:
    1. Use dietetic or diabetic foods as much as possible
    2. Substitute only among foods listed in the same exchange
    3. Food exchanges are not particularly important as long as you stay within your recommended calories
    4. Substitution within a food exchange for meal planning can only be done by a physician or dietitian

23. When visiting friends, Miss Van Houten was offered half a cup of blackberries. Since she does not care for blackberries, what would she be able to substitute for them?
    1. Ice milk
    2. Pineapple juice
    3. Cheddar cheese
    4. Pecans

24. For dinner one evening Miss Van Houten fries an egg in 1 teaspoon of margarine, has a biscuit with 1 teaspoon of butter, and drinks a cup of black coffee. Out of which exchange lists has she selected her meal?
    1. One milk, two bread, and one fat exchange
    2. One meat, one milk, one fruit, and one fat exchange
    3. One bread, one meat, and one vegetable exchange
    4. One meat, one bread, and two fat exchanges

25. Miss Van Houten remarks to you that in the late afternoon she frequently becomes shaky and feels very nervous. What would you suggest to her as a readily available source of carbohydrate that could get her over this hypoglycemic episode?
    ① Crackers
    ② Oranges
    ③ Bread and butter
    ④ Cereal

Situation: You are working the 3:00 to 11:00 PM shift on a medical-surgical unit at a small community hospital. Because the dietician is no longer available on shift, you must make decisions and answer questions concerning the diet therapy of patients.

26. Grant Justice is a patient with a diagnosis of chronic renal failure. Which of the following dinner selections would be best suited for Mr. Justice?
    ① Apple juice, 1 oz roast chicken, asparagus, sliced tomatoes, fruit cup, and tea with sugar
    ② Ground round steak, asparagus, bread and butter, fruit cup, and milk
    ③ Hamburger with tomato on a bun, potato chips, and a glass of chocolate milk
    ④ Liver, cottage cheese with peach half, deviled eggs, and coffee with cream and sugar

27. Elise Johnson is a postoperative patient who has just begun a clear liquid diet. Which of the following selections would she be allowed?
    ① Cream-of-mushroom soup, jello, and tea
    ② Chicken broth, lime sherbet, and apple juice
    ③ Beef bouillon, raspberry ice, and tea
    ④ Beef bouillon, orange juice, and cherry jello

28. James Tucker is a 35-year-old accountant who is hospitalized with ulcerative colitis. The acute flare-up of his condition has passed, and you would expect him to be placed on a diet:
    ① Low in residue and high in vitamins and protein
    ② High in residue and high in vitamins and protein
    ③ Low in fat and calories
    ④ Low in sodium and carbohydrates

29. Harrison Fuller, admitted with a diagnosis of suspected myocardial infarction, complains about the soft diet ordered by the physician. You explain to Mr. Fuller that the purpose of this diet is:
    ① To reduce the number of calories in his diet
    ② To decrease peristalsis within the digestive tract
    ③ To decrease irritation to the digestive tract
    ④ To reduce the work load on the heart

30. Curtis Wilber has a problem with atonic constipation probably caused by poor eating habits coupled with his dependence on laxatives. Which of the following menus would be best suited to helping Mr. Wilber overcome constipation?
    ① Ground beef patty, boiled potato, baked squash, and milk
    ② Beef stew with carrots and onions, coleslaw, rye bread, and tea
    ③ Macaroni and cheese, peach halves, vanilla ice cream, and milk
    ④ Baked chicken, macaroni, cooked carrots, custard, and coffee

31. The National Institute of Health, the American Heart Association, and the U.S. Surgeon General have issued similar dietary recommendations. Each has stated that the average person should:
    ① Decrease total calories in the diet
    ② Increase carbohydrates to approximately 30% of total caloric intake
    ③ Decrease dietary fat, especially polyunsaturated fats
    ④ Decrease total dietary fats, especially saturated fats

32. Among the four basic food groups, the milk group primarily supplies which nutrients?
    ① Vitamin C and calcium
    ② Calcium and protein
    ③ Iron and calcium
    ④ B complex vitamins and protein

33. A variety of diets have been used over the years to deal with gastrointestinal disorders. Which statement best describes current thinking concerning diet and peptic ulcer disease?
    ① Eat what you like but avoid foods that are especially irritating
    ② Milk and milk products should be the foundation of peptic ulcer diets
    ③ Food and drink containing caffeine, chocolate, and alcohol can be taken in unrestricted amounts
    ④ Physicians are strongly encouraging compliance with the bland diet for conditions such as peptic ulcer

34. Which of the following statements about diabetes mellitus and diet are correct?
    ① The best kinds of carbohydrates to include are refined, simple carbohydrates
    ② The use of any alcoholic beverage is absolutely prohibited
    ③ The food choices available are extremely limited
    ④ Include high-fiber foods in menu planning

35. Which of the following statements is true?
    ① Blood cholesterol levels of 250 to 300 mg/dl are considered ideal
    ② Of the factors an individual can control, diet has the greatest effect on blood cholesterol levels
    ③ A high ratio of low-density lipoprotein (LDL) to high-density lipoprotein (HDL) is considered desirable
    ④ Lowering blood cholesterol levels requires both medication and dietary adjustments

36. The food guide pyramid recently introduced by the U.S. Department of Agriculture:
    ① Places fruits and vegetables as the foundation of a healthy diet
    ② Graphically illustrates the approximate proportions of various foods needed for a healthy diet
    ③ Places meat, poultry, fish, dry beans, and nuts as the foundation of a healthy diet
    ④ Does not address placing fats, oils, and sweets in the diet

CHAPTER 6

Medical-Surgical Nursing

This chapter presents the nursing assessment of medical-surgical patients and is grouped according to the body system affected. Following the nursing process, frequent patient problems and recommended nursing care are identified and discussed. A selected group of major diagnoses, medical management, and nursing care plans are included. Although assessment of each system's functioning and problems is isolated, the student must remember that total patient assessment is necessary each time a patient is given care. Before studying this chapter, the student should have completed a review of Chapters 2 and 3, dealing with nursing fundamentals and anatomy and physiology, repsectively. Nursing assessment, care, and responsibility for the patient before and after surgery, diagnostic testing, and nursing care procedures are discussed. Medications, the specific nursing responsibilities they entail, and their adverse effects are addressed in Chapter 4, Pharmacology.

The Musculoskeletal System

Musculoskeletal disorders may be acute or chronic. Acute problems are usually related to simple injuries. Chronic disorders may be more distressing to the patient because of loss of mobility and changes in self-image. The nurse needs to possess good skills in observation, positioning the patient safely, and use and care of equipment. The nurse is probably the most important health care provider in preventive care associated with complications of immobility.

NURSING ASSESSMENT

A. Nursing observations
   1. General appearance
   2. Age
   3. Vital signs
   4. Loss of height
   5. Abnormal gait
   6. Impaired neurovascular status
   7. Comparisons between affected and nonaffected sides
   8. Absence of extremity
   9. Deformity
   10. Limb nonalignment
   11. Loss or inability to move body part
   12. Diminished handgrip
   13. Limited range of motion (ROM)
   14. Abnormal spinal curvature
   15. Bony joint enlargement
   16. Joint pain
   17. Presence of warmth, redness, or edema over skin
   18. Ability to perform activities of daily living (ADL)
   19. Capillary refill
   20. Assistive devices; casts
B. Patient description (subjective data)
   1. Pain with or without movement
   2. Weakness
   3. Fatigue
   4. Feeling of joint stiffness
   5. Anorexia
   6. Weight loss or weight gain
   7. Limited movement/gait difficulty
   8. Recent injury

DIAGNOSTIC TESTS/METHODS

A. Serum laboratory studies
   1. Complete blood count (CBC): an aid in determining anemia or the presence of infection
   2. Erythrocyte sedimentation rate (ESR): elevation is evidenced during inflammatory processes
   3. Rheumatoid factor: a protein found in the blood of most persons afflicted with rheumatoid arthritis
   4. Uric acid: high concentration is found in persons who have gout
   5. Lupus erythematosus (LE) cell
      a. A cell identified in persons with lupus
      b. Normally there are no LE cells in the blood
B. Procedures
   1. Roentgenogram (x-ray): a film to determine the presence of a deformity, fracture, or tumor of the skeletal system
   2. Aspiration: withdrawal of fluid from a joint to obtain a specimen for diagnostic purposes
   3. Bone biopsy: removal and examination of bone tissue
   4. Myelogram: x-ray examination of the spinal cord after injection with radiopaque dye
   5. Bone scan: isotope imaging of the skeleton
   6. Computerized tomography (CT): use of roentgen rays to provide accurate images of thin cross sections of the body
   7. Magnetic resonance imaging (MRI): aid for the diagnosis of musculoskeletal conditions through the

clear differentiation of various types of tissue, such as bones, fat, and muscle

8. Arthroscopy: endoscopic examination that allows for direct visualization of a joint

C. Nursing intervention for myelogram

1. After procedure, have patient remain flat in bed 12 to 24 hours before allowing him or her to resume usual activities
2. Encourage fluids to 2000 to 3000 ml every 24 hours
3. Observe for alterations in normal motor and sensory states
4. Observe for nausea and vomiting

FREQUENT PATIENT PROBLEMS AND NURSING CARE

A. Disturbance in self-concept; body image related to immobility

1. Provide atmosphere of acceptance
2. Express empathy, warmth, and friendliness
3. Encourage acceptance of self-limitations
4. Encourage self-performance

B. Impairment of skin integrity; potential breakdown related to immobility/assistive devices

1. Change the patient's position frequently
2. Keep the skin clean, dry, and lubricated
3. Massage bony prominences
4. Provide sheepskin or polyurethane foam pad

C. Potential joint contracture related to incorrect body alignment

1. Place hands, feet, and knees in the natural position of function
2. Provide sandbags to protect against poor alignment of body part
3. Assist in performance of active and passive ROM exercises
4. Provide trapeze over the patient's bed
5. Avoid knee Gatch position/pillow under knee

D. Potential respiratory secretion congestion related to ineffective airway clearance

1. Change the patient's position frequently
2. Encourage coughing and deep breathing
3. Observe for coughing, fever, and green-yellow sputum

E. Potential thrombus and emboli related to impaired physical mobility/edema

1. Encourage patient to move lower extremities
2. Encourage adequate hydration
3. Avoid use of knee Gatch/pillow under knee
4. To avoid release of emboli, never rub legs

F. Bone pain related to bone fracture or disease

1. Inspect and palpate the painful site looking for inflammation, edema, bruising, tenderness, and skin warmth
2. Support the affected body part
3. Apply warm, moist compress to affected body part where prescribed
4. Give prescribed analgesic
5. Evaluate effectiveness of pain relief measures

G. Potential limited ROM related to cast or traction confinement, joint pain, stiffness, or inflammation

1. Explain the reason for and intended effect of ROM exercises

2. Maintain body alignment
3. Provide total exercising of muscles and joints except if severe pain or inflammation is present; contraindicated if recent surgery was performed on or near the joint

H. Alteration in comfort: pain related to cast

1. Massage the area around the cast
2. Pad rough edges
3. Provide a scratching device
4. Inspect the skin for irritation
5. Observe for cyanosis of the extremity in a cast
6. Observe for complaints of numbness and tingling of extremity

I. Self-care deficits (feeding, bathing, and hygiene) related to impaired physical mobility

1. Assist with ADL
2. Provide self-care aids/devices
3. Teach self-care activities

MAJOR MEDICAL DIAGNOSES
Rheumatoid Arthritis

A. Definition: a chronic, systemic disease in which inflammatory changes occur throughout the body's connective tissue destroying joints internally; joints most involved are hands, wrists, elbows, knees, and ankles

B. Pathology: cause is unknown; related theories include microorganisms, viruses, and genetic predisposition

C. Signs and symptoms

1. Subjective
   a. Sore, stiff, swollen joint(s)
   b. Fatigue
   c. Weakness
   d. Malaise
   e. Loss of appetite
2. Objective
   a. Low-grade fever
   b. Weakened grip
   c. Anemia
   d. Weight loss
   e. Subcutaneous nodes
   f. Enlarged lymph nodes
   g. Joint deformity
   h. Muscle atrophy
   i. Limited ROM
   j. Edema and tenderness of joint
   k. Extraarticular symptoms: lung, heart, blood vessels, muscle, eye, and skin

D. Diagnostic tests/methods

1. Elevated ESR
2. Slightly elevated white blood cell (WBC) count
3. Presence of serum rheumatoid factors
4. Synovial fluid aspiration
5. X-ray film reveals joint deformity
6. Low hemoglobin and hematocrit

E. Treatment

1. Antiinflammatory agents, analgesics, corticosteroids, gold salts, and immunosuppressive drugs
2. Heat applications such as paraffin dip, hot packs, and warm tub baths or showers for analgesia or muscle relaxation
3. Surgical intervention to prevent deformities or remove damaged joints

4. Physical therapy to maintain optimal function
F. Nursing intervention
   1. Provide undisturbed periods of rest
   2. Use firm mattress, foot boards, splints, and sandbags to maintain proper body alignment
   3. Encourage self-performance activities such as combing hair, feeding self, and brushing teeth
   4. Provide ROM exercises within limits of pain tolerance

Osteoarthritis

A. Definition: a local joint disorder affecting weight-bearing joints; results in disintegration of the cartilage covering the ends of bones
B. Pathology: cause is unknown; predisposing factors include aging, joint trauma, and obesity
C. Signs and symptoms
   1. Subjective
      a. Pain after exercise; relieved by rest
      b. Morning stiffness
      c. Muscle spasms
      d. Reduced strength
   2. Objective
      a. Limited ROM
      b. Crepitant joint
      c. Prominent bony enlargement
D. Diagnostic tests: x-ray studies reveal joint abnormalities
E. Treatment
   1. Weight reduction to relieve strain
   2. Heat and massage for aching and stiffness
   3. Physical therapy to maintain optimum level of functioning
   4. Drugs to relieve symptoms
      a. Analgesics
      b. Antiinflammatory agents
      c. Steroids
   5. Surgical intervention to prevent deformity, relieve inflammation, delay progression, or replace affected joint
F. Nursing intervention
   1. Encourage patient to express feelings concerning disorder
   2. Provide moist heat, massage, and prescribed exercise, if ordered, to relax muscle and relieve stiffness or discomfort

Gouty Arthritis (Gout)

A. Definition: a disorder in which excessive amounts of uric acid are retained in the blood
B. Pathology
   1. Cause is related to a disorder of purine metabolism
   2. Uric acid crystals are deposited in the joints and cartilage and form lumps (tophi)
   3. Deposits cause local irritation and an inflammatory response
   4. Men older than 30 years of age are most commonly affected
C. Signs and symptoms
   1. Subjective
      a. Acute pain, swelling, and inflammation of great toe (most affected joint)
      b. Headache

c. Malaise
d. Anorexia
e. Pruritus
   2. Objective
      a. Skin over joint is swollen, warm, and red
      b. Limited ROM
      c. Tophi located in cartilage of ears, hands, and feet
D. Diagnostic tests/methods
   1. Elevated serum uric acid level
   2. Elevated ESR and WBC count
E. Treatment
   1. Dietary restriction of foods high in purines
   2. Uricosuric drugs to increase uric acid excretion
   3. Allopurinol to inhibit uric acid formation
   4. Colchicine to reduce pain and relieve swelling
   5. Alkaline ash diet to increase urinary pH
F. Nursing intervention
   1. Instruct patient to avoid foods high in purine content: liver, kidney, sweetbreads, sardines, and brains
   2. Encourage physical activity to promote optimal muscular and skeletal function
   3. Place bed cradle to prevent pain of part by linen pressure
   4. Encourage fluid intake of 2000 to 3000 ml daily to avoid renal calculi unless contraindicated
   5. Instruct patient to limit alcohol intake, which may precipitate an acute attack
   6. Instruct patient to avoid salicylates because of antagonistic actions of uricosuric drugs

Systemic Lupus Erythematosus (SLE)

A. Definition: a chronic multisystem inflammatory disorder involving the connective tissues, such as the muscles, kidneys, heart, and serous membranes; may affect the skin, lungs, and nervous system
B. Pathology
   1. Cause is unknown; is believed to be an autoimmune disorder
   2. Inflammation produces fibroid deposits and structural changes in connective tissue of organs and blood vessels
   3. Results in problems with mobility, oxygenation, and elimination
C. Signs and symptoms
   1. Subjective
      a. Abdominal, joint, and muscle pain
      b. Weakness; fatigue
      c. Depression
   2. Objective
      a. Low-grade fever
      b. Weight loss
      c. Butterfly skin rash over bridge of nose and cheeks, which increases with exposure to the sun
      d. Anemia
      e. Alopecia
D. Diagnostic tests
   1. Positive LE test
   2. Elevated ESR
   3. Increased gamma globulin levels
   4. Positive antinuclear antibody titer
   5. High anti-DNA test

E. Treatment
   1. Corticosteroids, analgesics, and medications for anemia
   2. Avoidance of exposure to sunlight
F. Nursing intervention
   1. Provide emotional support to patient and family in coping with poor prognosis
   2. Encourage alternative activity and planned rest periods
   3. Instruct to avoid persons with infections, undue exposure to sunlight, and emotional stress, which can cause exacerbations
   4. Encourage intake of foods high in iron content: liver, shellfish, leafy vegetables, and enriched breads and cereals

Scleroderma (Progressive Systemic Sclerosis)

A. Definition: fiberlike changes in the connective tissue throughout the body caused by collagen deposits and subsequent fibrosis
B. Pathology
   1. An insidious, chronic, progressive disorder usually beginning in the skin
   2. Skin becomes thick and hard; fingers and toes become fixed in a position
   3. Other disorders that occur are difficulty in swallowing, impaired gastrointestinal (GI) mobility, cardiac and renal problems, and osteoporosis
C. Signs and symptoms
   1. Subjective
      a. Sweating of hands and feet
      b. Stiffness of hands
      c. Muscle weakness
      d. Joint pain
      e. Dysphagia
   2. Objective
      a. Increased pigmentation or dyspigmentation
      b. Dilated capillaries of lips, fingers, face, and tongue
D. Diagnostic tests/methods
   1. Positive LE cell test
   2. False-positive syphilis test
E. Treatment
   1. Skin care to prevent formation of decubiti
   2. Physical therapy
   3. Analgesics for joint pain
   4. Corticosteroids
F. Nursing intervention
   1. Provide emotional support to patient and family in promoting physical and psychologic needs
   2. Encourage moderate exercise to promote muscular and joint function
   3. Force fluids
   4. Avoid cold temperatures
   5. Plan rest periods

Polyarteritis Nodosa

A. Definition: a collagen disease that results in inflammation and necrosis in the walls of small- to medium-sized arteries
B. Pathology
   1. Impairment of artery supply alters organ systems
   2. Most involved structures are muscles, kidneys, liver, and GI tract
C. Signs and symptoms
   1. Subjective
      a. Prolonged fever
      b. Malaise
      c. Weakness
      d. Weight loss
   2. Objective
      a. Palpable nodules along arterial walls
      b. Subcutaneous nodules
      c. Hematuria
D. Diagnostic tests/methods
   1. Positive rheumatoid factor
   2. Elevated ESR
E. Treatment: corticosteroids
F. Nursing intervention
   1. Provide emotional support to patient and family in dealing with poor prognosis
   2. Provide comfort measures for relief of symptomatic pain
   3. Encourage balanced food intake for weight loss
   4. Encourage moderate exercise, when able, to maintain muscle tone and slow development of disability

Osteomyelitis

A. Definition: bone inflammation caused by direct or indirect invasion of an organism
B. Pathology: bacteria enter bloodstream through an open fracture, open wound, or by secondary invasion from blood-borne infection from a distant site such as bone or infected tonsils
C. Signs and symptoms
   1. Subjective
      a. Tenderness over the bones
      b. Painful movement; limited mobility
      c. Malaise
   2. Objective
      a. Fever
      b. Chills
      c. Heat, swelling, and redness of the skin over the bone
      d. Signs of sepsis
      e. Wound drainage
D. Diagnostic tests/methods
   1. Positive blood cultures
   2. Elevated ESR
   3. Elevated WBC count
   4. X-ray film may not reveal abnormalities for 5 to 10 days from onset
E. Treatment
   1. Antibiotic therapy
   2. Drainage from abscess with continuous irrigation of wound
   3. Surgical removal of necrotic bone
F. Nursing intervention
   1. Use strict aseptic technique when changing dressings
   2. Keep affected limb in proper alignment with pillows and sandbags
   3. Maintain drainage and secretion precautions for disposal of dressings

4. Provide a high-calorie, high-protein diet and adequate hydration
5. Provide undisturbed rest periods
6. Move affected body part gently, because of severe pain

Osteoporosis

A. Definition: metabolic bone disorder in which bone mass is decreased
B. Pathology
   1. Common in postmenopausal women
   2. May be result of deficit of estrogen and androgens, prolonged immobilization, insufficient calcium intake or absorption, or endocrine disorder
   3. Sites usually affected are vertebrae, pelvis, and femur
C. Signs and symptoms
   1. Subjective: backache; worsens with sitting, standing, coughing, and sneezing
   2. Objective
      a. Kyphosis
      b. Loss of height
      c. Pathologic fractures
D. Diagnostic test: x-ray film reveals bone demineralization and compression of vertebrae
E. Treatment
   1. Physical activity and exercise to prevent disuse atrophy
   2. Estrogen replacement to provide calcium balance
   3. Diet high in protein and calcium
   4. Vitamin D supplements
   5. Support of spine with brace or corset
F. Nursing intervention
   1. Encourage use of walker or cane to stabilize balance when ambulating
   2. Encourage fluid intake of 2000 to 3000 ml daily, unless contraindicated, to avoid formation of renal calculi
   3. Give instruction on those foods high in protein and calcium content
   4. Emphasize need to follow prescribed daily activity and exercise
   5. If confined to bed, give passive and active ROM exercises
   6. Teach safety measures to protect from fractures

Osteogenic Sarcoma

A. Definition: a tumor located in the bone composed of cells derived from connective tissue
B. Pathology
   1. Highly malignant tumor metastasizing through the lymph nodes to the lungs
   2. Affects children, adolescents, and young adults
   3. Usually occurs in shaft of long bones, especially affecting the knee
C. Signs and symptoms
   1. Subjective: pain
   2. Objective:
      a. Restricted ROM
      b. Swelling
      c. Weight loss
      d. Anemia

D. Diagnostic tests/methods
   1. X-ray examination to reveal lesion in the extremity and chest; CT scan
   2. Biopsy examination to evaluate cells
   3. Frozen section for rapid diagnosis of possible malignant lesion
E. Treatment
   1. Chemotherapeutic agents to reduce and retard growth
   2. Radiation therapy to destroy malignant tissue
   3. Amputation of affected limb or resection of tumor
F. Nursing intervention
   1. Provide emotional support to patient and family to reduce fear and anxiety
   2. Provide diet high in protein and caloric content
   3. If patient undergoes amputation procedure, follow special nursing actions (refer to amputations)
   4. If patient is receiving radiotherapy
      a. Provide noninfectious environment
      b. Avoid ointments, lotions, powders, and washing of port (treated) areas
      c. Do not remove markings on skin
      d. Observe site for redness, swelling, itching, and drying

Osteomalacia

A. Definition: a disorder in which widespread softening and demineralization of bones occur
B. Pathology
   1. Possible causes
      a. Vitamin D deficiency resulting from poor dietary intake of vitamin D
      b. Body's inability to absorb or use vitamin D
      c. Lack of ultraviolet rays
   2. The effect of parathyroid hormone on bone resorption and calcium absorption is decreased
   3. Most affected bones are spine, pelvis, and lower extremities
C. Signs and symptoms
   1. Subjective
      a. Rheumatic-type pain
      b. Weakness
   2. Objective
      a. Waddling gait
      b. Spontaneous fractures
      c. Bone deformities
D. Diagnostic tests/methods
   1. Reduced calcium and phosphorus serum levels
   2. X-ray examination reveals fracturelike lines of affected bones
E. Treatment
   1. Therapeutic doses of vitamin D
   2. High dietary intake of calcium and phosphorus
F. Nursing intervention
   1. Change patient's position gradually
   2. Teach good body mechanics
   3. Encourage intake of foods high in calcium: meat, shellfish, and dark green, leafy vegetables
   4. Emphasize need to maintain weight in normal range
   5. Instruct on avoidance of heavy lifting

Osteitis Deformans (Paget's Disease of Bone)

A. Definition: an inflammatory condition in which certain bones become soft, thick, and deformed
B. Pathology
   1. Cause is unknown: occurs mainly in men in middle age or older
   2. Disease disturbs new bone tissue with bones becoming enlarged and coarse in texture
C. Signs and symptoms
   1. Subjective
     a. Bone pain; worsens at night
     b. Tenderness on pressure of the bones
     c. Back pain
     d. Headache from enlarged skull
     e. Deafness or blindness caused by pressure from overgrowth of bone
   2. Objective
     a. Pathologic fractures
     b. Decrease in height
     c. Bowing of femur and tibia
     d. Enlarged skull
D. Diagnostic tests/methods
   1. Skeletal x-ray film reveals bone enlargement and denseness
   2. Elevated serum alkaline phosphate value
   3. Urinary excretion of hydroxyproline is increased
E. Treatment
   1. Androgen therapy for men; estrogen therapy for women to reverse hypercalciuria, if present
   2. Salicylates for pain
F. Nursing intervention
   1. Observe for stress fractures
   2. Emphasize need for maintenance of normal weight
   3. If fracture occurs and patient becomes immobilized
     a. Limit calcium intake to avoid renal calculi
     b. Provide high fluid intake to avoid hypercalcemia

Herniated Nucleus Pulposus (Slipped Disk or Rupture of Intervertebral Disk)

A. Definition: protrusion of the nucleus pulposus, which compresses the nerve roots of the spinal cord
B. Pathology
   1. Site usually affected is between L4 and L5, L5 and sacrum, C5 and C6, and C6 and C7
   2. Causes may be straining of the spine in an unnatural position, degenerative changes, heavy lifting when bending from the waist, and accidents
C. Signs and symptoms
   1. Subjective
     a. Cervical disk
       (1) Stiff neck
       (2) Shoulder pain descending down the arm into the hand
       (3) Numbness of arm and hand
     b. Lumbosacral disk: low-back pain radiating down the posterior thigh
   2. Objective
     a. Cervical disk: sensory disturbances of the hand
     b. Lumbosacral disk
       (1) Difficulty in ambulating
       (2) Lasègue's sign: pain in back and leg while raising heel with knee straight
       (3) Numbness of leg and foot
D. Diagnostic tests/methods
   1. X-ray examination to reveal narrowing disk space
   2. Myelogram to localize site
   3. Electromyography
   4. CT scan of the spine
   5. MRI of spine
E. Treatment
   1. Cervical traction (cervical disk); traction to lower extremities (lumbosacral disk)
   2. Bed rest, heat application, and analgesics
   3. Surgical intervention
     a. Laminectomy: removal of a portion of the vertebra and excision of the ruptured portion of the nucleus pulposus
     b. Spinal fusion: permanent binding of the vertebrae
     c. Chemonucleolysis: dissolving of the affected disk through the injection of chymopapain
F. Nursing intervention
   1. Encourage patient to verbalize feelings related to immobility, fears, and future impairment
   2. Observations for traction
     a. Check that it is hanging free and has not fallen or become caught in bed grooves
     b. Observe for frayed cords and loosened knots
   3. Give back care to promote circulation and relax muscles
   4. Maintain proper body alignment
   5. Provide diet high in fiber with adequate hydration to avoid constipation and straining
   6. Instruct patient on principles of body mechanics
   7. If patient has myelogram procedure
     a. Position flat for period prescribed by physician
     b. Encourage adequate hydration
   8. If patient undergoes surgical intervention, follow general postoperative nursing actions
     a. Observe for leakage of cerebrospinal fluid on surgical dressing; reinforce dressing until inspected by physician
     b. Change position by log rolling to prevent motion of spinal column
     c. Provide straight-backed chair for patient to sit; feet must be on floor
     d. Discharge instructions include
       (1) Avoid heavy lifting and climbing stairs
       (2) Avoid riding in car
       (3) Avoid forward flexion of head (cervical laminectomy)

Fractures

A. Definition: a break in the continuity of bone that may be accompanied by injury of surrounding soft tissue, producing swelling and discoloration
B. Pathology
   1. Most fractures are a result of trauma; pathologic fractures result from disorders such as osteoporosis, malnutrition, bone tumors, and Cushing's syndrome
   2. Types of fractures
     a. Closed (simple): skin is intact over the site
     b. Open (compound): break in skin is present over

the fracture site; the ends of the bone may or may not be visible

c. Complete: fracture line extends completely through the bone

d. Incomplete (partial): fracture line extends partially through the bone; one side breaks while the opposite side bends

e. Comminuted: more than one fracture with bone fragments either crushed or splintered into several pieces

f. Green-stick: splintering of one side of a bone (most often seen in children because of soft bone structure)

g. Impacted: one bone fragment is driven into another bone fragment

C. Signs and symptoms
  1. Subjective
     a. Pain on movement of body part
     b. Tenderness
     c. Loss of function
     d. Muscle spasms
  2. Objective
     a. Deformity
     b. Edema
     c. Bruising
     d. Crepitus

D. Diagnostic test: x-ray examination to confirm location and direction of fracture line

E. Treatment
  1. Reduction of the fracture consists of pulling the broken bone ends to correct alignment and regain continuity; usually a cast is applied or the part may be placed in a traction device
     a. Closed reduction: manual manipulation to bring ends into contact
     b. Open reduction: surgical intervention to cleanse the area and attach devices to hold the bones in position
  2. Cast application to immobilize, support, and protect the part during the healing process
  3. Traction to apply a pulling force in two directions to realign the bones
     a. Skin traction is temporarily applied: light weights that are attached to the skin with strips of adhesive tape
        (1) Buck's extension: exerts a straight pull on the limb; used for fractures of upper and lower leg, hip dislocation, and pelvic injuries
        (2) Bryant's traction: vertical extension of lower extremities, hip flexed 90 degrees, knees extended, and buttocks clear of the bed (see Fig. 9-14, p. 293) for reduction of femur or hip dislocation in very young children
        (3) Russell traction: a sling is placed behind the knee to create an upward pull of the knee, and at the same time a horizontal force is exerted on the tibia and fibula; used for fractures of femurs
     b. Skeletal traction provides continuous reduction by the attachment of a device to the bone

(1) Kirschner wires or Steinmann pins are surgically inserted through the skin and bone; a traction bow or stirrup is attached to the wire or pin to exert a longitudinal pull and control rotation

(2) Crutchfield tongs are inserted into parietal areas of the skull to obtain hyperextension; used for spinal fractures

(3) Halo traction-halo loop for alignment of cervical area; loop is attached to a halo vest or cast

F. Nursing intervention
  1. Provide emergency nursing care of fractures (refer to Chapter 11)
  2. Provide nursing care for the patient with a cast
     a. Observe for circulatory impairment of limb: color, temperature, pulse, and motor function
     b. Elevate extremity in cast on pillow
     c. Promote drying of cast by exposing it to air
     d. Inspect for skin irritation under edges of cast: apply lotion, pad edges, and apply tape to edge of cast
     e. If drainage is present on the cast, measure and note
     f. Observe for possible infection: increased temperature, foul odor from cast, edema, and "hot spots" over the cast
     g. Observe for complications of pulmonary embolisms, fat embolism, and compartment syndrome
     h. Educate patient on home cast care
  3. Provide nursing care for the patient in traction
     a. Inspect and maintain ropes, knots, and pulleys; taut rope rides easily over pulleys; knots should not slip and should be unobstructed
     b. Inspect and maintain weights: hang freely, off the floor and free of bedding
     c. Observations for skin traction
        (1) Inspect skin condition at distal ends of bandages (wrist and heel) for possible skin breakdown
        (2) Ensure that tapes do not encircle a limb, are applied smoothly, and are applied on skin that is free of irritation
        (3) Assess circulatory status: color, pulses, warmth, and sensation
     d. Observations for skeletal traction
        (1) Inspect insertion points daily for signs and symptoms of infection
        (2) Provide dressing change or wound care aseptically to prevent infection
        (3) Inspect pins, wires, and skeletal apparatus for sharp ends that may catch on bed linen
        (4) Assess neurovascular status
     e. Examine and give skin care to all pressure points on which the patient rests
     f. Provide foot support to prevent foot drop, especially for patients with Russell traction or Buck's extension
     g. Observe for thrombophlebitis, especially for the patient with Russell traction because of pressure to the popliteal space

h. Encourage diet high in protein and vitamins to promote healing

i. Encourage 2000 to 3000 ml fluid intake daily to prevent complications such as constipation, renal calculi, and urinary tract infections

j. Encourage patient to perform ROM and isometric exercises

k. Maintain proper position and good alignment

Fractured Hip

A. Definition: fracture of the hip joint

B. Pathology

    1. Site of fracture

        a. Inside the joint (intracapsular or neck of the femur)

        b. Outside the joint (extracapsular or base of the neck of the femur)

    2. Elderly women experience high incidence because of osteoporosis

C. Signs and symptoms

    1. Subjective: pain

    2. Objective

        a. Leg appears shorter than nonaffected extremity

        b. Foot points upward and outward on affected side

        c. Edema

        d. Discoloration

D. Diagnostic test: x-ray study confirms discontinuity of the bone

E. Treatment

    1. Russell traction or Buck's extension: before open reduction to prevent muscle spasms if surgery is not contraindicated

    2. Closed reduction with application of hip spica cast if the fracture occurred in the intertrochanteric site

    3. Open reduction and implantation of a prosthesis to replace head and neck of femur or fixation device to secure fragments of the fracture

        a. Austin Moore prosthesis

        b. Neufeld nail and screws

        c. Smith-Petersen nail

F. Nursing intervention

    1. Provide nursing care for the patient in traction as outlined previously in section on Fractures

    2. Be aware of coexisting problems such as diabetes or cardiac, vascular, or neurologic disorders

    3. Considerations for the geriatric patient

        a. Complications of immobility

        b. Reduced tolerance to drugs

        c. Delayed healing because of nutritional problems related to the elderly

    4. Keep side rail up and provide trapeze to facilitate movement

    5. Encourage patient to participate in activities of daily living: eating, bathing, and combing hair

    6. Provide postoperative care

        a. Inspect dressings and linen for drainage and bleeding

        b. Provide trochanter roll to prevent external rotation of legs

        c. Provide and maintain proper alignment; adduction, external rotation, or acute flexion of the hip can dislocate hip before it is healed

d. Encourage quadriceps-setting exercises

e. Assist the patient to learn to use walker, ambulating with a non–weight-bearing technique

Arthroplasty

A. Definition: replacement of a joint, which may be necessary to restore function, relieve pain, and correct deformity

B. Pathology: arthritic changes damage the joint, resulting in impaired mobility, pain, and deformity; hip, knee, elbow, and shoulder are commonly affected

C. Signs and symptoms

    1. Subjective

        a. Pain

        b. Limited ROM

        c. Limited weight-bearing ability

    2. Objective

        a. Limited ROM

        b. Edema and skin character changes around affected joint

D. Diagnostic tests/methods

    1. X-ray studies confirm joint changes and damage

    2. Arthroscopy provides direct visualization and inspection of joint changes

E. Treatment: a prosthetic device used to replace the articulating joint surfaces (hip, knee, shoulder, elbow, and fingers)

F. Nursing intervention

    1. Proper positioning postoperatively (e.g., if hip is replaced, maintain affected leg in abduction)

    2. Wound care: monitor drains, note blood loss, and monitor dressing status

    3. Monitor continuous passive ROM machine, if used for knee replacement

    4. Assist with prescribed activity and encourage prescribed exercise

    5. Monitor pain; provide pain control

    6. Assess neuromuscular function

    7. Monitor skin integrity

Amputation

A. Definition surgical removal of part or all of an extremity

B. Pathology

    1. Majority of amputations result from blood vessel disorders causing inadequate oxygen supply to the tissue

    2. Other indications for amputation are gas gangrene, malignant tumors, septic wounds, severe trauma, and burns

    3. Usually a skin flap is constructed for prosthetic equipment

C. Signs and symptoms

    1. Subjective

        a. Gas gangrene and septic wounds: pain

        b. Peripheral vascular diseases

            (1) Pain

            (2) Tingling

    2. Objective

        a. Gas gangrene and septic wounds

            (1) Fever

            (2) Edema

            (3) Foul odor

      (4) Bronze or blackened wound
      (5) Necrosis
  b. Peripheral vascular diseases
      (1) Edema
      (2) Pallor
      (3) Cyanosis
      (4) Diminished pulses
      (5) Hyperpigmentation
      (6) Ulcer formation

D. Diagnostic tests/methods
  1. Oscillometry
  2. Arteriography
  3. Skin temperature studies
  4. X-ray examination

E. Treatment
  1. Psychologic preparation
  2. Rehabilitation preparation
  3. Nutritional status buildup
  4. Prosthetic device

F. Nursing intervention
  1. Provide preoperative care
    a. Encourage expression of feelings by providing honesty concerning loss of limb
    b. Explain to the patient the possibility of experiencing pain in the amputated limb (called phantom limb pain)
    c. Explain to the patient that he or she will undergo a program of exercises that includes strengthening of upper extremities, transferring from bed to chair, and ambulating with a walker or crutches
  2. Provide postoperative care
    a. Provide routine postoperative care
    b. Monitor for bleeding and have a large tourniquet available to apply around the residual limb in the event of hemorrhage
    c. Apply elastic (Ace) bandages in a crisscross or figure-8 pattern only
    d. Elevate the residual limb 8 to 12 hours on a pillow; remove after 12 hours to prevent hip contracture; place in prone position 1 hour out of every 4 hours to prevent hip contractures
    e. Prevent outward rotation by placing trochanter roll along the outer side of the residual limb
    f. Instruct the patient not to hang the residual limb over the edge of the bed, wheelchair, chair, or handrail of his or her crutches to avoid residual limb contracture
    g. When conditioning of the residual limb is ordered, begin by having the patient push the residual limb against a pillow and progress to pushing against a firmer surface
    h. Teach the patient to massage the residual limb to soften the scar and improve vascularity
    i. Use TENS (transcutaneous electrical nerve stimulator) for relief of phantom limb pain
    j. Encourage progressive ambulation and physical therapy

The Respiratory System

All cells of the body are dependent on adequate oxygenation and removal of carbon dioxide for health. The respiratory system is dependent on central nervous system regulation and on the cardiovascular system for blood supply. Respiratory distress or dysfunction may be secondary to disease in another system. Many pulmonary diseases are chronic. Therefore it is essential that the nurse make a complete respiratory assessment of all patients and include this in nursing care planning, even when the primary diagnosis is unrelated to the respiratory system.

The following are terms used to describe respirations:

bradypnea   slow respirations
Cheyne-Stokes   periods of apnea alternating with rapid respirations
DOE   dyspnea on exertion
dyspnea   difficulty breathing; may be subjective or objective
Kussmaul breathing   fast, deep, and labored respirations
orthopnea   difficulty breathing in a supine position; relieved by sitting up
paroxysmal nocturnal dyspnea   transient episodes of acute dyspnea that occur a few hours after falling asleep
SOB   short of breath
tachypnea   rapid respirations
wheeze   sound as air moves out through bronchi and bronchioles that have been narrowed by spasm, swelling, and secretions

NURSING ASSESSMENT

A. Nursing observations (objective data)
  1. Respirations
    a. Rate
    b. Depth
    c. Characteristics, and any difficulty
  2. Oxygen deprivation (note any)
    a. Restlessness
    b. Yawning
    c. Anxiety
    d. Drowsiness
    e. Confusion
    f. Disorientation
  3. Cough
    a. Frequency
    b. Relationship to activity and precipitating factors
    c. Production of sputum
    d. Describe completely (e.g., dry, productive, nonproductive, hoarse, barking, moist, or hacking)
  4. Lung sounds (adventitious)
    a. Crackles
    b. Wheezes
    c. Friction rub
  5. Sputum (note the following)
    a. Consistency (e.g., thick, tenacious, watery, or frothy)
    b. Amount (e.g., scant, moderate, or copious)
    c. Color (e.g., white, yellow, pink, rust, blood tinged, or green)
    d. Odor
  6. Skin color
    a. Pallor, ashen, or ruddy
    b. Cyanosis (bluish discoloration): observe lips, nail beds, and mucous membranes
  7. Skin
    a. Temperature
    b. Diaphoresis
  8. Vital signs
    a. Pulse: note rate, quality and characteristics

b. Blood pressure

c. Temperature (rectal)

9. Nasal discharge

10. Voice: huskiness

B. Patient description (subjective data)

1. Cough

2. Pain

3. Difficulty breathing

4. Fatigue or weakness

5. Sputum

C. Patient history

1. Use of extra pillows needed to sleep

2. Respiratory illness or difficulty

3. Injuries

4. Use of medications or respiratory aids

5. Smoking

DIAGNOSTIC TESTS/METHODS

A. Chest x-ray examination: a picture of lung tissue from different angles; based on a knowledge of normal anatomy and usual changes in disease, diagnosis of many conditions can be made (e.g., tumors, pneumonia); there is no preparation and no special care or observations after x-ray examination

B. Bronchoscopy

1. Direct inspection of the trachea and bronchi through a scope passed via the nose or mouth; with this procedure specimens are obtained for biopsy and culture; foreign bodies can be removed (e.g., fish bones)

2. Nursing responsbilities: provide general preparation as that for a surgical procedure (see Chapter 2); after procedure monitor vital signs, provide oral hygiene, and observe for cough and blood-streaked sputum; do not allow patient to eat or drink until gag reflex returns

C. Bronchogram

1. Visualization of bronchial tree through x-ray examination after introducing radiopaque dye; patient is given sedative and antispasmodic

2. Nursing responsibilities: provide postural drainage to aid in removal of dye; encourage deep breathing and coughing; do not allow patient to eat or drink until gag reflex returns

D. CT scan: produces clear, anatomic images of the chest cavity

E. Ultrasound: image of area is created by high-frequency sound; used for specific data relative to lung capacities

F. MRI: image created by magnetic resonance, a noninvasive procedure

G. Thoracentesis

1. Needle aspiration of fluid from pleural cavity (space); local anesthesia is used

2. Nursing responsibilties: maintain proper positioning; support and reassure patient during the procedure; monitor vital signs during and after the procedure

H. CBC: WCB count changes from normal values indicate type of infection

I. Arterial blood gases

1. Measurement of the partial pressure of oxygen and carbon dioxide in the blood; arterial puncture is performed

2. Nursing care: once the blood sample is obtained, apply constant pressure to the site for 5 minutes; apply pressure dressing; inspect site frequently for hematoma and pain

J. Culture and sensitivity

1. Throat or nasopharynx

2. Sputum

a. Identifies organisms and specific medication to which patient will respond

b. Nursing responsibilities: obtain before starting antibiotics; first sputum in the morning usually has the most organisms

K. Sputum analysis

1. Acid-fast bacillus (AFB): determines presence of mycobacterium tuberculosis

2. Cytology: assists in the diagnosis of lung carcinoma

L. Pulmonary function tests: determine extent of respiratory difficulty and evaluate function of respiratory system; measure vital capacity, tidal volume, and total lung capacity; no special preparation or nursing care after testing

M. Lung scan—Positron emission tomography (PET): radioisotopes are inhaled or administerd intravenously; a scanning device records the pattern of radioactivity; used in diagnosing vascular diseases (e.g., pulmonary embolism); no special preparation or nursing care

N. Biopsy examination

1. Removal of a small amount of tissue to identify disease; biopsy may be of a lymph node to determine if the disease has spread into the lymphatic system

2. Nursing care: provide general preoperative and postoperative care (see Chapter 2)

FREQUENT PATIENT PROBLEMS AND NURSING CARE

A. Activity intolerance related to fatigue and weakness: body cells' demand for oxygen is not met; the patient tires easily and becomes short of breath

1. Protect from exertion; provide care

2. Plan care to include rest periods

3. Leave bed in low position

4. Leave call bell and all personal belongings within easy reach

5. Provide oxygen with humidity as ordered

6. Limit conversation

B. Potential for injury related to dizziness: caused by diminished oxygen to the brain cells

1. Provide all care as in preceding list

2. Maintain safety; use side rails

3. Make neurologic assessment every 4 hours (q4h)

C. Altered oral mucous membrane related to mouth breathing

1. Force fluids if allowed

2. Provide oral hygiene q2h

3. Lubricate lips

D. Altered breathing pattern related to orthopnea

1. Place a pillow longitudinally under back

2. Provide table with pillow for headrest in extreme difficulty

3. Use footboard to prevent slipping down in bed

4. Semi- to high-Fowler's position

E. Ineffective airway clearance; impaired gas exchange related to dyspnea and coughing

1. Oxygen therapy: maintain safety of equipment and proper care and observations

2. Organize care and work efficiently to conserve patient's energy
3. Plan rest periods
4. Position in semi- to high-Fowler's position; use two pillows
5. Provide soft diet and small, frequent feedings
6. Avoid gas-forming foods
7. Prevent constipation and straining
8. Use rectal thermometer
9. Make accurate observations about cough and sputum
10. Obtain specimens as needed
11. Provide tissues and bag for disposal in easy reach
12. Provide sputum cup if needed
13. Change position q2h
14. Encourage deep breathing
15. Force fluids q2h
16. Provide oral hygiene q2h
17. Provide postural drainage if ordered (see Chapter 2)
18. Give expectorants as ordered (see Chapters 2 and 4)

F. Anxiety related to dyspnea, fatigue, and weakness
1. Maintain quiet environment
2. Remain calm
3. Explain everything slowly and carefully
4. Provide physical and mental rest
5. Answer call lights promptly
6. Provide frequent contacts
7. Offer realistic encouragements
8. Provide restful diversion (e.g., music)
9. Encourage patients to express feelings and concerns

G. Alteration in nutrition, less than body requirements, related to dry mouth from mouth breathing, foul taste and odor from sputum, and fatigue; may affect desire for food
1. Make mealtime pleasant
2. Provide oral hygiene before each meal
3. Remove used tissues and sputum cups
4. Request food preferences
5. Give small, frequent, attractively served meals

MAJOR MEDICAL DIAGNOSES
Sinusitis

A. Definition: inflammation of one or more of the sinuses of the frontal, ethmoid, sphenoid, or maxillary bones; secretions become infected; is acute but becomes chronic if not treated or leads to complications: septicemia, meningitis, brain abscess
B. Cause: results from the spread of organisms from the nose or trapped secretions interfering with drainage (e.g., nasal polyps or edema from allergy)
C. Signs and symptoms
1. Pain and headache
2. Nasal secretions, possibly purulent and blood tinged
3. Elevation of temperature; mild leukopenia
D. Diagnostic tests/methods
1. Patient history and physical assessment
2. X-ray examination
E. Treatment
1. Irrigation and inhalation of steam
2. Antibiotics and decongestants (see Chapter 4)
3. Surgery (e.g., Caldwell-Luc [infected maxillary sinus is removed through an incision under the upper lip] or ethmoidectomy)

F. Nursing intervention
1. Administer nonnarcotic analgesics or nasal constrictors (see Chapter 4)
2. Provide moist steam
3. Provide hot wet pack
4. Give general preoperative and postoperative care (see Chapter 2); note specific orders for care or observations

Epistaxis (Nosebleed)

A. Definition: bleeding from the nose
B. Cause: may be spontaneous, related to direct trauma, or a result of a systemic diseases (e.g., hypertension or blood dyscrasias); may be caused by local irritation from chronic infections or low-humidity environment
C. Sign: bleeding
D. Diagnostic tests/methods: patient history and physical examination
E. Treatment (only if bleeding cannot be stopped)
1. Nasal packing
2. Cauterization of site with 10% silver nitrate stick
3. Epinephrine spray
4. Treatment of systemic disease
5. Hemostatic agents
F. Nursing intervention
1. Maintain patent airway (direct patient to breathe through mouth); have suction available
2. Control bleeding: pinch nose firmly with fingers on soft part of nose; position in high-Fowler's with head forward
3. Instruct patient to expectorate blood (swallowing will cause vomiting)
4. Apply ice or cold compresses to nasal area to constrict blood vessels
5. Monitor vital signs
6. Avoid hot liquids
7. Provide oral hygiene

Deviated Septum

A. Definition: airway obstruction caused by deflection of bone and cartilage in the nasal septum
B. Causes
1. Trauma
2. Congenital
C. Diagnostic test/methods
1. Patient history
2. Physical assessment
3. X-ray examination
D. Treatment: surgery—submucous resection (SMR), performed through the mucous membrane within the nares; bone and cartilage are removed
E. Nursing intervention
1. Provide general preoperative and postoperative care (see Chapter 2)
2. Before surgery inform patient that nasal packing will be in place 24 to 48 hours; nasal-breathing will not be possible; there will be a temporary loss of smell; sneezing must be avoided; and there will be pain, discoloration, and swelling around the eyes
3. Maintain airway; place patient on side or in semi-Fowler's position; monitor respirations
4. Provide oral hygiene every 1 to 2 hours

5. Provide ice compresses; note bleeding on dressing; inspect back of throat for trickle of blood
6. Use rectal thermometer
7. Provide liquid diet when tolerated; encourage fluids; prevent constipation
8. Discourage forceful coughing

Polyps

A. Definition: grapelike swellings of tissue; nasal polyps obstruct breathing and block sinus drainage (see sinusitis)
B. Treatment: surgical removal

Laryngitis

A. Definition: an inflammation and swelling of the mucous membrane lining of the larynx
B. Cause: local irritation (e.g., smoking or spread of infection from elsewhere in the upper respiratory tract)
C. Signs and symptoms
   1. Hoarseness
   2. Pain
   3. Loss of voice
   4. Cough
D. Diagnostic tests/methods
   1. Physical assessment
   2. Patient history
E. Treatment and nursing intervention
   1. Rest voice; provide alternate means of communication
   2. Removal of cause
   3. Provide moist steam inhalations
   4. Administer astringent or antiseptic spray (see Chapter 4)

Carcinoma of the Larynx

A. Description: squamous cell carcinoma grows, spreads, and metastasizes; the rate of growth is determined by location of the lesion in the larynx
B. Causes: related to heavy smoking, chronic laryngitis and vocal abuse, and alcohol consumption
C. Signs and symptoms
   1. Hoarseness
   2. Signs of metastasis: pain, lump in throat, difficulty swallowing, dyspnea, and enlarged, painful lymph nodes
   3. Anxiety concerning surgery; confirmation of diagnosis; disfigurement
D. Diagnostic tests/methods
   1. Patient history
   2. Visual examination (laryngoscopy)
   3. Biopsy examination
E. Treatment: Surgery
   1. Removal of larynx (laryngectomy) (partial or complete)
   2. Radical neck dissection: wide excision including lymph nodes, epiglottis, thyroid cartilage, and muscle tissue; a permanent tracheostomy is performed
   3. Radiotherapy with surgery
F. Nursing intervention
   1. Provide general preoperative and postoperative care (see Chapter 2)
   2. Immediate postoperative care
      a. Maintain patent airway; patient may have a permanent tracheostomy (see nursing care and suctioning of a patient with a tracheostomy—Chapter 2); there will be a shorter tube (laryngectomy tube); place patient in semi-Fowler's position
      b. Observe dressing qh; connect wound drains to suction as ordered; prevent movement of head
   3. Continued postoperative care
      a. Provide method of communication (e.g., magic slate), leave call bell close to hand, and answer promptly in person
      b. Assist and be supportive as alternate methods of speech are learned (e.g., esophageal speech or use of mechanical voice box)
      c. Provide high-calorie, high-protein diet (may require tube feedings at first)
      d. Arrange for a visit from someone who has had a similar operation and satisfactory rehabilitation

Pneumonia

A. Description: an inflammation of the lungs or part of the lung (e.g., left lower lobe [LLL] pneumonia) secretions fill the alveolar sacs, which is a good medium for bacterial growth; the inflammation spreads to adjacent sacs; spaces of the lung consolidate with thick exudate; irritation may cause bleeding, and sputum has the characteristic rusty color; exchange of air is difficult and, in advanced conditions, not possible
B. Causes: bacterial infections and viruses are spread by respiratory secretions (droplets); chemical irritation; fungi and other organisms; patients with poor health and low natural resistance to infection are more susceptible (e.g., the elderly, those with chronic illness, and immunocompromised individuals)
C. Signs and symptoms
   1. Dyspnea, short of breath, pain on inspiration, shallow breathing, signs of air hunger, orthopnea, and oxygen deprivation
   2. Marked elevation in temperature
   3. Cough: painful and dry at first, then productive with copious amounts of thick sputum (color according to organism)
D. Diagnostic tests/methods
   1. Patient history
   2. Physical assessment with auscultation of chest
   3. Chest x-ray examination
   4. Sputum culture and sensitivity
   5. CBC
E. Treatment
   1. Specific and broad-spectrum antibiotics (see Chapter 4)
   2. Antipyretics, analgesics (codeine), expectorants, and bronchodilators (see Chapter 4)
   3. Intravenous (IV) fluids; force oral fluids
   4. Oxygen with humidity; incentive spirometer
F. Nursing intervention
   1. Provide optimum rest: provide care; help patient conserve energy; schedule rest periods; limit conversation; keep personal items and call bell within easy reach; alleviate anxiety
   2. Maintain oxygen with humidity
   3. Isolate as indicated, especially patients with oral and

nasal secretions; provide for proper disposal (see Isolation Technique, Chapter 2)
4. Liquefy secretions: force fluids (3000 ml daily or more); observe and document production of sputum; suction as necessary
5. Provide oral hygiene q2h
6. Monitor vital signs q4h; use rectal thermometer; monitor lung sounds
7. Assist with loosening of secretions: have patient turn, cough, and deep breathe q2h (splint chest if painful); observe and document cough
8. Maintain adequate nutrition: provide liquid-to-soft diet high in protein and calories
9. Maintain IV fluids and medication schedule to ensure continued blood levels
10. Position for comfort (high-Fowler's or lying on affected side)

Pleurisy

A. Description: inflammation of the pleural membranes (local or diffuse); may or may not have fluid exudate; when fluid is present, the condition is pleural effusion, when purulent, the condition is empyema
B. Cause: infections (e.g., pneumonia, lung abscess, or trauma)
C. Signs and symptoms
1. Sharp pain on inspiration (referred to shoulder, abdomen, or affected side)
2. Dyspnea and cough
3. Anxiety
4. Elevation of temperature
D. Diagnostic tests/methods
1. Chest x-ray examination
2. Patient history
3. Physical assessment including auscultation of chest
4. Examination of pleural fluid obtained via thoracentesis
E. Treatment (according to cause)
1. Analgesics and antibiotics
2. Drainage of fluid: thoracentesis, then chest tubes to underwater seal drainage with suction
3. Oxygen if dyspnea is severe; alleviate pain by turning patient to affected side
F. Nursing intervention: see plan for patient with chest tubes (the box to the right); provide diet high in protein, calories, minerals, and vitamins; alleviate anxiety

Pneumothorax/Hemothorax

A. Description
1. Pneumothorax: air in pleural space (see Chapter 3) allowing for partial or complete collapse of the lung
2. Hemothorax: blood in pleural space
B. Causes
1. May be spontaneous
2. Trauma (e.g., knife wound or fractured rib that punctures lung)
3. Postoperative (e.g., where the thoracic cavity has been entered)
C. Signs and symptoms
1. Sudden, sharp chest pain (when spontaneous)
2. Anxiety: diaphoresis, rapid pulse, and rapid respirations

Patient with Chest Tubes

Description

Drainage tubes are inserted between ribs into the pleural cavity to allow for drainage of secretions, blood, or air; the tube(s) is attached to an underwater seal system to allow for expansion of the lung and to prevent air from entering the pleural cavity; the drainage system may or may not be attached to suction

Indications

Chest surgery
Stab wounds of the chest
Pleural effusion
Spontaneous pneumothorax

Nursing intervention

Do complete assessment of the respiratory system q2h; place patient in semi-Fowler's position; provide oxygen with humidity
Prevent complications of immobility: have patient turn, deep breathe, and cough q2h; encourage patient to ambulate as ordered and as condition allows; splint chest to cough
Force fluids to liquefy secretions; provide tissues and bag for proper disposal; provide sputum cup
Provide oral hygiene q2h
Anticipate pain, medicate as needed, observe respirations 30 minutes after administration of sedative or analgesic
Observe underwater seal system qh
  Drainage color and amount
  Rise and fall of water in bottle (or suction) going to patient
  Bubbling (if connected to suction)
Alleviate anxiety

---

3. Vertigo
4. Decreased blood pressure
5. Decreased breath sounds
6. Dyspnea
D. Diagnostic tests/methods
1. Patient history and physical assessment
2. Chest x-ray examination
E. Treatment
1. Closure of wound with airtight dressing
2. Aspiration of fluids and air; water-seal drainage
3. Analgesics
4. Thoracentesis
F. Nursing intervention
1. Provide nursing care and observations as necessary for primary diagnosis
2. Place patient in high-Fowler's position
3. Monitor vital signs
4. Administer oxygen
5. Provide nursing care for a patient with chest tubes as described in the box above

Influenza

A. Description: acute disease that may occur as an epidemic; recovery is usually complete; no permanent immunity results; complications and death may occur in patients with chronic or debilitating conditions, especially cardiac or pulmonary

B. Cause: virus
C. Signs and symptoms
 1. Headache, chest pain, nuchal rigidity, and muscle ache
 2. Elevated temperature
 3. Coughing, sneezing, dry throat, nasal discharge, and herpetic lesions
 4. Gastrointestinal symptoms: nausea, vomiting, and anorexia
 5. Weakness
D. Diagnostic tests/methods: patient history and physical assessment
E. Treatment
 1. Prevention with vaccines
 2. Symptomatic
F. Nursing intervention
 1. Provide rest, assist with care; provide quiet environment and dim lighting
 2. Force fluids
 3. Relieve symptoms: provide antipyretics, analgesics

Pulmonary Tuberculosis

A. Description: a chronic, progressive infection; alveoli are inflamed, and small nodules are produced called primary tubercles; the tubercle bacillus is at the center of the nodule (these become fibrosed); the area becomes calcified and can be identified on x-ray film; the person who has been infected harbors the bacillus for life; it is dormant unless it becomes active during physical or emotional stress
B. Cause: *Mycobacterium tuberculosis,* Koch's bacillus, an acid-fast bacillus (AFB) spread by droplets from an infected person
C. Signs and symptoms
 1. Malaise; patient is easily fatigued
 2. Chest pain, cough, and hemoptysis (coughing up blood from the respiratory tract)
 3. Elevation of temperature and night sweats
 4. Anorexia and weight loss
 5. Anxiety, fear of chronic disease, and fear of public rejection
D. Diagnostic tests/methods
 1. Patient history and physical assessment
 2. Chest x-ray examination
 3. Sputum specimen for AFB; aspiration of gastric fluid for AFB if unable to obtain specimen
 4. Tuberculin skin testing (e.g., tine or Mantoux test)
E. Treatment
 1. Antituberculin drugs for 18 to 24 months (see Chapter 4)
 2. Rest (physical and emotional)
 3. Diet high in carbohydrates, proteins, and vitamins (especially B_6)
 4. Surgical resection of affected lung tissue or involved lobe (only when necessary)
F. Nursing intervention
 1. Provide rest; assist with or provide care; plan rest periods; limit conversation; leave personal items in easy reach
 2. Prevent transmission: ensure respiratory isolation; provide tissues and bag for disposal; encourage proper use of tissues; insist on patient covering mouth and nose when coughing or sneezing

3. Provide frequent, small meals and nutritious snacks
4. Avoid chills; keep skin dry and clean; protect from drafts, especially at night
5. Allay fears of patient and family about transmission: encourage proper adherence to drug maintenance; explain how organism is carried, transmitted, and destroyed (nurse must be aware that a tuberculin test is recommended for all contacts with a person with tuberculosis (TB); a positive test result does not mean the disease has manifested but indicates that the organism has entered the body and that the body has produced antibodies at some point

Chronic Obstructive Pulmonary Disease

Chronic obstructive pulmonary disease (COPD) includes chronic and frequently progressive pulmonary disorders that affect expiratory air flow; asthma, chronic bronchitis, and pulmonary emphysema may occur independently or together.

Asthma

A. Description: spasms of the bronchial muscle occur; edema and swelling of the mucosa produce thick secretions; air flow is obstructed; air enters and is trapped; a characteristic wheeze accompanies attempts to exhale through narrowed bronchi; breathing is labored; coughing is attempted, but patient fails to expectorate satisfactory amounts; patient experiences great anxiety; the attacks last 30 to 60 minutes, often with normal breathing between attacks; if attack is difficult to control, and is resistant to all forms of treatment, it is called *status asthmaticus*
B. Causes
 1. Recurrent respiratory infection
 2. Allergic reaction
 3. Physical or emotional stress may provoke attack in a person with asthma
C. Signs and symptoms
 1. Shortness of breath, expiratory wheeze, labored respirations, and diaphoresis
 2. Thick, tenacious sputum (after acute attack)
 3. Anxiety or feeling of suffocation
D. Diagnostic tests/methods: patient history and physical examination
E. Treatment
 1. Removal of cause (source of allergy) or desensitization
 2. Low-flow, humidified oxygen
 3. Bronchodilators, mast cell inhibitors, corticosteroids, or sedatives (see Chapter 4)
F. Nursing intervention
 1. Reduce anxiety: provide time to listen; do not leave patient alone during attack
 2. Remove cause: keep environment free from dust and other allergens
 3. Provide continuous humidity as ordered
 4. Force fluids; maintain IV as ordered
 5. Position for maximum comfort and breathing: have patient sit in high-Fowler's position with arms supported by over-bed table
 6. Prevent secondary infections: avoid staff and visitors with upper respiratory infections

7. Teach abdominal breathing
8. Do not allow smoking; refer patient for help in quitting

Chronic Bronchitis

A. Description: chronic, progressive infection accompanied by hypersecretion of mucus by the bronchioles; without treatment and prevention of acute attacks, the alveolar sacs and capillaries will extend and destruct
B. Causes
   1. Asthma
   2. Acute respiratory tract infections (e.g., pneumonia, influenza, smoking, and air pollution contribute to incidence)
   3. Familial tendency
C. Signs and symptoms
   1. Problems related to acute infection
   2. Cough, productive with thick, white sputum; sputum is blood tinged as disease progresses (cough is greatest on arising)
D. Diagnostic tests/methods
   1. Patient history
   2. Pulmonary testing to rule out other disease (e.g., tuberculosis or malignancy)
E. Treatment
   1. Prevent irritation of bronchial mucosa: encourage patient to discontinue smoking and change aggravating conditions in occupation or home environment
   2. Prevent upper respiratory tract infection: maintain optimum health, adequate rest, and high-protein, high-vitamin diet
   3. Provide bronchodilators, antibiotics, corticosteroids, and influenza vaccine during epidemics (see Chapter 4)
F. Nursing intervention
   1. Provide care to relieve patient problems (see discussion on frequent patient problems and nursing care outlined earlier in this chapter)
   2. Loosen, liquefy, and remove secretions: provide postural drainage and chest percussion as ordered; force fluids
   3. Involve patient and family in care and care planning
   4. Do not allow smoking; refer patient for help in quitting

Emphysema

A. Description: a chronic, progressive condition in which the alveolar sacs distend, rupture, and destroy the capillary beds; the alveoli lose elasticity, inspired air is trapped; inspiration is difficult and expiration is prolonged; the lung tissue becomes fibrotic; exchange of gases is not possible; anxiety increases; signs of oxygen deprivation are evident
B. Cause (see discussion on bronchitis)
C. Signs and symptoms
   1. Dyspnea on exertion (later, dyspnea on slightest exertion and orthopnea); inspiration is difficult; expiration is prolonged, accompanied by wheeze
   2. Chronic cough; productive, purulent sputum in copious amounts
   3. Difficulty talking: speaks in short, jerky sentences

4. Cerebral anoxia: is drowsy and confused; may become unconscious and go into coma
5. Barrel chest
6. Anorexia, weight loss, and weakness
D. Diagnostic tests/methods
   1. Patient history and physical examination
   2. Chest x-ray examination
   3. Pulmonary function tests
   4. Arterial blood gasses; CBC
   5. Sputum analysis
E. Treatment (see discussion on bronchitis)
F. Nursing intervention
   1. Loosen, liquefy, and remove secretions: provide postural drainage and chest percussion as ordered; force fluids; administer expectorants as needed
   2. Promote respiratory function: breathing exercises and coughing
   3. Administer oxygen; oxygen is administered in low concentrations only (1 to 2 L); oxygen can be dangerous when the carbon dioxide level of the blood is high; the respiratory center of the brain becomes accustomed to the low blood oxygen level; if oxygen increases, respiratory rate will slow significantly
   4. Prevent and control infections: administer antibiotics; avoid contact with people with upper respiratory tract infections; avoid smoking
   5. Provide rest: limit exertion of any type; provide care; minimize conversation; assist with all movements (e.g., turning and getting into chair)
   6. Include family in care and care plan; be understanding that this condition is chronic
   7. Teach pursed-lip breathing; abdominal breathing

Cancer of the Lung

A. Description: primary or secondary (from metastasis [e.g., from prostate]) malignant tumor; bronchogenic carcinoma is the most common primary tumor; is usually without symptoms until late stages when metastasis has occurred to brain, spinal cord, or esophagus; treatment is difficult in late stages and usually is symptomatic; prognosis is poor unless detected and treated early
B. Cause: exact cause is unknown, but strongly related to smoking, air pollution, and chemical irritants
C. Signs and symptoms (occur in late stages)
   1. Productive cough with blood-streaked sputum
   2. Dyspnea and chest pain
   3. Fatigue, anorexia, and weight loss
D. Diagnostic tests/methods
   1. CT scan; MRI
   2. Examination of sputum for cells
   3. Bronchial biopsy examination
E. Treatment
   1. Surgery: procedure depends on size and location of tumor (lobectomy or pneumonectomy)
   2. Radiation
   3. Chemotherapy
F. Nursing intervention
   1. Provide nursing care for symptoms (see discussion on frequent patient problems and nursing care earlier in chapter)
   2. Provide preoperative and postoperative nursing care (see Chapter 2)

a. Maintain patent airway; administer oxygen; have patient turn, cough, and deep breathe q2h; a patient with a pneumonectomy must not cough; do not turn on operative side until physician orders (prevent mediastinal shift)

b. Provide special care for a patient with chest tubes (rarely used, but still a possibility)

The Cardiovascular System

Diseases related to the cardiovascular system are the leading cause of death in the United States. Cardiovascular health problems occur across the age continuum. To reduce death and disability, three major objectives include early detection of the disease, appropriate treatment to control the disease progression, and reduction of predisposing factors by promoting screening, education, and patient care of cardiovascular health.

NURSING ASSESSMENT

A. Nursing observations
  1. Skin for temperature and color; jaundice, cyanosis, and pallor
  2. Auscultation of vascular bruits and murmurs
  3. Distended neck veins
  4. Thorax for precordial movement
  5. Abnormal heart sounds/dysrhythmias
  6. Extremities for club-shaped fingers and toes; presence of edema
  7. Irregular pulses
  8. Abnormal respirations
B. Patient description (subjective data)
  1. Chest pain during periods of physical and emotional stress; pain may radiate to arm or jaw
  2. Easily fatigued
  3. Dyspnea on exertion
  4. Palpitations
  5. Dizziness or actual fainting
  6. Hemoptysis
  7. Family history of heart disease and hypertension

DIAGNOSTIC TESTS/METHODS

A. Electrocardiogram (ECG)
  1. A tracing of the electrical activity of the heart
  2. A tool used to identify abnormal cardiac rhythms (dysrhythmias) and coronary atherosclerotic heart disease
  3. Reassure the patient that the ECG is recording the electrical impulses of the heart and is not delivering any electrical impulses to the body
B. Stress test
  1. A procedure designed to detect cardiac ischemia that develops during exercise or exertion
  2. A heart tracing (ECG) is recorded and monitored while a patient performs an activity such as stair climbing, pedaling a stationary bicycle, or walking on a treadmill
C. Blood tests
  1. Complete blood count (CBC): analyzes components of the blood
    a. Low hemoglobin and hematocrit indicate anemia
    b. Elevated WBC count indicates inflammation/infection

  2. Erythrocyte sedimentation rate (ESR): may indicate inflammation
  3. Blood urea nitrogen (BUN) and creatinine: to detect the effects of heart disease on the kidneys
  4. Serum enzymes and isoenzymes (serum glutamic-oxaloacetic transaminase [SGOT], creatine phosphokinase [CPK], and lactate dehydrogenase [LDH]): will elevate in a myocardial infarction
  5. Serum lipids: elevated blood lipids have been associated with coronary disease
  6. Blood cultures: if bacterial endocarditis is suspected
  7. Coagulation studies: useful in monitoring anticoagulant therapy
  8. Serum electrolytes: detect imbalances in sodium, potassium, and calcium
  9. Arterial blood gases: monitor oxygenation and acid-base balance
D. Urinalysis: to determine the effects of heart disease on the kidney
E. Holter monitoring
  1. Portable monitor designed and equipped to record the patient's heartbeat during a 24-hour period; a written record of the patient's activity is kept simultaneously; helpful in determining dysrhythmias
  2. Assist the patient in the recording of activity
F. Coronary angiography
  1. A roentgenogram of the coronary circulation facilitated by the introduction of contrast medium into the artery to outline the vessel and determine the extent of the disease process
  2. After the study the patient must be observed for bleeding from the puncture site and have a cardiovascular status check of the involved area (pulses and skin temperature)
G. Chest x-ray examination: a standard chest roentgenogram is used to determine heart size and shape
H. Echocardiography (ultrasound cardiography)
  1. Echoes from sound waves are used to study the movements and dimensions of cardiac structures; determines abnormalities
  2. Information derived includes size of cardiac structures
I. Radionuclide studies
  1. Tracing material is injected intravenously, and the radioactivity emitted over a body part is recorded
  2. Size, shape, and filling of the heart chambers can be recorded; heart damage can also be evaluated
J. Cardiac catheterization
  1. A cardiac catheter is introduced through a vein or artery and is advanced through the system; pressures of the heart chambers and pulmonary arteries are recorded and blood is analyzed; a contrast dye can be injected for visualization of certain structures to detect defects
  2. Patient may feel a warm flushing sensation on injection of the dye; some patients experience chest pain
  3. Patient observations after examination: monitor bleeding at the insertion site, check pulses and skin warmth in the involved area, and check heart rate and rhythm
K. Oscillometry: a noninvasive test that measures the amplitude of pulsations over an artery

FREQUENT PATIENT PROBLEMS AND NURSING CARE

A. Pain related to decreased cardiac output; overactivity
   1. Evaluate and record onset, duration, and intensity
   2. Note any associated symptoms (nausea, vomiting, dyspnea, etc.)
   3. Monitor vital signs and record
   4. Give vasodilators as prescribed; monitor for effectiveness and observe for side effects
   5. If pain is unrelieved in 15 minutes by drugs or rest, notify physician
   6. Reinforce patient teaching regarding diet, drugs, planned exercise, and stress management
   7. Record reactions to treatment and nursing care

B. Ineffective breathing pattern related to dyspnea
   1. Monitor vital signs and record
   2. Note character and rate of respirations
   3. Elevate the head of the bed at least 30 degrees
   4. Help patient assume an orthopneic position when necessary
   5. Auscultate chest and note the presence of abnormal lung and heart sounds
   6. Monitor oxygen therapy
   7. Monitor intake and output
   8. Record reactions to treatment and nursing care
   9. Give diuretics, cardiotonics, and bronchodilators as prescribed and monitor for side effects
   10. Note color, character, and amount of sputum

C. Decreased cardiac output related to dysrhythmias
   1. Monitor vital signs and record
   2. Note and report any changes in the vital signs
   3 Auscultate chest, noting any abnormal heart sounds and report abnormalities
   4. Give antidysrhythmic drugs as prescribed and monitor for side effects
   5. Monitor for and report any associated symptoms

D. Impaired tissue perfusion related to edema
   1. Note and record location and degree
   2. Elevate legs
   3. Change positions when in bed
   4. Note degree of pitting
   5. Note "weeping" of skin areas
   6. Monitor for skin breakdown
   7. Give prescribed diuretics and cardiotonics
   8. Note the presence of tenderness in the upper quadrant of the abdomen
   9. Note the presence of ascites
   10. Note daily weight
   11. Record intake and output
   12. Limit fluid intake as prescribed
   13. Reinforce teaching for reduction of dependent edema

E. Fatigue/activity intolerance related to reduced cardiac reserve
   1. Encourage progressive ambulation
   2. Encourage progressive resuming of activites of daily living
   3. Provide for planned activity and rest periods
   4. Monitor for signs of fatigue
   5. Stop activity at the first sign of intolerance
   6. ROM exercises
   7. Provide prescribed diet
   8. Reinforce patient instruction of planned exercise

F. Alteration in tissue perfusion related to decreased cardiac output
   1. Observe for presence of postural hypotension
   2. Assist patient to dangle legs over the side of the bed before standing
   3. Instruct patient to get up slowly
   4. Assess patient's pulse when standing

G. Fluid volume excess related to decreased cardiac output
   1. Note daily weight; report weight changes
   2. Record intake and output
   3. Monitor serum electrolytes
   4. Limit fluids as prescribed
   5. Provide salt-restricted diet if ordered
   6. Give diuretic medication as prescribed
   7. Reinforce instructions regarding diet, drugs, and weight control

H. Alteration in tissue perfusion related to hypertension
   1. Monitor vital signs and report changes
   2. Provide sodium-restricted diet as prescribed
   3. Provide cholesterol-controlled diet if prescribed and monitor for side effects
   5. Instruct in the avoidance of risk factors (smoking, stress, and obesity)
   6. Reinforce teaching in the areas of diet, weight control, avoidance of risk factors, and home monitoring of blood pressure

MAJOR MEDICAL DIAGNOSES
Arteriosclerosis-Atherosclerosis

A. Definition
   1. Arteriosclerosis: a process in which the arterial walls harden, thicken, and lose their elasticity, resulting in restricted blood flow
   2. Atherosclerosis: one form of arteriosclerosis; fatty plaques form on the intima (inner layer) of the arteries

B. Pathology
   1. The underlying mechanism is the formation of fatty plaque deposits in the arteries
   2. The plaque increases in size and ultimately obstructs blood flow to vital areas

C. Arteriosclerosis is associated with the following health problems
   1. Coronary artery disease
   2. Angina pectoris
   3. Myocardial infarction
   4. Hypertension
   5. Peripheral vascular disease
   6. Cerebrovascular accidents (strokes)

D. Signs and symptoms vary, depending on the arteries affected by the sclerosing process
   1. Extremity involvement
      a. Cramping pain (intermittent claudication)
      b. Numbness and tingling
      c. Reduced circulation causing ulceration or pain
      d. Outward changes: skin pallor, cool skin, reduced or absent pulses, loss of leg hair, and skin ulceration
   2. Coronary involvement
      a. Chest pain
      b. Dyspnea

c. Palpitations

d. Fainting (syncope)

e. Fatigue

E. Diagnostic tests/methods

1. Patient history and physical examination

2. Arteriograms

3. ECG

4. Oscillometry

F. Treatment

1. Dietary restriction of fat and cholesterol

2. Vasodilating drugs

3. Cholesterol-lowering drugs

4. Elimination or reduction of risk factors

   a. Smoking

   b. Obesity

   c. Stress

   d. Lack of exercise

5. Weight management

6. Planned exercise

7. Prevention of pressure on extremities

8. Use of special devices such as bed cradles

9. Bypass surgery or removal of plaques may be considered

G. Nursing intervention

1. Assess and document signs and symptoms

2. Protect the extremity from trauma

3. Monitor protective devices (bed cradles, pads, etc.)

4. Provide skin care to ulcerated areas or areas affected by reduced circulation

5. Monitor pulses and skin character of involved extremities

6. Report changes in the involved extremities

   a. Absence of pulse

   b. Cyanosis

   c. Increased pain

   d. Temperature change (coldness)

7. Monitor for signs and symptoms of infection in ulcerated areas

8. Provide slow, progressive physical activity as prescribed

9. Give prescribed diet

10. Administer prescribed drugs

11. Relieve pain from ischemia

12. Avoid cold and provide adequate warmth to prevent vasoconstriction

13. Avoid clothing that impairs circulation

14. Educate patient and family regarding avoidance of risk factors, dietary management, medication, and activity

Angina Pectoris

A. Definition: episodes of acute chest pain resulting from insufficient oxygenation of myocardial tissue, caused by decreased blood flow to the area

1. Episodes occur most frequently during periods of physical or emotional exertion

   a. Exercise

   b. Eating a heavy meal

   c. Environmental temperature extremes

2. Episodes seldom last more than 15 minutes

B. Causes

1. The major cause is atherosclerosis

2. Narrowed coronary arteries obstruct blood flow; thus oxygen carried by the blood cannot sufficiently meet tissue demands, particularly during periods of exertion

C. Signs and symptoms

1. Substernal chest pain, usually brought on by exertion

2. Radiation of pain to the jaw or an extremity

3. Dyspnea

4. Anxiety or feeling of impending doom

5. Tachycardia

6. Diaphoresis

7. Sensation of heaviness, choking, or suffocation

8. Indigestion

D. Diagnostic tests/methods

1. Patient history and physical examination

2. ECG

3. Holter monitoring

4. Coronary angiography

5. Stress testing

6. Chest x-ray examination

7. Serum lipid and enzyme values

E. Treatment

1. Relief of chest pain through the use of vasodilating drugs (e.g., nitrates, beta blockers, calcium channel blockers), sedatives, and analgesics

2. Dietary restriction of fat and cholesterol

3. Planned exercise

4. Weight management

5. Stress management

6. If conservative measures are unsuccessful, coronary bypass surgery or an angioplasty may be considered

F. Nursing intervention

1. Assess and document signs and symptoms and reactions to treatment

2. Administer vasodilating medication and monitor for side effects

3. Instruct patient to inform the nursing staff at the onset of an anginal attack

4. Provide emotional support and assurance

5. Provide prompt relief of pain

6. Monitor vital signs, particularly during an attack

7. Educate patient and family regarding diet, activity, drug therapy, and avoidance of risk factors

Hypertension (High Blood Pressure)

A. Definition: characterized by persistent elevation of blood pressure in which the systolic pressure is above 140 mm Hg and the diastolic pressure is above 90 mm Hg

1. Primary hypertension (essential): a persistent elevation of blood pressure without an apparent cause

   a. Actual cause is unknown

   b. Primarily, small blood vessels are affected; peripheral resistance increases; and blood pressure rises

   c. Constricted blood vessels eventually cause damage to organs that rely on a blood supply from these vessels

2. Secondary hypertension: a persistent elevation of blood pressure associated with another disease state

   a. Renal disease

   b. Toxemia

   c. Adrenal dysfunction

d. Atherosclerosis
e. Coarctation of the aorta

B. Predisposing factors
1. Smoking
2. Obesity
3. Heavy salt and cholesterol intake
4. Heredity
5. Aggressive, hyperactive personality
6. Age: develops between 30 and 50 years of age
7. Sex: primarily men over 35 years of age and women over 45 years of age
8. Race: blacks have twice the incidence of whites
9. Birth control pills and estrogens

C. The heart, brain, kidney, and eyes can be damaged if the hypertensive state continues without correction

D. Signs and symptoms may be insidious and vague; a person can have the disorder and not know it
1. Tinnitus
2. Light-headedness
3. Blurred vision
4. Irritability
5. Fatigue
6. Tachycardia and palpitations
7. Occipital, morning headaches
8. Nosebleeds (epistaxis)
9. Dyspnea on exertion

E. Diagnostic tests/methods
1. Patient history and physical examination
2. Series of resting blood pressure readings
3. Routine urinalysis, BUN, and serum creatinine to screen for renal involvement
4. Serum electrolytes to screen for adrenal involvement
5. Blood sugar levels to screen for endocrine involvement
6. Lipid profile
7. Chest x-ray examination
8. ECG
9. Holter monitoring
10. Funduscopic eye examination

F. Treatment
1. Lowering blood pressure through the use of antihypertensive drugs
2. Sodium-restricted diet
3. Cholesterol-controlled diet
4. Weight management
5. Stress management
6. Reduction or elimination of smoking
7. Planned exercise

G. Nursing intervention
1. Assess and document signs and symptoms and reactions to treatments
2. Administer prescribed medication
3. Observe for and report drug-related side effects
4. Monitor weight every day (qd) to evaluate initial diuretic therapy
5. Monitor intake and output to evaluate initial diuretic therapy
6. Monitor vital signs, particularly blood pressure, under the same conditions qd
7. Provide planned activity and rest periods
8. Provide prescribed diet
   a. Calorie controlled
   b. Sodium restricted
   c. Cholesterol controlled
9. Educate patient and family
   a. Drug therapy and side effects
   b. Dietary restrictions; weight management
   c. Elimination of risk factors, such as smoking
   d. Activity
   e. Blood pressure monitoring
   f. Need for participation and compliance of the prescribed regimen

Myocardial Infarction (Heart Attack)

A. Definition: the obstruction of a coronary artery or one of its branches
1. The obstruction results in the death of the myocardial tissue supplied by that vessel
2. The myocardial tissue dies because of oxygen deprivation (Fig. 6-1)
3. The heart's ability to regain or maintain its function depends on the location and size of the area of infarction

B. A myocardial infarction can occur whenever a coronary artery or branch of the artery becomes occluded by a thrombus, emboli, or the atherosclerotic process.

C. Signs and symptoms
1. "Crushing" chest pain lasting longer than 15 minutes and unrelieved by rest or drugs
2. Shortness of breath
3. Nausea and vomiting
4. Tachycardia
5. Diaphoresis and pallor
6. Temperature rise after 48 hours
7. Elevation of the cardiac enzymes
8. Dysrhythmias
9. Anxiety

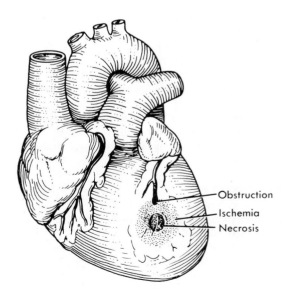

FIG. 6-1. Myocardial infarction: areas of ischemia and necrosis. (From Billings DM, Stokes LG: *Medical-surgical nursing: common health problems of adults and children across the life span*, St Louis, 1986, Mosby.)

D. Diagnostic tests/methods
   1. Patient history and physical examination
   2. ECG
   3. Cardiac enzyme studies (SGOT, LDH, CPK-MB)
   4. Chest x-ray examination
E. Treatment
   1. Analgesic drugs to relieve pain
   2. Oxygen to relieve respiratory distress
   3. Vasopressor drugs to prevent circulatory collapse (cardiogenic shock)
   4. Cardiac monitoring to detect dysrhythmias
   5. Hemodynamic monitoring: internal monitoring of the blood pressure and pulmonary artery pressure
   6. Bed rest with progressive activity to allow the damaged myocardium to heal
   7. Intravenous (IV) fluids to provide for IV drug administration
   8. Cardiopulmonary resuscitation in the event of cardiac standstill (arrest)
   9. Pacemaker insertion
   10. Anticoagulant therapy
   11. Thrombolytic therapy to dissolve blood clot and restore blood flow
F. Nursing intervention
   1. Provide pain relief
   2. Provide ongoing assessment and documentation of symptoms and reactions to treatment
   3. Administer and monitor oxygen
   4. Record vital signs qh during the acute period
   5. Record intake and output qh during the acute period
   6. Provide best rest during the acute period and progressive activity as prescribed
      a. Apply antiembolism stockings
      b. Allow patient out of bed to use bedside commode (less taxing to the cardiovascular system)
      c. Monitor pulse during periods of activity
   7. Avoid activities that produce straining (Valsalva's maneuver) to avoid taxing the cardiovascular system
      a. Administer stool softeners as prescribed
      b. Caution patient against straining when attempting a bowel movement
   8. Provide diet as prescribed
      a. May start out on liquids and then progress
      b. Sodium and cholesterol may be restricted
      c. Caffeine may be restricted
   9. Give prescribed antidysrhythmics and monitor for side effects
   10. Give prescribed cardiotonics and diuretics and monitor for side effects
   11. Monitor for complications
      a. Cardiogenic shock: circulatory collapse caused by decreased cardiac output; the vital organs are not being perfused
         (1) Monitor vital signs every 15 minutes
         (2) Record intake and output qh
         (3) Report changes in rate, rhythm, and conductivity
         (4) Observe and report signs and symptoms of restlessness, diaphoresis, pallor, low blood pressure, and tachycardia
         (5) Administer and monitor prescribed vasopressors and antidysrhythmics

         (6) Administer oxygen as prescribed
         (7) Provide cardiac and hemodynamic monitoring (hemodynamic monitoring refers to the internal monitoring of blood pressure and pulmonary artery pressure)
      b. Pulmonary edema: left ventricle failure (pumping mechanism) caused by strain on a diseased heart; cardiac output (the amount of blood pumped out by the heart to the body per minute) is reduced, resulting in lung congestion
         (1) Observe and report symptoms of anxiety, dyspnea, orthopnea, frothy, pink-tinged sputum, rales, decreased urine output, and dependent edema
         (2) Record vital signs every 15 minutes
         (3) Record intake and output qh
         (4) Place bed in high-Fowler's position
         (5) Administer cardiotonics and diuretics as prescribed and monitor for side effects
         (6) Administer and monitor oxygen therapy
         (7) Use rotating tourniquets: to reduce the circulatory volume to the right side of the heart
         (8) Be prepared to administer analgesics to allay anxiety and reduce respiratory rate
         (9) Provide emotional support to patient and family

Congestive Heart Failure

A. Definition: failure of the pumping mechanism of the heart resulting in an insufficient blood supply to meet the body's needs
B. Causes
   1. The underlying mechanism in congestive heart failure (CHF) involves the failure of the pumping mechanism of the heart to respond to the metabolic changes of the body
   2. The end result is a heart that cannot supply a sufficient amount of blood in relation to the body's needs and to the amount of blood returning to the heart (venous return); pressure builds up in the vascular beds on the affected side of the heart
C. CHF is described in terms of left-sided or right-sided failure, depending on which side is affected
D. Signs and symptoms are divided into left-sided failure and right-sided failure, although both sides may be affected
   1. Left-sided failure leads to pulmonary congestion
      a. Dyspnea
      b. Orthopnea
      c. Nonproductive cough that worsens at night
      d. As severity of failure increases, frothy, blood-tinged sputum is noted
      e. Anxiety and restlessness
      f. Fatigue
   2. Right-sided failure may follow left-sided failure and results in systemic venous congestion
      a. Weight gain caused by fluid accumulation in the tissues
      b. Dependent edema in the form of ankle edema or sacral edema
      c. Ascites caused by the collection of fluid in the

abdominal cavity; ascites may also hinder respiration

   d. Fatigue

   e. Gastrointestinal symptoms such as nausea, vomiting, and anorexia

   f. Decreased urine output

E. Diagnostic test/methods

   1. Patient history and physical examination including the findings of edema, abnormal heart sounds, and the presence of rales with dyspnea (orthopnea)

   2. Chest x-ray examination

   3. ECG

   4. Arterial blood gas studies

   5. Liver function studies

   6. Renal function studies

F. Treatment

   1. Drug therapy: digitalization, diuretics, and sedatives

   2. Recording of weight qd

   3. Monitoring intake and output

   4. Oxygen therapy

   5. Rotating tourniquets (seldom used)

   6. Restricting fluids

   7. Restricting dietary sodium

   8. Bed rest with progressive activity

   9. Elevate the head of the bed on blocks

   10. Monitor vital signs

G. Nursing intervention

   1. Provide ongoing assessment and documentation of signs, symptoms, and reactions to treatment

   2. Monitor oxygen therapy

   3. Record vital signs every 15 minutes to 2 hours during the acute phase

   4. Record intake and output qh during the acute phase

   5. Weigh patient qd

   6. Administer and monitor prescribed cardiotonics, diuretics, and sedatives; observe for side effects

   7. Determine the amount of activity that produces the least discomfort to the patient

   8. Monitor for dependent edema

     a. Ankle edema when sitting upright

     b. Sacral edema when in supine position

   9. Raise the head of the bed as prescribed

   10. Observe for complications of bed rest

     a. Have patient turn, cough, and take deep breaths

     b. Apply antiembolism stockings

   11. Provide emotional support to the patient and family

   12. Provide a diet low in sodium if prescribed

   13. Educate the patient and family concerning dietary management, drug therapy, and activity

   14. Restrict fluids as ordered

Valvular Disease

A. Valvular dysfunction results in either stenosis or insufficiency of the heart valves

   1. Valvular stenosis results from cardiac infections; the valve leaflets (cusps) become fibrotic and thicken and may even fuse together, thus hindering blood flow

   2. Valvular insufficiency occurs in much the same way as valvular stenosis; after repeated infections the valve leaflets (cusps) become inflamed and scarred and no longer close completely; the incomplete closure allows blood to leak from the left ventricle into the left atrium during systole

B. Blood flow through the heart is altered, resulting in decreased cardiac output, systemic and pulmonary congestion, and dilation of the heart chambers

C. Causes

   1. Rheumatic heart disease is the primary cause of valvular dysfunction

   2. Other causes include syphilis, bacterial endocarditis, and congenital malformations

D. Signs and symptoms

   1. Mitral stenosis

     a. Dyspnea on exertion

     b. Orthopnea

     c. Pink-tinged sputum

     d. Fatigue

     e. Palpitations

     f. Heart murmur

   2. Mitral insufficiency

     a. Fatigue

     b. Dyspnea or exertion

     c. Heart murmur

     d. Orthopnea

     e. Pulmonary congestion

   3. Aortic stenosis

     a. Fatigue

     b. Angina

     c. Syncope

     d. Heart murmur

     e. Congestive heart failure

   4. Aortic insufficiency

     a. Palpitations

     b. Dyspnea

     c. Fatigue

     d. Orthopnea

     e. Anginal pain occurring even at rest

E. Diagnostic tests/methods

   1. Patient history and physical examination; a murmur is a common finding of the examination

   2. ECG

   3. Chest x-ray examination: to determine heart size

   4. Cardiac catheterization: may reveal pressure changes

   5. Echocardiogram: provides information concerning structure and function of valves

   6. Laboratory studies

F. Treatment

   1. Mitral stenosis

     a. Antibiotics administered prophylactically to prevent recurrences of causative agents

     b. Drug therapy: diuretics, cardiotonics, and antidysrhythmics

     c. Restricted sodium diet

     d. Planned activity and avoidance of symptom-producing activity

     e. Surgical correction of the defect

       (1) Mitral commissurotomy: the fused valve leaflets are separated, and the mitral opening may be dilated

       (2) Valve replacement: diseased valve is replaced with a prosthetic valve

   2. Mitral insufficiency

     a. Planned exercise and avoidance of symptom-producing activity

     b. Sodium-restricted diet

c. Drug therapy: diuretics, cardiotonics, antidysrhythmics, and vasodilators
d. Surgical correction
   (1) Valvuloplasty: repair of the existing valve
   (2) Valve replacement
3. Aortic stenosis
  a. Prevention of infective endocarditis
  b. Treatment of symptoms
  c. Drug therapy: diuretics, nitrates, and cardiotonics
  d. Sodium-restricted diet
  e. Valve replacement

G. Nursing intervention
1. Assess and document signs and symptoms and reaction to treatments
2. Administer prescribed medication and observe patient for side effects
3. Provide a calm, quiet environment
4. Allow patient and family to verbalize their anxieties and fears
5. Monitor vital signs and report changes
6. Weigh the patient qd
7. Provide the prescribed diet
  a. Nutritionally well balanced
  b. Sodium restricted to prevent fluid retention
8. Progressive activity as prescribed
  a. Consider the patient's limitations
  b. Provide rest periods
9. Monitor intake and output if diuretics are used
10. Educate patient and family concerning diet, drugs, activity, and need for compliance
11. Vocational counseling may be needed if the patient has a demanding job

Inflammatory Disorders of the Heart

A. Definition: diseases resulting from acute or chronic inflammation of the lining of the heart and valves caused by bacteria or viruses, trauma, or other factors
1. Pericarditis: an inflammation of the pericardium
  a. The result is a loss of elasticity or fluid accumulation within the pericardial sac
  b. Heart failure and cardiac tamponade may result
2. Myocarditis: an inflammation of the myocardium
  a. The result is impairment of contractility
  b. Myocardial ischemia and necrosis may result
3. Endocarditis: an inflammation of the inner lining of the heart and valves associated with a streptococcal infection
4. Rheumatic heart disease
  a. Usually associated with rheumatic fever
  b. Rheumatic fever is an inflammatory process that can affect all the layers of the heart
  c. Cardiac impairment results from swelling and scarring of valve leaflets, leading to valvular changes (mitral insufficiency, aortic insufficiency, and pericarditis)

B. Signs and symptoms
1. Chest pain
2. Dyspnea
3. Chills and intermittent fever
4. Weakness and fatigue
5. Diaphoresis
6. Anorexia
7. Dysrhythmias
8. Elevated cardiac enzymes
9. Friction rubs (auscultatory sound created by the rubbing together of two serous surfaces)
10. Presence of Aschoff bodies (collection of cells and leukocytes in the interstitial layers of the heart)
11. New heart murmur or an abnormal heart sound
12. Existing streptococcal infection
13. Cardiac enlargement
14. Joint involvement

C. Diagnostic tests/methods
1. Patient history and physical examination
  a. History of recent infections
  b. History of heart disease
2. ECG
3. Chest x-ray examination
4. Cardiac enzyme studies
5. Blood cultures
6. Echocardiogram: to assess valvular disease and vegetation (growth of scar tissue)
7. Laboratory studies: CBC, electrolytes, ESR
8. Radionuclide studies: to assess heart structure and heart damage

D. Treatment
1. Identification and elimination of the infecting agent
2. Drug therapy: antibiotics, cardiotonics, antiinflammatory agents, analgesics, and corticosteroids
3. Blood cultures
4. Rest and planned activity
5. Well-balanced diet
6. Prevention of exposure to other infectious agents

E. Nursing intervention
1. Assess and document signs and symptoms and reactions to treatment
2. Maintain a calm, quiet environment
3. Administer prescribed drugs and monitor for side effects
4. Evaluate the patient's understanding of the disease process and the need for compliance
5. Alleviate pain
6. Allay patient's and family's fears and anxieties
7. Monitor vital signs and report changes
8. Observe for signs and symptoms of complications (tachycardia, dyspnea, and orthopnea)
9. Educate patient concerning the illness, diet, drugs, activity, avoidance of infections, dental care, vocational counseling, and compliance to the regimen

Peripheral Vascular Disease

Peripheral vascular disease refers to vascular disorders exclusive of those affecting the heart. The underlying factor in peripheral vascular disease is the arteriosclerotic process. Blood flow is slowed because of vessels that are narrowed or obstructed. The lack of normal blood flow causes tissue changes (see arteriosclerosis under assessment of the cardiovascular system). Vascular disease related to the lower extremities is discussed in this section.

NURSING ASSESSMENT

A. Nursing observation
1. Skin of the lower extremities
  a. Redness (hyperemia) of the leg when in a dependent position

b. Cold or blue feet
c. Varicose veins
d. Sparse hair distribution
e. Lesions or stasis ulcers
f. Edema
g. Dermatitis or brown pigmentation of the skin
2. Delayed capillary filling
3. Diminished or absent pulses
   a. Rigidity (hardness) of the vessels
   b. Palpable vibration of the vessels (thrill)
4. Assess major arteries for bruits (an auscultatory sound taking the form of a buzzing or humming sound)
5. Differences in leg circumference
6. Thickening of nail beds
B. Patient description (subjective data)
1. Leg cramps
2. Aching calves
3. Leg numbness
4. Leg pain occurring during exercise (claudication)
5. Loss of sensation in the leg(s)
6. Past or present history
   a. Alcohol excess
   b. Diabetes mellitus
   c. Hypertension
   d. Thrombophlebitis

DIAGNOSTIC TESTS/METHODS

A. Chest x-ray examination for abnormalities
B. Oscillometry: a noninvasive test that measures the amplitude of pulsations over an artery
C. Doppler ultrasonography: a device that emits sound waves that can be used to measure the amount of blood flow through a vessel
D. Arteriography: Used to determine the location and extent of the disease process
E. Venography: radiographic study used to determine the location and size of a blood clot, vessel distention, and development of collateral circulation
F. Trendelenburg test
1. Used to determine valvular competency
2. The leg is elevated to 90 degrees, and a tourniquet is placed around the thigh
3. The patient stands, and the vein-filling pattern is observed
4. Normally the veins fill slowly from below in 20 to 30 seconds; the rate of filling should not greatly accelerate when the tourniquet is removed
G. Lung scan
1. Used to assess the presence of pulmonary embolism and lung damage.
2. An intravenous, radiographic isotope is injected into the patient
3. Pulmonary circulation is assessed with a scanning device
4. The patient also inhales a radioactive gas and is scanned to determine lung distribution of this gas
H. Arterial blood gas analysis: used to assess the adequacy of ventilation
I. X-ray examination of the abdomen: may show evidence of an aneurysm

J. Blood tests
1. CBC: for routine evaluation
2. ESR: used to determine the presence of an inflammatory process
3. Coagulation studies (platelet count, bleeding time, prothrombin time [PT], and partial thromboplastin time [PTT]: used to determine the existence of blood disorders

FREQUENT PATIENT PROBLEMS AND NURSING CARE

A. Pain related to intermittent claudication
1. Evaluate and record onset, duration, and intensity
2. Provide rest during the episode
3. Determine the amount of exercise the patient can tolerate before claudication occurs
4. Assess for and report claudication occurring without activity
5. Educate the patient to avoid exposure to cold and maintain warmth
B. Fluid volume excess related to edema of the lower extremities/decreased cardiac output
1. Note and record location and degree
2. Instruct patient to avoid activity that places the legs in a dependent position for prolonged periods
3. Instruct patient to avoid wearing constricting clothing around the legs
4. Monitor for skin breakdown
5. Elevate legs
C. Impaired skin integrity related to stasis ulcers
1. Note location and character of ulceration
2. Maintain bed rest with leg elevation
3. Perform prescribed wound care
4. Instruct patient to avoid trauma to the legs
5. Instruct patient in proper skin care measures
6. Reinforce patient teaching in the area of drugs, diet, activity, and skin care

MAJOR MEDICAL DIAGNOSES
Arteriosclerosis Obliterans

A. Definition: a chronic arteriooclusive disease
1. Progresses slowly and insidiously
2. The medial and intimal layers of arteries become inflamed and thrombosed
3. There is loss of vessel elasticity, and plaques obstruct blood flow
4. Vessels primarily affected are the femoral and carotid arteries
B. Causes
1. Associated with atherosclerotic process
2. Predisposing factors include hypertension, smoking, hyperlipidemia, obesity, and a positive family history
C. Signs and symptoms
1. Intermittent claudication
2. Pain in the legs at rest
3. Impotence
4. Paresthesia
5. Pallor or blanching on elevation of leg
6. Hyperemia (redness) or dusky appearance of the leg(s) when dependent
7. Loss of hair on extremities
8. Absent or diminished pulses

D. Diagnostic tests/methods
1. Patient history and physical examination
2. Oscillometry
3. Doppler ultrasonography
4. Arteriography
5. Laboratory studies
E. Treatments
1. Protection of extremity from injury
2. Prevention and control of infection
3. Drug therapy: vasodilators, analgesics, and antibiotics
4. Weight-reduction diet if patient is obese
5. Bed rest
6. Avoidance of smoking
7. Surgical management: endarterectomy (removing the obstructing plaque) or a bypass graft
F. Nursing intervention
1. Assist the patient in obtaining body warmth and warmth to the extremity
   a. Warm room
   b. Warm bath
   c. Warm clothes such as socks
2. Avoid applying direct heat to the affected part
3. Protect the affected part from trauma and pressure
   a. Use bed cradle
   b. Assess skin lesions and monitor for signs of infection
   c. Caution patient against wearing anything that constricts
4. Give prescribed drugs and monitor for side effects
5. Assess the affected part qd
   a. Assess skin color, temperature, and circulation
   b. Monitor for pain
6. Provide emotional support
7. Educate the patient and family regarding
   a. Hygiene and avoidance of infection
   b. Rest and planned exercise
   c. Protection from injury
   d. Diet
   e. Drugs
   f. Improvement of circulation

Buerger's Disease (Thromboangiitis Obliterans)

A. Definition: an inflammatory process primarily affecting arteries that causes occlusion, thrombosis, and ultimately ischemia
1. Medium-sized distal arteries of the legs are primarily affected
2. Veins can also be affected
B. Causes
1. Exact cause is unknown
2. Associated with smoking
3. Men in the 25- to 40-year age group who smoke are at risk
4. Familial tendency
C. Signs and symptoms
1. Coldness of the extremities
2. Diminished or absent pulses
3. Numbness and tingling
4. Cramping pain (intermittent claudication)
5. Pain at rest, not associated with activity
6. Skin ulceration

7. Aggravation of symptoms by exposure to cold environment
8. Change in appearance of extremities
9. Muscle atrophy
10. Slow-healing cuts
11. Gangrene
12. Sensitivity to cold
D. Diagnostic tests/methods
1. Patient history and physical examination
2. Oscillometry
3. Doppler ultrasonography
4. Arteriography
5. Laboratory studies
6. ECG
7. Chest x-ray examination
E. Treatment
1. Restricting smoking
2. Drug therapy: vasodilating drugs, analgesics, and anticoagulants
3. Moderate exercise
4. Avoidance and treatment of infection
5. Protection from trauma
6. Sympathectomy (disruption of nerve impulses to a particular area)
7. Nerve blocks (use of drug injections to block nerve impulses)
8. Amputation, as a last resort
F. Nursing intervention
1. Support the patient in his effort to stop smoking
2. Give prescribed vasodilators, analgesics, and anticoagulants; monitor for side effects
3. Document location and character of pain
4. Assist the patient in maintaining warmth
5. Educate the patient and family concerning drug therapy, activity, and avoidance of smoking, exposure to cold, constricting clothing, and trauma

Raynaud's Disease

A. Definition: a peripheral vascular disease affecting digital arteries
1. Disease occurs primarily in women
2. Exposure to environmental cold, emotional stress, or tobacco use produces spasms of the arteries
3. Hands and arms are usually affected
B. Cause
1. Exact cause is unknown
2. Associated with collagen diseases in women
C. Contributing factors
1. Pressure to the fingertips such as that encountered by typists and pianists
2. Use of hand-held vibrating equipment on a regular basis
D. Signs and symptoms
1. Numbness and tingling
2. Blanching of digits and cyanosis
3. Hyperemia
4. Coldness
5. Dryness and atrophy of the nails
6. Pain
7. Punctate (small holes) lesions of the fingertips
8. Eventual gangrene of the fingertips

E. Diagnostic tests/methods
1. Patient history and physical examination
2. Doppler ultrasonography
3. Arteriography
4. ECG
5. Chest x-ray examination

F. Treatment
1. Drug therapy with vasodilators
2. Sympathectomy: in advanced cases
3. Elimination of smoking
4. Avoidance of stressful situations
5. Avoidance of exposure to cold

G. Nursing intervention
1. Document location and characteristics of pain
2. Observe affected areas qd
3. Administer prescribed vasodilators and analgesics; monitor for side effects
4. Instruct patient to avoid activities that precipitate spasms
5. Instruct patient to avoid exposing the hands to the cold without proper protection
6. Support patient's effort to give up smoking
7. Offer emotional support and allay anxiety
8. Educate patient and family concerning drug therapy, avoidance of cold, protection from trauma/infection, and prevention of spasms

Aneurysms

A. Definition: the enlargement or ballooning of an artery, usually caused by trauma, congenital weakness, arteriosclerosis, or infection; aorta is most frequently affected artery

B. Causes
1. Causes are varied, but the prime culprit is arteriosclerosis; plaque formation causes degenerative changes leading to loss of vessel elasticity, weakness, and dilation
2. Syphilis
3. Infections
4. Congenital disorder
5. Trauma

C. Signs and symptoms
1. Abdominal
a. Increased blood pressure
b. Visible or palpable pulsating mass
c. Pain or tenderness in the abdominal area
2. Thoracic
a. Dyspnea
b. Dysphagia
c. Hoarseness or cough
d. Severe chest pain
3. Ruptured aneurysm
a. Anxiety
b. Restlessness
c. Pain
d. Diminished pulses
e. Hypotension and shock

D. Diagnostic tests/methods
1. Patient history and physical examination
2. Chest x-ray examination
3. Abdominal x-ray examination
4. Ultrasonography

5. Angiography/arteriography
6. Routine ECG
7. Laboratory studies

E. Treatment
1. Conservative measures
a. Drug therapy: antihypertensives, pain relievers, and negative inotropic agents
b. Correct hydration and electrolyte imbalances
c. Decreased activity
2. Surgical repair
a. Resection and replacement with a prosthesis of Teflon or Dacron
b. Resection and replacement with a graft

F. Nursing intervention
1. Provide immediate postoperative care
a. Assess vital signs and peripheral pulses every 15 minutes; then decrease the frequency as ordered
b. Record intake and output qh
c. Compare extremities for warmth and color
d. Administer IV fluids at prescribed rate
e. Relieve pain with prescribed analgesic
f. Monitor oxygen therapy
g. Give prescribed prophylactic antibiotics as ordered
h. Assess level of consciousness every 1 to 2 hours
i. Auscultate lung sounds and bowel sounds at least q4h
j. Monitor for dysrhythmias
k. Have patient turn, cough, and deep breathe at least q2h
2. Other postoperative considerations
a. Provide antiembolism stockings
b. Provide emotional support and allay anxiety
c. Encourage early ambulation as prescribed
d. Instruct patient to observe for changes in the extremities such as color and warmth
e. Instruct patient on assessments of peripheral pulses

Phlebitis and Thrombophlebitis

A. Definition: inflammatory disorders of the veins
1. Phlebitis: inflammation of a vein
2. Thrombophlebitis: inflammation of a vein with clot formation

B. Causes
1. The inflammation and clot formation are associated with venous stasis, vessel damage, and enhanced blood coagulability
2. Situations that produce venous stasis include immobility, prolonged periods of standing, wearing confining clothing, and increased abdominal pressure

C. Signs and symptoms
1. Redness and pain along vein path
2. Elevation of temperature
3. Swelling
4. Positive Homans' sign (pain on dorsiflexion of the foot)
5. Area is sensitive to the touch

D. Diagnostic tests/methods
1. Patient history and physical examination
2. Doppler ultrasonography

3. Venography
4. Laboratory studies: CBC, ESR, and coagulation studies
5. Lung scan to rule out pulmonary embolism

E. Treatment
1. Bed rest
2. Anticoagulant therapy
3. Warm, moist packs to the affected leg (some physicians prefer ice packs to the area)
4. Antiembolism stockings
5. Elevation of affected extremity
6. Surgical intervention is required in only a small percentage of patients

F. Nursing intervention
1. Assess and document signs and symptoms
2. Administer analgesics as ordered and monitor for side effects
3. Elevate leg as ordered; avoid the use of a knee gatch or pillow under the affected knee; avoid crossing legs
4. Apply warm, moist heat as ordered
5. Assess thigh and calf measurements qd
6. Monitor vital signs q4h
7. Maintain bed rest as ordered
8. Apply antiembolism stockings on unaffected leg
9. Avoid massaging calf of affected leg
10. Avoid constrictive clothing
11. Monitor anticoagulant therapy
12. Monitor for bleeding tendencies
   a. Bleeding gums
   b. Epistaxis
   c. Bruising easily
   d. Melena
   e. Petechiae
13. Monitor hemoglobin and hematocrit levels
14. Educate patient and family concerning drug therapy, avoiding activities that aggravate the existing state, and monitoring for signs and symptoms of complications
15. Monitor patient for complications such as an embolism

Embolism

A. Definition: a blood clot circulating in the blood
B. Causes
1. The clot may be a fragment of an arteriosclerotic plaque, or it may have originated in the heart
2. If large, an embolism may lodge in a vessel bifurcation and obstruct the flow of blood to vital organs or tissues
3. Most emboli arise from deep vein thrombi; the embolis travels in the bloodstream until it lodges in a narrowed area, usually the lungs
C. Signs and symptoms: depend on the area involved
1. Pain at the site
2. Shock
3. Areas supplied by the involved vessel evidence pallor, coldness, numbness, tingling, and cyanosis
4. Sudden onset of dyspnea
5. Cough and hemoptysis
6. Chest pain
7. Tachycardia

8. Tachypnea
D. Diagnostic tests/methods
1. Patient history and physical examination
2. Lung scan
3. Chest x-ray examination
4. Arterial blood gases
E. Treatment
1. Oxygen therapy
2. IV fluids
3. IV anticoagulants
4. Analgesics
5. Thrombolytic agents
F. Nursing intervention
1. Assess and document signs and symptoms and reactions to treatments
2. Monitor vital signs
3. Monitor arterial blood gas reports
4. Administer prescribed analgesic and monitor for side effects
5. Administer anticoagulants as prescribed and monitor for bleeding tendencies
6. Monitor oxygen therapy
7. Give ROM exercises
8. Provide antiembolism stockings
9. Educate patient and family concerning drug therapy, monitoring for bleeding tendencies, and restriction of activities

Varicose Veins

A. Definition: dilated, tortuous leg veins resulting from blood back-flow caused by incomplete valve closure; this leads to congestion and further enlargement
B. Causes
1. Basic cause of varicosities is unknown
2. Predisposing factors: heredity, pregnancy, obesity, and aging
C. Signs and symptoms
1. Leg fatigue and aching
2. Leg cramping and pain
3. Heaviness in the legs
4. Dilated veins
5. Ankle edema
D. Diagnostic tests/methods
1. Patient history and physical examination
2. Venography
3. Trendelenburg test
E. Treatment
1. Rest with elevation of legs
2. Exercise
3. Support stockings
4. Avoid prolonged standing, sitting, and crossing the legs
5. Weight management
6. Surgical vein stripping/ligation; vein sclerosing
F. Nursing intervention
1. After surgery check legs for color, movement, temperature, and sensation
2. Provide leg exercises as prescribed
3. Reinforce the importance of weight management
4. Instruct the patient to avoid prolonged sitting and standing
5. Avoid constrictive clothing

The Hematologic System

Disorders of hemopoiesis refer to problems of the blood-forming tissues. These include the blood cells, bone marrow, spleen, and lymph system. This discussion includes descriptions of the anemias, leukemia, and acquired immunodeficiency syndrome.

NURSING ASSESSMENT

A. Nursing observations
   1. Mouth ulcerations
   2. Incoordination
   3. Tachycardia
   4. Tachypnea
   5. Hypotension
   6. Pallor and jaundice
   7. Pruritus
   8. Smooth tongue
B. Patient description (subjective data)
   1. Weakness and fatigue
   2. Irritability
   3. Anorexia
   4. Nausea and vomiting
   5. Dyspnea
   6. Bleeding from the mouth and nose
   7. Numbness, tingling, and burning of the feet
   8. Headache
   9. Incoordination
   10. Easy bruising
   11. Nonhealing cuts
   12. Swollen, tender lymph nodes

DIAGNOSTIC TESTS/METHODS

A. Red blood cell (RBC) count
   1. RBCs are formed in the bone marrow
   2. RBCs transport oxygen to cells and take carbon dioxide to the lungs
   3. Circulating RBC counts elevate in conditions such as anemia and hypoxia
   4. The blood study is used in routine screenings
B. Erythrocyte indexes (mean cell volume, mean cell hemoglobin concentration, and mean cell hemoglobin)
   1. Aid in describing the anemias
   2. Provide a relationship between the number, size, and hemoglobin content of the RBCs
C. Hemoglobin and hematocrit levels
   1. Provide an index to the severity of the anemia
   2. Hematocrit refers to the number of packed RBCs found in 100 ml of blood
   3. Hemoglobin is the oxygen-carrying component of the RBC and is more reliable in determining the severity of the anemia
D. Reticulocyte count
   1. Provides information concerning the cause of the anemia
   2. Indicates whether the anemia is a result of diminished production or excessive loss or destruction of RBCs
E. Sedimentation rate
   1. Not specific to anemias
   2. Elevated ESR suggests the presence of an underlying disease process; therefore further workup may be indicated

F. Serum iron
   1. Helpful in classifying the anemia
   2. Useful in differentiating an acute from a chronic disorder
G. Total iron-binding capacity (TIBC): helpful in classifying the anemia and differentiating between an acute and a chronic disorder
H. Serum bilirubin
   1. Useful in evaluating the degree of RBC hemolysis
   2. Bilirubin is formed from the hemoglobin of destroyed RBCs
   3. Elevations may indicate the increased destruction of RBCs caused by a particular disease process
I. Schilling test
   1. Used in classifying anemias, particularly a vitamin B_{12} disorder
   2. Helps differentiate between an intrinsic factor deficiency and an intestinal absorption disorder
   3. Patient preparation
      a. The patient may be instructed to take nothing by mouth (NPO) before the test
      b. Oral radioactive vitamin B_{12} is administered
      c. Nonradioactive parenteral dose is given 2 hours later
      d. Urine collection follows
      e. A third of the vitamin appears in the urine; little or no radioactivity in the urine suggests a gastrointestinal malabsorption problem
      f. Procedure may be repeated with the addition of intrinsic factor to the oral vitamin B_{12}
      g. Nonabsorption of B_{12} without intrinsic factor but absorption with the intrinsic factor is suggestive of pernicious anemia
   4. Nursing intervention
      a. Explain the basic procedure to the patient
      b. Maintain NPO
      c. Collect the urine at the specified time
J. Vitamin B_{12} level
   1. Used to help classify the anemias
   2. Provides an index for determining the adequacy of B_{12} levels and the need for further evaluation
   3. Vitamin B_{12} is important for normal hematopoiesis
K. Serum folate level
   1. Folic acid is another important factor in hematopoiesis
   2. Useful in classifying the anemias
L. Gastric analysis
   1. Nasogastric tube is inserted and then histamine is injected to stimulate gastric secretions
   2. Gastric contents are aspirated and analyzed
   3. Achlorhydria (absence of hydrochloric acid) is a feature of pernicious anemia
M. Sickle cell preparation
   1. The reaction of the blood specimen in hypoxia is observed
   2. Sickling of cells in hypoxia suggests sickle cell trait or sickle cell anemia
N. Hemoglobin electrophoresis
   1. An electric field separates the specimen into the various types of hemoglobin present
   2. Hemoglobins S and A suggest sickle cell anemia or trait
   3. Hemoglobin F suggests thalassemia

O. Bone marrow biopsy
  1. Bone marrow aspiration provides information about blood cell production
  2. Test may be used in patients suspected of having leukemia, aplastic anemia, and other hematologic disorders
  3. Sample of marrow may be obtained from the sternum, iliac crest, vertebrae, or vertebral body
  4. Procedure
    a. The skin over the designated area is prepared and anesthetized
    b. The needle is inserted into the center of the bone, and a small amount of marrow is aspirated
  5. Nursing intervention
    a. Allay patient's anxiety before examination
    b. Assist with the marrow as instructed
    c. Place patient in a comfortable position after the procedure
    d. Monitor pain status (soreness remains for several days)
    e. Monitor puncture site for bleeding
P. WBC count and differential
  1. Determines the total number of leukocytes
  2. The differential helps analyze each type of WBC and determine if the amount present is in proper proportion
  3. Aids in the diagnosing of infection and blood disorders such as leukemia
Q. Platelet count
  1. Evaluates adequacy of platelet levels
  2. If platelet levels drop below a certain level, spontaneous hemorrhage is possible
R. Serum for HIV: determines the presence of the AIDS virus
S. Lymphangiography: radiologic examination used to detect lymph node involvement

FREQUENT PATIENT PROBLEMS AND NURSING CARE

A. Activity intolerance related to weakness and fatigue
  1. Provide planned activity and rest periods
  2. Monitor for signs of fatigue
  3. Reinforce patient teaching of planned activity and exercise
  4. Assist patient with activities of daily living
  5. Assess vital signs as ordered
B. Potential alteration in tissue perfusion related to hypotension
  1. Observe for evidence of postural hypotension
  2. Assist patient to dangle legs over the side of the bed before standing
  3. Instruct patient to get up slowly
  4. Assess patient's pulse when standing
C. Ineffective breathing pattern related to dyspnea on exertion
  1. Note the degree or kind of activity that causes dyspnea
  2. Note character and rate of respirations during the episodes
  3. Instruct the patient to stop the activity and relax when dyspnea is experienced
  4. Assist the patient in planning activities so that dyspnea will not occur

  5. Reinforce patient teaching regarding planned exercise and rest periods
D. Impaired swallowing caused by ulcerations of the mouth and tongue
  1. Assess the ulcerated areas qd
  2. Provide mouth care with a soft-bristle brush or cotton swab
  3. Offer soothing mouthwashes every 2 to 4 hours
  4. Instruct the patient to avoid ingesting food or drink that may aggravate the ulcers
E. Fluid volume deficit related to hemorrhage
  1. Assess for signs of bleeding
    a. Tarry stools
    b. Hematuria
    c. Bleeding gums
    d. Bleeding tendency
    e. Petechiae
    f. Epistaxis
  2. Protect from trauma and injury
  3. Avoid parenteral injections
  4. Have patient use soft-bristle brush for mouth care
  5. Monitor vital signs at least q4h
  6. Monitor hemoglobin and hematocrit values
  7. Encourage intake of fluids and the prescribed diet
F. High risk for infection related to interference with the immune system
  1. Prevent exposure to others with infection
  2. Monitor for signs and symptoms of infection
  3. Give prescribed drugs and monitor for side effects
  4. Place in protective isolation if ordered

MAJOR MEDICAL DIAGNOSES
Anemia Caused by Decreased RBC Production

A. Normally there is a balance between RBC production and RBC destruction; however, alterations do occur that significantly affect RBC production
  1. Iron deficiency anemia
    a. Results from insufficient dietary intake of iron, which is needed for the formation of hemoglobin and RBCs
    b. Other causes: malabsorption, blood loss, and hemolysis
  2. Pernicious anemia
    a. Caused by a lack of intrinsic factor in the GI tract
    b. Intrinsic factor is needed for the absorption of vitamin B_{12}
    c. Anemia usually results from a loss of the mucosal surface of the GI tract, which secretes intrinsic factor
    d. Patients undergoing total gastrectomies and small bowel resections are at risk
  3. Folic acid deficiency anemia
    a. Folic acid is required in the synthesis of DNA, which in turn is necessary for the production of RBCs
    b. Common causes: poor diet (lacking in green, leafy vegetables, citrus fruits, liver, grains, and dried beans), malabsorption, and drugs that interfere with the absorption of folic acid
  4. Thalassemia
    a. Unlike the other three anemias, thalassemia is a genetic disorder resulting in abnormal hemoglobin synthesis

b. The main problem is an inadequate production of normal hemoglobin; hemolysis is a secondary problem
c. People of Mediterranean ancestry are at risk
d. Mild forms of this anemia (thalassemia minor) may be asymptomatic
e. Patients with a more severe hemolytic form (thalassemia major) may experience hepatomegaly, splenomegaly, jaundice, and bone marrow hypertrophy

B. Signs and symptoms
1. Skin changes
   a. Pallor
   b. Jaundice
   c. Pruritus
   d. Dermatitis
2. Eye and visual disturbances
   a. Blurred vision
   b. Scleral icterus
3. Mouth
   a. Glossitis
   b. Smooth tongue
   c. Ulcerations of the mucosa
4. Cardiovascular
   a. Tachycardia
   b. Murmurs
   c. Angina
   d. Congestive heart failure (CHF)
   e. Hypotension
5. Respiratory
   a. Tachypnea
   b. Dyspnea on exertion
   c. Orthopnea
6. Neurologic
   a. Dizziness
   b. Headaches
   c. Irritability
   d. Depression
   e. Incoordination
   f. Impaired thought processes
7. Gastrointestinal (GI)
   a. Nausea and vomiting
   b. Anorexia
   c. Hepatomegaly
   d. Splenomegaly
8. General
   a. Weight loss
   b. Weakness and fatigue
   c. Bone pain
   d. Numbness, tingling, and burning of the feet

C. Diagnostic tests/methods
1. Patient history and physical examination
2. Routine chest x-ray examination
3. Routine ECG
4. Schilling test
5. Gastric analysis
6. CBC
7. Bone marrow aspiration or biopsy
8. Serum iron level

D. Treatment
1. Iron therapy
2. Increase dietary iron intake
3. Vitamin B_{12} replacement (pernicious anemia)
4. Folic acid replacement
5. Use of hematinics
6. Blood transfusions (thalassemia)

E. Nursing intervention
1. Assess and document signs and symptoms and reactions to treatments
2. Provide planned activity alternated with rest periods
3. Assist patient with activities of daily living to avoid fatigue
4. Monitor supplemental oxygen therapy in use
5. Administer prescribed drugs and monitor for side effects
6. Monitor blood transfusions
7. Provide oral hygiene, particularly if mouth ulcers are present
8. Provide the prescribed diet
9. Instruct patient to get up from bed or chair slowly to avoid dizziness
10. Instruct patient on avoiding and preventing exposure to infection
11. Support patient and allay anxiety
12. Educate patient and family concerning drugs, diet therapy, and planned activity

Anemia Caused by RBC Destruction

A. Definition: a process in which RBCs are being destroyed faster than they are produced
B. Known causes of RBC destruction
1. Snake venom
2. Infections
3. Drugs or chemicals
4. Heavy metals or organic compounds
5. Antigen-antibody reaction
6. Splenic dysfunction
7. Congenital causes
   a. Thalassemia: a group of hereditary hemolytic anemias characterized by a defect or defects in one or more of the hemoglobin polypeptide chains
   b. Sickle cell anemia: see Chapter 9, Pediatric Nursing
   c. Spherocytosis: A hemolytic anemia characterized by spherocytes (small, globular erythrocytes without the characteristic central pallor) in the blood; the abnormal cells are destroyed by the spleen
   d. Glucose-6-phosphate dehydrogenase (G6PD) deficiency: a hemolytic disorder brought on by stressors such as infection, certain drugs, acidosis, and toxic substances; individuals with this genetic disorder are relatively symptom free until they experience the stressor that initiates the hemolytic process

C. Signs and symptoms
1. Anemia
2. Jaundice
3. Splenomegaly
4. Hepatomegaly
5. Weakness and fatigue
6. Skin pallor
7. Anorexia

8. Weight loss
9. Dyspnea
10. Tachycardia
11. Tachypnea
12. Hypotension
13. Cholelithiasis (gallstones): caused by excessive bilirubin

D. Diagnostic tests/methods
1. Patient history and physical examination
2. Laboratory studies
3. Routine chest x-ray examination
4. Routine ECG
5. Bone marrow biopsy
6. Renal studies to monitor kidney status

E. Treatment
1. Identify the causative agent
2. Blood or blood product replacement
3. Supportive care
4. Genetic counseling
5. Splenectomy to halt the destruction of abnormal RBCs by the spleen
6. Maintain renal function
7. Maintain fluid and electrolyte balance

F. Nursing intervention
1. Assess and document signs and symptoms and reactions to treatment
2. Monitor vital signs as ordered and report abnormalities
3. Allay fears and anxieties
4. Provide planned exercise and rest periods
5. Caution patient to get up slowly from the bed or chair to avoid postural hypotension
6. Assist patient with activities of daily living
7. Monitor intake and output
8. Monitor laboratory studies
9. Encourage intake of fluids
10. Provide prescribed diet
11. Administer prescribed drugs and monitor for side effects
12. Educate patient and family concerning drugs, diet, activity, and compliance to the prescribed regimen

Aplastic Anemia (Hypoplastic)

A. Definition: a failure of the bone marrow to produce adequate amounts of erythrocytes, leukocytes, and platelets

B. Exact cause is unclear (idiopathic)
1. May be congenital
2. Related to radiation exposure
3. Results from a disorder that suppresses bone marrow (cancer)
4. Exposure to toxic substances may be a contributing factor

C. Signs and symptoms
1. General symptoms of anemia; refer to the preceding outlines in this section
2. Susceptibility to infection
3. Fever
4. Bleeding tendencies

D. Diagnostic tests/methods
1. Patient history and physical examination
2. Laboratory studies, particularly WBC count and platelet count; a reduced WBC count predisposes

patient to infection; a low platelet count predisposes patient to a bleeding disorder
3. Bone marrow biopsy examination to evaluate blood cell production
4. Routine chest x-ray examination
5. Routine ECG

E. Treatment
1. Identify the causative agent
2. Supportive care
3. Administration of blood or blood products
4. Hydration with IV fluids
5. Protect from injury and infections
6. Prevent hemorrhage
7. Splenectomy
8. Bone marrow transplant

F. Nursing intervention
1. Assess and document signs and symptoms and reactions to treatment
2. Monitor vital signs at least q4h
3. Monitor for and report signs of bleeding
4. Give prescribed medication and monitor for side effects
5. Avoiding fatiguing the patient; provide planned exercise and rest periods
6. Prevent injury and exposure to infection
7. Neutropenic precautions may be necessary
8. Monitor supplemental oxygen if ordered
9. Provide and encourage the prescribed diet
10. Allay fears and anxiety
11. Provide oral hygiene, avoiding aggravation of bleeding gums
12. Provide skin care using protective devices and frequent repositioning
13. Educate patient and family concerning drug therapy, diet, planned activity, avoidance of injury and infection, monitoring for bleeding tendencies, and compliance with the regimen

Leukemia

A. Definition: a disorder of the hematopoietic system characterized by an overproduction of immature WBCs
1. As the disease progresses, fewer normal WBCs are produced
2. The abnormal cells continue to multiply and eventually infiltrate and damage the bone marrow, spleen, lymph nodes, and other organs

B. Classification of leukemias
1. Two major categories are acute and chronic
   a. Acute leukemia has a rapid onset; cells in this phase are young, undifferentiated, and immature
   b. Chronic leukemia has a gradual onset; cells are mature and differentiated
2. Further classification: identifying the type of WBC involved
   a. Acute granulocytic leukemia: the myeloblasts proliferate; myeloblasts are the precursors of granulocytes
   b. Acute lymphoblastic leukemia: immature lymphocytes proliferate in the bone marrow
   c. Chronic granulocytic leukemia: excessive neoplastic granulocytes are found in the bone marrow

d. Chronic lymphocytic leukemia: characterized by inactive, mature-appearing lymphocytes

C. Leukemia is considered a neoplastic process; cause is unknown

D. Predisposing factors
1. Familial tendency
2. Viral origin
3. Exposure to chemicals
4. Exposure to radiation

E. Once leukemia is diagnosed, the aim of therapy is to prolong survival by attaining a state of remission
1. Management of acute leukemia is aggressive
2. Management of chronic leukemia aims to control the disorder and maintain remission
3. All forms of leukemia are fatal if untreated

F. Signs and symptoms
1. General symptoms of anemia
2. Decreased resistance to infection
3. Fever
4. Bleeding tendencies
5. Enlarged lymph nodes
6. Splenomegaly
7. Hepatomegaly
8. Elevated WBC count
9. Low platelet count and low hemoglobin and hematocrit levels
10. Poor appetite
11. Mouth ulcers
12. Diarrhea

G. Diagnostic tests/methods
1. Patient history and physical examination
2. Laboratory studies to evaluate peripheral blood
3. Bone marrow biopsy
4. Routine chest x-ray examination
5. Routine ECG
6. Lymph node biopsy examination

H. Treatment
1. Drug therapy: chemotherapeutic agents, analgesics, sedatives, and antibiotics
2. Radiation therapy
3. Bone marrow transplants are still under investigation
4. Hydration with IV fluids
5. Replacement of blood and blood products
6. Monitoring renal status
7. Protection against infection (neutropenic precautions if needed)
8. Prevention of hemorrhage

I. Nursing intervention
1. Assess and document signs and symptoms and reactions to treatment
2. Prevent patient from being exposed to infection
   a. Screen visitors
   b. Monitor WBC counts
3. Avoid fatigue
   a. Provide planned exercises and rest periods
   b. Assist patient with activities of daily living
4. Monitor for bleeding tendencies
5. Administer blood or blood components as ordered and monitor for side effects
6. Monitor intake and output
7. Encourage intake of fluids
   a. Keep fluids at the bedside
   b. Provide patient with favorite fluids

8. Administer prescribed medication as ordered and monitor for side effects
   a. Analgesics and sedatives
   b. Antiemetics
9. Monitor IV fluids
   a. Monitor the IV site for infiltration
   b. Monitor rate
10. Allay anxieties and fears
11. Monitor vital signs at least q4h and report abnormalities
12. Monitor supplemental oxygen if ordered
13. Provide and encourage the prescribed diet
14. Provide oral hygiene, which avoids aggravation of bleeding and drying of the mouth
15. Provide skin care to include the use of protective devices and frequent repositioning
16. Educate patient and family concerning drug therapy, diet, activity, monitoring for bleeding tendencies, avoidance of injury and infection, and compliance with the regimen

Acquired Immunodeficiency Syndrome (AIDS)

A. Definition: a viral disorder that disrupts the balance of T-lymphocytes and ultimately destroys them, rendering the body incapable of defending itself against infection; course is progressive and fatal

B. Causes
1. The virus is spread by sexual contact; sharing of infected needles by drug abusers; and blood and blood products
2. Infected mothers can pass on the virus to the unborn baby
3. The virus may also enter the body when contaminated blood or body fluids come in contact with broken skin surfaces
4. Symptoms may occur 2 to 6 weeks after exposure; seroconversion may not occur until 8 to 12 weeks or longer

C. Signs and symptoms (vary with each patient; may harbor the virus, but be asymptomatic for months)
1. Swollen lymph glands
2. Recurrent fever; night sweats
3. Weight loss; diminished appetite
4. Chronic diarrhea
5. Fatigue
6. White patches or lesions in the mouth
7. Presence of opportunistic infections such as *Pneumocystis carinii* (pneumonia) and Kaposi's sarcoma (purplish skin lesions)
8. Dry cough; shortness of breath

D. Diagnostic tests/methods
1. Patient history and physical examination
2. Serum for HIV
3. Presence of opportunistic infections
   a. *Pneumocystis carinii* pneumonia
   b. Kaposi's sarcoma
4. Bronchial biopsy
5. Lumbar puncture
6. CT scan
7. Enzyme-linked immunosorbent assay (ELISA); detects antibodies for HIV; false positives may occur
8. Western blot test: used to confirm the results of a positive ELISA test; detects HIV antibodies

E. Treatment
1. Treatment is instituted according to the symptoms
2. Protect the patient from opportunistic infections
3. Vaccines are still in experimental stages (e.g., azidothymidine [AZT] interferes with replication of HIV virus/may slow disease process)
4. Nutritional support
F. Nursing care
1. Assess and document signs and symptoms and reactions to treatment
2. Monitor vital signs
3. Monitor arterial blood gas, CBC, and platelet count
4. Administer prescribed medication and monitor for side effects
5. Employ blood and body fluid precautions
a. Wear protective clothing (gloves, masks, goggles, gowns, etc.) as needed for the procedure
b. Wash hands thoroughly
c. Label specimens accordingly
d. Dispose of contaminated articles properly
6. Plan activity followed by rest periods
7. Encourage physical independence
8. Monitor oxygen therapy
9. Monitor pain status and provide analgesia and comfort measures
10. Support patient and allay anxiety
11. Educate the patient and family concerning mode of spread, protective measures, and home care

The Gastrointestinal System

The GI system provides a means by which food and fluid enter the body and are converted into elements that help maintain the human organism. It is important to note that other systems of the body influence this system. The endocrine system, central nervous system, and autonomic nervous system all serve as regulators to the GI system.

NURSING ASSESSMENT

A. Nursing observations
1. Gingivitis
2. Stomatitis
3. Hematemesis
4. Stool changes: melena, clay-colored, or frothy stool
5. Constipation or diarrhea
6. Hemorrhoids
7. Distention
8. Jaundice
9. Edema
10. Dark urine
B. Patient description (subjective data)
1. Nausea and vomiting
2. Difficulty chewing
3. Dysphagia
4. Appetite change: increase or decrease
5. Weight changes
6. Indigestion and dyspepsia
7. Intolerance to certain foods
8. Pain
9. Gas
10. Changes in bowel habit
11. Bruising easily
12. Medical history of GI-related problems
13. Family history of GI-related problems

DIAGNOSTIC TESTS/METHODS

A. Patient history and physical examination
B. Examination of stool
1. Examination of stool for occult (hidden) blood
2. Fecal analysis: analysis of stool for mucus, pus, blood, parasites, and fat content
3. Nursing intervention
a. Instruct the patient in the proper collection of the specimen
b. Take the specimen to the laboratory promptly
C. Radiographic examination
1. Upper GI series
a. Patient ingests contrast medium (barium), and the movement of the medium through the esophagus and into the stomach is observed by fluoroscopy; x-ray films are also taken
(1) Aids in identification of esophageal and stomach pathology
(2) Nursing intervention
(a) Explain procedures to the patient
(b) Patient is usually NPO before the examination
(c) Enemas or cathartics may be given before and after the examination
(d) Allay patient's anxiety
2. Lower GI series (barium enema)
a. The filling of the colon with barium is observed by fluoroscopy; x-ray films of the colon are also taken
b. Aids in the detection of abnormalities or defects in the colon such as lesions, polyps, tumors, and diverticula
c. Nursing intervention
(1) Explain procedures to the patient
(2) Patient is usually NPO before the examination
(3) Enemas or cathartics may be given before and after the examination
(4) Allay patient's anxiety
3. Gallbladder series (oral cholecystography)
a. Patient is given an oral radiographic dye to ingest the evening before the examination
b. The gallbladder is visualized to detect gallstones and obstruction of the biliary tract
c. Nursing intervention
(1) Explain procedures to the patient
(2) Administer the radiographic dye as prescribed
(3) Maintain NPO after the dye is given
(4) Allay patient's anxiety
4. Cholangiography
a. Aids in the visualization of the biliary duct system
b. Three methods
(1) Intravenous cholangiography (IVC): a radiographic dye is administered intravenously, and x-ray films are taken
(2) Percutaneous transhepatic cholangiography: under fluoroscopy a cannula is inserted into the liver and bile duct; a radiographic dye is injected into the duct, and filling is observed
(3) Operative or T-tube cholangiography: contrast medium is instilled into the common

bile duct, cystic duct, or gallbladder using a fine needle or catheter during surgery or via an existing T-tube postoperatively

 c. Nursing intervention

  (1) Explain procedures to the patient

  (2) Maintain NPO as ordered

  (3) Monitor the patient for bleeding or bile leakage if the percutaneous approach was used

 5. Barium swallow: barium contrast study used to detect esophageal abnormalities

D. Endoscopy

 1. Endoscopy of the upper GI tract (esophagoscopy, gastroscopy, gastroduodenoscopy, esophagogastroduodenoscopy)

  a. Visualization of the esophagus, stomach, or duodenum with a lighted scope

  b. Useful in detecting inflammation, ulceration, tumors, and other lesions

  c. Nursing intervention

   (1) Explain procedures to the patient

   (2) Obtain signed consent

   (3) Maintain NPO as ordered

   (4) Administer preoperative medication as ordered

   (5) After the examination, maintain NPO until the gag reflex returns

 2. Colonoscopy/sigmoidoscopy

  a. Visualization of the internal structures of the colon with a fiberoptic scope

  b. Lesions, tumors, and polyps may be visualized, and a biopsy may be performed

  c. Nursing intervention

   (1) Explain procedures to the patient

   (2) Prepare patient with enemas and cathartics as ordered

   (3) After the examination, observe for rectal bleeding and signs of perforation (malaise, distention, and tenesmus)

E. Ultrasonography

 1. Noninvasive test that uses echoes from sound waves to visualize deep structures of the body

 2. No special preparation is needed

 3. Useful in detecting masses, fluid accumulation, cysts, tumors, etc.

F. Scans (liver and pancreas)

 1. Assessment of size, shape, and position of the organ

 2. Radionuclide is injected intravenously, and a scanning device picks up the radioactive emissions, which are recorded on paper

 3. Nursing intervention

  a. No preparation is required for liver scanning

  b. Fasting and dietary preparation may be ordered for pancreatic scanning

  c. Explain procedures to the patient

  d. Allay patient's anxiety

G. Computerized tomography (CT scan)

 1. Noninvasive, radiologic imaging technique that takes exposures of the body or body part at different depths

 2. No special preparation is necessary

H. Liver biopsy

 1. Invasive procedure in which a needle is inserted into the liver through a small incision in the skin and a sample of liver tissue is obtained

 2. The incision is usually made on the right side, at the sixth, seventh, eighth, or ninth intercostal space

 3. Nursing intervention

  a. Obtain signed consent

  b. Explain procedure to the patient

  c. Take baseline vital signs

  d. Provide assistance during the procedure

  e. After the procedure monitor the vital signs every 15 minutes to 1 hour; carry out prescription for bed rest (position flat or on the right side), assess the site and monitor for complications

I. Laboratory studies

 1. Serum amylase

  a. Measures the secretion of amylase by the pancreas

  b. Useful in diagnosing pancreatitis

 2. Serum lipase

  a. Measures the secretion of lipase by the pancreas

  b. Useful in diagnosing pancreatitis

 3. Serum bilirubin and spot urine amylase: indicates the liver's ability to conjugate and excrete bilirubin

 4. Coagulation studies (PT and PTT): useful in analyzing hemostatic functions

 5. Liver enzyme studies (SGOT, serum glutamic-pyruvic transaminase [SGPT], and LDH): elevations usually indicate liver damage

 6. Hepatitis-associated antigen (HAA): presence suggests hepatitis

 7. Ammonia levels: elevated in advanced liver disease

 8. Urine amylase: elevated amylase levels indicate pancreatic dysfunction

J. Gastric analysis

 1. Gastric contents are analyzed primarily for hydrochloric acid content

 2. Acidity (pH), volume, and cytology may also be determined

K. D-xylose tolerance test

 1. This study evaluates absorption

 2. Xylose in water is given orally

 3. A urine collection of several hours follows; the amount of D-xylose in the urine is measured

 4. Abnormal amounts of D-xylose in the urine indicate a malabsorption problem

 5. Nursing intervention

  a. Explain procedure to the patient

  b. Maintain NPO before the examination

  c. Give patient instructions on collecting the urine

FREQUENT PATIENT PROBLEMS AND NURSING CARE

A. Pain related to stomatitis

 1. Give soft, bland foods

 2. Encourage intake of fluids that do not aggravate the condition

 3. Encourage the use of soothing mouth rinses

 4. Administer topical medication as prescribed

B. Impaired swallowing related to gingivitis

1. Give mouth irrigations as prescribed
2. Offer soft, bland foods and liquids
3. Instruct the patient in the benefit of good oral hygiene and professional dental cleaning

C. Potential fluid volume deficit related to nausea and vomiting
   1. Observe character and quantity of emesis
   2. Observe for associated symptoms
   3. Observe for precipitating factors
   4. Administer antiemetics as prescribed
   5. Offer ice chips
   6. Maintain cool environment
   7. Apply a cool compress to the neck and forehead for comfort
   8. Offer sips of clear liquids such as 7-Up
   9. Reduce environmental stimuli such as noise, unpleasant odors, and unpleasant sights
   10. Encourage rest and deep breathing
   11. Serve patient's favorite foods
   12. Limit food servings
   13. Provide mouth care after episodes of emesis

D. Impaired swallowing related to dysphagia
   1. Provide patient with favorite foods arranged attractively
   2. Provide soft, bland foods that can easily be chewed
   3. Provide small, frequent feedings
   4. Avoid irritating food and fluid
   5. Monitor intake
   6. Administer topical medication as ordered

E. Alteration in nutrition, less than body requirements, related to anorexia
   1. Assess status of the anorexia
   2. Monitor intake of food and fluid
   3. Determine patient's food likes and dislikes
   4. Prepare patient for meals
      a. Relieve pain
      b. Provide mouth care
      c. Assist patient to a comfortable position
      d. Use patient screen for privacy
      e. Remove unpleasant stimuli from patient's view
   5. Prepare food tray
      a. Serve food at the proper temperature
      b. Make the tray attractive
      c. Serve appropriate quantities (large quantities may reduce the appetite)

F. Potential fluid volume deficit related to diarrhea
   1. Document character, consistency, and number and appearance of stools
   2. Assess for associated symptoms
   3. Monitor intake and output
   4. Administer antidiarrheals as prescribed and monitor for side effects
   5. Cleanse the anal area to avoid excoriation
   6. Avoid milk and milk products
   7. Increase fluid intake to at least 3000 ml daily
   8. Monitor vital signs at least q4h
   9. Identify symptoms of electrolyte imbalance
   10. Monitor laboratory reports for electrolyte values

G. Constipation related to decreased peristalsis/activity
   1. Administer enemas, stool softeners, and cathartics as ordered
   2. Force fluids to at least 3000 ml daily
   3. Provide hot drinks to stimulate peristalsis
   4. Encourage a diet high in fiber
   5. Check for an impaction
   6. Encourage exercises
   7. Instruct patient concerning proper diet, increased fluid intake, exercise, and avoidance of laxative abuse

MAJOR MEDICAL DIAGNOSES
Esophagitis

A. Definition: an inflammation of the esophagus; more common in middle age
B. Causes
   1. Inflammation of the esophagus may be brought on by irritants (food and tobacco), bacteria, or trauma (also see hiatal hernia)
   2. Fungal: *Candida*
   3. Reflux esophagitis: an incompetent lower esophageal sphincter allows a reflux of gastric contents into the esophagus
   4. Malignancy
   5. Prolonged nasogastric intubation
   6. Repeated vomiting

C. Signs and symptoms
   1. Heartburn (epigastric distress)
   2. Pain with eructation or regurgitations
   3. Dysphagia
   4. Pain associated with ingestion of citrus liquids, alcohol, or hot or cold fluid
   5. Symptoms aggravated by recumbency
   6. Bleeding

D. Diagnostic tests/methods
   1. Patient history and physical examination
   2. Barium swallow
   3. Esophagoscopy and biopsy
   4. Routine chest x-ray examination

E. Treatments
   1. Avoid food and fluids that aggravate the symptoms
   2. Administer antacids, analgesics, and sedatives
   3. Elevate head of bed on shock blocks
   4. Maintain bland diet
   5. Surgery may be necessary if conservative measures fail
      a. Fundoplication: plication (making tucks) in the fundus of the stomach around the lower end of the esophagus
      b. Vagotomy and pyloroplasty: interruption of the impulses carried by the vagus nerve to reduce gastric secretions; the pylorus is also surgically manipulated to provide a larger conduit between the stomach and the duodenum

F. Nursing intervention
   1. Assess signs and symptoms and reactions to treatments
   2. Provide small, frequent feedings of bland, low-roughage foods
   3. Discourage intake of food close to bedtime
   4. Administer medication as prescribed and monitor for side effects
   5. Place in semi-Fowler's position

Esophageal Varices

A. Definition: dilated vessels that occur at the lower end of the esophagus

B. Causes
1. Dilation of these vessels is usually a complication arising from cirrhosis of the liver
2. Veins in the lower esophagus become distended as a result of increased portal pressure; the varices may rupture, causing hemorrhage and subsequent shock

C. Signs and symptoms
1. Usually no signs and symptoms appear until the varices become ulcerated
2. Hematemesis and coffee-ground emesis
3. Melena
4. Tachycardia
5. Hypotension
6. Low hemoglobin and hematocrit levels

D. Diagnostic tests/methods
1. Patient history and physical examination: history of alcoholism may exist
2. Fiberoptic endoscopy
3. Laboratory studies: hemoglobin, hematocrit, and liver function studies
4. Angiography
5. Barium swallow
6. CT scan
7. Ultrasound

E. Treatment
1. Blood and blood product replacement
2. Control of bleeding through ice water lavages, insertion of Sengstaken-Blakemore tube, and vitamin K therapy
3. Laboratory studies to monitor bleeding status and effectiveness of treatments
4. Hydration with IV fluids
5. Monitor intake and output
6. Surgery if needed to control bleeding
7. Injection of the bleeding varices with a sclerosing agent to control the bleeding

F. Nursing intervention
1. Provide ongoing assessment of signs and symptoms and reactions to treatment
2. Monitor vital signs at least q4h and monitor vital signs every half hour if bleeding is occurring
3. Record intake and output qh if varices are bleeding
4. Monitor fluids: assess the site, and monitor flow rate
5. Give prescribed medication as ordered and monitor for side effects
6. Allay patient's anxieties and fears
7. Assess all emesis and stool for the presence of blood
8. Monitor laboratory studies and inform physician of incoming laboratory test values
9. Keep head of bed elevated
10. Monitor the Sengstaken-Blakemore tube if in use; keep scissors taped to the head of the bed in case of emergency
11. Note the character of respirations

Hiatal Hernia

A. Definition: a protrusion of the proximal area of the stomach through a weakened area of the diaphragm into the thoracic cavity (Fig. 6-2)

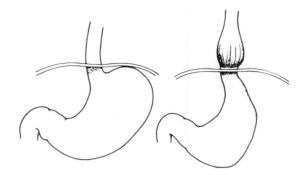

FIG. 6-2. Hiatal hernia shows protrusion of the proximal area of the stomach through the diaphragm into the thoracic cavity. (From Given BA, Simmons SJ: *Gastroenterology in clinical nursing*, ed 4, St Louis, 1984, Mosby.)

B. Causes
1. Congenital weakness
2. Increased abdominal pressure
3. Trauma
4. Relaxation of the musculature
5. Gastric reflux may flow into the esophagus, causing inflammation and ulceration

C. Signs and symptoms
1. Heartburn (pyrosis)
2. Sternal pain after a heavy meal
3. Regurgitation
4. Feeling of fullness
5. Dysphagia
6. Dyspnea

D. Diagnostic tests/methods
1. Patient history and physical examination
2. Upper GI series (barium swallow)
3. Esophagoscopy
4. Routine chest x-ray examination

E. Treatment
1. Conservative
   a. Elevation of the head of the bed on shock blocks
   b. Bland diet with frequent small feedings
   c. Avoidance of caffeine, alcohol, and chocolate
   d. Drug therapy with anticholinergics and antacids
   e. Weight management
   f. Avoidance of activities that increase intraabdominal pressure
2. When conservative measures fail, surgery is indicated: fundoplication—"wrapping" the upper part of the stomach around the esophageal sphincter to prevent reflux
   a. Nasogastric tube
   b. IV therapy
   c. Drug therapy with analgesics and antiemetics
   d. Monitor vital signs
   e. Monitor intake and output

F. Nursing intervention
1. Assess and document signs and symptoms and reactions to treatments

2. Administer prescribed drugs and monitor for side effects
3. Monitor vital signs at least every shift and more often if surgery was performed
4. Monitor intake and output if surgery was performed
5. Provide the prescribed diet
6. Inform the physician if gastric reflux is reported by the patient after surgery
7. Educate patient and family concerning drug therapy, diet, activities to avoid, and the need for compliance

Gastritis

A. Definition: an inflammation in the mucosal lining of the stomach; the condition may be acute or chronic
B. Gastritis may be caused by bacteria, drugs, or toxins that cause the lining of the stomach to become inflamed and edematous
C. Signs and symptoms
   1. Nausea and vomiting
   2. Anorexia
   3. Epigastric tenderness
   4. Feeling of fullness
   5. Cramping
   6. Diarrhea
   7. Fever
D. Diagnostic tests/methods
   1. Patient history and physical examination
   2. Identification of a causative agent
   3. Laboratory studies
   4. Stool culture
   5. Endoscopy with biopsy
   6. Gastric analysis
E. Treatment
   1. Supportive care
   2. Bed rest
   3. NPO if nausea or vomiting is severe
   4. Hydration with IV fluids
   5. In severe cases a nasogastric tube is inserted
   6. Drug therapy: antiemetics, antacids, and H_2 receptor antagonists
   7. Progressive diet when acute symptoms subside
   8. Restriction of smoking
F. Nursing intervention
   1. Assess and document signs and symptoms and reactions to treatments
   2. Monitor vital signs at least q4h
   3. Monitor intake and output
   4. Provide the prescribed diet
   5. Administer medication as prescribed and monitor for side effects
   6. Note amount and character of emesis and diarrhea
   7. Monitor IV fluids
   8. Educate patient and family concerning drug therapy, diet, activities, and any restrictions

Cancer of the Stomach

A. Cancer can develop anywhere in the stomach
B. Causes
   1. Exact cause is unknown
   2. Familial tendency is suspected
   3. Predisposing conditions: chronic gastric ulcers and gastritis
C. Signs and symptoms
   1. Loss of appetite; early satiety
   2. Weight loss
   3. Weakness and fatigue
   4. Pain
   5. Melena
   6. Anemia
   7. Hematemesis
   8. Dizziness
   9. Indigestion or dysphagia
   10. Constipation
D. Diagnostic tests/methods
   1. Patient history and physical examination
   2. Laboratory studies
   3. Stool analysis
   4. Gastric analysis
   5. Barium studies
   6. Gastroscopy
E. Treatment
   1. Preoperative therapy
      a. Correct nutritional deficiencies
      b. Treat anemias
      c. Blood replacement
      d. Gastric decompression with a nasogastric tube
   2. Surgery: removal of the cancerous lesion or tumor along with a margin of normal tissue
   3. Radiation therapy and chemotherapy may be used if the patient is not expected to undergo surgery
      a. Combination therapy has a better response rate
      b. Single-agent therapy has proved to be of little value
F. Nursing intervention
   1. Preoperative care
      a. Support the patient and family
      b. Assess and document signs and symptoms and reactions to treatments
      c. Provide and encourage the prescribed diet
      d. Monitor vital signs at least q8h
      e. Monitor blood and fluid replacement therapy
      f. Provide preoperative teaching
   2. Postoperative care (immediate)
      a. Have patient turn, cough, and breathe deeply
      b. Monitor nasogastric suctioning and tube patency
      c. Monitor vital signs as ordered
      d. Record intake and output
      e. Administer prescribed medication and monitor for side effects
      f. Assess dressing
      g. Assess for bowel sounds
      h. Encourage early ambulation and ROM exercises to prevent thrombosis
      i. Provide antiembolism stockings
      j. Relieve pain with drugs and supportive measures
   3. Postoperative period
      a. Provide six to eight small feedings
      b. Weigh patient qd while in hospital to monitor weight loss
      c. Reduce fluids taken with meals if not tolerated
      d. Educate patient and family concerning drug therapy, dietary restrictions, activity, wound care, and compliance with the regimen

Peptic Ulcers

A. Definition: ulcerations in the mucosal lining of the distal esophagus, stomach, or small intestine (duodenum or jejunum); duodenal ulcers are more common than gastric ulcers, and men are more prone to ulcers than women
B. Cause: exact cause is unknown
C. Predisposing factors
   1. Stress
   2. Smoking
   3. Heavy caffeine ingestion
   4. Ingestion of certain drugs
D. Signs and symptoms
   1. Loss of appetite
   2. Weight loss or gain
   3. Pain (gnawing, burning)
   4. Melena
   5. Anemia
   6. Hematemesis; coffee-ground emesis
   7. Occasional nausea or vomiting
   8. Dark, tarry stools
E. Diagnostic tests/methods
   1. Patient history and physical examination
   2. Gastroscopy and duodenoscopy
   3. Barium studies
   4. Gastric analysis
   5. Laboratory studies
F. Treatment
   1. Conservative
     a. Rest
     b. Drug therapy: antacids, anticholinergics, histamine receptor antagonists, sedatives, and analgesics
     c. Elimination of smoking and caffeine
     d. Reduction of stress
     e. Bland diet with small, frequent feedings
     f. In acute situations the patient may be NPO and have nasogastric tube inserted
   2. Surgical intervention
     a. Closure if perforation has occurred
     b. Pyloroplasty and vagotomy if the gastric outlet is obstructed
     c. Total or partial resection of the stomach to remove the ulcerated area(s)
G. Nursing intervention
   1. Conduct ongoing assessment of signs and symptoms and reactions to treatments
   2. Monitor vital signs at least q4h
   3. Administer the prescribed medication and monitor for side effects
   4. Provide the prescribed diet
   5. Provide physical and emotional rest
   6. Monitor for signs and symptoms of complication (perforation, hemorrhage, and obstruction)
   7. Instruct patient regarding elimination of smoking, avoidance of certain foods, and reduction of stress
   8. Educate patient and family concerning drug therapy, diet and dietary restrictions, avoidance of stress, and the need for compliance with the prescribed regimen

Obstruction

A. Definition: a mechanical or neurologic abnormality inhibiting the normal flow of gastric or intestinal contents
B. Obstructions may result from scar tissue formation, cancer, or strangulated hernias; all are mechanical barriers to the normal flow of gastric or intestinal contents
C. A neurologic obstruction, in the form of a paralytic ileus, causes interference with innervation, thus hindering normal peristaltic activity
D. Signs and symptoms
   1. Abnormal pain and distention
   2. Projectile vomiting
   3. Nausea
   4. Possible absence of bowel sounds or increase in bowel sounds
   5. Cramping
   6. Abdomen may be tense (distended)
   7. Obstipation (chronic constipation)
E. Diagnostic tests/methods
   1. Patient history and physical examination
   2. Flat plate of the abdomen
   3. Laboratory studies
F. Treatment
   1. Surgery is the treatment for mechanical obstructions
   2. Gastric or intestinal decompression to decrease nausea and vomiting
   3. Hydration with IV therapy
   4. Prophylactic antibiotics
   5. Monitor intake and output
   6. Supportive care
G. Nursing intervention
   1. Assess and document signs and symptoms and reactions to treatments
   2. Monitor vital signs at least q4h
   3. Record intake and output
   4. Monitor the decompression tube and assess quantity and character of drainage
   5. Provide mouth care while patient is intubated
   6. Administer prescribed medication and monitor for side effects
   7. Maintain NPO
   8. Monitor the states of distention and hydration
   9. Provide routine postoperative care if patient undergoes surgery

Crohn's Disease (Regional Enteritis)

A. Definition: an inflammatory disease affecting primarily the small bowel and also possibly the large bowel; the intestinal lining ulcerates, and scar tissue forms; bowel becomes thick and narrow
B. Cause is unknown; stricture, obstruction, and perforation can occur as a result of this disorder; malabsorption of fluid and nutrients is also associated with this disorder
C. Signs and symptoms (aggravated by illness/stress)
   1. Abdominal pain and cramping
   2. Diarrhea
   3. Weight loss
   4. Fever
   5. Anemia
   6. Weakness and fatigue
   7. Anorexia
   8. Abdominal tenderness
D. Diagnostic tests/methods
   1. Patient history and physical examination
   2. Laboratory studies: CBC, electrolytes, clotting studies

3. Stool examination
4. Endoscopy
5. Proctosigmoidoscopy and biopsy examination
6. Barium studies

E. Treatment
1. Drug therapy: sedatives, antidiarrheals, antibiotics, steroids, hematinics, anticholinergics, and analgesics
2. Hydration with IV therapy
3. Correct nutritional deficiencies
4. Provide symptomatic relief
5. In severe cases the patient may be NPO, have a nasogastric tube, and require blood transfusions
6. High-calorie, high-protein, low-residue diet
7. Surgery is indicated if there is fistula formation, bleeding, perforation, or obstruction

F. Nursing intervention
1. Assess and document signs and symptoms and reactions to treatments
2. Monitor vital signs q4h
3. Record intake and output
4. Provide and encourage the prescribed diet
5. Assist with activities of daily living
6. Monitor the number, amount, and character of stools
7. Monitor hydration status
8. Assess for abdominal distention
9. Maintain skin integrity and monitor for anal excoriation
10. Provide support to the patient
11. Administer prescribed medication and monitor for side effects
12. Educate patient and family concerning drug therapy, dietary restrictions, and compliance

Ulcerative Colitis

A. Definition: an inflammatory disorder of the large bowel; the inflammatory process begins in the distal segments of the colon and ascends
1. The mucosa ulcerates, bleeds, and becomes edematous and thickens
2. Perforations and abscesses can occur
3. The colon eventually loses its elasticity, and its absorptive ability is reduced

B. Cause is unknown, although it has been associated with stress, autoimmune factors, and food allergies

C. Signs and symptoms
1. Abdominal cramping pain with diarrhea
2. Nausea
3. Dehydration
4. Cachexia
5. Weight loss
6. Anorexia
7. Bloody diarrhea
8. Anemia

D. Diagnostic tests/methods
1. Patient history and physical examination
2. Laboratory studies reveal anemia and electrolyte imbalance: CBC, electrolytes
3. Stool examination
4. Proctosigmoidoscopy
5. Barium studies

E. Treatment
1. Drug therapy: sedatives, antidiarrheals, antibiotics, steroids, hematinics, anticholinergics, and analgesics

2. Correction of malnutrition
3. Hydration with IV therapy
4. Colectomy with ileostomy if other medical treatment fails
5. Provide symptomatic relief
6. Monitor weight
7. Monitor intake and output
8. Parenteral hyperalimentation may be necessary
9. Psychotherapy

F. Nursing intervention
1. Assess and document signs and symptoms and reactions to treatments
2. Provide emotional as well as physical rest
3. Monitor number, amount, and characteristics of stools
4. Provide skin care measures to avoid anal excoriation
5. Monitor intake and output
6. Monitor vital signs q4h
7. Weigh patient qd
8. Increase intake of fluids
9. Provide the prescribed diet
10. Administer prescribed medication and monitor for side effects
11. Assess bowel sounds q4h
12. Assist with activities of daily living
13. Provide emotional support
14. Educate patient and family concerning drug therapy, dietary restrictions, avoidance of stress, and compliance with the prescribed regimen

Diverticulosis/Diverticulitis

A. Definition: *diverticulum*—an outpouching of the mucosa of the colon
1. Diverticulosis: the existence of diverticula in the large intestine
2. Diverticulitis: an inflammation of the diverticulum

B. Cause of diverticulosis is unknown; theories include a congenital weakness of the colon, colon distention, constipation, and inadequate dietary fiber

C. Signs and symptoms
1. Abdominal cramps
2. Lower-quadrant tenderness
3. Constipation or constipation alternating with diarrhea
4. Fever
5. Occult bleeding
6. Elevated WBC count

D. Diagnostic tests/methods
1. Patient history and physical examination
2. Laboratory studies
3. Stool examination for occult blood
4. Sigmoidoscopy
5. Colonoscopy
6. Barium studies

E. Treatment
1. High-residue diet
2. Drug therapy: bulk laxatives, antibiotics, stool softeners, and anticholinergics
3. In more severe cases the patient may be NPO and require IV therapy
4. Surgery: colon resection for obstruction and hemorrhage

F. Nursing intervention
   1. Assess and document signs and symptoms and reactions to treatments
   2. Provide increased roughage in the diet
   3. Increase intake of fluids
   4. Administer prescribed medication and monitor for side effects
   5. Instruct patient to avoid activity that increases intraabdominal pressure (straining at stool, lifting, bending, and wearing restrictive clothing)
   6. Educate patient and family concerning drug therapy, dietary restrictions, and avoidance of constipation and activity that increases intraabdominal pressure

Colon/Rectal Cancer and Polyps

A. Definition: the cancerous process can invade the large intestine; cancer of the colon and rectum may take the form of well-defined tumor or cancerous polyp: a polyp is pouchlike structure projecting from the wall of the bowel; polyps may be cancerous or benign
B. Cause of colon cancer is unknown; persons with colon polyps, lesions, diverticula, or ulcerative colitis are monitored closely for malignant changes in the bowel
C. Signs and symptoms
   1. Changes in bowel pattern
   2. Rectal bleeding
   3. Changes in the shape of stool
   4. Weakness and fatigue
   5. Weight loss
   6. Rectal pain
   7. Abdominal pain
   8. Anemia
D. Diagnostic tests/methods
   1. Patient history and physical examination
   2. Laboratory studies
   3. Barium studies
   4. Proctosigmoidoscopic examination
E. Treatment
   1. Surgical resection of the affected area/creation of a colostomy if necessary
   2. Chemotherapy
   3. Radiation therapy
   4. Supportive therapy
F. Nursing intervention (also see nursing care plan for cancer of the stomach)
   1. Assess and document signs and symptoms and reactions to treatments
   2. Monitor vital signs at least q4h and more often during the postoperative periods
   3. Record intake and output
   4. Monitor dressings and wound drainage
   5. Relieve pain
   6. Administer prescribed medication and monitor for side effects
   7. Provide psychologic support
   8. Monitor colostomy site
   9. Monitor perineal area if drain or packing has been inserted
   10. Assist patient with sitz baths if ordered
   11. Assist patient with activities of daily living as needed
   12. Monitor hydration status
   13. Encourage increased fluid intake

14. Educate patient and family concerning drug therapy, diet, activities, colostomy care, and adaptation to everyday activity

Hemorrhoids

A. Definition: varicosities or dilated vessels in the rectal and anal area
B. Cause: hemorrhoids result from increased abdominal pressure such as that during pregnancy and from prolonged periods of sitting and standing; constipation and obesity are also predisposing factors
C. Signs and symptoms vary from no symptoms at all to pain, itching, and bleeding
D. Diagnostic tests/methods
   1. Patient history and physical examination
   2. Digital examination
   3. Proctoscopy
E. Treatment
   1. Symptomatic relief in mild cases
      a. Topical medication to shrink the mucous membrane
      b. Stool softeners and laxatives to keep stool soft and avoid straining
      c. Sitz baths to relieve pain
      d. High-fiber diet to keep stools soft
   2. Rubber-band ligation of internal hemorrhoids: the constriction impairs circulation; the tissues become necrotic and slough off
   3. Hemorrhoidectomy: the surgical excision of hemorrhoids
      a. Removal may be by clamp, excision, or cautery
      b. Postoperative treatments are similar to those identified previously for symptomatic relief
F. Nursing intervention
   1. Assess and document signs and symptoms and reactions to treatments
   2. Alleviate pain with analgesics, positioning, and sitz baths
   3. Administer prescribed medication and monitor for side effects
   4. Monitor vital signs at least q4h
   5. Monitor dressings for drainage
   6. Monitor voiding after surgery
   7. Assist with gradual return to activity
   8. Encourage increased fluid intake
   9. Provide patient with rationale for avoiding constipation and prolonged sitting and standing
   10. Educate patient and family concerning drug therapy, high-fiber diet, activity, and avoidance of constipation

Cholelithiasis/Cholecystitis

A. Definition:
   1. Cholelithiasis: the presence of gallstones in the gallbladder or biliary tree
   2. Cholecystitis: an inflammation of the gallbladder usually associated with the presence of gallstones
B. Cause
   1. Cholelithiasis is believed to be precipitated by chemical changes in bile
      a. Bile stasis, infections of the gallbladder, and metabolic changes can precipitate stone formation

b. Stones may lodge in the biliary tree, causing obstruction and biliary colic (Fig. 6-3)

2. Cholecystitis: may be brought on by cholelithiasis or the presence of an organism in the gallbladder

C. Signs and symptoms
   1. Indigestion after a meal high in fat
   2. Nausea and vomiting
   3. Flatulence
   4. Belching
   5. Right upper-quadrant pain radiating to the back or shoulder
   6. Fever
   7. Jaundice
   8. Clay-colored stools
   9. Dark-colored urine
   10. Elevated WBC count

D. Diagnostic tests/methods
   1. Patient history and physical examination
   2. Laboratory studies
   3. Oral cholecystography
   4. IV cholangiography
   5. Ultrasound of gallbladder

E. Treatment
   1. Hydration with IV fluids
   2. Drug therapy: analgesics, antibiotics, and antispasmodics
   3. Drug therapy to dissolve stones has been effective in certain patients
   4. Low-fat diet
   5. Lithotripsy (use of shock waves to disintegrate gallstones) has been attempted in patients having few stones
   6. Surgical removal of the gallbladder (cholecystectomy) or gallstones (cholecystostomy)

F. Nursing intervention
   1. Assess and document signs and symptoms and reactions to treatments
   2. Administer prescribed medication and monitor for side effects
   3. Alleviate pain and promote comfort
   4. Monitor IV therapy
   5. Provide the prescribed diet
   6. Monitor the state of hydration
   7. Assess vital signs at least q4h
   8. Provide postoperative care: monitor dressing, nasogastric tube, and T tube (tube is inserted into the common bile duct during surgery if the common bile duct is explored) (Fig. 6-4)
   9. Educate patient and family concerning drug therapy, dietary restrictions, and wound care if surgery was performed

Hepatitis

A. Definition: inflammation of the liver
B. Causes
   1. Drugs or chemicals (toxic hepatitis)
   2. Viral origin (hepatitis A [HAV] and B [HBV])

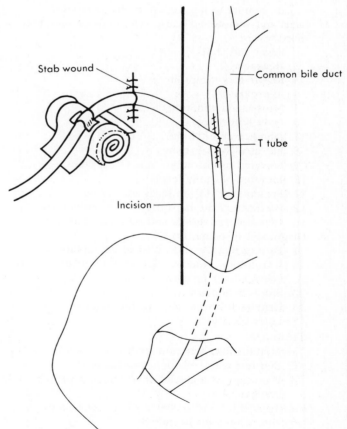

FIG. 6-4. Placement of a T tube in the common bile duct after bile duct exploration. (From Given BA, Simmons SJ: *Gastroenterology in clinical nursing,* ed 4, St Louis, 1984, Mosby; adapted from Shafer et al: *Medical-surgical nursing,* ed 6, St Louis, 1975, Mosby.)

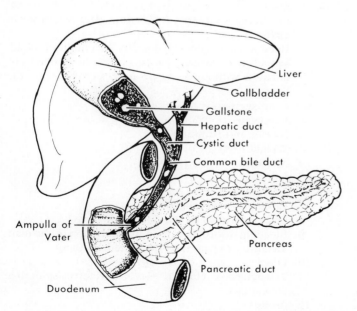

FIG. 6-3. Common sites of gallstones. (From Given BA, Simmons SJ: *Gastroenterology in clinical nursing,* ed 4, St Louis, 1984, Mosby.)

3. Multiple blood transfusions (hepatitis non-A or non-B)

C. The most common forms of HAV and HBV
  1. HAV: infectious hepatitis
    a. Transmitted by the fecal-oral route
    b. Incubation period is approximately 2 to 7 weeks
    c. May be spread by contaminated food, water, milk, and shellfish
  2. HBV: serum hepatitis
    a. Associated with contaminated needles and syringes
    b. Transmitted through blood or blood products and pricking of the skin with contaminated equipment
    c. May also be spread through feces, urine, saliva, and semen
    d. Patients are prone to exacerbations and complications (cirrhosis) from the disease
    e. Incubation period is approximately 6 to 26 weeks
  3. Non-HAV, non-HBV
    a. Name given to forms of hepatitis caused by a virus genetically different than hepatitis A or B
    b. Associated with blood transfusions, particularly from paid donors
    c. No specific antigen is associated with the form
    d. Similar to hepatitis B in characteristics

D. Signs and symptoms: (early symptoms of HAV may be more severe)
  1. Fever and chills
  2. Headache
  3. Respiratory symptoms
  4. Anorexia
  5. Nausea and vomiting
  6. Liver tenderness
  7. Jaundice and itching
  8. Elevated liver enzymes
  9. Elevated prothrombin time (PT) values
  10. Elevated bilirubin levels
  11. Presence of HAV in feces and serum
  12. Presence of the hepatitis surface antigen HB_s Ag
  13. Clay-colored stools and dark-colored urine

E. Diagnostic tests/methods
  1. Patient history and physical examination
  2. Laboratory studies: hepatitis-associated antigen (HAA); liver profile
  3. Stool examination
  4. Urinary bilirubin and urobilinogen
  5. Liver biopsy

F. Treatment
  1. Monitor liver function studies
  2. Bed rest with bathroom privileges
  3. High-calorie, high-carbohydrate, high-protein, moderate-fat diet
  4. Topical lotions to alleviate dry, itchy skin
  5. Hydration with IV therapy
  6. Administration of vitamin K preparations
  7. Monitor for bleeding tendencies and progression of the illness
  8. Blood and body fluid precautions
  9. Passive immunity

G. Nursing intervention
  1. Assess and document signs and symptoms and reactions to treatments
  2. Monitor skin, stool, and urine color
  3. Promote balanced activity and rest periods
  4. Maintain blood and body fluid precautions
  5. Monitor IV therapy
  6. Assess intake and output
  7. Monitor vital signs at least q4h
  8. Provide and encourage the prescribed diet
  9. Support the patient and family
  10. Administer prescribed medication and monitor for side effects
  11. Monitor for bleeding tendencies
  12. Educate patient and family concerning drug therapy, the prescribed diet, activity level, and monitoring for complications

Cirrhosis

A. Definition: cell degeneration occurring in the liver wherever scar tissue replaces normally functioning tissue
B. Cirrhosis is a complication of alcoholism, hepatitis, biliary disease, and certain metabolic disorders
C. Whatever the cause of the liver destruction, the course of cirrhosis is the same
  1. Liver parenchyma dies and regenerates, and fibrous tissue (scarring) occurs
  2. This alteration in structure progresses in the liver, causing problems in hepatic blood flow and normal liver function; in time the liver fails
D. Major complications of cirrhosis
  1. Portal hypertension: hypertension resulting from the obstruction of normal blood flow through the portal system; the obstruction is caused by changes in the liver from the cirrhotic process
  2. Esophageal varices (refer to esophageal varices at the beginning of this section)
  3. Ascites: the accumulation of fluid in the peritoneal or abdominal cavity, which is a later symptom in cirrhosis
  4. Hepatic coma (encephalopathy): a condition of advanced liver disease; blood enters the general circulation without being properly detoxified by the liver
E. Signs and symptoms
  1. Headache
  2. Nausea and vomiting
  3. Weight loss
  4. Anorexia
  5. Jaundice
  6. Abdominal pain
  7. Fatigue and weakness
  8. Liver enlargement and fibrosis
  9. Bleeding disorders caused by disruption in the manufacture of vitamin K–dependent factors
  10. Edema
  11. Telangiectasis (blood vessels develop a spiderlike appearance)
  12. Ascites
  13. Esophageal varices
  14. Hepatic coma

F. Diagnostic tests/methods
   1. Patient history and physical examination
   2. Laboratory studies to assess liver function
   3. Liver scan
   4. Liver biopsy
G. Treatment
   1. Rest with activity as tolerated
   2. Nutritious diet with protein level determined by liver functioning
   3. If ascites is present, restrict fluid and sodium, monitor weight, and monitor intake and output
   4. Monitor for complications such as ascites, esophageal varices, and hepatic coma
   5. Drug therapy to reduce ammonia levels, prevent bleeding, reduce edema, and provide comfort
H. Nursing intervention
   1. Assess and document signs and symptoms and reactions to treatments
   2. Administer prescribed medication and monitor for side effects
   3. Provide and encourage the prescribed diet
   4. Promote comfort
   5. Monitor vital signs at least q4h and report abnormalities
   6. Monitor status of ascites
      a. Record weight
      b. Assess measurements of extremities and abnormal girth
      c. Monitor intake and output
   7. Provide planned exercise and rest periods
   8. Assist patient with activities of daily living
   9. Monitor skin status and take measures to prevent skin breakdown
   10. Protect against infection
   11. Provide diversional activity
   12. Offer emotional support
   13. Provide ongoing assessment for evidence of hepatic encephalopathy
      a. Monitor for symptoms of lethargy, confusion, twitching, tremors, sweetish breath odor, fever, and increasing somnolence
      b. Eliminate dietary protein
      c. Administer prescribed drugs and enemas to reduce ammonia levels
      d. Monitor IV fluids
      e. Give narcotics and sedatives cautiously
   14. Also see care of patient with esophageal varices at the beginning of this section
   15. Educate patient and family concerning home-bound care

Pancreatitis

A. Definition: an acute or chronic inflammation of the pancreas
B. Pancreatitis is associated with biliary disease, infections, drug toxicity, nutritional deficiencies, and ingestion of alcohol
C. The digestive enzymes of the pancreas are released into the pancreatic tissue, causing inflammation
   1. As the condition progresses, ischemia, duct obstruction, and necrosis may occur

   2. Bleeding occurs if tissue necrosis affects vessels
   3. Pancreatic abscesses may occur if bacteria invade the necrotic tissue
   4. In chronic pancreatitis the tissue becomes fibrotic and normal function is compromised
D. Signs and symptoms
   1. Acute pancreatitis
      a. Epigastric pain that radiates to the back
      b. Eating tends to aggravate pain
      c. Patient may assume a side-lying position with knees bent for comfort
      d. Nausea and vomiting
      e. Low-grade fever
      f. Hypotension
      g. Tachycardia
      h. Jaundice
      i. Elevated WBC count
      j. Shock: if there is blood vessel or tissue erosion
   2. Chronic pancreatitis
      a. Abdominal pain
      b. Weight loss
      c. Steatorrhea (foul-smelling, foamy stool)
      d. Diabetes mellitus if beta function is affected
E. Diagnostic tests/methods
   1. Patient history and physical examination
   2. Laboratory tests, particularly electrolytes, amylase, lipase, and liver enzymes
   3. Pancreatic scan and sonography
   4. Visualization of the pancreatic duct (endoscopy)
   5. X-ray studies
F. Treatment
   1. Control of pain
   2. Hydration with IV fluids
   3. Correction of any bleeding
   4. Nasogastric tube and NPO to reduce pancreatic secretions
   5. Drug therapy: analgesics, antibiotics, steroids, vitamins, and pancreatic extracts
   6. Diet that does not stimulate pancreatic secretions
   7. Control of blood glucose levels if beta cells are affected
G. Nursing intervention
   1. Assess and document signs and symptoms and reactions to treatments
   2. Administer prescribed medication and monitor for side effects
   3. Provide the prescribed diet
   4. Explain dietary restrictions to patient
   5. Monitor vital signs at least q4h
   6. Monitor IV therapy
   7. Promote comfort and relieve pain
   8. Provide emotional support
   9. Assess intake and output
   10. Relieve nausea and vomiting if present
   11. Note color, character, and amount of urine and stool
   12. Monitor jaundice if present
   13. Monitor the nasogastric tube and secretions
   14. Educate patient and family concerning drug therapy, diet and dietary restrictions, avoidance of alcohol, monitoring steatorrhea, blood glucose monitoring (glucometer), and compliance with the regimen

Cancer of the Pancreas

A. Cancer of the pancreas can affect any portion of the pancreas, including the beta cells; metastasis readily occurs to adjacent structures
B. Cancerous tissue impairs normal pancreatic function, primarily by causing obstruction and hindering the flow of pancreatic secretions
C. Signs and symptoms
   1. Early symptoms may be vague
      a. Nausea and vomiting
      b. Anorexia
      c. Weight loss
      d. Weakness and fatigue
   2. Later symptoms
      a. Pain
      b. Jaundice
      c. Diabetes mellitus
D. Diagnostic tests/methods
   1. Patient history and physical examination
   2. Laboratory studies
   3. Pancreatic scan and sonography
   4. X-ray studies
   5. Visualization of the pancreatic duct
E. Treatment
   1. Supportive therapy
   2. Surgical excision: Whipple's procedure may be performed removing the head of the pancreas, lower portion of the common bile duct, distal portion of the stomach, and the duodenum
   3. Palliative surgery: to restore bile and pancreatic output
   4. Chemotherapy
F. Nursing intervention: see cancer of the stomach

Appendicitis

A. Definition: inflammation of the appendix
B. Signs and symptoms
   1. Right lower-quadrant pain
   2. Nausea and vomiting
   3. Anorexia
   4. Fever
   5. Elevated WBC count
C. Diagnostic tests/methods
   1. Patient history and physical examination
   2. Laboratory tests, particularly a WBC count
   3. Routine urinalysis
D. Treatment
   1. Supportive therapy
   2. Immediate surgical removal (appendectomy)
E. Nursing intervention
   1. Assess and document signs and symptoms and reactions to treatments
   2. Monitor IV fluids
   3. Provide comfort measures such as an ice pack to the abdomen and analgesia
   4. Administer prescribed drugs and monitor for side effects
   5. Monitor vital signs as ordered
   6. Encourage progressive ambulation after surgery
   7. Monitor the dressing and operative site after surgery
   8. Educate patient and family concerning drug therapy, activity restrictions, and care of the operative site

Peritonitis

A. Definition: infection and subsequent inflammation of the peritoneal membrane by trauma or bacterial invasion
B. The inflammation may be localized or widespread and affect the organs of the abdominal cavity; adhesions, abscesses, and obstructions may occur
C. Signs and symptoms
   1. Nausea and vomiting
   2. Abdominal pain
   3. Abdominal rigidity and distention
   4. Fever
   5. Paralytic ileus
   6. Fluid and electrolyte imbalance
   7. Elevated WBC count
   8. Constipation; diarrhea
D. Diagnostic tests/methods
   1. Patient history and physical examination
   2. Laboratory tests including a WBC count, electrolytes, and blood cultures
E. Treatment
   1. Identification of the causative agent
   2. Intestinal decompression
   3. Hydration with IV therapy
   4. Pain control
   5. Drug therapy: analgesics and antibiotics
   6. Monitoring vital signs
   7. Monitoring intake and output
   8. Controlling the spread of infection
F. Nursing intervention
   1. Assess and document signs and symptoms and reactions to treatment
   2. Assess vital signs every 1 to 2 hours during the acute period
   3. Monitor intake and output
   4. Administer prescribed medication and monitor for side effects
   5. Provide comfort and relief of pain
   6. Assess bowel sounds
   7. Maintain NPO during the acute period
   8. Maintain nasogastric tube and monitor output during the acute period
   9. Support patient and allay anxieties
   10. Place patient in semi-Fowler's position
   11. Have patient turn, cough, and deep breathe at least q2h

Hernias

A. Definition: a protrusion of an organ or structure through the wall of the containing cavity
B. Hernias may occur around the umbilical area, inguinal area, diaphragm, femoral ring, and at the site of an incision
C. Hernias are categorized as
   1. Reducible: can be returned to its normal position
   2. Irreducible: cannot be returned to the normal position
   3. Incarcerated: obstruction of intestinal flow
   4. Strangulated: blood supply is cut off (occluded)— surgical emergency
D. Causes
   1. Congenital weakness in the containing wall
   2. Weakness in containing wall is related to straining and the aging process

3. Trauma
4. Increased intraabdominal pressure (obesity or pregnancy)
E. Signs and symptoms
1. Protrusion of a structure without symptoms
2. Appearance of a protrusion when straining or lifting
3. In certain instances there may be pain
4. If the intestine is obstructed, there may be distention, pain, nausea, and vomiting
F. Diagnostic methods: patient history and physical examination
G. Treatment
1. Surgery is the treatment of choice
a. Herniorrhaphy: surgical repair of the hernia
b. Hernioplasty: the surgical reinforcement of the weakened area
2. Use of a truss (a support worn over the hernia to keep it in place)
H. Nursing intervention
1. Assess and document signs and symptoms and reactions to treatments
2. Assess vital signs every shift before surgery
3. Report any symptoms of coughing, sneezing, or upper respiratory tract infection noted before surgery because this will weaken the surgical repair
4. Apply ice packs as ordered to control pain and swelling
5. Monitor voidings following inguinal hernia repair
6. Educate patient and family concerning care of the operative site, activity restrictions, and avoidance of constipation

The Neurologic System

Pathology of the central nervous system (CNS) arises from injuries, new growths, vascular insufficiency, infections, and as complications secondary to other diseases. Patient problems are related to interference with normal functioning of the affected tissue.

The following terms are used in describing the patient with a neurologic impairment:

anesthesia   complete loss of sensation
aphasia   loss of ability to use language
  auditory/receptive aphasia   loss of ability to understand
  expressive aphasia   loss of ability to use spoken or written word
ataxia   uncoordinated movements
coma   state of profound unconsciousness
convulsion   involuntary contractions and relaxation of muscle
delirium   mental state characterized by restlessness and disorientation
diplopia   double vision
dyskinesia   difficulty in voluntary movement
flaccid   without tone—limp
neuralgia   intermittent, intense pain along the course of a nerve
neuritis   inflammation of a nerve or nerves
nuchal rigidity   stiff neck
nystagmus   involuntary, rapid movements of the eyeball
papilledema   swelling of optic nerve head
paresthesia   abnormal sensation without obvious cause, with numbness and tingling
spastic   convulsive muscular contraction
stupor   state of impaired consciousness with brief response only to vigorous and repeated stimulation
tic   spasmodic, involuntary twitching of a muscle
vertigo   dizziness

NURSING ASSESSMENT

A. Nursing observations
1. Mental status: drowsiness or lethargy, ability to follow commands
2. Level of consciousness (LOC): ability to be aroused in response to verbal and physical stimuli; ranges from awake and alert to "coma"; Glasgow Coma Scale is the usual guide for assessing and describing the degree of conscious impairment, based on three determinants:
a. Eye opening
b. Motor response
c. Verbal response
3. Orientation
a. Time: knows month or year
b. Place: has general knowledge of where patient is (e.g., hospital)
c. Person: knows own name; able to name relative or friend
4. Behavior: is it appropriate for the situation
5. Emotional response: is it appropriate for the situation
6. Memory: capability for early and recent recall
7. Speech: presence of aphasia, appropriate speech, words distinct or slurred
8. Vital signs: temperature, pulse, respirations, and blood pressure
9. Ability to follow simple directions
10. Eyes
a. Pupillary reaction to light: the pupils are periodically assessed with a flashlight to evaluate and compare size, configuration, and reaction. Differences between both eyes and from previous assessments are compared for similarities and differences
b. Movement of lids and pupils
11. Motor function: coordination, gait, balance, posture, strength, and functioning
12. Bladder and bowel control
13. Ears for drainage
14. Facial expression for symmetry
15. Sensation for
a. Pain
b. Light
c. Smell
B. Patient description (subjective data)
1. History of head injury, loss of consciousness, vertigo, weakness, headache, sleep problems, paralysis, seizures, or diplopia
2. Complaints of pain, numbness, problems with elimination, memory loss, difficulty concentrating, drowsiness, or visual problems
3. Medications taken
C. History from family
1. Medical
2. Activities of daily living (ADL)
3. Behavior

DIAGNOSTIC TESTS/METHODS

A. Computerized tomography (CT; CAT scan): computer analysis of tissues as x-rays pass through them; has replaced many of the usual tests; no special preparation or care after test

B. Lumbar puncture (spinal tap)
1. Description: under local anesthesia a puncture is made at the junction of the third and fourth lumbar vertebrae to obtain a specimen of cerebrospinal fluid; cerebrospinal fluid pressure can be measured; this procedure is also used to inject medications (e.g., spinal anesthesia) and in diagnostic x-ray examination to inject air or dye (e.g., myelogram)
2. Nursing intervention
a. Monitor vital signs
b. Keep patient supine 4 to 8 hours
c. Observe for headache and nuchal rigidity

C. Cerebral angiography
1. Description: intraarterial injection of radiopaque dye to obtain an x-ray film of cerebrovascular circulation
2. Nursing intervention after procedure
a. Related to dye: observe for allergic reaction: urticaria, decreased urinary output, respiratory distress, and difficulty swallowing
b. Related to injection site
(1) Provide ice pack and bed rest
(2) Monitor vital signs
(3) Have tracheostomy set available
(4) Observe for pain, tenderness, and bleeding

D. Electroencephalography (EEG)
1. Description: electrodes are placed on unshaven scalp with tiny needles and electrode jelly
2. Nursing intervention
a. Anticipate patient's fears about electrocution; do not give stimulants/depressants before test
b. Wash hair and scalp after procedure to remove jelly
c. Patient may resume all previous activities

E. Brain scan
1. Description: after an IV injection of a radioisotope, abnormal brain tissue will absorb more rapidly than normal tissue; this can be detected with a Geiger counter to diagnose brain tumors
2. Nursing intervention
a. No observations
b. Patient may resume all previous activities

F. Magnetic resonance imaging (MRI)
1. Description: MRI uses a combination of radio waves and a strong magnetic field to view soft tissue (does not use x-rays or dyes); produces a computerized picture that depicts soft tissues in high-contrast color
2. Nursing intervention
a. Before the procedure, instruct the patient to remain perfectly still in the narrow cylinder-shaped machine
b. Inform the patient that there will be no pain or discomfort, but there is no room for movement during the MRI
c. No specific care or observations are necessary after the procedure

G. Myelography (MEG)
1. Description: injection of a radiopaque dye into the subarachnoid space via a lumbar puncture; performed to locate lesions of the spinal column or ruptured vertebral disk
2. Nursing intervention after the procedure
a. Maintain bed rest
b. Monitor vital signs
c. Force fluids
d. Observe for headache, pain in neck, and dizziness

H. Position emission tomography (PET scan)
1. The patient inhales or is injected with a radioactive substance
2. The computer can diagnose and determine level of functioning of an organ
3. Exposure to radiation is minimal and no special care is indicated

I. Skull x-ray examination: no preparation; no nursing care or observations indicated afterward

FREQUENT PATIENT PROBLEMS AND NURSING CARE

A. Impaired physical mobility related to progression of primary disease
1. Give specific care and assessment as required
2. Perform neurologic assessment every 2 to 4 hours
3. Initiate all nursing care measures to prevent complications of immobility

B. Potential for injury/infection related to "fixed eyes" (no blinking)
1. Protect with eye shields
2. If needed remove dried exudate with warm saline solution and mineral oil
3. Close eyes
4. Inspect for inflammation

C. Ineffective breathing pattern related to neuromuscular impairment
1. Maintain patent airway, suction as needed, and elevate head 20 to 30 degrees
2. Have tracheostomy set available
3. Provide oxygen with humidity
4. Monitor vital signs q2h
5. Provide oral hygiene q2h
6. Lubricate lips

D. High risk for alteration in body temperature related to neuromuscular impairment
1. Assess rectal temperature q2h
2. Use external heating and cooling (e.g., hypo-hyperthermia machine)

E. High risk for aspiration related to neuromuscular impairment
1. Maintain NPO
2. Position patient on side; turn q2h
3. Provide nasogastric tube feedings
4. Monitor IV fluids

F. High risk for injury related to restlessness, involuntary motions, or seizures
1. Maintain safety (e.g., padded side rails)
2. Follow precautions, care, and observations for a patient with seizures
3. Restrain *only* as necessary

G. Altered patterns of urinary elimination related to neuromuscular impairment

1. Oliguria
   a. Provide indwelling catheter care
   b. Monitor intake and output qh
2. Incontinence
   a. Wash, dry, and inspect skin as needed
   b. Implement measures to prevent decubitus ulcers
   c. Implement bladder training
H. Bowel incontinence/constipation related to neuromuscular impairment
   1. Incontinence
      a. Wash, dry, and inspect skin as needed
      b. Implement measures to prevent decubitus ulcers
      c. Provide bowel training
   2. Constipation
      a. Record bowel movements
      b. Provide stool softeners, laxatives, and enemas as ordered
      c. Check for impaction; disimpact as needed
I. Fear/anxiety related to pain; complications; surgery; possible disfigurement, disability, or dependency; fatal prognosis
   1. Explain everything (actions) carefully
   2. Encourage patient to express feelings
   3. Report to health team

SPECIAL SITUATIONS

A. The patient in coma
   1. Unconscious state in which the patient is unresponsive to verbal or painful stimuli; this occurs with many primary diseases; the patient is dependent on the nurse for maintenance of all basic human needs, nourishment, bathing, elimination, respiration, prevention of complications, and assessment and provision of care for problems (A to I in the preceding outline)
   2. Nursing intervention
      a. Include family in nursing care and care planning as much as possible
      b. Note level of consciousness (LOC) (see nursing assessment of the neurologic patient) every 15 minutes if LOC decreases; assess every 1, 2, or 4 hours as LOC improves
      c. Demonstrate respect in patient's presence
      d. Provide a quiet, restful environment
      e. Speak to patient; use proper name; introduce self, and explain all care before starting
      f. Provide privacy
B. The patient with paralysis
   1. Paraplegia (tetraplegia): paralysis of the lower extremities from sudden injury (e.g., automobile accident) or progressive degenerative disease (e.g., multiple sclerosis) to the spinal cord; there may be no motion or sensory function or reflexes; there may be uncontrollable muscle spasms; perspiration ceases and then becomes profuse; there is a loss of bladder and bowel control; sexual dysfunction, anxiety, fear, depression, anger, and embarrassment are major patient problems; patient may be totally dependent
   2. Quadriplegia (tetraplegia): paralysis of all four extremities from sudden injury (e.g., diving accident) or progressive degenerative disease (e.g., amyo-

trophic lateral sclerosis [ALS]); symptoms and patient problems include those encountered with paraplegia, as well as autonomic dysreflexia
   3. Nursing intervention
      a. Take measures to prevent complications of immobility
      b. Provide bowel and bladder training
      c. Prevent deformity: maintain joint mobility and correct alignment
      d. Force fluid intake
      e. Provide high-protein diet
      f. Encourage independence according to ability
      g. Communicate and work closely with the physiatrist, physical therapist, occupational therapist, and other members of the rehabilitation team
      h. Include family in nursing care and planning

MAJOR MEDICAL DIAGNOSES
Increased Intracranial Pressure (IICP)

A. Description: fluid accumulation or a lesion takes up space in the cranial cavity, producing IICP; the brain is gradually compressed, or life-sustaining functions cease; may be sudden or progress slowly
B. Causes: tumors, hematoma, edema from trauma, and abscesses from infections
C. Signs and symptoms: related to primary diagnosis
   1. Headache, restlessness, and anxiety
   2. Vomiting: recurrent, projectile, and not related to nausea or meals
   3. Change in pupil response to light
   4. Seizures
   5. Respiratory difficulty: irregular, Cheyne-Stokes, or Kussmaul breathing
   6. Blood pressure elevates, with wide pulse pressure
   7. Pulse increases at first then slows to 40 to 60 beats/min, regular and strong
   8. Altered LOC: becomes lethargic, speech slows, becomes confused, and shows decreased level of response
   9. Visual disturbances: diplopia and blurred vision
   10. Progressive weakness or paralysis
   11. Loss of consciousness, coma, and death
D. Diagnostic tests/methods: neurologic assessment by physician and nurse
E. Treatment: depends on cause
   1. Surgical intervention (craniotomy)
   2. Steroids, anticonvulsants, mannitol, dexamethasone (Decadron), or urea to decrease edema
F. Nursing intervention
   1. Elevate head to semi-Fowler's position; never place in Trendelenburg's position
   2. Monitor vital signs every 15 minutes
   3. Prevent aspiration; place patient on side
   4. Maintain airway; O_2 therapy as necessary
   5. Observe pupillary response (usually unequal and may not react to light)
   6. Report any change in LOC immediately
   7. Provide special care and observation when a patient has a seizure
   8. Provide care and safety for an unconscious patient
   9. Monitor IV fluids closely to prevent overhydration

Convulsive Disorders

A. Description: frequently a convulsion or seizure is not a disease but a symptom of a neurologic disorder; epilepsy is a disease characterized by a disposition for seizures; the following are types of seizures
   1. Generalized or grand mal: there may be a premonition or sign (aura); the individual cries out, loses consciousness, and enters a tonic phase (the body is rigid, and the jaw is clenched); then there is a clonic phase, with jerking movements of muscles, cessation of respirations, and fecal and urinary incontinence; lasts 1 to 2 minutes followed by a short period of unresponsiveness
   2. Partial or petit mal: loss of consciousness that lasts 5 to 30 seconds, during which time normal activities may or may not cease; there may be amnesia concerning this time
   3. Jacksonian (motor): a focal seizure that may be limited to jerky movements of one extremity; may precede a grand mal seizure
B. Causes:
   1. May be secondary to another condition: cerebrovascular accident (CVA), head injury, brain tumor, markedly elevated temperature, toxins, or electrolyte imbalance
   2. Epilepsy may have no known cause; onset usually is in childhood, usually before 30 years of age
C. Patient problems
   1. Related to primary disease
   2. Fear of injury
   3. Anxiety related to a chronic, lifelong disease
   4. Embarrassment
   5. Fear of public rejection
   6. Side effects of drug therapy
D. Diagnostic tests/methods
   1. Specific tests to identify lesions
   2. EEG, CT scan, and MRI
E. Treatment
   1. Treat and remove cause, if known
   2. Anticonvulsant drugs (see Chapter 4)
F. Nursing intervention
   1. Provide accurate observation and documentation including: aura, time of onset, whether seizure is general or focal, specific parts of body involved, eye movement, loss of consciousness, bowel and bladder control, condition after seizure, memory loss, weakness, and any injury caused by seizure
   2. Encourage patient to wear medical identification tag
   3. Have suction available
   4. Secure seizure stick and airway for easy accessibility
   5. During generalized (grand mal) seizure
      a. Insert seizure stick between teeth before seizure (do not force)
      b. Maintain airway
      c. Prevent head injury
      d. Place patient on side if possible
      e. Protect extremities from injury by guiding movements
      f. Do not restrain
      g. Loosen clothing
      h. Remove pillows
      i. Maintain safety until fully conscious

Transient Ischemic Attacks (TIAs)

Altered cerebral tissue perfusion related to a temporary neurologic disturbance
A. Manifested by sudden loss of motor or sensory function
B. Lasts for a few minutes to a few hours
C. Caused by a temporarily diminished blood supply to an area of the brain
D. Patient is at high risk for developing a stroke
E. Medical management is indicated (control of hypertension, low-sodium diet, possible anticoagulant therapy, stop smoking)
F. Nursing care would include close observation and assessment; specific care based on treatment

Cerebrovascular Accident (CVA) (Stroke)

A. Description: decreased blood supply to a part of the brain caused by rupture, occlusion, or stenosis of the blood vessels; onset may be sudden or gradual; symptoms and patient problems depend on location and size of area of brain with reduced or absent blood supply (left CVA results in right-sided involvement often associated with speech problems; right CVA results in left-sided involvement often associated with safety/judgment problems)
B. Causes: increased incidence with aging
   1. Atherosclerosis
   2. Embolism
   3. Thrombosis
   4. Hemorrhage from a ruptured cerebral aneurysm
   5. Hypertension
C. Signs and symptoms
   1. Altered level of consciousness
   2. Change in mental status: decreased attention span, decreased ability to think and reason, difficulty following simple directions
   3. Communication: motor or sensory aphasia, difficulty reading, writing, speaking, or understanding
   4. Bowel or bladder dysfunction: retention, impaction, or incontinence
   5. Seizures
   6. Limited motor function: paralysis, dysphagia, weakness, hemiplegia, loss of function, or contractures
   7. Loss of sensation/perception
   8. Headaches and syncope
   9. Loss of temperature regulation and elevated temperature, pulse, and blood pressure
   10. Absent gag reflex (aspiration)
   11. Unusual emotional responses: depression, anxiety, anger, verbal outbursts, and crying; emotional lability
   12. Problems related to immobility (see Chapter 2)
D. Diagnostic tests/methods
   1. Physical assessment and patient or family history
   2. EEG, CT scan, lumbar puncture, or cerebral angiography
E. Treatment
   1. Remove cause, prevent complications, and maintain function; rehabilitation to restore function
   2. Provide antihypertensives, anticoagulants, and stool softeners (see Chapter 4)
   3. Surgical removal of clot or repair of aneurysm
F. Nursing intervention
   1. Maintain bed rest; provide complete care; use turning sheet, foot board, firm mattress, pillows; and tro-

chanter rolls to maintain proper body aligment; anticipate needs and leave things within reach (e.g., call bell)

2. Reposition patient q2h; provide passive and active ROM exercises; place patient in chair as soon as allowed; use flotation mattress or sheepskin
3. Provide bath, inspect, and provide nursing measures to prevent decubitus ulcers
4. Provide oxygen with humidity; have patient cough and take deep breaths q2h if possible; maintain airway; suction as needed; prevent aspiration; keep head turned to side; place in semi-Fowler's position
5. Ensure adequate nutrition and fluid and electrolyte balance; provide nasogastric/gastrostomy tube feeding; maintain IV fluids; provide soft diet when tolerated; use total parenteral nutrition (TPN)
6. Establish means of communication: call bell, pad and pencil, and nonverbal gestures; use simple commands; speak slowly, explain all care; provide speech therapy
7. Be nonjudgmental about personality changes; encourage family participation; provide diversional activities; praise accomplishments realistically
8. Assess LOC; maintain safety in environment; use side rails; restrain only as necessary
9. Observe for IICP
10. Monitor vital signs q4h
11. Ensure elimination; check for impaction; monitor bowel movements; monitor intake and output; provide indwelling catheter care; then conduct bowel and bladder training
12. Provide care, safety, and precautions for a patient with seizures
13. Provide support for family
14. Schedule physical and occupational therapy as soon as possible
15. Provide nursing measures to prevent complications of immobility (see Chapter 2)
16. Encourage self-care

Brain Tumor

A. Description: a benign or malignant growth that grows and exerts pressure on vital centers of the brain, depressing function and causing increased pressure
B. Cause: unknown
C. Signs and symptoms: individual, depending on location and size
   1. Personality changes, fear, and anxiety
   2. Headaches, dizziness, and visual disturbance (e.g., double vision)
   3. Seizures
   4. Pituitary dysfunction
   5. Signs of IICP
   6. Local paresthesia or anesthesia
   7. Aphasia
   8. Problems with coordination
D. Diagnostic tests/methods
   1. Patient history and physical examination
   2. Neurologic assessment including EEG, CT scan, angiography, and MRI
E. Treatment: surgical removal if possible (craniotomy), frequently combined with radiotherapy and chemotherapy
F. Nursing intervention

1. Perform neurologic assessment and documentation
2. Provide safety and assist with care as needed
3. Be nonjudgmental about personality changes; encourage the patient to express feelings
4. Provide postoperative care
   a. Anticipate and provide care as needed to maintain airway
   b. Provide safety and observation during a seizure
   c. Regulate body temperature
   d. Position on unoperated side
   e. Elevate head only under medical order
   f. Inspect dressing every 30 minutes for hemorrhage or drainage (leakage of cerebrospinal fluid)
   g. Make neurologic assessment qh until patient is stable and then q4h; observe for IICP
   h. Provide care for the patient in coma as indicated earlier in this section

Head Injuries

A. Description: trauma resulting in a fracture to the skull, either a simple break in the bone or bone fragmentation that penetrates the brain tissue; can also cause hemorrhage, concussion, or contusion
   1. Cerebral concussion: injury to the head; patient may be dazed or unconscious for a few minutes; some functions (e.g., memory) may be impaired for as long as several weeks
   2. Cerebral contusion: head injury causing bruising of brain tissue; person experiences stupor, confusion, or loss of consciousness; if severe, may go into coma
   3. Cerebral laceration: a break in continuity of brain tissue
B. Cause: blow to the head (e.g., from a fall or automobile accident
C. Signs and symptoms: individual, according to location and extent of blow
   1. Nausea and vomiting
   2. Lethargy: increasing loss of consciousness to impending coma
   3. Disorientation
   4. Drainage of cerebrospinal fluid from ear or nose
   5. Convulsions
   6. Problems related to IICP
D. Diagnostic tests/methods
   1. Patient history and physical/neurologic assessment
   2. X-ray examination
   3. Angiography
   4. CT scan
   5. PET
E. Treatment
   1. Anticonvulsions
   2. Maintenance of fluid balance
   3. Surgery
F. Nursing intervention
   1. Provide care as discussed for a patient with IICP (see previous outline)
   2. Neurologic assessment qh
   3. Maintain airway
   4. Give care as required for the unconscious patient if necessary
   5. Take precautions for a patient with seizures
   6. Observe for serous or bloody discharge from ears/nose

Multiple Sclerosis

A. Description: a chronic, progressive disease of the brain and spinal cord; lesions cause degeneration of the myelin sheath and interfere with conduction of motor nerve impulses; there are periods of remissions and exacerbations; onset occurs in young adults; it has an unpredictable progression
B. Cause: unknown; exacerbates with stress
C. Signs and symptoms vary with individual
1. Ataxia
2. Paresthesia
3. Weakness and loss of muscle tone
4. Loss of sense of position
5. Vertigo
6. Blurred vision, diplopia, nystagmus, patchy blindness that may progress to total blindness
7. Inappropriate emotions: euphoria/apathy/depression
8. Dysphagia
9. Slurred speech
10. Bladder and bowel dysfunction: incontinence or retention
11. Sexual dysfunction: impotence, diminished sensation
12. Spasticity as disease progresses
D. Diagnostic tests/methods
1. Patient history and physical neurologic assessment
2. CT scan
3. MRI
4. Examination of cerebrospinal fluid (CSF)
E. Treatment: symptomatic—corticosteroids during acute exacerbations
F. Nursing intervention
1. Provide care to prevent complications of immobility (see Chapter 2)
2. Encourage patient to maintain independence
3. Encourage patient to participate in care plan
4. Encourage high-caloric, high-vitamin, high-protein diet; provide nutrition that can be swallowed easily
5. Provide bowel and bladder training (may have indwelling catheter)
6. Provide diversional activities
7. Provide safety
8. Allow time for patients to express concerns about disabilities and dependencies: be supportive
9. Avoid precipitating factors that cause exacerbations (fatigue, cold, infections)
10. Patient/family education

Parkinson's Disease

A. Definition: a progressive, degenerative disease causing destruction of nerve cells in the basal ganglia of the brain caused by a deficiency of dopamine; limbs become rigid, fingers have characteristic pill-rolling movement, and head has to-and-fro movement; the patient has a bent position and walks in short, shuffling steps; facial expression becomes blank with wide eyes and infrequent blinking (Parkinson's mask); intelligence is not affected
B. Cause: unknown
C. Signs and symptoms
1. Tremor
2. Voluntary movement is slow and difficult; coordination is poor (ataxia)

3. Impaired chewing and eating; excessive salivation and drooling
4. Speech is slow and patient is soft spoken; written communication is difficult
5. Excessive sweating
6. Emotional changes: depression, paranoia, and eventually confusion
7. Dependency
D. Diagnostic tests/methods
1. Patient history and physical assessment
2. Neurologic assessment
E. Treatment: many patients respond to drug therapy, and the disease is controlled with medication for the remainder of their lives; others have no response, and the disease progresses to a state of invalidism and immobility (usually treated with a combination of drugs) (see Chapter 4)
F. Nursing intervention
1. Encourage patient to maintain independence as much as possible in hygiene and dressing; include patient in planning all aspects of care as much as possible
2. Encourage participation in previous work and social and diversional activities (avoid social withdrawal)
3. Help patient avoid embarrassment while eating; use straws, wipe drooling saliva, use bib, and keep clothing clean; use utensils with large handles for easy grip
4. Recommend a soft diet or one of a consistency the patient is able to chew
5. Provide diversion (activity therapy)
6. Encourage daily exercises as tolerated, especially walking; take safety measures
7. Encourage patient to avoid fatigue
8. Help patient to avoid frustration; emphasize capabilities rather than limitations
9. Reinforce speech, physical, and occupational therapy treatment protocols
10. Administer stool softeners to avoid constipation
11. Provide bowel and bladder training
12. Be patient when patient is slow or clumsy
13. Establish a means of communication
14. Enhance cognitive skills (reorient frequently)
15. Prevent pneumonia; force fluids; turn patient when in bed and encourage patient to be out of bed as much as possible
16. Provide mouth care q4h
17. Encourage family participation in all aspects of rehabilitation

Spinal Cord Impairment

The vertebral column houses the spinal cord. A small cartilage disk acts as a cushion between the vertebrae. All sensory and motor nerves to the neck, trunk, and extremities branch out from the spinal cord. The degree of disability and patient problems is related to the location of the body controlled by the injured or diseased nerves.

Herniated Intervertebral Disk

A. Description: a portion of the cartilage disk protrudes and compresses the nerves; continued pressure can cause degeneration

B. Causes
   1. Straining
   2. Lifting
C. Signs and symptoms
   1. Pain usually radiating over the buttock and down the leg
   2. Weakness of ankle and knee; tingling; numbness
   3. Complications of immobility
D. Diagnostic tests/methods
   1. CT scan
   2. X-ray examination
   3. Myelogram (identifies level of herniation)
   4. MRI
E. Treatment
   1. Bed rest with traction
   2. Muscle relaxants, antiinflammatory drugs, and narcotic analgesics
   3. Brace
   4. Surgery
      a. Laminectomy: with the patient under general anesthesia, first the lamina, or arch of the vertebra, is removed and then the disk; dangers include injury to motor roots, which can result in paralysis, and clot formation that will exert pressure on the spinal cord
      b. Spinal fusion (performed with laminectomy): a graft from the posterior iliac crest is taken and used as a bridge between the laminae; this supports the spinal column; after surgery patient may be in cast for immobilization to promote healing; recovery is slow (4 to 5 weeks)
F. Nursing intervention
   1. Provide bed rest; give care as indicated to prevent complications of immobility (may be allowed to be out of traction at specific times [e.g., during meals or to use the bathroom])
   2. Provide heat, either moist or dry, before surgery as ordered
   3. Provide firm mattress; use bed board
   4. Use fracture bedpan if bed rest is prescribed for patient
   5. Anticipate and medicate for pain
   6. Provide general preoperative and postoperative care (see Chapter 2)
      a. Follow specific orders related to operative procedure: movement, turning, raising head, and early ambulation
      b. Keep patient off operative site; turn patient side to side to prone position (when allowed); maintain proper alignment at all times; use log-rolling technique
      c. Medicate for pain
      d. Provide care for the patient in a body cast
      e. Provide care and observation to donor site; maintain asepsis
      f. Communicate and work with physical therapist when ordered

Spinal Cord Lesion

A. Description: a growth compressing the spinal cord; may be benign or malignant; interferes with nerve function
B. Cause: unknown
C. Signs and symptoms: individual, according to area involved
D. Diagnostic tests/methods
   1. Patient history
   2. Myelography
   3. Neurologic assessment
E. Treatment: Surgical removal
F. Nursing intervention: See care of a patient with a laminectomy (in preceding outline)

Spinal Cord Injuries

A. Description: complete or partial severing of the spinal cord; if severing is complete, there is permanent paralysis of body parts below site of injury; when there is partial damage, edema may cause a temporary paralysis
B. Cause: accident (e.g., automobile, shooting, or diving)
C. Signs and symptoms: individual, according to level of spinal cord involved
   1. Respiratory distress
   2. Paralysis
D. Diagnostic tests/methods: physical examination
E. Treatment
   1. Immobilization: Crutchfield tongs, halo traction, back brace, or body cast
   2. Surgery
F. Nursing intervention
   1. See care of a patient with paralysis in the preceding section
   2. Maintain airway and respiratory function
   3. See emergency care of a patient with a spinal cord injury (Chapter 11)

The Endocrine System

A disturbance in one of the secreting glands may affect the regulation of another gland; therefore the patient may also experience multiple problems and needs. Some of these disturbances affect the patient's appearance, personality, and activity level. Because of this the nurse must be emotionally supportive to the patient and family. The nurse must also provide patient teaching because some patients must have lifelong hormonal drug therapy related to endocrine deficiencies.

NURSING ASSESSMENT

A. Nursing observations
   1. General appearance
   2. Vital signs
   3. Weight
   4. Skin
      a. Color
         (1) Pallor
         (2) Flushed
         (3) Yellow pigmentation
         (4) Bronze pigmentation
         (5) Purple striae over obese areas
      b. Temperature
      c. Dry
      d. Moist
      e. Excess diaphoresis
      f. Poor wound healing
   5. Hair
      a. Dry

b. Brittle
c. Thin
6. Nails
   a. Dry
   b. Thin
   c. Thick
7. Musculoskeletal
   a. Muscle mass distribution
   b. Fat distribution
   c. Change in height
   d. Changes in body proportions: enlarged ears, nose, jaws, hands, and feet
   e. Diminished muscle strength
8. Central nervous system
   a. Personality changes
   b. Alterations in consciousness
      (1) Listlessness
      (2) Slowed cognitive ability
      (3) Stupor
      (4) Seizures
      (5) Confusion
      (6) Coma
   c. Slowed, hoarse speech
   d. Reflexes
      (1) Trousseau's sign
      (2) Chvostek's sign
9. Eyes
   a. Periorbital edema
   b. Protruding eyeball (exopthalmos)
   c. Drooping eyelids (ptosis)
10. Gastrointestinal system
    a. Anorexia
    b. Polyphagia
    c. Polydipsia
    d. Constipation
    e. Diarrhea
    f. Nausea and vomiting
11. Cardiovascular system
    a. Hypertension
    b. Hypotension
    c. Tachycardia
    d. Bradycardia
12. Respiratory system
    a. Tachypnea
    b. Acetone breath
    c. Kussmaul-Kien respirations
13. Renal system
    a. Polyuria
    b. Oliguria
14. Reproductive system
    a. Menstrual disturbances
    b. Libido disturbances
    c. Galactorrhea (excess mammary gland secretion in females)
    d. Gynecomastia (increased breast tissue in males)
B. Patient description (subjective data)
   1. Pain
      a. Headache
      b. Skeletal pain
      c. Back pain
      d. Muscle spasms
   2. Appetite
      a. Anorexia

b. Polyphagia
3. Weakness
4. Numbness
5. Tingling
6. Mood swings
7. Nausea
8. Intolerance to heat or cold
9. Polydipsia
10. Polyuria, nocturia, and dysuria
11. Decreased libido and impotence
12. Frequent infections

DIAGNOSTIC TESTS/METHODS

A. Serum laboratory studies
   1. Protein bound iodine (PBI)
      a. The thyroid hormone, thyroxine, contains iodine that binds itself to blood proteins; therefore, the function of the thyroid gland is evaluated by measuring the amount of this iodine
      b. Factors that may alter test findings
         (1) Ingestion of drugs or administration of dyes containing iodine
         (2) Mercurial diurectics or estrogen
         (3) Pregnancy
   2. Iodine 131 uptake (radioactive iodine thyroid uptake)
      a. Measures the amount of radioactive iodine that has concentrated in the thyroid gland after ingestion of the iodine preparation
      b. Test findings may be altered by recent ingestion of iodides or use of radiographic dyes
      c. A normal thyroid gland removes 15% to 50% of iodine from bloodstream
   3. Basal metabolic rate (BMR): measures the amount of oxygen consumed by the body while the patient is in a state of complete mental and physical rest
   4. T_3 (triiodothyronine): measures thyroid function indirectly by evaluating whether radioactive triiodothyronine binds to a serum specimen
   5. T_4 (thyroxine): measures the amount of thyroxine in the circulation
   6. Thyroid-stimulating hormone (TSH) radioimmunoassay: indicator of thyroid-stimulating hormone production based on pituitary function; measures TSH levels
   7. Fasting blood sugar (FBS)
      a. Measures the amount of glucose in the bloodstream during a fasting period
      b. No food is permitted for 12 hours before the test
      c. Normal value: 80 to 120 mg/dl
   8. Postprandial blood sugar
      a. Evaluates the patient's ability to dispose of blood glucose after a meal
      b. Normal value: 80 to 120 mg/dl serum
   9. Glucose tolerance test (GTT)
      a. Determines patient response to a measured dose of glucose
      b. Normal value: blood glucose climbs to a peak of 140 mg/dl serum in the first hour and returns to normal by the second or third hour
   10. Serum potassium
       a. Measures the amount of K in the bloodstream
       b. Normal range: 3.5 to 5.0 mEq/L

11. Serum sodium
    a. Measures the amount of Na in the bloodstream
    b. Normal range: 135 to 145 mEq/L
12. Total serum calcium
    a. Measures the amount of Ca in the bloodstream
    b. Normal range: 4.8 to 5.2 mEq/L (9 to 11 mg/dl)
13. Serum ketones: determines the amount of ketones produced by the metabolism of fat
14. Blood pH
    a. Measures the acid-base status of the blood
    b. Normal arterial blood findings: pH 7.35 to 7.45
    c. Normal venous blood findings: pH 7.31 to 7.41
15. Serum phosphorus: measures the amount of serum phosphorus in the bloodstream
16. Adrenocorticotropic hormone (ACTH) stimulating test (or glucocorticoid stimulating test)
    a. Evaluates the changes in adrenocortical function produced by the administration of ACTH
    b. ACTH is administered intramuscularly (IM) or intravenously (IV)
    c. For the IM methods a blood specimen is obtained 1 hour after the administration of ACTH
    d. For the IV method a 24-hour urine specimen is collected and analyzed
17. Cortisone suppression test: used to differentiate between Cushing's syndrome and Cushing's disease
18. Plasma cortisol
    a. Hormonal study of the adrenal cortex
    b. Low levels are seen in Addison's disease
    c. Elevated levels indicate Cushing's syndrome
19. Plasma cortisol response to ACTH
    a. Hormonal study of the adrenal cortex
    b. Patient's blood specimen is drawn in a fasting state and examined for plasma cortisol levels
    c. Next ACTH is administered IM, and a second blood sample is withdrawn
    d. A rise in the plasma cortisol level in the second specimen is normal
20. Urine 17-ketogenic steroids
    a. Measures adrenocortical function
    b. Urine specimen is collected for a 24-hour period and should be kept cold
B. Urine laboratory studies
   1. Twenty-four-hour quantitative sugar specimen
      a. An evaluation of the patient's glucose loss over a 24-hour period
      b. Normally the urine is free of sugar
      c. Nursing implications
         (1) Have the patient void and discard the specimen at the beginning of the 24-hour period
         (2) Save all urine voided in a container provided by the laboratory
         (3) At the end of the 24 hours, have the patient void again and save the specimen in the container
   2. Urine pH
      a. Measures the acid-base balance of the urine
      b. Normal range: pH 4.8 to 7.5
   3. Quantitative urinary calcium: measures the amount of Ca in a 24-hour urine specimen after a period of Ca deprivation

4. Vanillylmandelic acid (VMA) test
   a. Determines the amount of urinary excretion of the end product of catecholamine metabolism
   b. Factors that may alter test findings
      (1) Ingestion of coffee, tea, chocolate, bananas, vanilla-containing food, or aspirin
      (2) Stress
C. Scans
   1. Thyroid scan: radionucleotide study of the thyroid to determine function
   2. CT scan: used to visualize cross sections of tissue

FREQUENT PATIENT PROBLEMS AND NURSING CARE

A. Self-esteem disturbance related to body image
   1. Observe the patient for loss of appetite, insomnia, disinterest in self, and unwillingness to discuss alteration in body image
   2. Encourage patient to express feelings
   3. Encourage communication with significant other
B. Altered nutrition, less than body requirements, related to noncompliance with therapeutic diet
   1. Observe the patient for diet intolerance such as refusal to eat, complaints of foods, and eating of foods that are contraindicated
   2. Explain to the patient and family the reason for and intended effect of therapeutic diet and necessity of maintaining it until discontinued by physician
   3. Instruct the patient and family on prescribed food selection
C. Knowledge deficit related to prescribed medication
   1. Explain to the patient and family the dosage and method of administering prescribed drugs
   2. Provide information about the purpose of the drug and potential side effects
   3. Describe symptoms that should be reported to the physician
   4. Explain where therapeutic supplies may be obtained
   5. Evaluate the patient's response to teaching
D. High risk for injury related to toxic effects of iodine preparations. Discontinue iodides if evidence of the following exists
   1. Swelling of buccal mucosa
   2. Excessive salivation
   3. Swelling of neck glands
   4. Skin eruptions
E. High risk for injury related to hypoglycemia
   1. Observe for complaints of headache, nervousness, hunger, dizziness, pallor, and sweating (diaphoresis)
   2. Assess vital signs
   3. Give quick-acting carbohydrate
      a. Orange juice
      b. Coca-cola
      c. Granulated sugar
      d. Crackers
      e. Hard candy
   4. If patient is unconscious: give instant glucose (buccally); glucagon (SC); IV glucose
   5. Have laboratory withdraw serum specimen for glucose assessment
   6. Assess reason for reaction after situation has been controlled

a. Length of time since last meal
b. Correct amount of food eaten or meal omitted
c. Correct dosage of insulin
d. Kinds of activities or situation before reaction

F. High risk for injury (seizures) related to hypocalcemia
1. Observe for complaints of numbness, tingling, cramping, or spastic movements of extremities
2. Emergency treatment requires administration of IV calcium
3. Prevent airway obstruction
a. Keep seizure stick at bedside
b. Provide suction machine at bedside
c. Provide tracheostomy set at bedside
4. Prevent injury by putting padding along side rails, easing patient to floor, or removing constrictive clothes
5. Monitor and record vital signs
6. Note frequency, time, level of consciousness, and length of seizure

MAJOR MEDICAL DIAGNOSES
Hyperpituitarism

A. Definition: overproduction of growth hormone by the anterior pituitary gland
B. Pathology
1. Increased activity of the gland usually results from a secreting pituitary tumor
2. Two major disorders arise from hypersecretion
a. Gigantism: develops in children; hypersecretion before the growth plate closes, results in bone and tissue growth
b. Acromegaly: a disorder in adults caused by hypersecretion after closure of the epiphyses of the long bones
C. Signs and symptoms
1. Subjective
a. Headache
b. Visual disturbances
c. Weakness
2. Objective
a. Coarse facial features: enlarged ears, nose, lips, tongue, and jaws
b. Broad hands, fingers, and feet
c. Palpable, enlarged visceral organs
d. Disturbances in carbohydrate metabolism, menstruation, and libido
e. Gynecomastia in the male; galactorrhea in the female
f. Symmetrical bone overgrowth (gigantism)
g. Increased heights: 8 to 9 ft (gigantism)
D. Diagnostic tests/methods
1. X-ray studies of jaws, sinuses, hands, and feet
2. Changes in physical appearance
3. CT scan to identify tumor
4. Cerebral arteriography to identify tumor
5. Growth hormone assay
E. Treatment
1. Surgical intervention: hypophysectomy (excision of the pituitary gland); excision of tumor with laser
2. Irradiation of the pituitary gland
3. Medication to treat symptoms related to other hormonal disturbances as a result of hypersecretion

F. Nursing intervention
1. Assist the patient to accept altered body image emphasizing person's value as an individual
2. Explain the basis for altered sexual functioning
3. Emphasize need for lifelong medical follow-up
4. If the patient has undergone hypophysectomy
a. Follow nursing care as for the patient who has undergone intracranial surgery
b. Observe for potential postoperative complications
(1) Adrenal insufficiency
(2) Hypothyroidism
(3) Diabetes insipidus

Hypopituitarism (Simmonds' Disease)

A. Definition: total absence of all pituitary secretions
B. Pathology: occurs after destruction of the pituitary gland by surgery, infection, injury, hemorrhage, or tumor
C. Signs and symptoms
1. Subjective
a. Lethargy
b. Loss of muscle strength
c. Weakness
d. Menstrual irregularities
2. Objective
a. Emaciation
b. Pallor
c. Dry, yellow skin
d. Diminished axillary and pubic hair
e. Decreased muscle size
f. Increased susceptibility to infection
D. Diagnostic tests/methods
1. T_3 and T_4
2. Urine 17-ketogenic steroids
E. Treatment
1. Replacement hormones
2. Surgical ablation if tumor is present in pituitary gland
F. Nursing intervention
1. Emphasize need for lifelong medical follow-up
2. Teach the patient self-administration of drug: purpose, proper dosage, and potential side effects
3. Follow nursing care as for the patient who has undergone intracranial surgery

Hyperthyroidism (Graves' Disease and Thyrotoxicosis)

A. Definition: overactivity of the thryoid gland with hypersecretion of T_4
B. Pathology
1. Metabolic rate is increased, resulting in a high amount of energy and oxygen expenditure
2. May be caused by decreased production of thyroid-stimulating hormone (TSH) by malfunctioning pituitary gland; which results in high T_4 serum concentration
3. May be attributed to enlarged thyroid gland caused by decreased iodine intake
C. Signs and symptoms
1. Subjective
a. Polyphagia
b. Hyperexcitability/personality changes
c. Heat intolerance

  d. Insomnia
  e. Amenorrhea
  f. Diarrhea/constipation
  g. Increased appetite
  h. Fatigue/weakness
  2. Objective
  a. Weight loss
  b. Exophthalmos
  c. Excessive sweating
  d. Increased pulse rate
  e. Fine hand tremors
  f. Warm, flushed skin
  g. Elevated blood pressure
  h. Bruit over thyroid
D. Diagnostic tests: increased laboratory values of T_3, T_4, ^{131}I uptake, PBI, and BMR confirm hyperthyroidism; thyroid scan
E. Treatment
  1. Medication to inhibit T_4 production
  2. Radioactive iodine to destroy thyroid gland cells to decrease T_4 secretion
  3. Drugs to control tachycardia and hyperexcitability
  4. Subtotal or total thyroidectomy
F. Nursing intervention
  1. Teach the patient and family signs and symptoms of hypothyroidism when patient is receiving thyroid-inhibiting drugs
  a. Increased body weight
  b. Sensitivity to cold
  c. Fatigue
  d. Dry skin, hair, and nails
  e. Slow, hoarse speech
  f. Constipation
  2. Encourage adequate nutrition for increased energy expenditure
  a. High-calorie, high-vitamin, and high-carbohydrate intake
  b. Between-meal snacks
  c. Increased fluid intake
  d. Avoidance of caffeine
  3. Plan undisturbed rest periods to restore energy: provide cool, quiet, nonstressful environment
  4. Advise the patient to elevate the head of bed while recumbent to improve eye drainage
  5. If the patient has undergone surgery
  a. Place patient on back in a low-Fowler's or semi-Fowler's position to avoid strain on sutures
  b. Observe dressing for hemorrhage or constriction of the throat; examine back of neck for pooling
  c. Keep tracheostomy set at bedside in event of respiratory obstruction caused by hemorrhage, edema of glottis, laryngeal nerve damage, or tetany
  d. Encourage patient to cough and expectorate secretions from throat and bronchi
  e. Observe for signs of thyroid storm (may occur as a result of gland manipulation during surgery): fever, tachycardia, and restlessness
  f. Observe for signs of tetany (may occur if parathyroids are accidentally removed); numbness and tingling around mouth, carpopedal spasms, convulsions

Hypothyroidsm

A. Definition: absence or decreased production of T_4 by the thyroid gland
B. Pathology
  1. The disorder causes a depression of metabolic activity, resulting in physical and mental sluggishness
  2. There are three classifications of hypothyroidism
  a. Cretinism: total absence of T_4 from birth
  b. Hypothyroidism without myxedema: mild thyroid failure in older children and adults
  c. Hypothyroidism with myxedema: a severe form of gland failure in adults
C. Signs and symptoms
  1. Subjective
  a. Lethargy
  b. Fatigues easily
  c. Cold intolerance
  d. Constipation
  2. Objective
  a. Increased body weight with loss of appetite
  b. Coarse facial features
  c. Slow, hoarse speech
  d. Dry skin, hair, and nails
  e. Bradycardia
  f. Impaired memory
  g. Slowed thought process
  h. Personality changes
D. Diagnostic tests: decreased laboratory values of T_3, T_4, ^{131}I uptake, PBI, and BMR confirm hypothyroidism; thyroid scan
E. Treatment: thyroid-replacement drugs
F. Nursing intervention
  1. Educate the patient on self-administration of drug: purpose, proper dosage, and potential side effects
  2. Emphasize need for lifelong medical follow-up
  3. Teach the patient and family signs and symptoms of hyperthyroidism when receiving thyroid-replacement drugs: chest pain, tachycardia, nervousness, headache, excessive sweating, heat intolerance, and weight loss
  4. Encourage decreased caloric intake to avoid weight gain
  5. Encourage application of emollients to sooth dry skin

Hyperparathyroidism

A. Definition: oversecretion of parathormone by the parathyroid gland(s)
B. Pathology
  1. Results in calcium loss from the bones and an increased secretion of calcium and phosphorus by the kidneys
  2. Usually the result of a parathyroid tumor
C. Signs and symptoms
  1. Subjective
  a. Fatigue
  b. Thirst; poor appetite
  c. Nausea
  d. Back pain
  e. Skeletal pain
  f. Pain on weight bearing
  g. Constipation
  h. Visual disturbances

2. Objective
   a. Pathologic features
   b. Vomiting
   c. Kidney stones composed of calcium phosphate
D. Diagnostic tests
   1. Quantitative urinary calcium
   2. Total serum calcium
   3. Serum phosphorus
   4. X-ray film to reveal skeletal changes
E. Treatment: surgical resection of parathyroid gland
F. Nursing intervention
   1. Observe for postoperative conditions (refer to postoperative nursing interventions under diseases of the thyroid gland: hyperthyroidism)
   2. Observe for tetany: tingling of hands and feet, facial muscle spasms, and muscle twitching
   3. Protect from accidents: position carefully, keep bed low, keep side rails up, and assist to ambulate
   4. Explain rationale for low-calcium, low-phosphorus diet
   5. Encourage adequate hydration and dietary fiber to avoid constipation

Hypoparathyroidism

A. Definition: undersecretion of parathormone by the parathyroid glands
B. Pathology
   1. Insufficiency of parathormone causes a decrease of the serum calcium level and slows bone resorption
   2. Serum phosphorus value rises
   3. Increased neuromuscular irritability results in tetany
C. Signs and symptoms
   1. Subjective
      a. Lethargy
      b. Painful muscle spasms
      c. Tingling of hands and feet
      d. Visual disturbances
   2. Objective
      a. Dry skin, hair, and nails
      b. Respiratory distress caused by laryngeal spasms
      c. Convulsions
D. Diagnostic tests/methods
   1. Quantitative urinary calcium
   2. Total serum calcium
   3. Positive Trousseau's sign (spasms of fingers and hands after application of blood pressure cuff to arm)
   4. Presence of Chvostek's sign (hyperactivity of facial muscle in response to tapping near the angle of the jaw)
   5. X-ray studies reveal increased bone density
E. Treatment
   1. Calcium replacement in chronic cases
   2. Calcium gluconate IV for emergency treatment
   3. Diet high in calcium and low in phosphorus
   4. Vitamin D preparation
F. Nursing intervention
   1. Keep endotracheal tube and tracheostomy set at bedside at all times when caring for patients with acute tetany
   2. Promote rest with a quiet, calm, and low-lit environment
   3. Explain need for diet high in calcium but low in phosphorus: avoid milk, cheese, and egg yolks

4. Emphasize importance of lifelong medical follow-up; serum calcium level should be assessed at least three times a year

Diabetes Mellitus

A. Definition: insufficiency or absence of insulin production by pancreatic islets, creating a disturbance in carbohydrate metabolism as well as a deficiency in protein and fat conversion
B. Pathology
   1. Develops when there is a persistent deficiency of insulin
   2. May be caused by trauma, infection, or tumor of the pancreas or increased insulin requirements attributable to obesity, pregnancy, infection, or stress
   3. Those at risk: women over 40 years of age and individuals who are obese or who have a familial tendency to diabetes
   4. Two classifications
      a. Type I (formerly juvenile diabetes): rapid onset with no production of insulin; affects children and adolescents; is controlled with insulin
      b. Type II (formerly adult onset): gradual onset; may be controlled by diet, oral hypoglycemic drugs, or insulin injection
   5. Lack of insulin disrupts transportation of glucose into cells, and cells become energy exhausted; cells must use proteins and fats as a compensatory mechanism
   6. Blood sugar level becomes elevated because of lack of insulin in the cells
   7. Cellular dehydration occurs because blood sugar pulls water from the cells into the bloodstream
   8. Glucose builds up in urine, creating osmotic pull; kidneys cannot reabsorb water
C. Signs and symptoms
   1. Subjective
      a. Polyuria and nocturia
      b. Polydipsia
      c. Polyphasia
      d. Weakness
   2. Objective
      a. Hyperglycemia
      b. Glycosuria
      c. Ketosis
      d. Retarded wound healing
D. Diagnostic tests/methods
   1. Presence of polyuria, polydipsia, and polyphasia
   2. Family and medical history
   3. Laboratory studies: FBS, postprandial blood sugar, and GTT
   4. Twenty-four hour urine quantitative sugar specimen
E. Treatment
   1. Drug therapy for hyperglycemia; refer to Chapter 4, Pharmacology, for indicated nursing actions
   2. Therapeutic diet low in calories and carbohydrates to correct and avoid obesity
      a. American Diabetes Association (ADA) food exchange list widely prescribed by physicians (see Appendix J)
      b. Consists of classifying foods into lists: milk, fruit, vegetables, bread, meat, and fat
      c. Identifies content by protein, carbohydrates, fats, and calories of each food group

F. Nursing intervention
1. Assist patient in adjusting to condition: allow verbalization of feelings, offer reassurance, and give support at patient's own pace
2. Emphasize need to comply with diet and eat meals at prescribed times
3. Instruct the patient and family on signs of impending hypoglycemia: diaphoresis, pale, cold, and clammy skin, nervousness, hunger, mental confusion; give orange juice, sugar, or hard candy
4. Encourage prompt treatment of minor injuries or irritation to skin
5. Emphasize importance of continued medical follow-up, regular vision examinations, and foot care
6. Patient teaching should include
   a. Self–blood glucose level testing with Chemstrip bG or glucometer
   b. Self-injection of insulin: selection of equipment, sites of injection, rationale for rotation, accurate withdrawal of insulin, injection technique, and peak action time of insulin
   c. How to use food exchange list and make substitutions
   d. Instructions on foot care: hygiene, proper trimming of toe nails, proper fit of shoes and stockings, and treatment of minor abrasions
   e. Relationship between exercise and blood glucose
7. Instruction to patient and family on signs and symptoms of impending ketoacidosis: hot, dry, flushed skin, polydipsia, fruity odor of breath, nausea, and abdominal pain
8. Administration of insulin by way of pump
   a. Method of needle insertion and filling of syringe
   b. Instruction on site rotation and needle change q48h
   c. Remove pump and cover needle and tubing for bathing

Diabetic Coma (Ketoacidosis)

A. Definition: excess glucose and acid (ketones) in the bloodstream
B. Pathology
1. A response to insufficient insulin levels
2. Fats are mobilized for energy; fatty acids are rejected by muscles, resulting in buildup of acids in the bloodstream
3. Body's buffer system becomes exhausted
C. Signs and symptoms
1. Subjective
   a. Weakness
   b. Polydipsia
   c. Abdominal pain
   d. Nausea
   e. Headache
   f. Polyphagia
2. Objective
   a. Hot, dry, flushed skin
   b. Listlessness and drowsiness
   c. Kussmaul's respirations
   d. Sweet or acetone breath
   e. Hypotension
   f. Confusion

g. Polyuria
h. Nausea/vomiting
i. Coma
D. Diagnostic tests
1. Elevated serum glucose level
2. Elevated serum and urinary ketones
3. Lowered blood pH
E. Treatment
1. Insulin replacement
2. Correct electrolyte and pH imbalance
3. Fluid replacement
F. Nursing intervention
1. Give insulin as ordered; have another person check to prevent error
2. Monitor and record vital signs and intake and output
3. Test for glucose and acetone levels; record on diabetic flow sheet
4. Position patient with head of bed elevated 30 degrees
5. Maintain patent airway
6. Give oral care q4h and when required (prn); keep lips and mouth moist
7. Assess level of consciousness
8. Observe patient for signs of hypoglycemia: pale, cool, clammy skin, lethargy, and hypotension
9. Instruct patient and family on factors and signs of impending ketoacidosis
10. Explain importance of balance among diet, exercise, and insulin
11. Before discharge provide diabetic alert band or chain

Hypoglycemia (Insulin Shock)

A. Definition: abnormally low level of glucose in the bloodstream
B. Pathology
1. Accelerated glucose is removed from the serum
2. May be caused by overproduction or overdosage of insulin
3. Omission of a meal or too little food eaten by a patient receiving insulin
4. Too much exercise without extra food; rapid onset
C. Signs and symptoms
1. Subjective
   a. Hunger
   b. Weakness
   c. Visual disturbances
   d. Tingling lips and tongue
   e. Nervousness
2. Objective
   a. Pale, moist skin
   b. Tremors
   c. Tachycardia
   d. Hypotension
   e. Muscle weakness
   f. Disorientation
   g. Coma
D. Diagnostic test: lowered serum glucose level
E. Treatment
1. Sweetened fluids or sugar given orally; oral glucose preparations
2. Glucagon subcutaneously or IM
3. Glucose IV

F. Nursing intervention
1. Give medications as ordered
2. Monitor and record vital signs and intake and output
3. Patient teaching should include
   a. Always carry and ingest quick-acting carbohydrate when initial signs appear; fruit juices, sweetened sodas, granulated sugar, or hard candy
   b. Prevent medication error by having another person check dosage
   c. Record each administration of medication to avoid duplication
   d. Always wear medical identification tag
   e. Remember to eat a regular meal after raising glucose level to prevent a rebound effect

Diabetes Insipidus

A. Definition: water metabolism disorder related to hyposecretion of antidiuretic hormone (ADH) by the posterior pituitary lobe
B. Pathology
1. Renal tubules are unable to reabsorb water, resulting in elimination of large amounts of water
2. Hyposecretion may occur in conjunction with lung cancer, head injuries, pituitary tumor, myxedema, or encephalitis
3. Other causes may be due to malfunctioning, surgical removal, or atrophy of the pituitary gland
C. Signs and symptoms
1. Subjective
   a. Polydipsia
   b. Polyuria
2. Objective
   a. Signs of dehydration (loss of skin turgor, dry skin and mucous membranes, and cracked lips)
   b. Low specific gravity (sp gr) (1.001 to 1.006)
   c. Increased fluid intake (5 to 40 L/24 hr)
   d. Increased urine output (5 to 25 L/24 hr)
   e. Electrolyte imbalance
D. Diagnostic method: restriction of fluid intake to observe changes in urine volume and concentration
E. Treatment: vasopressin replacement
F. Nursing intervention
1. Monitor and record intake and output
2. Monitor specific gravity
3. Weigh patient daily

Primary Hyperaldosteronism (Conn's Syndrome)

A. Definition: hypersecretion of aldosterone by the adrenal cortex
B. Pathology
1. Usually caused by a tumor(s), which results in renal retention of sodium and excretion of potassium
2. Leads to inability of kidneys to concentrate urine (acidify)
C. Signs and symptoms
1. Subjective
   a. Headache
   b. Polyuria and polydipsia
   c. Paresthesia
2. Objective
   a. Hypertension with postural hypotension
   b. Signs of kidney damage: flank pain, chills, fever, and increased frequency of voiding

   c. Low specific gravity
D. Diagnostic tests
1. Low serum potassium level
2. Elevated serum sodium value
3. Elevated urinary aldosterone level
4. Increased urine pH
5. X-ray study reveals cardiac hypertrophy caused by chronic hypertension
E. Treatment: surgical removal of adrenal tumor
F. Nursing intervention
1. Monitor and record blood pressure, specific gravity, and intake and output
2. Identify and explain diet high in potassium and low in sodium
3. Provide fluids to meet excessive thirst
4. If the patient has undergone adrenalectomy
   a. Protect the patient from exposure to infections
   b. Follow general postoperative nursing actions
5. Once patient is convalescent, teach the patient self-administration of drugs: purpose, proper dosage, and potential side effects
6. Before discharge obtain medical identification tag

Cushing's Syndrome

A. Definition: hyperactivity of the adrenal cortex
B. Pathology
1. Excessive cortisol is secreted
2. Disorder results from abnormal growth of cortices or tumor to one of the glands
3. May occur because of pituitary gland dysfunction, causing excessive production of adrenocorticotropic hormone (ACTH)
C. Signs and symptoms
1. Subjective
   a. Weakness
   b. Bruises easily
   c. Amenorrhea
   d. Decreased libido
   e. Changes in secondary sex characteristics
2. Objective
   a. Fat deposits to face, back of neck, and abdomen
   b. Decreased muscle mass on limbs
   c. Unusual growth of body hair
   d. Purple striae over obese areas
   e. Impaired wound healing
   f. Hypertension
   g. Mood lability
D. Diagnostic tests
1. Increased plasma cortisol levels
2. ACTH stimulating test
3. Cortisone suppression test
E. Treatment
1. Drugs to inhibit cortisol production
2. Bilateral adrenalectomy
3. Resection of pituitary gland
4. Potassium supplements
5. Diet with sodium restriction
F. Nursing intervention
1. Assist patient in adjusting to altered body image
2. Place in noninfectious environment
3. Maintain diet low in calories, carbohydrates, and sodium and high in potassium
4. Weigh patient daily

5. Monitor glucose and acetone levels
6. Follow general postoperative nursing actions if patient undergoes adrenalectomy
7. Once the patient is convalescent, instruct on self-administration of replacement hormones and drugs: proper dosage, purpose, and potential side effects

Addison's Disease

A. Definition: hypofunction of adrenal cortex
B. Pathology
   1. As a result of dysfunction, adrenal cortex shrinks and atrophies
   2. Disorder usually originates within itself or may result from destruction of the adrenal cortex
   3. Results in disturbances of sodium and potassium
C. Signs and symptoms
   1. Subjective
      a. Weakness and fatigue
      b. Anorexia and nausea
      c. Depression
      d. Diarrhea
      e. Abdominal pain
   2. Objective
      a. Weight loss
      b. Hypotension
      c. Hypoglycemia
      d. Bronze or tan skin pigmentation
      e. Susceptibility to infection
      f. Dysrhythmias
D. Diagnostic tests
   1. Eight-hour IV ACTH test
   2. Plasma cortisol response to ACTH
   3. Low serum sodium level
   4. High serum potassium level
E. Treatment
   1. Replacement of adrenal cortex hormones
   2. Restoration of sodium and potassium balance
   3. Diet high in sodium and low in potassium, with adequate fluids
F. Nursing intervention
   1. Monitor and record vital signs and intake and output
   2. Weigh patient daily
   3. Observe for sodium imbalance: increased body weight, pitting edema, puffy eyelids, coughing and diaphoresis
   4. Observe for potassium imbalance: lethargy, flaccid muscles, anorexia, hypotension, and dysrhythmias
   5. Provide small, frequent feedings
   6. Observe for hypoglycemia: weakness, clammy skin, tremors, and mental confusion
   7. Before discharge obtain medical identification tag
   8. Emphasize need for compliance to diet and medication regimen
   9. Observe for addisonian crisis (causes: stress, surgery, trauma, infection, withdrawal of medication): hypotension, asthenia, abdominal pain, confusion, shock, and vascular collapse
   10. Teach patient to avoid infections and stressful situations

Pheochromocytoma

A. Definition: hyperactivity of the adrenal medulla
B. Pathology: caused by tumor in adrenal medulla, resulting in increased secretion of epinephrine and norepinephrine
C. Signs and symptoms
   1. Subjective
      a. Headache
      b. Visual disturbances
      c. Nervousness
      d. Heat intolerance
   2. Objective
      a. Hypertension (blood pressure may be as high as 220/140)
      b. Orthostatic hypotension
      c. Tachycardia
      d. Hyperglycemia
      e. Blanching of skin
      f. Weight loss
      g. Dysrhythmias
      h. Diaphoresis
D. Diagnostic tests
   1. Chemical and pharmacologic drug tests to differentiate from hypertension or hyperthyroidism
   2. X-ray studies to reveal adrenal medullary tumor
   3. Twenty-four hour urine collection for vanillylmandelic acid (VMA) and metanephrines
   4. Arteriography
   5. CT scan
   6. Intravenous pyelogram
E. Treatment
   1. Surgical excision of tumor
   2. Drugs to control hypertension and dysrhythmias
F. Nursing intervention
   1. Monitor blood pressure q4h and record
   2. Plan undisturbed rest periods: cool, quiet, nonstressful environment
   3. Encourage adequate hydration: record intake and output
   4. If patient undergoes adrenalectomy, follow general postoperative nursing actions: observe for adrenal crisis—falling blood pressure, tachycardia, elevated temperature, restlessness, convulsions, and coma
   5. Patient teaching should include
      a. Self-administration of medications: purpose, proper dosage, and potential side effects
      b. Signs of impending adrenal crisis
      c. Avoidance of exposure to infection; report symptoms of infections to physician
      d. Avoidance of stressful situations
      e. Emphasize need for adequate rest and good nutrition
   6. Provide medical identification tag

The Urinary System

The urinary system regulates the composition and volume of the blood. It excretes metabolic wastes and fluids and maintains fluid and electrolyte balance and acid-base balance. Malfunction of this system has generalized effects on the body's normal physiology. Frequently patients are older and have chronic medical problems (e.g., cardiac); these must be considered when nursing care is planned (e.g., many diagnoses and procedures require additional fluids as a natural irrigation; increased fluids might be contraindicated in the patient with a cardiac condition). Problems of the male reproductive system are discussed in this section.

The following terms are used to describe urine output:

anuria   absence of urine output
bacteriuria   bacteria in the urine
dribbling   voiding without stream, in small amounts, frequently or constantly
dysuria   painful or difficult urination
enuresis   involuntary voiding while asleep
frequency   voiding often and in small amounts
hematuria   blood in the urine
hesitancy   cannot immediately empty full bladder when the desire is present
incontinence   partial or complete inability to control urine output
micturition   voiding, urination
nocturia   awakening to void
oliguria   diminished urine production
overflow incontinence   leakage of urine in small amounts while bladder remains full and distended
polyuria   excessive production and excretion of urine
residual urine   urine remaining in the bladder after voiding
retention   inability to excrete urine from bladder
urgency   an intense stimulus to void (may cause incontinence)
voiding   micturition, elimination of urine

NURSING ASSESSMENT

A. Nursing observations
 1. Observe bladder for distention: lower abdominal area will be rigid, tense, swollen, and sensitive to the touch
 2. Assess urine: amount, color, odor, opacity (clear or cloudy), presence of sediment, mucus, or clots
 3. Check catheter (if indwelling) for drainage and meatus for irritation or secretions
 4. Check genitals (scrotum, labia and anal area) for irritation, rashes, and lesions
 5. Monitor fluid and electrolyte balance
 6. Check eyes, extremities, and scrotum for edema
 7. Monitor vital signs: note elevation of temperature and blood pressure
 8. Note problems or disabilities related to aging
B. Patient description (subjective data)
 1. Change in voiding habits
 2. Problems with elimination
 3. Urethral discharge
 4. Burning on voiding
 5. Pain: suprapubic or flank
C. Obtain patient history regarding
 1. Normal urinary and bowel elimination habits
 2. Medical problems with the urinary system (e.g., stones or sexually transmitted diseases [STDs])
 3. Medical problems with other body systems; trauma
 4. Medications
 5. Diet
 6. Food or medication allergies
 7. Decreased urinary stream
 8. Pain or spasms: what precipitated this and what relieved it
 9. Discharge
 10. Edema

DIAGNOSTIC TESTS/METHODS

A. Blood studies
 1. Blood urea nitrogen (BUN): normal level 10 to 20 mg/dl; urea is an end product of protein metabolism and is excreted by the kidneys in urine; an increase indicates impaired renal function
 2. Creatinine: normal level 0.5-1.3 mg/dl; elevation indicates decreased renal function
 3. Acid and alkaline phosphatase: normal value varies with laboratory; increase may indicate metastasis to bone or liver; nurse must assess for bone fracture or liver pathology
 4. Albumin: globulin ratio is usually 2:1; a change indicates damage to nephron and loss of albumin in the urine; patient retains fluid and has edema
B. Urine studies
 1. Routine urine: a single voided specimen to observe and compare to known normal specimens; results give information about renal function and systemic health
 2. Specific gravity (sp gr): normal value 1.010 to 1.030; change indicates dehydration or inadequate kidney function; a single voided specimen is required
 3. Urine culture and sensitivity (see Chapter 2)
 4. Phenosulfonphthalein test (PSP): after an IV injection of PSP dye, urine specimens are collected to measure amounts excreted; delay in excretion indicates renal disease; nurse collects specimens as directed by laboratory
 5. Creatine: 24-hour urine collection to measure creatinine excreted; oral fluids are encouraged (see Chapter 2: collecting a 24-hour specimen)
C. X-ray procedures
 1. Kidneys, ureter, bladder (KUB): an abdominal x-ray study that gives baseline information about size, shape, and placement of organs; flatus and stones are visualized; no preparation or care after procedure is required
 2. Intravenous pyelogram (IVP): an IV injection of a radiopaque dye that is rapidly excreted by the kidney; this tests renal function, and the x-ray films outline renal pelvis, ureters, bladder, and urethra; nursing responsibilities: keep NPO before procedure; after procedure observe for allergic reaction to dye; note voiding
 3. Retrograde pyelogram: visualization of upper genitourinary (GU) tract by injecting radiopaque dye through ureteral catheters to locate obstruction (e.g., stone or tumor); nursing implications: preparation is the same as for preoperative preparation (see Chapter 2); after procedure monitor vital signs, anticipate pain and administer analgesics, note voiding, and observe urine
 4. Cystoscopy: a direct visualization of the bladder and urethral orifices; a cystoscope is inserted through the urethra into the bladder; the bladder is distended with sterile solution; stones, tumors, and polyps can be diagnosed; urine can be observed entering the bladder from each ureter to evaluate renal function; instruments may be passed through the cystoscope to crush stones, take biopsy specimens, or pass catheters into ureters; nursing responsibilities: provide

general preoperative and postoperative care (see Chapter 2); after procedure determine what was done during procedure; assess urinary function; observe urine; provide care and observation of a patient with indwelling catheter (see Chapter 2)

FREQUENT PATIENT PROBLEMS AND NURSING CARE

A. Incontinence (types: urge, total, stress, reflex, and functional) related to catheter use, infection, tissue damage, immobility
   1. Minimize embarrassment; provide privacy
   2. Wash, dry, and inspect skin and take measures to prevent decubitus ulcers (pressure sores)
   3. Provide bladder training
B. Impaired skin integrity related to retention of metabolic wastes and resulting toxicity (uremia)
   1. Urea is excreted through the skin, causing odor and pruritus: provide frequent and thorough skin care; wash and pat dry; use weak vinegar solution to dissolve uric acid crystals
   2. Confusion and disorientation; may progress to state of unconsciousness and coma; provide all care; maintain safety (see earlier discussion of comas under The Neurologic System)
   3. Nausea and vomiting: provide mouth care q2h
   4. Renal failure: see nursing care for patient with chronic renal failure
C. Pain related to bladder spasms: bladder spasms caused by catheter irritation are intermittent in the suprapubic area, radiating to the urethra
   1. Assess type, location, and severity of pain
   2. Check catheter for obstruction; irrigate as ordered
   3. Administer medication as ordered (antispasmodics, see Chapter 4)
   4. Reassure patient that spasms are not abnormal
D. Fluid volume deficit related to dehydration
   1. Use hydration methods (force fluids)
   2. Monitor intake and output
E. Potential for infection/injury (hematuria) related to surgery and/or pathogens
   1. Monitor signs and symptoms; vital signs
   2. Administer medication as ordered
   3. Note characteristics of urine at each voiding
   4. Force fluids if not contraindicated
   5. Report clots
   6. Maintain patency and gravity drainage of catheters
   7. Assess for signs of anemia (weakness and fatigue)
   8. Provide nursing care and safety as indicated
   9. Reassure patient that blood-tinged urine is not unusual after instrumentation or surgery
F. Urinary retention related to surgery
   1. Take nursing measures to assist patient with voiding (see Chapter 2)
   2. Monitor intake and output
   3. Force fluids if not contraindicated
G. Anxiety related to sexual dysfunction, impending surgery, and/or possible change in body image and/or function
   1. Provide time to listen to patient express feelings
   2. Explain all care and procedures; reassure often

   3. Be honest; provide privacy; avoid embarrassing situations
   4. Praise patient's progress toward discharge goals

MAJOR MEDICAL DIAGNOSES
Cystitis

A. Definition: inflammation of the bladder mucosa; is difficult to cure; recurs and may be chronic
B. Pathology: is usually a bacterial infection
   1. May be secondary to infection elsewhere in urinary system (e.g., urethritis)
   2. Contamination during catheterization or instrumentation
   3. An obstruction causing urinary stasis in the bladder (e.g., enlarged prostate or urethral stricture)
C. Signs and symptoms
   1. Burning, dysuria, urgency, frequency, nocturia, hematuria, and pyuria
   2. Low-back pain and bladder spasms
   3. Elevation of temperature
D. Diagnostic tests/methods
   1. Patient history and assessment
   2. Urine culture
E. Treatment: systemic medications, urinary antiseptics, antibiotics, sulfonamides, and antispasmodics (see Chapter 4)
F. Nursing intervention
   1. Force fluids: 3000 ml daily over that of dietary intake unless contraindicated
   2. Provide and supervise proper perineal care
   3. Provide diet that acidifies urine (e.g., cranberry juice)
   4. Monitor temperature and administer antipyretics as ordered
   5. Provide sitz baths

Urethritis

A. Definition: inflammation of the urethra; may develop scar tissue and stricture, causing obstruction, cystitis, and nephritis
B. Pathology
   1. Prostatis: injury during instrumentation or catheterization
   2. Gonococcus infection
C. Signs and symptoms
   1. Urgency
   2. Frequency
   3. Dysuria
   4. Burning on urination
   5. Purulent discharge
D. Diagnostic tests/methods
   1. Patient history and physical examination
   2. Culture of discharge
E. Treatment
   1. Antibiotics
   2. Dilatation for stricture
F. Nursing intervention
   1. Sitz baths
   2. Isolation as indicated
   3. Demonstrate and supervise thorough hand washing
   4. Care of Foley catheter

Pyelonephritis

A. Definition: infection of the kidney; may be acute or become chronic; kidney becomes edematous, mucosa is inflamed, and multiple abscesses may form; the kidney will become fibrotic, and uremia may develop

B. Pathology
   1. Ascending infection from an infection lower in the GU tract
   2. Staphylococcal or streptococcal infection carried in the blood

C. Signs and symptoms
   1. Markedly elevated temperature (102° to 105° F); shaking, chills
   2. Nausea and vomiting
   3. Dysuria, burning, frequency, pyuria, and hematuria
   4. Flank pain and tenderness in kidney
   5. Increased WBC count

D. Diagnostic tests/methods
   1. Urine culture and sensitivity
   2. Patient history and physical examination
   3. IVP

E. Treatment: urinary antiseptics and specific antibiotics (see Chapter 4); follow-up care for at least 1 year

F. Nursing intervention
   1. Prevent dehydration: force fluids and maintain IV therapy
   2. Provide rest and conserve energy
   3. Prevent chill; keep skin dry and clean
   4. Provide mouth care q2h
   5. Provide soft diet
   6. Provide and assist with pericare; demonstrate proper technique and hand washing
   7. Anticipate pain: administer analgesics and local heat
   8. Administer antiemetic as needed
   9. Control temperature: administer antipyretics and sponge baths as ordered

Calculi (Lithiasis)

A. Definition: formation of stones in the urinary tract caused by deposits of crystalline substance that normally remain in solution and are excreted in the urine; may be found in the kidney, ureters, or bladder; vary in size from renal calculi that can be as large as an orange or as small as grains of sand; can obstruct urine flow, causing chronic infection, backflow, hydronephrosis, and gradual destruction of kidney; many small stones pass spontaneously

B. Cause
   1. Infection
   2. Urinary stasis
   3. Dehydration and concentration of urine
   4. Metabolic diseases (e.g., gout)
   5. Immobility (see dangers of immobility, Chapter 2)
   6. Familial tendency

C. Signs and symptoms
   1. Pain (can be extreme) radiates down flank to pubic area
   2. Frequency and urgency
   3. Hematuria and pyuria
   4. Diaphoresis, nausea, vomiting, and pallor (related to pain)

D. Diagnostic tests/methods: x-ray studies—KUB, IVP; urine studies

E. Treatment: depends on location—stones are removed; normal urine production and elimination are restored; recurrence is prevented
   1. Cystoscopy and crushing of stones (litholapaxy)
   2. Dislodging ureteral stone by passing ureteral catheter
   3. Surgery to remove ureteral or kidney stone
      a. Pyelolithotomy: removal of stones from renal pelvis
      b. Nephrolithotomy: incision through kidney and removal of stone
      c. Ureterolithotomy: removal of ureteral calculus
      d. Transcutaneous shock wave lithotripsy: ultrasonic waves used to disintegrate renal calculi

F. Nursing intervention
   1. Provide general preoperative and postoperative nursing care (see Chapter 2)
   2. Supervise and explain diet restrictions as ordered according to type of stone
   3. Provide analgesics as ordered
   4. Observe, describe, and strain all urine
   5. Maintain gravity drainage: never clamp ureteral or nephrostomy catheters
   6. Observe patency of catheters: never irrigate renal or ureteral catheters
   7. Record output from each catheter separately; immediately report scanty output from one tube
   8. Force fluids (but keep NPO if there is nausea, vomiting, or abdominal distention)

Hydronephrosis

A. Definition: an accumulation of fluid in the renal pelvis; there is distention of the renal tubules, calyces, and pelvis; renal tissues are destroyed from pressure; leads to uremia (azotemia)

B. Pathology
   1. Congenital defective drainage; blockage from stones or scar tissues
   2. Reflux (backup) from obstructed bladder neck in benign prostatic hypertrophy

C. Signs and symptoms
   1. Related to cause
   2. Infection
   3. Flank tenderness and pain

D. Diagnostic tests/methods
   1. Patient history and physical examination
   2. Blood serum tests (urea/creatinine)
   3. IVP

E. Treatment
   1. Remove cause
   2. Provide for adequate urinary drainage (e.g., bladder catheter or nephrostomy tube)
   3. Antibiotics

F. Nursing intervention
   1. Provide rest
   2. Provide medication and care as needed for symptoms (e.g., elevation of temperature or pain)
   3. Assess for and provide care as indicated for patient with uremia

Bladder Tumors

A. Definition: benign or malignant lesions that ulcerate into the mucous membrane; bladder capacity is decreased; benign tumors tend to recur and become malignant
B. Pathology
  1. Related to cigarette smoking and exposure to dyes (industrial)
  2. Chronic bladder irritation (e.g., stones or infection)
  3. Related to aging
C. Signs and symptoms
  1. Painless, gross hematuria
  2. Anemia
  3. Signs of bladder infection: dysuria, frequency, urgency, and chills
D. Diagnostic tests/methods
  1. Patient history and physical examination
  2. X-ray studies: IVP and KUB
  3. Cystoscopy and biopsy examination
E. Treatment
  1. Removal of the tumor through cystoscopy if benign
  2. Surgery
    a. Partial cystectomy
    b. Cystectomy: total removal of the bladder and provision for urinary diversion (see the following outline)
    c. Radiation
    d. Chemotherapy
F. Nursing intervention: give according to method of treatment (see specific sections)

Urinary Diversion

A. Definition: surgical intervention to allow for urinary elimination; the bladder is removed; the procedure is permanent
  1. Ileal conduit (ileal passageway): a small segment of ilium is separated from the intestine and the distal end is brought out of the abdomen to form a stoma; the ureters are implanted into this ileal pouch; urine flows continuously from the renal pelvis through the ureters into the ileal pouch and into a collecting bag
  2. Ureterointestinal implant: the ureters are anastomosed into the sigmoid colon or rectum; urine is mixed with feces, and evacuation is controlled from the anal sphincter
  3. Cutaneous ureterostomies: the ureters are implanted on the abdomen, forming one or two stomas that drain urine continuously into drainage bags
B. Indication: cancer of the bladder
C. Patient problems (depends on procedure)
  1. Susceptibility to infection
  2. Anxiety or depression about diagnosis and change in body image
  3. Inability to control elimination
  4. Embarrassment
  5. Odor if urine leaks onto skin
D. Nursing intervention (varies with procedures)
  1. Provide general preoperative and postoperative care (see Chapter 2)
  2. Provide time to listen to patient fears and anxieties
  3. Assess fluid and electrolyte imbalance
  4. Maintain integrity of the skin: clean, inspect, and change drainage bag as needed

  5. Prevent infection: maintain asepsis; force fluids; patient must know when to seek medical attention for pain or elevation of temperature
  6. Do not give patient laxatives or enemas (rectal implant)
  7. Arrange a visit from a person who has undergone a similar procedure (with permission of physician and patient)
  8. Elimination of odor in drainage bags; use weak solution of vinegar

Kidney Tumor

A. Definition: most tumors of the kidney are malignant; no early symptoms are presented
B. Cause: unknown
C. Signs and symptoms (only in late stages)
  1. Hematuria with no pain
  2. Low-grade temperature
  3. Weight loss
  4. Anemia
  5. Symptoms related to metastasis (e.g., bone pain)
D. Diagnostic tests/methods
  1. Renal arteriogram: IVP and KUB
  2. Renal biopsy examination
  3. CT scan, MRI
E. Treatment
  1. Surgery: radical nephrectomy
  2. Radiation
  3. Chemotherapy
F. Nursing intervention
  1. Provide nursing care for individual symptoms (see above)
  2. Provide general nursing care: before and after surgery, during radiation, and for a patient receiving chemotherapy (see specific discussions)

Acute Renal Failure (Renal Shutdown)

A. Definition: sudden damage to the kidneys causing cessation of function and retention of toxins, fluids, and end products of metabolism; patient may recover, or disease may become chronic or be fatal
B. Causes: blood transfusion reaction, shock, toxins, burns, or trauma
C. Signs and symptoms
  1. Lethargy, headache, and drowsiness; convulsion; may go into coma
  2. Nausea, vomiting, and diarrhea
  3. Sudden oliguria or anuria
  4. Increased bleeding time
D. Diagnostic tests/methods
  1. Patient history and physical examination
  2. Blood serum tests
E. Treatment
  1. Removal of cause
  2. Peritoneal dialysis
  3. Hemodialysis
F. Nursing intervention
  1. Provide nursing observations and care as indicated for primary problem
  2. Provide care and observations as indicated for patient with chronic renal failure (see following outline)

3. Provide nursing care as indicated for a patient receiving peritoneal dialysis (see later outline)
4. Provide nursing care as indicated for a patient receiving hemodialysis (see later outline)
5. Offer emotional support

Chronic Renal Failure (End-Stage Renal Disease)

A. Definition: progressive kidney damage; the nephron deteriorates; the kidneys stop functioning; this is the final stage of many chronic diseases (e.g., hypertension)
B. Causes
   1. Glomerulonephritis, pyelonephritis, polycystic kidney, or urinary tract obstruction, diabetes
   2. Essential hypertension
   3. Lupus erythematosus
C. Signs and symptoms
   1. Malaise
   2. Nausea and vomiting
   3. Anemia
   4. Oliguria
   5. Hyperkalemia
   6. Twitching (from low serum calcium and increased phosphorus levels)
   7. Hypertension (from fluid retention)
   8. Very susceptible to infection: delayed wound healing and ulcers in the mouth
   9. Bleeding tendency
   10. Uremic frost: urea is excreted in perspiration onto the skin, and small crystals can be seen; this causes severe pruritus
   11. Headaches and visual disturbances, disorientation, convulsions, coma, and death
D. Diagnostic tests/methods
   1. Patient history and physical examination
   2. Serum blood tests
   3. Kidney function tests; BUN; creatinine level
   4. X-ray studies
E. Treatment
   1. Remove (treat) cause
   2. Hemodialysis
   3. Peritoneal dialysis
   4. Kidney transplant
F. Nursing intervention
   1. Monitor fluid balance: weigh patient daily; record intake and output
   2. Maintain asepsis: provide catheter care, prevent infections, and encourage frequent hand washing; do not expose patient to staff or visitors with upper respiratory tract infections
   3. Conserve energy: provide care, maintain rest periods
   4. Provide safety: place side rails up (see earlier discussion on care of patient in coma under section on The Neurologic System)
   5. Relieve pruritus: wash patient frequently with tepid water; a weak solution of vinegar dissolves uric acid; handle skin gently; use skin lotion; cut nails; apply calamine lotion
   6. Assist with administration of transfusion
   7. Provide oral hygiene every 1 to 2 hours; use cotton swabs and antiseptic mouth wash; apply mineral oil to lips
   8. Provide soft, high-carbohydrate, low-potassium, low-sodium, low-protein diet in small feedings
   9. Restrict fluids as ordered
   10. Anticipate cardiac arrest: monitor vital signs
   11. Assess LOC: orient as necessary
   12. Provide nursing care and precautions as indicated for a patient with seizures (see earlier discussion of convulsive disorders in this chapter).
   13. Provide nursing measures to prevent dangers of immobility (see Chapter 2)
   14. Anticipate and prevent bleeding
      a. Observe stool, urine, sputum, and vomitus
      b. Monitor vital signs
      c. Use soft swab for mouth care
      d. Avoid injections if possible

Peritoneal Dialysis

A. Description: toxins, end-products of metabolism and fluids, are removed from the blood through the peritoneal membrane; a catheter is passed into the peritoneal cavity; dialyzing fluid, which is similar to plasma, is instilled by gravity into the abdominal cavity, and the catheter is clamped; toxins and electrolytes, which are in greater concentration in the blood vessels of the peritoneal membrane, pass into the dialyzing fluid; after 1 hour the catheter is unclamped, and the fluid drains out by gravity
B. Patient problems
   1. Potential for infection related to dialysis procedure
   2. Self-care deficit related to discomfort and immobility
C. Nursing intervention
   1. Record baseline vital signs; complete assessment; carefully measure fluid instilled/drained
   2. Maintain surgical asepsis; prevent peritonitis
   3. Assist patient with self-care activities

Hemodialysis

A. Description: blood leaves the patient through an arterial cannula and travels through coils placed in a solution; dialysis takes place, and the detoxified blood returns to the patient's venous circulation; a surgically created arteriovenous fistula (connection) is necessary for repeated dialysis
B. Patient problems
   1. Self-esteem disturbance related to threatened self-image
   2. Powerlessness related to dependency on machine
   3. Potential for infection related to the hemodialysis procedure
   4. Anxiety related to lifelong, life-threatening disease
C. Nursing intervention
   1. Maintain surgical asepsis
   2. Assess bruit patency
   3. Provide emotional support; alleviate anxiety
   4. Provide patient teaching

Kidney Transplant

Removal of the diseased kidney and transplantation of a normal kidney is sometimes performed for patients with advanced renal failure.

The Male Genitourinary System
Benign Prostatic Hypertrophy (BPH)

A. Description: the prostate gland slowly enlarges (hypertrophies) and extends upward into the bladder; outflow of urine is obstructed; the urinary stream is smaller, and voiding is difficult; a pouch is formed in the bladder as the gland continues to enlarge; stasis of urine occurs; obstruction causes gradual dilation of ureters and kidneys; may cause hydronephrosis; when obstruction is complete, there is acute urinary retention

B. Cause: unknown; increased incidence with age, usually over 50 years of age; related to smoking

C. Signs and symptoms
  1. Dysuria, frequency, nocturia, urgency, retention, burning on urination, and decreased force of stream
  2. Urinary tract infection
  3. Acute urinary retention

D. Diagnostic tests/methods
  1. Patient history and assessment; palpation through rectal examination
  2. IVP, cystoscopy, and retrograde pyelography
  3. Urine culture
  4. BUN
  5. Serum creatinine

E. Treatment
  1. Immediate
    a. Bladder drainage with indwelling catheter
    b. Decompression
    c. Antibiotics as indicated
    d. Suprapubic cystotomy and insertion of catheter for long-term drainage
  2. Surgery: type depends on patient's age and size of enlargement
    a. Transurethral resection of the prostate (TURP): an instrument is passed through the urethra to the prostate; under direct visualization, small pieces of the obstructing gland are removed with electric wire; the bleeding points are cauterized; there is no incision; bleeding is a common postoperative problem
    b. Suprapubic (transvesicle) prostatectomy: a low incision is made over the bladder; the bladder is opened, and the prostatic tissue is removed through an incision into the urethral mucosa; two drainage tubes are inserted (a cystotomy tube and a Foley catheter); these are connected to a continuous bladder irrigation setup
    c. Retropubic prostatectomy: a low abdominal incision is made; the bladder is not entered
    d. Perineal prostatectomy: the gland is removed through an incision in the perineum; the entire gland and capsule are removed
    e. Bilateral vasectomy may be performed with a prostatectomy to reduce risk of epididymitis

F. Nursing intervention
  1. On admission, complete assessment related to
    a. Aging
    b. Possible infection
    c. Anxiety
    d. Medical problems associated with aging: diabetes, cardiovascular, hearing, sight, and gastrointestinal
  2. Force fluids if not contraindicated; monitor intake and output
  3. Maintain gravity drainage
  4. Provide general preoperative and postoperative care (see Chapter 2)
  5. Provide specific postoperative care; depends on the procedure performed
    a. Maintain gravity drainage
    b. Keep irrigation flowing (note clots); maintain a closed, continuous irrigation
    c. Maintain asepsis; change dressing when wet (may need order); there may be fecal incontinence if a perineal prostatectomy was performed
    d. Monitor vital signs; hematuria is expected; report frank bleeding or clots
    e. Use oral thermometer (no rectal treatments)
    f. Encourage patient to avoid straining; force fluids; provide stool softeners
    g. Observe for bladder spasms; note if catheter is draining freely; irrigate by syringe as ordered; administer antispasmodics
    h. Administer analgesic as needed for postoperative pain
    i. Monitor intake and output; record all drainage tubes separately

Cancer of the Prostate

A. Definition: a malignant tumor; it has no symptoms until it has become large or metastasized

B. Cause: unknown; increased incidence with age (all men older than 40 years should have rectal examinations yearly)

C. Signs and symptoms
  1. Early tumor has no symptoms
  2. Frequency, nocturia, and dysuria
  3. Back pain
  4. Symptoms from metastasis

D. Diagnostic tests/methods
  1. Rectal examination
  2. Biopsy examination
  3. Acid phosphatase

E. Treatment: surgery
  1. Radical perineal prostatectomy (removal of prostate, capsule, and seminal vesicles)
  2. Bilateral orchiectomy (removal of both testicles)
  3. TURP
  4. Estrogen therapy

F. Nursing intervention
  1. See nursing intervention for a patient with BPH
  2. Be supportive as concerns are expressed about a malignancy and feminization from estrogens; answer questions; refer problems to physician

Hydrocele

A. Definition: a cystic mass filled with fluid that forms around the testicle

B. Causes
  1. Infection
  2. Trauma

C. Signs and symptoms
  1. Swelling of testicle
  2. Discomfort in sitting and walking

D. Diagnostic tests/methods: assessment

E. Treatment
  1. Aspiration (usually only in children)

2. Surgery: hydrocelectomy
F. Nursing intervention
   1. Provide usual preoperative and postoperative care (see Chapter 2)
   2. Provide scrotal support
   3. Anticipate drainage; maintain asepsis; change dressing as ordered

Cancer of the Testes

A. Definition: an uncommon malignancy; usually no symptoms are present until metastasis occurs; can be diagnosed early only by examination and finding a hard, nontender mass; age of incidence is usually in early 30s
B. Treatment
   1. Surgery: orchiectomy
   2. Radiotherapy
   3. Chemotherapy
   4. Possibly radical: lymph node dissection
C. Nursing intervention: related to treatment selected

Sexually Transmitted Infectious Diseases (STDs)
Syphilis

A. Description: caused by a spirochete, *Treponema pallidum;* appears in three stages; transmitted through sexual contact or warm blood
   1. Primary stage: after an incubation period of 10 to 60 days (usually 3 weeks), during which there are no symptoms, an ulcer or chancre appears at the site of entry; it contains many organisms and is highly infectious; there may be minor local discomfort or mild generalized symptoms (e.g., headache or lymph node enlargement); without treatment it heals in 3 to 5 weeks
   2. Secondary stage: 3 weeks later it appears as a mild rash on skin (usually palms of hands and soles of feet) and as papules on mucous membranes; all lesions contain organisms and are highly contagious; symptoms may be mild or generalized (e.g., bone pain, sore throat, hair loss in patches, or lymph node changes); lasts a few weeks and becomes dormant if not treated; patient is infectious for about 1 year
   3. Third or latent stage: 10 to 30 years later the spirochetes, which have been deposited in tissues and organs are in lesions (gummas); these destroy the tissue; common sites are the CNS, eyes, and the aorta
B. Signs and symptoms: relate to organ involved (e.g., aortic aneurysm)
C. Diagnostic tests/methods
   1. Primary stage: microscopic examination of smear
   2. Second and third stages: blood serum tests (e.g., VDRL and Wassermann)
D. Treatment: penicillin or tetracycline

Gonorrhea

A. Definition: a highly communicable disease; there is inflammation of the urethra and spread to other organs of the genital tract; incubation period is 3 to 4 days
B. Cause: *Neisseria gonorrhoeae,* transmitted by sexual contact
C. Signs and symptoms
   1. Female patients may have no early symptoms or purulent vaginal discharge, dysuria, or urgency; un-

treated, it may spread to other organs in the pelvic cavity (see discussion of pelvic inflammatory disease [PID] in the following section)
   2. Male patients have purulent urethral discharge and burning on urination; may develop urethral stricture; epididymitis, prostatitis
D. Diagnostic tests/methods
   1. Patient history and physical examination
   2. Smear or culture
E. Treatment: penicillin or tetracycline

Herpes Genitalis

A. Description: fluid-filled vesicles on genitalia form crusts, causing generalized symptoms such as elevated temperature; pain; may have no symptoms; there are recurrent episodes; problems arise in pregnancy; is believed to predispose to cervical cancer
B. Cause: herpesvirus hominis type 2 HSV
C. Treatment: symptomatic; topical antiviral agents (acyclovir [Zovirax]); no cure

Chlamydia Trachomatis

A. Definition: most common STD in the United States; causes symptoms similar to gonorrheal infections
B. Cause: *Chlamydia trachomatis*
C. Signs and symptoms
   1. Males: urethritis, dysuria, frequency, watery mucoid discharge; complications include epididymitis, prostatitis, infertility
   2. Females: often asymptomatic; mucopurulent cervicitis, dysuria, frequency, local soreness; complications include salpingitis, PID, ectopic pregnancy, and infertility
D. Diagnostic tests/methods: urogenital smear analysis for enzyme or antibody
E. Treatment: antibiotic therapy (doxycycline, tetracycline, erythromycin)

Condylomata Acuminata

A. Definition: also referred to as genital/venereal warts; often seen with other STDs such as gonorrhea and trichomoniasis; highly contagious
B. Cause: human papilloma virus (HPV)
C. Signs and symptoms: initially single, small papillary growths that grow into large cauliflower-like masses, profuse foul-smelling vaginal discharge, bleeding; may progress to genital and cervical dysplasia, cancer
D. Diagnostic tests/methods: inspection of urinary meatus, vulva, labia, vagina, cervix, penis, scrotum, anus, perineum; culture and biopsy
E. Treatment
   1. Cryotherapy with liquid nitrogen or cryoprobe
   2. Laser therapy
   3. Acid treatments
   4. Surgery
   5. Chemotherapy (5FU)

Trichomoniasis/Candidiasis

A. Definition: very common STD; symptoms frequently seen only in women
B. Cause: *Trichomonas vaginalis* and *Candida albicans,* respectively

C. Signs and symptoms: itching; discharge
D. Diagnostic tests/methods: culture and inspection of affected tissues
E. Treatment: antifungals; antiprotozoal drugs (metronidazole [Flagyl])

The Female Reproductive System

Childbearing is the major physiologic function of the female reproductive system. Disorders of this system are distressing to the patient because of interference with sexuality, conception, and self-image. The nurse plays an important role by clearly providing information to the concerned patient.

NURSING ASSESSMENT

A. Nursing observations
   1. General appearance
   2. Vital signs
   3. Weight
   4. Breasts
      a. Contour
      b. Skin dimpling
      c. Nodules
         (1) Size
         (2) Consistency
         (3) Mobile or fixed
      d. Nipples
         (1) Asymmetry
         (2) Retraction
         (3) Rash
         (4) Ulceration
         (5) Discharge
   5. External genitalia
      a. Irritation
      b. Redness
      c. Excoriation
      d. Bulge
   6. Introitus
      a. Irritation
      b. Redness
      c. Excoriation
      d. Nodules
   7. Discharge
      a. Color
      b. Malodor
      c. Consistency
B. Patient description (subjective data)
   1. Lower abdominal pain and cramping
   2. Backache
   3. Stress incontinence
   4. Urinary frequency and urgency
   5. Urine or fecal material draining from vaginal tract
   6. Breasts
      a. Tenderness
      b. Burning
      c. Swelling
      d. Pain
      e. Nipples
         (1) Tenderness
         (2) Burning
   7. External genitalia
      a. Itching
      b. Burning
   8. Introitus
      a. Burning
      b. Itching
      c. Tenderness
      d. Dyspareunia (painful intercourse)
   9. Menstrual cycle
      a. Duration of cycles
      b. Number of days between cycles
      c. Associated symptoms
         (1) Pain
         (2) Headache
         (3) Irritability
         (4) Depression
         (5) Insomnia

DIAGNOSTIC TESTS/METHODS

A. Serum laboratory studies
   1. Luteinizing hormone (LH)
      a. Stimulates progesterone secretion
      b. Diminished levels may relate to prolonged, heavy menses
      c. Elevated levels may result in short, scanty menses
   2. Follicle-stimulating hormone (FSH)
      a. Stimulates estrogen secretion
      b. Diminished levels may relate to bleeding between cycles
      c. Elevated levels may result in excessive uterine bleeding
   3. Thyroid function tests
      a. Used to rule out menstrual abnormality secondary to thyroid dysfunction
      b. Diminished thyroid hormone secretion may result in bleeding between cycles, irregular menses, or absence of menstrual flow
   4. Adrenal function tests
      a. Used to rule out menstrual abnormality secondary to adrenal dysfunction
      b. Elevated or decreased production of adrenal cortex hormone secretion may result in amenorrhea
B. Procedures
   1. Pelvic examination: to inspect and assess the external genitalia, perineal and anal areas, introitus, vaginal tract, and cervix
      a. Have patient empty bladder
      b. Place patient in the lithotomy position
      c. Flex and abduct patient's thighs
      d. Place patient's feet in stirrups
      e. Extend patient's buttocks slightly beyond the edge of the examining table
   2. Laparoscopy: visualization of the pelvic structures with a lighted laparoscope inserted through the abdominal wall
   3. Culdoscopy: visualization of the ovaries, fallopian tubes, and uterus with a lighted instrument inserted through the vaginal tract
      a. After procedure, position patient on abdomen to expel air
      b. Monitor for vaginal bleeding
      c. Instruct patient to abstain from intercourse, douching, and use of tampons until advised by physician

4. Colposcopy: visualization of the cervix with an instrument that magnifies tissue
5. Papanicolaou smear test (Pap smear): a sample of cervical scrapings is obtained for study under a microscope for evidence of malignant cell changes
   a. Follow nursing actions as in a pelvic examination
   b. Write patient's name on the frost side of the slide, handling edges only
   c. Smear the specimen on a glass slide
   d. Place a drop of a fixative, dry, and send to laboratory
   e. Reenforce importance of a Pap smear once a year
6. Cervical biopsy examination: removal of tissue to examine for presence of malignancy
   a. After procedure, advise patient to rest and avoid strenuous activity for 24 hours
   b. Leave packing in place until physician permits removal (usually 12 to 24 hours)
   c. Monitor for vaginal bleeding
   d. Instruct patient to abstain from intercourse, douching, and use of tampons until advised by physician
   e. Explain that there will be a malodorous discharge that may last 3 weeks; daily bath should help control this
7. Conization
   a. Removal of cone-shaped tissue of the cervix for analysis of cancerous cells
   b. Indicated for removal of diseased cervical tissue
   c. Nursing intervention
      (1) Maintain packing 12 to 24 hours
      (2) Monitor for bleeding
      (3) Instruct patient to abstain from intercourse, douching, and use of tampons until advised by physician
8. Schiller's test
   a. Application of a dye to the cervix to aid in detecting cancerous cells
   b. Normal vaginal cells will stain a deep brown
   c. Abnormal cells with not absorb the dye
   d. Nursing intervention: recommend to patient that a perineal pad be used to protect clothes from stain
9. Ultrasonography
   a. A sound frequency that reflects an image of the pelvic structures
   b. An aid in confirming ovarian and uterine tumors
10. Culture and sensitivity
    a. The culture of a specimen of exudate suspected of infection
    b. The sensitivity of an antibiotic to the microorganism
11. Dilatation and curettage (D & C)
    a. A diagnostic and therapeutic procedure
    b. The cervix is dilated to scrape the lining of the uterine cavity with a curet
    c. Nursing intervention
       (1) After procedure, provide sterile perineal pads and record amount of drainage
       (2) Encourage voiding to prevent urinary retention
       (3) Instruct patient to abstain from inter-

course, douching, and use of tampons until advised by physician
12. Mammography: an x-ray examination of the breasts to detect tumors
13. Thermography: infrared photography used to detect breast tumors
14. Xerography: an x-ray examination of the breasts and skin that provides good definition of the tissue

FREQUENT PATIENT PROBLEMS AND NURSING CARE

A. Anxiety related to modesty
   1. Keep the patient's body covered at all times
   2. Provide privacy
   3. Speak with the patient during the examination or procedure
B. Knowledge deficit related to understanding of menstruation
   1. Provide factual information related to the process of menstruation
   2. Describe abnormalities associated with menstruation
   3. Describe emotional changes associated with menstruation
   4. Teach menstrual hygiene
      a. Change perineal pad or tampon every 3 to 4 hours
      b. Remove napkin front to back
      c. Alternate sanitary napkins and tampons qd to prevent toxic shock syndrome or back flow of menstruation
C. Knowledge deficit related to menstrual abnormalities: explain what menstrual symptoms are considered abnormal
   1. Flow occurring more frequently than every 21 days
   2. Flow occurring less frequently than every 35 days
   3. Duration of less than 3 days
   4. Duration of more than 7 days
   5. Use of 12 or more perineal pads per 24 hours
D. Pain related to menstruation
   1. Assess location, duration, onset, and quality of pain
   2. Apply heating pad to the abdomen
   3. Provide warm liquids of patient's choice
   4. Provide massage to lumbar area
   5. Provide pain relief medication as ordered by physician
E. Knowledge deficit related to breast self-examination
   1. Recommend that breasts be examined 7 days after onset of menstruation every month (Fig. 6-5)
   2. Instruct patient on technique of breast self-examination
      a. Inspect breasts in front of mirror with arms at sides
      b. Observe breasts with arms raised above the head
      c. With hands on hips, lean forward and contract chest muscles
   3. Lying supine, palpate each breast with flat part of fingers and continue in a circular movement to nipple
   4. Observations of the breasts
      a. Size
      b. Symmetry
      c. Skin texture

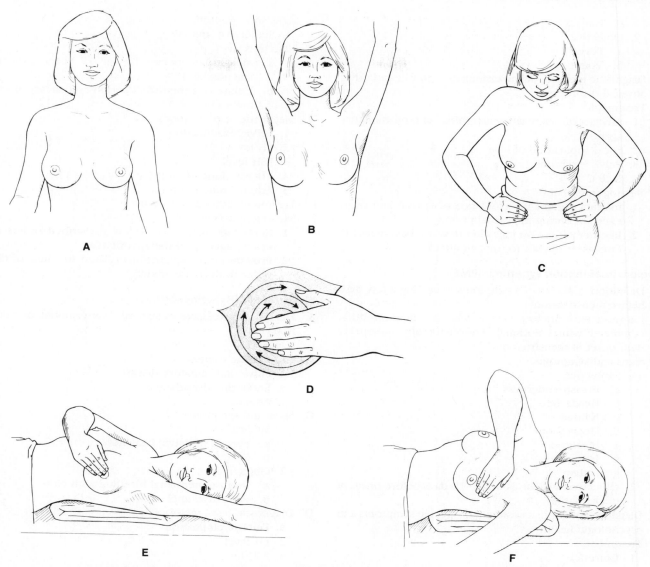

FIG. 6-5. Breast self-examination. **A,** Inspection. **B,** Inspection with arms raised. **C,** Inspection with muscles contracted. **D,** Circular pattern of palpation. **E,** Palpation of inner aspect of breast with arms raised. **F,** Palpation of outer aspect with arm lowered, (From Billings DM, Stokes LG: *Medical-Surgical nursing: common health problems of adults and children across the life span,* St Louis, 1986, Mosby.)

    d. Color
    e. Nipple position
    f. Nipple discharge
F. Knowledge deficit related to menopause
    1. Describe accompanying symptoms associated with menopause
       a. Irregular menses
       b. Hot flashes
       c. Night sweats
       d. Insomnia
       e. Depression
       f. Anxiety
    2. Onset is usually after age 40 years
    3. Explain that menopause does not interfere with sexuality
    4. Recommend use of lubricant before intercourse
    5. Recommend use of contraception for 6 months after the last menstrual period

MAJOR MEDICAL DIAGNOSES
Menstrual Abnormalities
Dysmenorrhea

A. Definition: intense pain at the time of menses
B. Cause: uterine spasms cause cramping of the lower abdomen
C. Signs and symptoms
    1. Subjective
       a. Headache, backache
       b. Abdominal pain
       c. Chills

d. Nausea
2. Objective
    a. Fever
    b. Vomiting
D. Diagnostic method: pelvic examination to rule out other physical disorders
E. Treatment
    1. Analgesics, such as nonsteroidal antiinflammatory agents
    2. Local application of heat
    3. Pelvic exercises
    4. D & C
F. Nursing intervention
    1. Instruct patient on avoidance of fatigue and overexertion during menstrual period
    2. Instruct patient on ingestion of warm beverages before onset of pain to prevent attack

Premenstrual tension syndrome (PMS)

A. Definition: a number of symptoms occurring a few days before menstruation
B. Cause: cause is unclear; may be related to fluid retention combined with emotional tension; usually disappears with onset of menstruation
C. Signs and symptoms
    1. Subjective
        a. Breast tenderness
        b. Headache
        c. Nausea
        d. Depression
        e. Insomnia
        f. Irritability
        g. Fatigue
    2. Objective: weight gain 2 to 10 days before onset of menstruation
D. Diagnostic method: assessment of specific symptoms and psychologic health
E. Treatment
    1. Diuretics
    2. Mild sodium restriction
    3. Mild tranquilizers
    4. Well-balanced diet
    5. Exercise
F. Nursing intervention
    1. Assist patient in working out a diet with decreased sodium content
    2. Instruct patient to decrease consumption of coffee, alcohol, and nicotine during latter half of menstrual cycle

Amenorrhea

A. Definition: absence of menstrual periods
B. Causes
    1. Diabetes
    2. Debilitating illness
    3. Malnutrition
    4. Obesity
    5. Extreme anxiety
    6. Anemia
    7. Oral contraceptives
    8. Chronic nephritis
    9. Tumors of the endocrine glands

C. Signs and symptoms
    1. Subjective: anxiety
    2. Objective
        a. Absence of menses by age 17 years (primary amenorrhea)
        b. Failure of a menstrual period (secondary amenorrhea)
D. Diagnostic tests/methods
    1. Pelvic examination
    2. LH level
    3. FSH level
    4. Thyroid function test
    5. Adrenal function test
E. Treatment: according to cause
F. Nursing intervention
    1. Encourage patient to follow prescribed orders to ensure success of therapeutic plan
    2. Provide clear explanations related to cause of disorder to decrease anxiety

Menorrhagia (Hypermenorrhea)

A. Definition: excessive menstrual flow (amount or duration)
B. Causes
    1. Uterine tumors
    2. Pelvic inflammatory disease
    3. Endocrine disturbances
    4. Anemia
C. Signs and symptoms
    1. Subjective
        a. Feeling of pelvic heaviness
        b. Fatigue
    2. Objective
        a. Profuse menstrual bleeding with clots
        b. Pale, tired appearance
D. Diagnostic tests/methods
    1. Pelvic examination
    2. LH level
    3. FSH level
    4. Thyroid function test
    5. Adrenal function test
    6. RBC count
E. Treatment
    1. According to cause
    2. D & C
F. Nursing intervention
    1. Encourage intake of foods high in iron content
    2. Encourage planned rest periods
    3. Instruct the patient to count number of pads used during an abnormal period
    4. Weigh each pad before and after use to estimate blood loss

Metrorrhagia

A. Definition: bleeding between menstrual intervals
B. Pathology
    1. Causes are similar to those of menorrhagia
    2. Break-through bleeding may occur with use of contraceptive pills
    3. May be early symptom of cervical cancer
C. Signs and symptoms
    1. Subjective

a. Feeling of pelvic heaviness

b. Fatigue

2. Objective

a. Spotting or bleeding between menstrual periods

b. Tired appearance

D. Diagnostic tests/methods

1. Pelvic examination

2. LH level

3. FSH level

4. Thyroid function test

5. Adrenal function test

6. RBC count

7. Pap smear

E. Treatment: according to cause

F. Nursing intervention

1. Instruct the patient on how to keep accurate records of bleeding episodes

2. Encourage continued medical follow-up because of possible cervical changes associated with cancer

Vaginitis

A. Definition: inflammation of the vaginal mucosa

B. Pathology

1. Invasion of virulent organisms permitted by changes in normal flora; pH becomes alkaline

2. Four classifications

a. Trichomoniasis: parasitic organism

b. *Candida albicans* (moniliasis): fungal organism

c. Atrophic (senile): occurs in postmenopausal women because of atrophy of vaginal mucosa

d. Simple: invasion by staphylococci, streptococci, or *Escherichia coli*

C. Signs and symptoms

1. Trichomoniasis: thick, white or yellow, frothy, malodorous discharge causing itching, burning, and excoriation of vulva

2. Monilial: thick or watery, white or yellow, curdlike discharge; mucosa becomes reddened

3. Atrophic: blood-flecked discharge with burning and itching of the vagina and dyspareunia

4. Simple: profuse, yellow mucoid discharge with irritation to vulva and urethra

D. Diagnostic tests/methods: culture and sensitivity; pelvic exam

E. Treatment

1. Trichomoniasis: metronidazole (Flagyl), floraquin tablets administered vaginally, and carbarsone suppositories administered rectally

2. Candidiasis: nystatin (Mycostatin) and gentian violet applied to vaginal mucosa

3. Atrophic: antibiotics and estrogen therapy

4. Simple: antibiotics and sulfonamide creams

5. Acetic acid douches

F. Nursing intervention

1. Reassure patient during vaginal examination to decrease anxiety

2. Instruct patient on perineal hygiene: cleansing front to back

3. In the event of trichomoniasis, instruct patient to abstain from intercourse or have partner wear a condom, because this infection can be transmitted

4. Advise patient that gentian violet causes staining of clothes; patient may wish to use perineal pads

Uterine Cancer (Endometrium)

A. Definition: new growth of abnormal cells in the uterine lining

B. Pathology

1. Spreads to cervix, fallopian tubes, ovaries, bladder, and rectum

2. Associated factors are women over 50 years of age, obesity, diabetes, and hypertension

3. Prognosis is good if identified in early stages

C. Signs and symptoms

1. Subjective

a. Postmenopausal bleeding

b. Bleeding between cycles

c. Bleeding after intercourse

d. Watery vaginal discharge

2. Objective

a. Uterine enlargement

b. Suspicious Pap test results

D. Diagnostic tests/methods

1. D & C

2. Tissue biopsy examination

E. Treatment

1. Surgical intervention

a. Panhysterectomy (removal of uterus and cervix)

b. Oophorectomy (removal of ovaries)

c. Salpingectomy (removal of fallopian tubes)

2. Chemotherapy

3. Radiation

F. Nursing intervention: refer to section on cancer of the cervix

Uterine Fibroid Tumors

A. Definition: a benign tumor located in the uterus

B. Pathology

1. Develops slowly, symptoms occur only in relation to size, location, and number of tumors present

2. Occurs in 25% of women over 35 years of age

C. Signs and symptoms

1. Subjective

a. Menstrual disturbances

b. Backache

c. Frequent urination

d. Constipation

2. Objective; uterine enlargement

D. Diagnostic tests/methods

1. Pelvic examination

2. Laparoscopy

E. Treatment

1. Excision of the myoma is indicated for small tumors

2. Hysterectomy (removal of uterus) with preservation of ovaries is indicated for large tumors

F. Nursing intervention

1. Explain to patient that tumors may decrease in size after menopause

2. Encourage patient to verbalize concerns

3. If patient undergoes myomectomy, follow general postoperative nursing measures related to abdominal surgery

4. If the patient undergoes a hysterectomy, follow nursing interventions covered under cancer of the cervix

Endometriosis

A. Definition: tissue resembling the endometrial membrane grows in another location in the pelvic cavity
B. Pathology
   1. During menstrual period, endometrial cells are stimulated by ovarian hormone
   2. Bleeding into surrounding tissue occurs, causing inflammation
   3. Condition may result in adhesions, fusion of pelvic organs, bladder dysfunction, stricture of bowel, or sterility
C. Signs and symptoms: Symptoms usually appear in women over 30 years of age
   1. Subjective
      a. Discomfort of pelvic area before menses, becoming worse during menstrual flow, and diminishing as flow ceases
      b. Dyspareunia
      c. Fatigue
   2. Objective: infertility
D. Diagnostic tests/methods
   1. Laparoscopy
   2. Culdoscopy
E. Treatment
   1. Hormonal therapy to suppress ovulation
   2. Surgical intervention: hysterectomy, oophorectomy, or salpingectomy
F. Nursing intervention
   1. Provide emotional support
   2. If patient is young, advise not to delay family because of risk of sterility
   3. Explain that hormonal drug may cause pseudopregnancy and irregular bleeding
   4. If patient is middle aged, advise her that menopause may stop progression of condition
   5. Follow general postoperative nursing actions if the patient undergoes surgical procedure
      a. Observe for vaginal hemorrhage, malodorous vaginal discharge, or vaginal discharge other than serosanguineous discharge
      b. Observe for urine retention, burning, frequency, or urgency to void
      c. Listen for renewed bowel sounds
   6. Patient teaching on discharge
      a. Heavy lifting, prolonged standing, walking, and sitting are contraindicated
      b. Sexual intercourse should be avoided until approved by physician

Pelvic Inflammatory Disease (PID)

A. Definition: inflammation of the pelvic cavity
B. Pathology
   1. Pathogenic organisms are introduced into the cervix
   2. PID may be confined to one or more structures: fallopian tubes, ovaries, pelvic peritoneum, pelvic veins, or pelvic tissue
   3. May result in adhesions, strictures, or sterility
   4. Most common causative organism: gonococcus
   5. Also caused by staphylococci or streptococci
C. Signs and symptoms
   1. Subjective
      a. Abdominal pain
      b. Pelvic pain
      c. Low-back pain
      d. Nausea
   2. Objective
      a. Malodorous, purulent discharge
      b. Fever
      c. Vomiting
D. Diagnostic tests/method: culture and sensitivity test and CBC; pelvic exam; laparoscopy
E. Treatment
   1. Antibiotic therapy
   2. Analgesics
F. Nursing intervention
   1. Provide nonjudgmental, accepting attitude
   2. Place patient in semi-Fowler's position to provide dependent pelvic drainage
   3. Apply heat to abdominal area if ordered to improve circulation and provide comfort
   4. Patient teaching should include
      a. Take shower instead of tub bath
      b. Perineal hygiene: wipe from front to back
      c. How to recognize if sexual partner is infected with gonococcus: discharge from penis of whitish fluid with painful urination
      d. Importance of routine physical examinations, because gonococcal infection is asymptomatic in females

Vaginal Fistula

A. Definition: tubelike opening between two internal organs
B. Pathology
   1. Causes include radiation therapy, gynecologic surgery, or traumatic childbirth
   2. Results in impaired blood supply and sloughing of tissue, leading to abnormal opening
   3. Four types affect female reproductive organs
      a. Ureterovaginal: between ureter and vagina; urine leaks into vagina
      b. Vesicovaginal: between bladder and vagina; urine leaks into vagina
      c. Urethrovaginal: between urethra and vagina; urine leaks into vagina
      d. Rectovaginal: between rectum and vagina; flatus and fecal matter leak into vagina
C. Signs and symptoms
   1. Subjective
      a. Leakage of urine, flatus, and fecal matter
      b. Pain in affected area
   2. Objective
      a. Excoriation
      b. Malodor
D. Diagnostic methods
   1. Symptoms and physical examination
   2. Patient history of radiation therapy
   3. Intravenous pyelogram (IVP)
   4. Cystoscopy
E. Treatment
   1. Small fistula may heal spontaneously
   2. Surgical excision
   3. Temporary colostomy for rectovaginal fistula
F. Nursing intervention
   1. Provide psychologic support: offer reassurance and acceptance

2. Encourage patient to verbalize feelings; express empathy
3. Observe vaginal discharge and record
4. Change perineal pad q4h and prn
5. Instruct on perineal hygiene
6. Provide sitz bath and irrigation solutions for hygiene if ordered
7. Follow general postoperative nursing actions if patient undergoes surgery
   a. Observe Foley catheter for drainage at all times
   b. Caution patient not to strain when having a bowel movement

Prolapsed Uterus

A. Definition: downward displacement of the uterus through the vaginal orifice
B. Pathology
   1. A result of weakened supporting muscles and ligaments of the pelvis
   2. Causes include childbirth injuries, repeated pregnancies with short intervals between, menopausal atrophy, and congenital weakness
C. Signs and symptoms
   1. Subjective
      a. Pain in lower abdomen
      b. Feeling of pressure within pelvis
      c. Stress incontinence
      d. Dyspareunia
      e. Backache
   2. Objective
      a. Urinary stasis
      b. Elongated cervix
D. Diagnostic methods
   1. Signs and symptoms
   2. Pelvic examination
E. Treatment
   1. Placement of a pessary in the vagina to support uterus
   2. Surgical suspension of the uterus
   3. Hysterectomy if condition is postmenopausal
F. Nursing intervention
   1. Approach unhurriedly, demonstrate calmness, and encourage expression of feelings to decrease anxiety
   2. Explain all procedures
   3. Follow general postoperative nursing actions
      a. Chart number of perineal pads used during 8-hour period
      b. Observe for hemorrhage
      c. Observe for vaginal discharge other than serosanguineous fluid
      d. Listen for renewed bowel sounds
      e. Observe for urinary retention and pelvic congestion

Cystocele and Rectocele

A. Definition
   1. Cystocele: abnormal protrusion of the bladder against the vaginal wall
   2. Rectocele: abnormal protrusion of part of the rectum against the vaginal wall
B. Pathology
   1. Result of weakened supporting muscles and ligaments of the pelvis
   2. Causes include childbirth injuries, repeated pregnancies with short intervals between, menopausal atrophy, and congenital weakness
C. Signs and symptoms
   1. Subjective
      a. Pelvic pressure; backache
      b. Stress incontinence and dysuria (cystocele)
      c. Constipation or incontinence of feces and flatus (rectocele)
   2. Objective
      a. Residual urine after voiding (cystocele)
      b. Hemorrhoids (rectocele)
D. Diagnostic methods
   1. Signs and symptoms
   2. Pelvic examination
E. Treatment
   1. Anterior colporrhaphy to adjust cystocele
   2. Posterior colporrhaphy to adjust rectocele
F. Nursing intervention
   1. Administer catheter care twice a day (bid) and prn
   2. Splint abdomen when coughing
   3. Place in low-Fowler's position or flat in bed to avoid pressure on suture line
   4. Explain to patient that she should respond to bowel stimuli to avoid suture strain
   5. After each bowel movement, clean perineum with warm water and soap; pat dry anterior to posterior
   6. Apply heat lamp, anesthetic spray, or ice packs if ordered to relieve discomfort
   7. Patient teaching includes
      a. Heavy lifting and prolonged standing, walking, and sitting are contraindicated
      b. Sexual intercourse should be avoided until approved by physician
      c. Pelvic exercises

Ovarian Tumors

A. Definition: a mass of tissue growing on the ovary; is usually asymptomatic until large enough to cause pressure
B. Pathology: two classifications
   1. Ovarian cyst: a benign condition but may transform to a malignancy; may be small containing clear fluid or may be filled with a thick yellow fluid; size varies
   2. Malignant tumors: usually a cancerous cell travels from another organ, and a secondary malignant site is established
C. Signs and symptoms
   1. Subjective
      a. Pelvic pain
      b. Menstrual disturbances
      c. Abdominal distention
      d. Constipation
      e. Dyspareunia
   2. Objective: palpable mass
D. Diagnostic tests/methods
   1. Culdoscopy
   2. Ultrasonography
   3. Biopsy examination
E. Treatment
   1. Cyst may be observed for regression in size
   2. Oophorectomy (removal of ovaries)
   3. Removal of all reproductive organs
   4. Estrogen replacement therapy
   5. X-ray therapy and chemotherapy

F. Nursing intervention
  1. If patient undergoes oophorectomy, follow general postoperative nursing care related to abdominal surgery
  2. If the patient undergoes surgery for removal of all abdominal reproductive organs, follow nursing intervention covered under cancer of the cervix
  3. Assist the patient in dealing with changes of body image

Cancer of the Cervix

A. Definition: new growth of abnormal cells in the neck of the uterus
B. Pathology
  1. Early stage is confined to epithelial cervical layer
  2. Will continue to invade surrounding area such as bladder and rectum
  3. Metastasizes to lungs, bones, and liver
C. Signs and symptoms
  1. Subjective
    a. Asymptomatic in early stage
    b. Menstrual disturbances
    c. Postmenopausal bleeding
    d. Bleeding after intercourse
    e. Watery discharge
  2. Suspicious Pap test result
D. Diagnostic tests/methods
  1. Pap smear
  2. Cervical biopsy examination
  3. Colposcopy
  4. Schiller's test
  5. Conization
E. Treatment
  1. Panhysterectomy (excision of uterus and cervix)
  2. Radiation in advanced case
  3. Chemotherapy
F. Nursing intervention
  1. Reassure patient and family that adjustment to illness can be slow
  2. Acknowledge that patient must adapt to illness according to her age, developmental stage, and past life experiences
  3. If patient is to receive internal radium implant
    a. Provide isolation
    b. Instruct patient to maintain supine or side-lying position
    c. Explain to patient and visitors that the amount of time spent with patient will be limited to avoid overexposure to radiation
    d. Provide high-protein, low-residue diet to avoid straining of bowels, which may dislodge implant
    e. Maintain high fluid intake: 2000 to 3000 ml daily
    f. Insert Foley catheter to prevent bladder distention
    g. Administer antiemetics as ordered
  4. If the patient undergoes surgery, follow general postoperative nursing actions
    a. Observe for vaginal hemorrhage, malodorous vaginal discharge, or any vaginal discharge other than serosanguineous discharge
    b. Observe for urinary retention
    c. Change perineal pads every 3 to 4 hours and prn
    d. Listen for renewed bowel sounds

Bartholin Cysts

A. Definition: a tumorlike capsule formed of retained secretions
B. Pathology
  1. May develop as a consequence of an earlier bacterial infection of these structures
  2. Formation of these cysts results from obstruction in the outlet of these glands
C. Signs and symptoms
  1. Subjective
    a. Pain on walking
    b. Dyspareunia
  2. Objective: mobile nodule
D. Diagnostic methods
  1. Pelvic examination
  2. Palpable nodule
E. Treatment
  1. Incision and drainage
  2. Antiseptic wound packing
F. Nursing intervention
  1. Reassure the patient that normal function of the gland will be regained after the procedure
  2. After surgery provide a sterile perineal pad q4h and prn
  3. Provide sterile wound care as ordered
  4. Instruct on perineal hygiene
  5. Provide sitz baths for increased circulation and comfort
  6. On patient's discharge from the hospital explain that the surgical wound is susceptible to bacterial infection until healing has taken place

Fibrocystic Breast Disease

A. Definition: fiberlike tumors of the breast tissue with cyst formation
B. Pathology
  1. Cause is unknown; possible hormonal imbalance
  2. Condition occurs during reproductive years and disappears with menopause
  3. A benign condition affecting 25% of women over 30 years of age
C. Signs and symptoms
  1. Subjective: breast tenderness and pain
  2. Objective: small, round, smooth nodules
D. Diagnostic tests/methods
  1. Mammography
  2. Thermomastography
  3. Xerography
E. Treatment
  1. Aspiration
  2. Biopsy examination to rule out malignancy
F. Nursing intervention
  1. Explain importance of monthly breast self-examination
  2. Encourage patient to seek medical evaluation if nodule forms because cystic disease may predispose to breast malignancy

Cancer of the Breast

A. Definition: small, painless, fixed lump most frequently located in the upper, outer portion of the breast
B. Pathology
  1. High-risk factors include women aged 30 to 50 years,

those who have not nursed, women with fibrocystic breast disease, those with a positive family history, those with early menarche and prolonged menstrual history; and women whose first pregnancy was after age 25 or who have never had children

   2. Sites of metastasis are lymph nodes, lungs, liver, brain, and bones
C. Signs and symptoms
   1. Subjective: nontender nodule
   2. Objective
      a. Enlarged axillary nodes
      b. Nipple retraction or elevation
      c. Skin dimpling
      d. Nipple discharge
D. Diagnostic tests/methods
   1. Mammography
   2. Thermography
   3. Xerography
   4. Breast biopsy examination
E. Treatment
   1. Lumpectomy: removal of the lump and partial breast tissue; indicated for early onset
   2. Mastectomy
      a. Simple mastectomy: removal of breast
      b. Modified radical mastectomy: removal of breast, pectoralis minor, and some of adjacent lymph nodes (the pectoralis major is preserved)
      c. Radical mastectomy: removal of the breast, pectoral muscles, pectoral fascia, and nodes
   3. Oophorectomy, adrenalectomy, or hypophysectomy to remove source of estrogen and those hormones that stimulate the breast
   4. Radiation therapy to destroy malignant tissue
   5. Chemotherapeutic agents to shrink and retard cancer growth
   6. Corticosteroids, androgens, and antiestrogens to alter cancer that is dependent on hormonal environment
F. Nursing intervention
   1. Provide atmosphere of acceptance, frequent patient contact, and encouragement in illness adjustment
   2. Introduce a person who has successfully undergone the same experience: arrange contact from Reach to Recovery representative
   3. Encourage grooming activities such as hair, nails, teeth, and skin
   4. Arrange attractive environment
   5. If the patient is receiving radiation or chemotherapy, explain and assist her with potential side effects
      a. Nausea and vomiting
      b. Anorexia
      c. Diarrhea
      d. Stomatitis
      e. Malaise
      f. Itching
      g. Hair loss (alopecia)
   6. If the patient has undergone surgical intervention, follow postoperative nursing actions
      a. Elevate affected arm above level of right atrium to prevent edema
      b. Drawing blood or administering parenteral fluids or taking blood pressure on affected arm is contraindicated
      c. Monitor dressing for hemorrhage; observe back for pooling
      d. Empty Hemovac and measure drainage q8h
      e. Assess circulatory status of affected limb
      f. Measure upper arm and forearm, bid, to monitor edema
      g. Encourage exercises of the affected arm when approved by physician; avoid abduction
         (1) Brushing hair
         (2) Squeezing ball
         (3) Feeding self
   7. Patient teaching on discharge
      a. Exercise to tolerance
      b. Sleep with arm elevated
      c. Elevate arm several times daily
      d. Avoid injections, vaccinations, and taking of blood pressure in affected arm
      e. Never allow blood to be drawn from or IV started in affected arm

Paget's Disease of the Breast

A. Definition: cancer of the nipple
B. Pathology
   1. Rare occurrence affecting women over 40 years of age
   2. Spreads from nipple to areola to part of the breasts; ulcerates
C. Signs and symptoms
   1. Subjective
      a. Itching
      b. Swelling
   2. Objective
      a. Blistering
      b. Discharge
      c. Nipple retraction
D. Diagnostic method: biopsy examination
E. Treatment: mastectomy
F. Nursing intervention: refer to nursing intervention as previously outlined under cancer of the breast

The Integumentary System

The skin is the body's barrier and protection from the environment. It prevents loss of body fluids and protects tissues and organs from external injury and organisms. Temperature regulation, sensation, and excretion of small amounts of water and sodium chloride are functions of the skin. Maximum health and healing of the skin are maintained by proper nutrition, hydration, electrolyte balance, exercise, and rest. Problems arise from systemic allergies (e.g., food and medication, exposure to external irritants such as chemicals, plants, and cosmetics, exposure to sun, parasites, microorganisms, injury, and new growths).

The following terms are used to describe skin lesions:

atheroma fatty patch or thickening on skin
bleb blister filled with fluid
bulla large blister filled with fluid, as occurs with burns
comedo blackhead or acne
cyst sac or capsule containing fluid or semisolid material (e.g., sebaceous cyst of scalp)
erythema red area (e.g., sunburn)
excoriation abrasion of the outer layer of skin (e.g., friction trauma)

exudate fluid, usually containing pus, bacteria, and dead cells (e.g., fluid from infected wound)

fissure groove, crack, or slit as occurs with ulceration

furuncle painful erythematous raised lesion (e.g., boil)

hive solid, raised, and itchy area (wheal), usually the result of allergy

macule small, flat discolored area (e.g., freckle)

maculopapular multiple lesions consisting of both macules and papules (e.g., early chickenpox)

mole flat or raised pigmented growth (e.g., birthmark)

nevus congenital raised, pigmented growth (e.g., birthmark or mole)

nodule small, solid mass (e.g., swollen lymph node)

papule small, red, raised elevation (e.g., measles)

petechia red pinpoint hemorrhage; seen in some blood diseases

pustule small elevation on the skin containing purulent fluid (e.g., acne)

ulcer depression (e.g., open lesion on skin)

urticaria hives (e.g., blood transfusion reaction)

vesicle small sac containing serous or sanguineous fluid (e.g., pimple)

wheal raised lesion, usually accompanied by itching (e.g., mosquito bite)

NURSING ASSESSMENT

A. Nursing observations
1. Skin
   a. Color: any deviation from normal, (e.g., pallor, cyanosis, jaundice, or blanching)
   b. Turgor: evaluate hydration and elasticity
   c. Lesions and rashes: size, location, color, drainage, and crusts
   d. Skin temperature for inconsistency: areas cool or warm to the touch
   e. Cleanliness and hygiene
   f. Odor
   g. Pressure areas for existing or potential decubitus ulcers
2. Hair and scalp
   a. Unusual distribution or absence of scalp and body hair
   b. Texture: smooth or coarse
   c. Parasites: scalp and pubic
3. Nails
   a. Cleanliness
   b. Brittleness
   c. Length
B. Patient description (subjective data)
1. History to include onset, changes, and presence of itching, pain, or burning
2. Factors that make condition worse/better
3. Allergies
4. Recent changes in environment and diet
5. Medications taken
6. Concerns about appearance, change in body image, and disfigurement
7. Changes in activities or life-style caused by disease

FREQUENT PATIENT PROBLEMS AND NURSING CARE

A. Body image disturbance related to disfigurement
1. Show acceptance by being nonjudgmental
2. Plan time to allow patient to express feelings

B. Pain related to pruritus (itching)
1. Administer antipruritics and antihistamines (see Chapter 4)
2. Keep nails short
3. Use cotton bedding and clothing; avoid rough fabrics
4. Encourage use of gloves when sleeping
5. Bathe with tepid water; use minimal soap; pat dry using no friction
6. Give oil, medicated, or starch baths
C. Potential for infection/injury related to open lesions
1. Use aseptic technique in cleaning
2. Maintain isolation only if patient is infectious
3. Use dressings only when necessary and apply loosely with gauze and nonallergenic tape
D. Impaired skin integrity related to seborrhea: oily scalp with shedding of greasy scales
1. Give frequent shampoos
2. Use medicated shampoos; rinse thoroughly

MAJOR MEDICAL DIAGNOSES
Contact Dermatitis

A. Definition: an inflammatory response of the skin with redness, edema, thickening of the skin, and frequent scaling; there may be vesicles and papules
B. Cause: an allergic reaction or unusual sensitivity when a substance comes in direct contact with the skin (e.g., poison ivy, soaps, cleaning agents, and fabrics)
C. Symptoms: pruritus; erythema
D. Diagnostic test/methods
1. Allergy testing
2. Patient history and assessment
E. Treatment
1. Systemic medication: antihistamines, antipruritics and corticosteroids (see Chapter 4)
2. Topical medication: corticosteroids (see Chapter 4)
3. Remove cause
F. Nursing intervention
1. Prevent scratching
2. Give tepid baths
3. Cut nails
4. Administer prn medications as soon as possible

Psoriasis

A. Definition: a chronic condition in which there are patches of inflammation that are red and covered with silvery scales that shed; these usually occur on elbows, knees, lower back, and scalp; they may cover the entire body
B. Cause: unknown, may be a family tendency, symptoms increase during stress and high anxiety; other related factors are alcoholism, trauma, and infection
C. Signs and symptoms
1. Pruritus, mild to severe
2. Depression related to appearance
D. Diagnostic methods: patient history and physical appearance
E. Treatment (individual)
1. Topical medication: coal tars and corticosteroids (see Chapter 4)
2. Systemic medication: corticosteroids and methotrexate (in severe cases) (see Chapter 4)
3. Exposure to ultraviolet light

4. Anxiolytics
5. Antimetabolites

F. Nursing intervention
   1. During bath gently remove scales with cloth or brush
   2. Occlusive dressing may be wrapped in plastic

Herpes Simplex (Cold Sore/Fever Blister) Type I

A. Definition: a group of blisters on a reddened base usually on or near mouth or genitalia
B. Cause: a viral infection precipitated by an upper respiratory tract infection or elevation of temperature from systemic infection; frequently related to emotional upset, menstrual cycle, or general immunosuppression
C. Signs and symptoms
   1. Pain and local discomfort
   2. Distress about appearance
D. Diagnostic methods: physical assessment
E. Treatment: lasts about 1 week; antiviral agents (acyclovir) administered topically or systemically
F. Nursing intervention: none indicated

Herpes Zoster (Shingles)

A. Definition: crops of vesicles and erythema following sensory nerves on face and trunk; higher incidence in the elderly
B. Cause: varicella zoster virus (chickenpox)
C. Signs and symptoms
   1. Severe pain
   2. Elevation of temperature
   3. Malaise
   4. Anorexia
   5. Pruritus
D. Diagnostic methods: physical examination; vesicles follow sensory nerve paths
E. Treatment: no specific treatment (symptomatic only); analgesics may be used for pain; usually subsides in 3 weeks (pain may last for months); antivirals, corticosteroids, antibiotics
F. Nursing intervention
   1. Keep patient in isolation while vesicles are present
   2. Apply topical lotions to lesions for itching
   3. Give baths or compresses for cooling and soothing
   4. Prevent scratching and secondary infection
   5. Anticipate pain: medicate as needed
   6. Provide small, frequent, well-balanced meals

Neoplasms

A. Definition: any new and abnormal growth; may be of varied size and location
B. Cause
   1. Benign: unknown
   2. Malignant: related to exposure to the sun and chemical and physical irritants, such as pipe smoking
C. Signs and symptoms: anxiety: related to diagnosis and change in physical appearance
D. Diagnostic test: biopsy examination; high cure rate with early detection
E. Treatment: see Table 6-1
F. Nursing intervention
   1. Assess all patients for skin lesions
   2. Discuss with patient the importance of reporting any changes in moles

Table 6-1. Classification of common tumors of the skin

Classification	Description	Treatment
Benign	Nevus, brown or black mole	Observe for changes: remove only if irritated or changes are observed
Premalignant or potentially malignant	Senile keratosis: brownish scaly spots on face and hands of aging persons	Surgical removal or topical medication or cryosurgery
	Leukoplakia: shiny white patches on mucous membranes of mouth and female genitalia	Removal of irritating teeth; oral hygiene. For genitalia: surgical excision; biopsy
	Moles (nevi) that bleed, grow, or are irritated or crusted	May become malignant and are surgically removed
	Black, smooth moles	
Malignant	Squamous cell carcinoma: begin as a warty growth and grow and become ulcerated; found on exposed surfaces of the body (tongue and lip)	Early surgical removal
	Basal cell carcinoma: a slow-growing tumor; results from exposure to sun	Chemosurgery, electrosurgery, or surgical removal
	Malignant melanoma: black tumor that metastasized	Widespread excision

3. Give general preoperative and postoperative care (see Chapter 2)
4. Provide general care for patient receiving radiotherapy (see Chapter 2)
5. Give general care for patient receiving chemotherapy (see Chapter 4)

G. Classification of common skin tumors (Table 6-1)

Burns

A. Definition: a wound in which the skin layers and underlying tissue is destroyed
B. Causes
   1. Heat (e.g., fire)
   2. Chemical (e.g., acids)
   3. Electrical (e.g., lightning or electrical wires)
   4. Radiation (e.g., sun)
   5. Mechanical (e.g., friction from rope)
C. Signs and symptoms: depend on depth (Table 6-2) and area involved
   1. Infection: there is destruction of the body's first line of defense
   2. Loss of body tissue (protein)
   3. Loss of fluid and electrolytes (edema)
   4. Pain

Table 6-2. Description of burns

Classification	Depth	Description	Possible cause
Superficial or shallow partial thickness	Epidermis	Red and dry; painful; may have edema; no scarring	Sunburn
Deep partial thickness	Epidermis and some dermis	Mottled, pink to red blisters; painful; leave scar	Hot oil
Full thickness partial	Epidermis, dermis, and subcutaneous tissue	Black or bright red eschar forms leathery covering; leaves scar; may have no pain	Fire
Full thickness deep	All of the above plus subcutaneous fat, fascia, muscle, and bone (nerve endings, hair follicles, and sweat glands are destroyed)	Black; there is no pain	Fire

5. Respiratory distress
6. Immobilization
7. Disfigurement
8. Impending shock

D. Diagnostic method: physical assessment
E. Treatment
   1. Respiratory evaluation, maintenance of airway, and possible tracheostomy; edema of lung tissue from smoke inhalation may cause increased secretions
   2. Replacement of fluids and electrolytes with IV solutions: plasma, blood, dextran, and electrolytes
   3. Emergency wound care: removal of foreign material; avoidance of contamination
   4. Prevention of infection: tetanus immune globlin and antibiotics
   5. Analgesics for pain (see Chapter 4)
   6. Prevention of shock: plasma expanders; keep patient warm; monitor vital signs, urine output
   7. Wound treatment method
      a. Open method exposure; wound heals by epithelialization of eschar; this method requires reverse isolation; eschar must be removed by debridement (cutting away) whirlpool baths, and escharotomy incision into eschar
      b. Topical medications (see Chapter 4)
      c. Grafts: to minimize infection and fluid loss; may be temporary since they are frequently rejected; this method allows for growth of new tissue underneath the protection of the graft
         (1) Autograft: transplantation of skin from patient's own body; care must also be given to donor site

         (2) Homograft (allograft): transplantation of tissue from living human
         (3) Heterograft: transplantation from animal (pig or cow)
         (4) Synthetic material used in grafting
      d. Cosmetic surgery may be performed during recovery phase

F. Nursing intervention
   1. Anticipate and prevent respiratory distress; maintain airway, monitor breathing qh then q4h (see Chapter 2); keep tracheostomy equipment available
   2. Maintain fluid balance: monitor IV fluids; monitor urine output qh through indwelling catheter; monitor sp gr qh; weigh patient qd
   3. Anticipate infection: maintain asepsis and reverse isolation; administer antibiotics; monitor temperature q2h; keep patient warm
   4. Anticipate pain: give frequent sedation as ordered, especially before dressing change (administered intravenously during early phase of treatment)
   5. Prevent dangers of immobilization (see Chapter 2); provide proper alignment to prevent deformities (may be uncomfortable or painful); prevent skin surfaces from touching; use turning frames and cradles
   6. To enhance tissue repair, diet must be high in calories (6000 calories qd) and high in protein; tube feeding or total parenteral nutrition may be necessary
   7. Anticipate shock: assess level of consciousness and mental status; monitor pulse rate and blood pressure
   8. Anticipate Curling's ulcer (stress ulcer): at the end of the first week assess for gastrointestinal distress or bleeding
   9. Be aware of anxiety: provide diversional activities; allow time for patient to verbalize feelings; encourage contact with family; involve patient as much as possible with planning and self-care; administer tranquilizers and sedation as necessary

The Eye

Sight is the most important sense to most people. Visual acuity is dependent on general good health, CNS regulation of movement and conduction, and condition of the structures of the eye. Changes in vision are frequently indicative of systemic disease; routine examination of the eye can provide information about diseases in other systems. The nurse must assess the eyes of each patient under his or her care. Although the incidence of blindness and visual impairment increases with age, most problems are seen in patients of all ages.

NURSING ASSESSMENT

A. Nursing observations
   1. Glasses, contact lenses, or false eyes
   2. Tearing, discharge (clear or purulent), and color of sclera (white, yellow, or pink)
   3. Accuracy and range of vision
   4. Edema of eyelids; crusting; blinking, rubbing; redness
   5. Clouded appearance over pupil; protrusion or bulging of eye(s); pupil response to light
   6. Squinting or drooping (ptosis) of lid
   7. Symmetry

B. Patient description (subjective data)
   1. Double vision (diplopia), decreased or absent vision in one or both eyes, or blurred or clouded vision
   2. Sensitivity to light (photophobia), spots, halos around lights, flashes of light, or problems seeing in the dark
   3. Eye fatigue, itching, pain, tearing, burning, or headache
C. Note patient history of
   1. Stumbling
   2. Trauma to face or eyes
   3. Contact lenses or eye medication
   4. Changes in vision and any related circumstances
   5. Any systemic medications taken

DIAGNOSTIC TESTS/METHODS

A. Ophthalmoscope: assessment of the interior of eye
B. Tonometer: measurement of intraocular pressure; increased pressure may indicate early glaucoma; recommended every 3 years for individuals between 35 and 40 years of age and on a yearly basis for individuals over 40
C. Fields of vision: testing to measure sight on one or both sides (peripheral vision)
D. Refraction: measurement of light refraction and lenses required for visual acuity
E. Slit lamp: examination of intraocular structures with a high-intensity light beam
F. Snellen chart: assessment of visual acuity

EYE CARE PROFESSIONALS

A. Ophthalmologist (also called oculist): a medical doctor who specializes in diagnosis, treatment, and surgery of the eyes, including the prescribing of glasses
B. Optometrist: educated and licensed to test for refractive problems; may prescribe and fit glasses; may, within limits, diagnose disease, prescribe medication, or treat eye diseases (laws vary among states)
C. Optician: fills prescription for corrective lenses as prescribed by physician; fits glasses properly

FREQUENT PATIENT PROBLEMS AND NURSING CARE

A. Anxiety/fear related to concerns about loss of vision, altered life-styles, ability to function, employment, plans for the future, and altered body image: allow time for the patient to express feelings
B. Potential for infection related to drainage
   1. Clean as necessary with normal saline solution
   2. Gently apply compresses to loosen if necessary
   3. Use aseptic technique; wipe from inner canthus to outer canthus
   4. If drainage is purulent, dispose of properly
C. High risk for injury related to need for corrective lenses
   1. Glasses must be kept clean and in a protective case
   2. Contact lenses are kept in a case with *R* and *L* to designate which eye the lens fits; obtain directions for soaking from patient
   3. If patient is dependent on lenses, obtain permission for patient to wear glasses or lenses when going for diagnostic tests
D. Potential injury related to photophobia
   1. Keep room dim and evenly lighted
   2. Keep blinds adjusted to avoid glare

THE VISUALLY IMPAIRED PATIENT
Low Vision

A. Definition: low vision refers to defects that cannot be corrected with lenses
B. Cause: disease of the eye itself, in the visual pathways to the brain, or in the receptors in the brain
C. Signs and symptoms: vision may be blurred and images distorted; vision may be clear only at close range; shades of color may not be distinguishable

Total or Legal Blindness

A. Definition: legal blindness is the ability to see at no more than 20 feet (6 m) what normally should be seen at a distance of 200 feet (60 m) (20/200); this may also refer to severe restrictions in peripheral fields of vision (after corrective lenses are used)
B. Pathology
   1. Degeneration, glaucoma, detached retina, or diabetic retinopathy
   2. Trauma or laceration
   3. Inflammation or optic neuritis
   4. Vascular or hypertensive retinopathy
   5. Neoplasms of the brain or eye
   6. Cataract
C. Patient problems
   1. Inability to care for self (dependency)
   2. Frustration
   3. Occupational hazards
   4. Boredom
D. Nursing intervention
   1. Allow as much independence as possible; help make use of existing vision; encourage use of any visual aids recommended by physician (e.g., special lenses, large-type books, and cane); provide reading material in braille for the patient who has learned this method
   2. Do not touch patient without talking; always address patient by name; introduce yourself; and tell patient when you are leaving the room
   3. Explain all care and treatments; encourage patient to participate in planning care
   4. At mealtime, indicate position of utensils and placement of food on dish by comparing it to numbers on a clock (e.g., "the potato is at 3 o'clock")
   5. Orient patient to room and entire unit; point out hazards and obstacles (doors and windows); explain location of furniture, bathroom, call bell, and telephone; keep things in the same place
   6. Leave bedside table, call bell, and personal items in close reach
   7. Maintain safety; keep unit uncluttered, floor clean and dry, bed in low position, and side rail(s) up as necessary; tell patient position of bed and side rails
   8. Guide the ambulatory patient by placing patient's arm on yours while walking slowly
   9. Provide diversion: radio and books on tapes; be aware of local agencies in your community; many libraries have braille books or tapes available

Refractive Disorders

A. Definition: inability of the refractory media to converge light rays and focus on retina (see Chapter 3)

1. Myopia (nearsightedness): the eyeball is too long; light rays focus at a point before reaching the retina
2. Hyperopia (farsightedness): the eyeball is shorter than normal; light rays focus beyond the retina
3. Presbyopia: a gradual loss of elasticity of the lens; there is decreased ability to focus on near objects
4. Astigmatism: unequal curve in the shape of the cornea or lens; vision is distorted

B. Cause: unknown; may be inherited
C. Symptoms: diminished or blurred vision
D. Diagnostic tests/methods
   1. Patient history
   2. Refraction
E. Treatment: corrective lenses (glasses or contact lenses)
F. Nursing intervention
   1. Encourage proper care of lenses
   2. Encourage follow-up checkups as indicated

Conjunctivitis

A. Definition: infection or inflammation of the conjunctiva
B. Causes: bacteria, usually *staphylococcus,* and allergens
C. Patient problems
   1. Very contagious (especially in young children)
   2. Purulent drainage and itching
D. Diagnostic method: physical assessment
E. Treatment: ophthalmic antibiotics (see Chapter 4)
F. Nursing intervention
   1. Prevent transmission to others: encourage frequent hand washing
   2. Provide warm compresses; cleanse eyelids; remove crusts before administering ophthalmic medications
      a. Discourage rubbing of eyes
      b. Isolate personal items (towels, washcloths, and pillowcases)

Cataract

A. Definition: the crystalline lens becomes clouded and opaque (not transparent)
B. Causes
   1. Trauma
   2. Congenital
   3. Related to diabetes
   4. High incidence in the elderly (senile cataracts)
   5. Heredity
   6. Infections
   7. Longtime exposure to the sun
C. Signs and symptoms
   1. Loss of vision
   2. Progressive blurring
   3. Haziness with eventual complete loss of sight
D. Diagnostic tests/methods
   1. Examination with ophthalmoscope
   2. Patient history
E. Treatment: surgical removal of opaque lens, usually on an outpatient basis; after surgery, corrective lenses are necessary (glasses, contact lenses, or surgical implantation of an artificial lens)
F. Nursing intervention
   1. Give general preoperative care (see Chapter 2)
   2. Provide nursing care as for the patient with low vision
   3. Postoperative management depends on surgical procedure; be careful to adhere to physician's order;

general principles: have patient avoid coughing, bending, or rapid head movements; provide bed rest for a specified time (usually 2 hours); keep patient flat or in low-Fowler's position; have patient deep breathe (avoid coughing); be sure patient avoids straining (give stool softener); help patient avoid vomiting (an antiemetic will be ordered; administer as needed); observe dressing; report pain or bleeding; position patient with unoperated side down

Glaucoma

A. Definition: intraocular pressure increases because of a disturbance in the circulation of aqueous humor (see Chapter 3); there is an imbalance between production and drainage as the angle of drainage closes
   1. Acute (closed-angle) glaucoma: dramatic onset of symptoms; immediate treatment is required, usually surgery
   2. Chronic (open-angle) glaucoma: symptoms progress slowly and are frequently ignored; if disease is not detected early, it may lead to permanent loss of vision
B. Pathology
   1. Familial tendency
   2. Related to age; incidence increases over 40 years of age
   3. Secondary to injuries and infections
C. Signs and symptoms
   1. Loss of peripheral vision, halos around lights, and permanent loss of vision (a leading cause of blindness)
   2. Pain, malaise, nausea, and vomiting
   3. Pupils fixed and dilated
D. Diagnostic tests/methods
   1. History of symptoms
   2. Measurement of visual fields
   3. Measurement of intraocular pressure
E. Treatment
   1. Miotics to decrease intraocular pressure (see Chapter 4)
   2. Surgery: iridectomy (an incision through the cornea to remove part of the iris to allow for drainage); laser trabeculoplasty (relieves excess intraocular pressure)
   3. Continued medical supervision
F. Nursing intervention
   1. Encourage patient to wear medical identification tag
   2. Administer eye medications on schedule
   3. Inform the patient to avoid drugs with atropine; discourage straining and lifting
   4. Give preoperative and postoperative care according to that for a patient with a cataract; pay careful attention to specifics in physician's orders

Detached Retina

A. Definition: the sensory layer of the retina pulls away from the pigmented layer; vitreous humor may leak into the space occupying the position the retina normally assumes
B. Cause: usually unknown and spontaneous; may be related to sudden blow to the head or follow eye surgery (e.g., removal of cataract)
C. Signs and symptoms
   1. Loss of vision in affected area (may be complete loss)

2. Visual disturbance (blurring)
3. Spots and flashes of light
D. Diagnostic tests/methods
1. Patient history and physical assessment
2. Retinal examination with ophthalmoscope
E. Treatment: depends on area of detachment
1. Bed rest
2. Prevention of extension of detachment
3. Mydriatics
4. Surgical intervention
F. Nursing intervention
1. Provide individual care according to location of detachment; physician's orders will be specific
2. Maintain absolute rest; restrict activity; patch eye to limit eye movement
3. Prepare patient for postoperative care: inform patient that both eyes may be patched and he or she may be unable to see
4. Postoperative care: position patient exactly as ordered; maintain eye patch(es); have patient deep breathe and avoid coughing; administer medication for pain; provide care as needed for a person with limited sight

The Ear

Hearing problems are not as obvious initially during assessment as are many other problems. Hearing loss may be misinterpreted. Many people associate hearing aids with dependency or disfigurement or signs of aging and refuse to wear them. Yet the sense of hearing contributes to well-being and safety. This assessment (hearing) must be made for each patient cared for.

NURSING ASSESSMENT

A. Nursing observations
1. Difficulty hearing or understanding verbal communication
2. Not responding to loud or sudden noises
3. Use of hearing aid, lip reading, or sign language
4. Drainage, dried secretion, or deformities of the ear
B. Patient description (subjective data)
1. Earache or headache
2. Difficulty hearing (or lack of hearing) in one or both ears
3. Itching, drainage, pressure or full feeling
4. Ringing, buzzing, popping, or echoes
5. Vertigo
6. Medications taken
C. Note history of
1. Ear infections
2. Ear surgery
3. Head injury
4. Medication taken

DIAGNOSTIC TESTS/METHODS

A. Audiometry: a hearing test to determine ability to discriminate sounds, voices, and degrees of loudness and pitch
B. Otoscopy: visual examination of the ear canal and tympanic membrane
C. Weber's test: a tuning fork is struck and placed midline on the patient's forehead; the patient is asked where the sound is heard; in this test of conduction, sounds should be heard equally well in each ear
D. Rinne test: the tuning fork is struck and placed on the mastoid process of the skull behind the ear; the fork is removed, and the patient indicates when the sound can no longer be heard; the still-vibrating fork is then placed near the external ear canal; normally the sound will be heard longer through air conduction than through bone

THE PATIENT WITH IMPAIRED HEARING

A. Definition
1. Conductive hearing loss occurs when injury or disease interferes with the conduction of sound waves to the inner ear (e.g., cerumen in canal)
2. Sensory hearing loss occurs when there is malfunction of the inner ear, auditory nerve, or auditory center in the brain (e.g., toxic effect to eighth cranial nerve from drugs [aspirin])
B. Patient problems
1. Inability to communicate
2. Inability to hear hazards in the environment (e.g., automobiles)
3. Frustration, anxiety, anger, and insecurity
4. Misinterpretation of communication
C. Treatment: according to cause: frequently none
D. Nursing intervention
1. Find out if a hearing aid can be fitted
a. Encourage patient to wear it
b. Test batteries for function
c. Make sure hearing aid is turned on
d. Protect hearing aid from breakage; ask patient or family about usual care and storage
2. Attract patient's attention before speaking
3. Do not touch patient until he or she is aware that you are in the room
4. Speak face to face; articulate clearly but not too slowly; move close to patient; avoid covering mouth with hand
5. Provide alternate methods of communication
a. Find out if patient lip-reads or uses sign language
b. Provide magic slate or pad and pencil
6. Nursing intervention after surgery
a. Give general preoperative and postoperative care (see Chapter 2)
b. Report drainage immediately
c. Observe for facial nerve injury: inability to close eyes or pucker lips
d. Anticipate vertigo: provide safety
e. Be sure patient avoids blowing nose
f. Note specific instructions from physician for positioning, activity, and diet

MAJOR MEDICAL DIAGNOSES
Ménière's Syndrome

A. Definition: a chronic disease with sudden attacks of vertigo and tinnitus (ringing in the ear) with progressive hearing loss; attacks last a few minutes to a few weeks; usually occurs in women over 50 years of age
B. Cause: unknown; related to fluid in cochlea—either increased production or decreased absorption
C. Signs and symptoms
1. Vertigo
2. Nausea and vomiting
3. Ringing in the ears and hearing loss
D. Diagnostic tests/method: patient history

E. Treatment
   1. Diuretics, low-sodium diet, and dimenhydrinate (Dramamine)
   2. Surgery: destruction of the labyrinth as a last resort
F. Nursing intervention
   1. Bed rest; position of comfort
   2. Maintain quiet and safety
   3. Low-sodium diet
   4. Provide specific nursing care as that for patient with limited hearing (see above)
   5. Provide general preoperative and postoperative care (see Chapter 2)
   6. Provide nursing care for patient after ear surgery (see preceding outline)

Mastoiditis

A. Definition: infection of the mastoid process; may be acute or chronic
B. Cause: extension of middle ear infection that was inadequately treated
C. Signs and symptoms
   1. Elevation of temperature
   2. Headache, ear pain, and tenderness over mastoid process
   3. Drainage from ear
D. Treatment
   1. Antibiotics
   2. Surgery
      a. Simple mastoidectomy: removal of infected cells
      b. Radical mastoidectomy: more extensive excision resulting in some degree of hearing loss
E. Nursing intervention
   1. See care of patient with impaired hearing
   2. Provide general preoperative and postoperative care (see Chapter 2)
   3. Provide nursing care for patient after ear surgery (see previous outline)

Otosclerosis

A. Definition: a progressive formation of new bone tissue around the stapes preventing transmission of vibrations to the inner ear
B. Cause: unknown
C. Signs and symptoms
   1. Loss of hearing
   2. Ringing or buzzing (tinnitus)
D. Treatment
   1. Hearing aid
   2. Surgery; stapedectomy (removal of diseased bone and replacement with prosthetic implant)

E. Nursing intervention
   1. Provide general care for patient who is hearing impaired (see previous outline)
   2. Give general preoperative and postoperative care (see Chapter 2)
   3. Follow specific orders from physician
   4. Provide general nursing care for patient after ear surgery (see previous outline)

Suggested Reading List

Billings DM, Stokes LG: *Medical-surgical nursing,* ed 2, St Louis, 1987, Mosby.

Brunner LS, Suddarth DS: *Textbook of medical-surgical nursing,* ed 6, Philadelphia, 1988, JB Lippincott.

Dittmar S: *Rehabilitation nursing,* St Louis, 1989, Mosby.

Gruendemann BJ, Meeker MG: *Alexander's care of the patient in surgery,* ed 8, St Louis, 1987, Mosby.

Hood GH, Dincher JR: *Total patient care: foundations and practices,* ed 8, St Louis, 1992, Mosby.

Hood GH, Dincher JR: *Workbook to accompany total patient care: foundations and practice of adult health nursing,* ed 8, St Louis, 1992, Mosby.

Kneedler JA, Dodge GH: *Perioperative patient care: the nursing perspective,* ed 2, Oxford, 1987, Blackwell Scientific.

Kron T: *The management of patient care: putting leadership skills to work,* Philadelphia, 1981, WB Saunders.

Long BC, Phipps WJ, Cassmeyer VL: *Medical-surgical nursing: a nursing process approach,* ed 3, St Louis, 1992, Mosby.

Luckmann J, Sorensen KC: *Medical-surgical nursing, a psychophysiologic approach,* ed 3, Philadelphia, 1987, WB Saunders.

Mason M, Bates G: *Basic medical-surgical nursing,* ed 5, New York, 1984, Macmillan.

Memmler RL, Wood DL: *Human body in health and disease,* ed 6, Philadelphia, 1987, JB Lippincott.

Mosby's medical, nursing & allied health dictionary, ed 3, St Louis, 1990, Mosby.

Nurses' Reference Library: Procedures, Springhouse, Pa, 1983, Intermed Communications.

Perry AG, Potter PA: *Clinical nursing skills and techniques,* ed 2, St Louis, 1990, Mosby.

Phipps WJ et al: *Medical-surgical nursing: concepts and clinical practice,* ed 4, St Louis, 1991, Mosby.

Physicians' desk reference, Montvale, NJ, Medical Economics (published annually).

Rosdahl CB: *Textbook of basic nursing,* ed 4, Philadelphia, 1985, JB Lippincott.

Scherer JC: *Introductory medical-surgical nursing,* ed 5, Philadelphia, 1991, JB Lippincott.

Thompson JM et al: *Mosby's clinical nursing,* ed 3, St Louis, 1993, Mosby.

Tucker SM et al: *Patient care standards: nursing process, diagnosis, and outcome,* ed 4, St Louis, 1992, Mosby.

Medical-Surgical Nursing Review Questions

Answers and rationales begin on p. 431.

Situation: Ms. Seville is a 22-year-old female with a diagnosis of rheumatoid arthritis. Over the past 2 years, she has had episodes of swollen joints and limited range of motion (ROM) of involved joints. Her presenting symptoms include anemia, weight loss, and pain, which is unrelieved by current medication regimen.

1. The nurse is aware that rheumatoid arthritis is a:
   ① Local joint disease
   ② Self-limited illness
   ③ Disease of striated muscles
   ④ Chronic and systemic disease
2. Ms. Seville's illness was being managed with rest, exercise, and medication. First-line pharmacologic management includes use of:
   ① Narcotic analgesics
   ② Muscle relaxants
   ③ Salicylates
   ④ Calcium channel-blocking agents
3. Ms. Seville takes large doses of an antiinflammatory medication that has a side effect of gastric irritation. Patient teaching should include instructions to:
   ① Avoid driving
   ② Take with food
   ③ Discontinue if CNS effects develop
   ④ Take on an empty stomach to enhance absorption

---

4. When caring for a patient in skin traction it is important for the nurse to:
   ① Encourage diet high in carbohydrates and vitamins
   ② Limit fluid intake to 1000 ml/day
   ③ Limit patient's activities to maintain effectiveness of traction
   ④ Assess circulatory status

Situation: You are caring for Mr. Jannal, a 63-year-old man. He had asthma as a child and has been treated for emphysema for the past 10 years. He continues to smoke two packs of cigarettes daily. He is admitted with a diagnosis of chronic obstructive pulmonary disease (COPD).

5. The symptoms of emphysema include:
   ① Pleuritic pain, hemoptysis, and tachypnea
   ② Slow respirations, dyspnea, and cyanosis
   ③ Dyspnea on exertion, cough, and fatigue
   ④ Cough, cyanosis, and Kussmaul's respirations
6. Fluid intake is encouraged for Mr. Jannal because the fluids will:
   ① Liquefy the secretions
   ② Soothe the mucous membranes
   ③ Prevent bronchospasms
   ④ Prevent fluid imbalance
7. Oxygen is ordered for dyspnea. The rate of administration should be:
   ① 1 to 2 L
   ② 3 to 4 L
   ③ 5 to 6 L
   ④ 7 to 8 L

8. The patient's symptoms from emphysema are caused by:
   ① A staphylococcal infection
   ② Allergy
   ③ Rupture of the alveoli
   ④ Spasm of the bronchi

Situation: Mrs. Robinson, 58 years of age, has been fatigued, has lost weight, and has had a cough for 1 month. When she had hemoptysis she sought medical attention and was admitted to the hospital with a diagnosis of tuberculosis (TB).

9. TB is:
   ① Idiopathic
   ② Infectious
   ③ Genetic
   ④ Congenital
10. Discharge instructions for Mrs. Robinson must include:
    ① Continuing medication for 2 years
    ② Resuming all previous activities
    ③ Postural drainage each morning
    ④ At-home isolation
11. Mrs. Robinson's daughter is anxious because she has a positive reaction to a tuberculin test; the nurse knows that this indicates:
    ① Presence of infection
    ② Presence of disease
    ③ Immunity to disease
    ④ Recovery from disease
12. The nurse noted relief of Mrs. Robinson's dyspnea when she was positioned in:
    ① Dorsal recumbent position
    ② Fowler's position
    ③ Sims' position
    ④ Supine position

---

13. In a patient recovering from orthopedic surgery or a patient with a fracture, the complication of osteomyelitis might be signaled through which of the following symptoms?
    ① Numbness and delayed capillary refill
    ② Edema, pain, and drainage
    ③ Chest pain and dyspnea
    ④ Paresthesia and bluish skin discoloration

Situation: Mr. Chin, a 23-year-old salesman, fractured his right tibia and fibula while skiing. He arrives on your unit following an open reduction and application of a long plaster cast.

14. Two hours after arriving on your unit, Mr. Chin complains of severe pain in his right leg. The best nursing action would be to:
    ① Administer the oral pain medication as ordered
    ② Turn the patient, rub his back, and straighten the linen
    ③ Evaluate the neurocirculatory status of the affected leg
    ④ Check the right leg to make sure that it is elevated and externally rotated

15. Signs and symptoms of an infection underneath a cast would include which of the following assessments of the affected extremity?
    ① Tingling and decreased sensation
    ② Full pulses and spontaneous capillary refill
    ③ Swelling and diminished motor function
    ④ Elevated temperature and the presence of a "hot spot" over the cast

Situation: Mr. Allen, 27 years of age, was admitted to the hospital with a fractured rib sustained during an automobile accident. In the emergency room he experienced sharp left-sided chest pain. A chest x-ray film showed a collapsed lung. A chest tube was inserted and connected to a water-seal drainage.

16. Mr. Allen asked why the tube was not passed through his nose into the lung. The correct response would be:
    ① "The air has entered a space outside of the lung tissue."
    ② "This method will not interfere with breathing."
    ③ "This is the method your physician uses."
    ④ "This method is used in an emergency."
17. While caring for Mr. Allen, the nurse:
    ① Changes the dressing
    ② Limits activity
    ③ Milks the chest tube
    ④ Keeps drainage at eye level
18. If the chest tube becomes dislodged from the water-seal drainage, the nurse must be prepared to:
    ① Tape it
    ② Remove it
    ③ Replace it
    ④ Clamp it
19. When Mr. Allen is out of bed:
    ① The chest tubes are clamped
    ② Anticipate pain
    ③ Water-seal drainage is lower than the chest
    ④ Dyspnea is expected
20. The physician removes Mr. Allen's chest tube. The incision must be:
    ① Kept dry and clean
    ② Covered with a pressure dressing
    ③ Exposed to the air
    ④ Cleaned four times daily (qid)
21. During morning care the nurse would be concerned if Mr. Allen:
    ① Complained of sharp chest pain
    ② Continued to cough and deep breathe
    ③ Wanted to get out of bed
    ④ Gave self-care in the bathroom

22. A significant postoperative complication following an amputation is:
    ① Depression
    ② Pneumonia
    ③ Hemorrhage
    ④ Phantom limb pain

Situation: Mr. Kowalski, a 58-year-old man with a history of coronary artery disease, is admitted with a complaint of chest pain that was unrelieved by nitroglycerin. The physician orders an ECG, and cardiac enzymes. The patient is placed in coronary care with the diagnosis of a myocardial infarction. A myocardial infarction protocol is implemented.

23. In the acute phase of Mr. Kowalski's myocardial infarction, supplemental oxygen is administered. The main goal of oxygen therapy is to:
    ① Increase oxygen supply to myocardial tissue
    ② Prevent ventricular fibrillation
    ③ Decrease anxiety and restlessness
    ④ Prevent shock
24. A concern for Mr. Kowalski is the development of cardiogenic shock. Signs of cardiogenic shock include:
    ① Hot, dry skin, rapid respirations, and mental confusion
    ② Bounding pulses, clammy skin, and fever
    ③ Hypotension, weak pulses, and clammy skin
    ④ Hypertension, shallow respirations, and chest pain
25. The nurse assesses Mr. Kowalski's breath sounds and hears fine crackles in the lower lung bases. This symptom may indicate:
    ① Dysrhythmias
    ② Pneumonia
    ③ An extension of the myocardial infarction
    ④ Lung congestion from heart failure
26. Which of the following interventions will the nurse anticipate implementing for Mr. Kowalski?
    ① Adjusting the bed to Trendelenburg's position
    ② Maintaining prescription of complete bed rest for at least 5 days
    ③ Providing clear, room-temperature liquids throughout hospitalization
    ④ Administering a stool softener to prevent straining with bowel movements
27. During the fifth day in coronary care, Mr. Kowalski develops dyspnea; has blood-tinged, frothy sputum, and becomes very anxious. These symptoms may indicate:
    ① Pulmonary edema
    ② Emphysema
    ③ Pulmonary embolism
    ④ Chronic obstructive pulmonary disease
28. After a 10-day stay in the coronary care unit, Mr. Kowalski is transferred to an intermediate care unit. Because he has been on extended bed rest, the nursing care plan includes monitoring for thrombophlebitis. The nurse is aware that symptoms of thrombophlebitis include:
    ① Numbness and tingling of an extremity
    ② Coldness and paleness of the involved area
    ③ Absence of pulses and reduced sensation
    ④ Pain and red streaking along the vein path

Situation: Mr. Haliburton is a 32-year-old, black male with primary hypertension. His physician has tried to control the hypertension using conservative management. Mr. Haliburton has been managed with a controlled-sodium diet, a mild diuretic, and a stress management regimen.

29. Management of hypertension is very important because of the effects that hypertension has on other organs. Organs most frequently affected by the hypertensive state include:

① Liver, lung, and stomach
② Heart, brain, and kidney
③ Liver, stomach, and colon
④ Brain, blood, and bladder

30. Symptoms of hypertension are vague and subtle. In assessing hypertensive patients, the nurse may observe symptoms of:
① Increased urination, fatigue, and blurred vision
② Nausea, vomiting, and nosebleeds
③ Chest pain, shortness of breath, and nervousness
④ Blurred vision, irritability, and occipital headaches

31. Mr. Haliburton may need a change in his medication regimen. Which one of the following medications is designed to lower blood pressure?
① Cimetidine (Tagamet)
② Ibuprofen (Motrin)
③ Digoxin (Lanoxin)
④ Hydrochlorothiazide (HydroDIURIL)

32. Should Mr. Haliburton's management include a diuretic, an important aspect of patient education would include:
① Drinking at least a quart of liquids a day
② Refraining from caffeine and caffeine-containing products
③ Maintaining a high-potassium diet
④ Avoiding spicy and high-fat, high-cholesterol foods

Situation: Ms. Thorpe is a 27 year old who entered the clinic with symptoms of nervousness, racing heart, and weight loss. Thyroid function studies were performed and a diagnosis of hyperthyroidism was made.

33. The nurse is aware that other symptoms of hyperthyroidism include:
① Dry skin, intolerance to cold, and slowed responses
② Urinary frequency, blurred vision, frequent infections
③ Increased sweating, hand tremor, and excitability
④ Constipation, depression, and brittle hair

34. The nurse notices that Ms. Thorpe's eyes evidence retraction of the upper lids (exophthalmos). The patient complains of dry eyes. An intervention for the nurse to consider is:
① Using artificial tears
② Administering mydriatic eye drops
③ Applying an antibiotic ointment
④ Recommending the prone position for sleep and rest

35. Which of the following diets would be best for Ms. Thorpe?
① Low-purine, high-fat, 1000-calorie diet
② High-protein, high-calorie, high-carbohydrate diet with snacks
③ Clear liquids in the form of six small feedings
④ 2-gram, low-sodium diet with an evening snack

36. Ms. Thorpe is nervous and anxious. She comes from a large, close-knit family. The family is hovering over her. An important aspect of care would include:
① Maintaining a calm, relaxed environment
② Encouraging visitors to help stimulate patient interactions
③ Placing her in a semiprivate room or ward to foster interaction and release tension
④ Provide for frequent interactions between the patient and the staff

37. Following a thyroidectomy, the accidental removal of the parathyroid glands would precipitate the symptoms of tetany. Nursing observations for evidence of tetany would include:
① Unrelenting headache and blurred vision
② Hypertension and somnolence
③ Painful muscle spasms of the hands and face
④ Blood-tinged urine and frequency

38. Damage to the laryngeal nerve may occur following a thyroidectomy. The nurse observes for symptoms of:
① Hoarseness
② Frothy sputum
③ Positive Chvostek's sign
④ Choking sensation

Situation: Mr. Wilkins is admitted to the hospital with cirrhosis of the liver related to alcohol abuse and malnutrition. He is jaundiced, has ascites, and has recently experienced dyspnea.

39. Mr. Wilkins' ascites is primarily caused by which of the following situations?
① Increased production of albumin
② Portal hypertension
③ Increased production of ammonia
④ Blockage of the common bile duct

40. Nursing observations of a patient with severe liver dysfunction with accompanying jaundice would include which of the following?
① Dark stools, yellow sclera, and dark urine
② Clay stools, yellow sclera, and blood-tinged urine
③ Clay stools, pruritus, and dark urine
④ Dark stools, pruritus, and amber urine

41. A paracentesis is to be performed to reduce the discomfort related to ascites. What nursing actions would the nurse anticipate in assisting with the procedure?
① Place patient in right lateral position to facilitate drainage
② Record amount and color of fluid removed
③ Prepare the area by cleansing with warm, soapy water and drape with sterile towels
④ Assist with the application of a simple sterile dressing after the procedure

42. Thirty percent of all patients with cirrhosis develop esophageal varices. Early management is directed toward treatment of bleeding. Treatment includes which of the following?
① Gastric lavage with room-temperature saline solution
② Use of Sengstaken-Blakemore tube and iced saline lavages
③ Administration of vasodilators, antibiotics, and antacids
④ Administration of platelets and refrigerated blood

43. Hepatic coma is a complication associated with cirrhosis. Measures to prevent hepatic coma include which of the following?
① Eliminate carbohydrates from the diet
② Eliminate protein from the diet
③ Give soapy enemas
④ Perform iced saline lavages

Situation: Mr. Lopez, 72 years of age, was admitted to the hospital yesterday with a diagnosis of cerebrovascular accident (CVA). His medical history includes hypertension treated by a low-sodium diet and diuretics. He was well until earlier in the morning when he had a severe headache, gradually became confused, and exhibited weakness. On admission he was unable to move his right arm and leg, and could not speak. During the night he became unresponsive.

44. Nursing care for Mr. Lopez must include:
    1. Communication assuming patient understanding
    2. Minimal conversation by nurse or family
    3. Continual sensory stimulation during daytime hours
    4. A well-lighted room with frequent noisy activity

45. The need for suctioning must be evaluated frequently because:
    1. A clear oropharynx will help patient to eat
    2. The sputum suctioned can be observed and sent to the pathology laboratory
    3. Aspiration of secretions may cause pneumonia
    4. The chest pain will be lessened

46. The nurse changes Mr. Lopez's position q2h. A major concern is:
    1. Placing him flat to prevent headache
    2. Placing him on his side, facing the door, for better observation
    3. Keeping a pillow under his head to maintain his airway
    4. Keeping him on his side to prevent aspiration

47. A priority in Mr. Lopez's nursing care is:
    1. Administration of stool softeners to prevent constipation
    2. Passive exercises to prevent deformities
    3. Forcing fluids to prevent renal calculi
    4. Observing pupillary reaction to light

48. Mr. Lopez is not blinking. His eyes should be cleansed with saline solution and covered with an eye patch to prevent:
    1. Conjunctivitis
    2. Corneal ulcers
    3. Ptosis
    4. Tearing

49. Nursing care plans for a patient in a coma include prevention of:
    1. Injury and convulsions
    2. Anxiety and aspiration
    3. Incontinence and paralysis
    4. Contractures and decubitus ulcers

50. As Mr. Lopez begins to recover, he receives speech therapy. Before the patient is able to speak, he can communicate by:
    1. Using nonverbal communication
    2. Speaking slowly and enunciating carefully
    3. Only nodding for "yes" and "no"
    4. Writing down what he wants to communicate

51. If the physician had indicated that Mr. Lopez had receptive aphasia, the nurse would anticipate that:
    1. Mr. Lopez would not understand the nurse
    2. The nurse would not understand Mr. Lopez
    3. Mr. Lopez must write to communicate
    4. Communication is not possible with Mr. Lopez

52. When assessing lung sounds, the nurse should ask the patient to assume which of the following positions for best results?
    1. Supine, without pillow
    2. Lying on either side, arms raised
    3. Dangling or sitting in chair, leaning slightly forward, arms in front, and hands on knees
    4. Semi-Fowler's, with pillow

53. When assessing lung sounds, the nurse should instruct the patient to breathe:
    1. Slowly and deeply, with mouth open
    2. Rapidly, in a panting manner
    3. With mouth closed
    4. Normally, no special directions

54. What is the best method for obtaining a sputum specimen for culture and sensitivity?
    1. Ask the patient to expectorate into a dry, sterile container several times during the day
    2. After awakening the patient, ask him or her to take three deep breaths, and at the end of the third breath, to cough deeply, bringing up sputum for the specimen
    3. Immediately before the patient retires for the evening, ask him or her to expectorate into the specimen container
    4. Always use a suction catheter for best results

55. When administering care to a patient with epistaxis the nurse knows that the patient should be positioned:
    1. Sitting up, head tilted forward
    2. Sitting up, head tilted backward
    3. Flat in bed, head to one side
    4. Semi-Fowler's in bed

---

56. Mr. Isaac is in the first day of care following a laryngectomy for carcinoma of the larynx. The nurse's top priority of care is to:
    1. Maintain communication
    2. Allay anxiety
    3. Monitor character of secretions
    4. Maintain patent airway

57. Gradually, Mr. Isaac is able to assume most of his own care, including coughing up his sputum, occasionally suctioning himself. However, he is frustrated about not being able to speak and having to write so much. What is the nurse's best intervention?
    1. Refer the situation to the physician; perhaps Mr. Isaac needs antianxiety medication
    2. Spend more time with Mr. Isaac; anticipate his needs
    3. Be available and reassure Mr. Isaac that he will feel better when he goes home
    4. Arrange a visit with a person who has had a laryngectomy and speaks with esophageal speech

---

58. Mrs. Simonelli, age 83, has left lower lobe pneumonia. She is receiving oxygen at 2 L/min through nasal cannula to:
    1. Rectify impaired gas exchange
    2. Counteract her fatigue
    3. Augment destroying the bacteria causing the pneumonia
    4. Reduce crackles evident in left lung

59. Mrs. Simonelli says, "I'm so tired. I can hardly find the energy to eat, much less do anything like walk." The best nursing response is:
    ① "I can feed you your meal."
    ② "You'll feel better soon. Don't worry."
    ③ "You're tired because you've been in bed for a long time. It's time you got moving and built up your strength."
    ④ "You're tired because the pneumonia makes it difficult for your body to use oxygen. As the infection clears, you will feel stronger."

60. Mr. O'Hara has been hospitalized with chronic obstructive pulmonary disease. You have been helping to implement his teaching plan, which aims to avoid rehospitalization because of complications. Which statement by Mr. O'Hara indicates understanding of your teaching?
    ① "I smoked my last cigarette 2 weeks ago."
    ② "I'm not going to take this medication if it makes me a little jittery."
    ③ "I'll just take a couple of whiffs of this inhaler when I feel I need it."
    ④ "My wife moved my bed downstairs in front of the TV so I don't have to get up."

Situation: Ms. Ortega is a 19-year-old woman with a diagnosis of Type I (juvenile onset) diabetes mellitus. She is hospitalized for insulin management and associated teaching.

61. The nurse is aware that cardinal symptoms of diabetes mellitus include:
    ① Headache, hypertension, and hyperglycemia
    ② Polyuria, polydipsia, and polyphagia
    ③ Lethargy, slowed mental processes, and hypotension
    ④ Clammy skin, tremors, and polyuria

62. Ms. Ortega is receiving Humulin R by sliding scale. Glucometer readings show a blood sugar of 250 mg/dl. Ms. Ortega will receive 6 units of Humulin R. Following subcutaneous administration, the nurse should monitor for symptoms of hypoglycemia at the peak time of insulin, which occurs _____ hours after the injection?
    ① 2 to 3
    ② 4 to 6
    ③ 7 to 8
    ④ 9 to 10

63. Ms. Ortega is now being managed on a split dose of 70/30 isophane insulin suspension (NPH insulin) at 7:30 AM and 4:30 PM. At 2:30 PM one afternoon, she calls the nurses' station stating that she is not feeling well. On observation, Ms. Ortega's skin is cool and clammy, her hands are shaking, and she appears very apprehensive. The glucometer blood sugar is 45 mg/dl. The most appropriate nursing intervention for Ms. Ortega's current symptoms is to provide the patient with:
    ① Four ounces of fruit juice
    ② Twelve ounces of diet drink
    ③ A large candy bar
    ④ A cube of sugar

64. Should Ms. Ortega lose consciousness during a hypoglycemic reaction, before food or drink can be administered by mouth, a suitable alternative would include:
    ① Administering intravenous (IV) insulin
    ② Sitting her up and placing small amounts of a beverage in her mouth
    ③ Placing crushed crackers in her mouth and making her swallow
    ④ Placing prepared glucose concentrate between the cheek and the gum and allowing it to absorb

65. Mr. Goldberg has a urinary tract infection. Which of the following nursing interventions should be part of his care plan?
    ① Minimize strenuous activity
    ② Catheterize every 6 hours if patient can't void on his own
    ③ Force fluids to 3000 ml/day unless contraindicated
    ④ Administer analgesics for dysuria

66. Why is it important for the nurse to use sterile technique in obtaining a urine specimen for culture and sensitivity?
    ① To prevent patient from exposure to other microorganisms
    ② To protect the nurse from infection by the patient
    ③ To ensure the cleanest specimen
    ④ To allow for a more accurate diagnosis

67. Mr. Furtado has entered the hospital with a diagnosis of possible kidney stone. He is complaining of acute pain. What would be the best nursing intervention?
    ① Administer analgesics as ordered by the physician
    ② Reassure Mr. Furtado that the pain will subside as soon as the stone reaches the bladder
    ③ Strain all urine; look for sediment
    ④ Provide rest for the patient

68. Which nursing observation alerts caregivers to the possibility of impending renal failure?
    ① Hypotension
    ② Oliguria
    ③ Hematuria
    ④ Confusion

69. Mr. Medeiros has returned from surgery for transurethral prostatic resection (TURP). His urinary catheter is draining bloody urine with small clots. The nurse should:
    ① Report the drainage to the physician immediately
    ② Irrigate the catheter immediately
    ③ Clamp the catheter for 20 minutes
    ④ Monitor the catheter drainage frequently

70. What nursing observations are particularly important in reviewing Mr. Medeiros' progress toward recovery and discharge?
    ① Voiding pattern, color, and clarity of urine
    ② Ability to cooperate with nursing staff
    ③ Ability for performing self-care activities
    ④ Mr. Medeiros' insistence on continuing to smoke

Situation: Mr. Thompson, a 46-year-old truck driver, feels a sharp pain in the lumbar area while unloading a truck. The pain continues and does not respond to analgesics or rest at home. He is admitted to the hospital with a diagnosis of ruptured intervertebral disk.

71. On admission the nurse assesses Mr. Thompson for:
    1. Relief when walking
    2. Pain radiating down one leg
    3. Respiratory difficulty
    4. Bowel and bladder incontinence

72. Conservative therapy is attempted. Nursing care includes:
    1. Complete bed rest and warm compresses
    2. Passive range-of-motion exercise to legs
    3. Ambulation tid
    4. Semi-Fowler's position and pillows under knees

73. A spinal fusion was performed. On return from the recovery room Mr. Thompson must:
    1. Ambulate as soon as possible
    2. Be placed in high-Fowler's position
    3. Stand to void after 8 hours
    4. Be logrolled for as long as 4 to 6 weeks

74. Mr. Thompson has glaucoma, which was diagnosed 6 years ago. He is treated with pilocarpine eye drops. Early patient problems of glaucoma are:
    1. Moving spots, flashes of light, and loss of vision in specific areas
    2. Eye pain, tearing, and purulent exudate
    3. Halos seen around lights, blurred vision, and headache
    4. Loss of vision, cloudy appearance, and difficulty reading

75. A priority in Mr. Thompson's care relative to his glaucoma is:
    1. Keep side rails up at all times
    2. Administer eye drops on time
    3. Encourage measurement of intraocular pressure every 3 years
    4. Provide reading aids

Situation: Mrs. Thorne is a 32-year-old housewife and mother of three young children. She is admitted with a 4-year history of multiple sclerosis.

76. Planning care for Mrs. Thorne will be most strongly influenced by which of these assessment findings:
    1. Vital signs
    2. Most recent cardiogram
    3. Motor strength and coordination
    4. Progression of paralysis

77. The main goal of nursing care for Mrs. Thorne is to:
    1. Assist with activities of daily living
    2. Keep her as independent and active as possible for as long as possible
    3. Prevent secondary infection
    4. Teach and encourage her to eat foods that are low in fat and protein

78. When assessing Mrs. Thorne, the nurse is likely to note the following signs and symptoms:
    1. Abnormal reflexes, ataxia
    2. Oliguria, diarrhea
    3. Tinnitus, cerumen
    4. Memory loss, confusion

79. As the disease progresses, Mrs. Thorne will:
    1. Have a high intolerance to medication
    2. Require multiple drugs used simultaneously
    3. Endure long periods before the illness responds to a particular medication
    4. Experience spontaneous remissions from time to time

80. Mrs. Thorne eventually loses control of her bowels and requires bowel training. Which of the following measures is likely to be effective?
    1. Limiting fluid intake to 1000 ml in 24 hours
    2. Setting a regular time for elimination
    3. Eating a diet low in roughage
    4. Avoiding use of patient bathrooms

81. Mrs. Thorne sometimes exhibits signs and symptoms of emotional distress. Her family should be informed that disturbances frequently associated with patients with multiple sclerosis are:
    1. Mood disorders
    2. Thought disorders
    3. Psychosomatic illnesses
    4. Drug-dependency problems

---

82. Miss Gorman is a sexually active 23 year old with a diagnosis of condylomata (genital warts). As you implement her teaching plan, you would include all of the following information *except*:
    1. Examination of sexual partner is necessary to prevent reinfection
    2. Specimens must be taken for analysis to rule out concurrent STDs
    3. Treatment is necessary because genital warts may predispose patient to cervical cancer
    4. Other than a minor annoyance, genital warts are harmless

83. Mr. Levesque is a sexually active 23 year old with dysuria and a watery mucous discharge from the urethra; the diagnosis is chlamydia. What statement by Mr. Levesque indicates his understanding of the teaching plan?
    1. "I think I've taken this medication before."
    2. "I can't wait for spring break at Daytona Beach."
    3. "My girlfriend's fine. She doesn't have any symptoms like I did."
    4. "I'll bring in my girlfriend tomorrow for an exam."

84. The incidence of melanoma is increasing at a rate higher than most other malignancies. Which of the following is *not* appropriate in a teaching plan for prevention and early detection of this disease?
    1. Use sunscreens to prevent sunburn, especially in children
    2. Routinely inspect all moles for abnormalities
    3. Family history of this disease is insignificant
    4. Have suspicious moles removed by a physician

85. The nurse describes skin lesions as maculopapular with occasional vesicles. This means:
    1. Red pinpoint hemorrhages
    2. Extended reddened areas with pus-filled blisters
    3. Red depressions with large blisters
    4. Flat, raised, small red lesions with small fluid-filled sacs

86. When caring for a patient who is visually impaired and independent in his activities of daily living, a goal in the care plan to maintain independence will be:
    1. The patient will remain in his room for safety
    2. The patient will allow the nurse to administer the daily insulin injection
    3. The patient will perform all hygiene by himself
    4. The patient will master the interpretation of braille

87. When administering eyedrops to the patient with glaucoma, the nurse knows the indicated medication is a _____ that _____ .
    1. Mydriatic; dilates the pupil
    2. Miotic; constricts the pupil
    3. Diuretic; reduces intraocular fluid
    4. Lubricant; moistens the eye

88. When assessing pupils and their response to light, darken the room and observe pupil size _____ .
    1. Before the light shines on them
    2. As soon as the light shines on them
    3. Ten seconds after shining light on them
    4. As you wave the flashlight over the eyes

89. Which intervention is most appropriate in the care plan for a patient with mild hearing impairment of the right ear?
    1. Provide alternate means of communication
    2. Speak loudly and enunciate slowly
    3. Touch patient before speaking to get his or her attention
    4. Approach patient from the left, speaking normally

Situation: Mr. Rodriguez, age 42, is admitted to the hospital. He has been undergoing outpatient peritoneal dialysis three times a week for endstage renal disease secondary to hypertensive nephrosclerosis. He is hypertensive, weak, and anorexic. He is scheduled for hemodialysis.

90. Mr. Rodriguez is to collect a 24-hour urine specimen, 9 AM Monday to 9 AM Tuesday. The nurse should instruct him to:
    1. Discard the urine voided at 9 AM on Monday and begin the specimen after that
    2. Begin the collection with urine voided at 9 AM on Monday
    3. Discard the urine voided at 9 AM on Tuesday and consider the urine collection completed
    4. Save the urine voided at 9 AM Monday and the urine voided at 9 AM on Tuesday and all urine voided in between these times

91. The nurse should explain to Mr. Rodriguez that the major difference between hemodialysis and peritoneal dialysis is that in peritoneal dialysis:
    1. The time needed for treatment is shorter
    2. There is no exchange of blood
    3. There is no loss of protein
    4. There are immediate results

92. While assessing a patient receiving peritoneal dialysis, the nurse is aware of the signs and symptoms that indicate infection. One indicator would be:
    1. Bleeding
    2. Cloudy or discolored returned peritoneal fluid
    3. A change in blood pressure
    4. Distention in bladder

93. The nurse understands that patients with renal failure have a bleeding tendency and that precautions must be taken. One such precaution is:
    1. Using a hard-bristle toothbrush for oral hygiene
    2. Having him shave with an electric razor
    3. Giving antiemetics routinely
    4. Administering aspirin for pain or temperature elevation

94. Mr. Rodriguez is at risk for an infection. The best nursing action for preventing transmission of hospital-acquired infections is:
    1. Administration of large doses of antibiotics
    2. Strict isolation
    3. Routine administration of vitamin C
    4. Careful handwashing

Situation: Miss Helen Green is a 45-year-old woman who has a diagnosis of open-angle chronic glaucoma.

95. The nurse explains to Miss Green that the chief aim of medical treatment in chronic glaucoma is:
    1. Controlling intraocular pressure
    2. Dilating the pupil to allow for an increase in the visual field
    3. Allowing for healing process by resting the eye
    4. Preventing secondary infections that may add to the visual problem

96. When assessing Miss Green, the nurse will observe for which of the following symptoms?
    1. Loss of peripheral vision
    2. Sudden loss of vision in one eye
    3. Purulent drainage
    4. Loss of night vision

97. To understand the treatment prescribed for Miss Green, the nurse must know the basis of the disease. Chronic glaucoma is caused primarily by:
    1. Obstruction to the circulation of aqueous humor at the angle of the anterior chamber of the eye
    2. Changes in the opacity of the lens
    3. Separation of the outer pigment epithelium and inner sensory layers of the retina
    4. Trauma to the optic nerve

98. Regarding patient assessment, the subjective data most indicative of glaucoma are:
    1. Eye pain and halos around lights
    2. Diplopia and myopia
    3. Mild loss of central vision and nausea
    4. Mild blurred vision and difficulty perceiving changes in color

99. Miss Green will receive pharmacologic treatment, including a prescription for a:
    1. Corticosteroid
    2. Miotic
    3. Mydriatic
    4. Antibiotic

100. Miss Green should be instructed to always have the following with her:
    1. Sugar cubes and medication
    2. Dark glasses and medication
    3. Identification card and dark glasses
    4. Medication and a medical identification tag

101. Acetazolamide (Diamox) is a drug used in the treatment of glaucoma because it:
    1. Increases the outflow of aqueous humor
    2. Constricts the pupil
    3. Decreases the rate of production of aqueous humor
    4. Acts as an osmotic diuretic

Situation: Carl Hawthorne is a 60-year-old man with a history of osteoarthritis. He is overweight and leads a sedentary life-style. Lately, his left hip has been particularly painful. His pain increases on weight bearing, and he has limited range of motion (ROM) in the left hip joint.

102. During the initial assessment of Mr. Hawthorne, an important piece of information for the nurse to obtain in planning his care is:
    1. Use of alcohol and tobacco
    2. Hobbies and interests
    3. Use of a cane, walker, or crutches
    4. Food likes and dislikes

103. Large weight-bearing joints are frequently involved in osteoarthritis. Common characteristics of involved joints include:
    1. Tenderness and crepitus
    2. Bilateral inflammation and immobility
    3. Pain resulting from destruction of supportive structures
    4. Fluid within the joint along with inflammatory tissue changes

104. An aim of disease management is control of symptoms. To help control joint strain, the nurse should teach Mr. Hawthorne the importance of:
    1. Exercising the involved joint
    2. Taking medication at the first sign of pain
    3. Applying intermittent heat application
    4. Weight reduction and maintenance

105. In severe cases of degenerative joint disease, a treatment that would facilitate pain reduction and improve joint function is:
    1. Arthrodesis
    2. Laparoscopy
    3. Arthroscopy
    4. Arthroplasty

106. After the patient has joint arthroplasty, the nurse is vigilant in monitoring for complications. In the immediate postoperative phase, which of the following assessments must be reported immediately?
    1. Nausea
    2. Neurocirculatory compromise
    3. Infiltration of intravenous fluids
    4. Inability to cough productively

Situation: Miss Farley, age 67, is admitted with a preliminary diagnosis of transient ischemic attack.

107. In assisting Miss Farley with daily care, the nurse must be especially observant for:
    1. Auras preceding seizures
    2. Decreasing visual fields
    3. Complaints of headache
    4. Any loss of motor or sensory function

108. When preparing Miss Farley for a CT scan without contrast medium, the nurse knows that:
    1. No special preparation is required
    2. All caffeine is withheld
    3. The patient must remain NPO for 6 to 8 hours before the test
    4. The patient must drink an opaque liquid

109. In which position should the nurse place a patient with increased intracranial pressure?
    1. Fowler's
    2. Head elevated 15 degrees to 30 degrees
    3. Side lying
    4. Flat, supine

110. To teach Miss Farley about her medications, the nurse must be familiar with which of the following medication regimens for transient ischemic attack (TIA)?
    1. Anticoagulants and aspirin
    2. Analgesics and corticosteroids
    3. Muscle relaxants and antihypertensives
    4. Vasodilators and antilipidemics

Situation: Bobby Garcia is a 19-year-old college student who is admitted to the hospital after having had recurring seizures. He sustained head injuries in a car accident several years ago. Bobby's seizure pattern suggests primary epilepsy.

111. Bobby states that he sees flashing lights just before the onset of a seizure. This phenomenon is known as:
    1. Aura
    2. Tetany
    3. Asterixis
    4. Anhidrosis

112. Bobby is out of bed, talking to his nurse, when he suddenly begins to have a seizure. To protect him from injury, the nurse might consider all of the following *except:*
    1. Restraining his movements
    2. Remaining with him during the episode
    3. Supporting his head if needed with a small pillow
    4. Inserting a seizure stick between the back teeth if the jaw is not clenched

113. Which is a commonly used medication to control grand mal seizures?
    1. Levothyroxine sodium (Synthroid)
    2. Phenytoin (Dilantin)
    3. Mannitol
    4. Prednisone

114. Bobby wants to know how long he must take his prescribed medication. The best reply by the nurse is:
    1. "Until you are discharged from the hospital."
    2. "Probably for the rest of your life."
    3. "If you are seizure free for 1 year, then your medicine can be stopped."
    4. "Until you can learn to avoid stressful situations."

115. The nurse caring for Bobby knows that oral care is essential when on long-term phenytoin (Dilantin) therapy because of:
    1. Formation of dental caries
    2. Gingival hypertrophy
    3. Eroding of the tooth enamel
    4. The possibility of xerostomia

Situation: Mr. Knight, 68 years of age, is admitted to the medical center. He has difficulty voiding and now has abdominal discomfort and is distended. His diagnosis is benign prostatic hypertrophy (BPH).

116. Mr. Knight appears fatigued. He tells you he woke up three times during the night. He states, "I feel I won't be able to get to the bathroom fast enough; then I can't begin to pass my urine. I have to wait." Your nurse's notes would state:
    ① Enuresis, dysuria, and oliguria
    ② Frequency, dribbling, and suppression
    ④ Polyuria, distention, and retention
    ④ Nocturia, hesitancy, and urgency

117. While reviewing Mr. Knight's chart, you note that the blood urea nitrogen (BUN) has increased greatly to 94 mg. You know that the normal range is 10 to 20 mg. The nursing care plan will include:
    ① Measures to prevent edema
    ② Measures to promote safety
    ③ Methods to force fluids
    ④ Thorough perineal care

118. After an intravenous pyelogram (IVP) the nurse observes for:
    ① Allergic reactions
    ② Urinary tract infection
    ③ Nausea and vomiting
    ④ Hematuria

119. Mr. Knight also has a diagnosis of cystitis. Nursing care for a patient with cystitis will usually include:
    ① Restricting fluids
    ② Monitoring fluids
    ③ Forcing fluids
    ④ Administering intravenous (IV) fluids

120. Mr. Knight was unable to void. An indwelling catheter was passed and:
    ① Connected to continuous bladder irrigation
    ② Removed when the bladder was empty
    ③ Urine specimens were taken for culture
    ④ Clamped and released qh for removal of 100 ml of urine

CHAPTER 7

Mental Health Nursing

The licensed practical/vocational nurse (LP/VN) requires a knowledge of mental health nursing principles in a variety of practice settings. Basic mental health concepts are useful in understanding the response to diseases and dysfunctions of both physical and social systems. Each person responds to disease and disorder in accordance with his or her own basic personality traits, past experiences, intelligence, and innate coping mechanisms. These concepts are explored and studied in mental health nursing.

HOLISM

A. Definition: a concept of health—holds that illness results from a complex interaction between the mind and body and the internal and external alterations that disturb the natural balance
B. Approaches to treatment: multifaceted approaches are used to treat disturbances, rather than simply relying on treatments aimed at specific symptoms; these approaches include the following dimensions
   1. Physical
   2. Psychologic
   3. Cultural
   4. Socioeconomic

MENTAL HEALTH CONTINUUM

A. Mental health and mental illness are seen as opposite poles on a continuum
B. The precise point at which an individual is deemed mentally ill is determined not only by the specific behavior exhibited but also by the context in which the behavior is seen
C. Some behaviors considered deviant in one setting are considered normal in another setting
D. Variations are based on the culture, the time or era, the specific personal characteristics of the individual, and many other variables
E. Behaviors of the mentally ill are exaggerations of normal human behaviors

MENTAL HEALTH

A. Definition: an individual's ability to manage life's problems and to derive satisfaction from living throughout various life stages
B. Persons may experience times of greater or lesser satisfaction with life and at times of lesser satisfaction, may seek the assistance of a therapist
C. No clear set of characteristics specific to mental health can be identified
   1. All behavior is considered meaningful and may be interpreted as the individual's effort to adapt or cope with the environment

2. At times some adaptations fail; others are continued long after the need for them has passed; still others may be directed to an undesired end

MENTAL ILLNESS

A. Definition: a pattern of behavior that is disturbing to the individual or to the community in which the individual resides
   1. The person who is mentally ill acts in ways that seem unrelated to the current reality
   2. Relationships with family and friends are disturbed
   3. The person's ability to work and to contribute to his or her own welfare may be impaired
   4. The person often experiences subjective discomfort
   5. The person may exhibit symptoms such as hallucinations or delusions
B. Historical perspective of mental illness
   1. Early history
      a. Mentally ill persons were thought to be possessed by supernatural forces
      b. Mentally ill persons were ostracized from society or mistreated in other ways
      c. Mentally ill persons were regarded as messengers of the gods or as divinely possessed
      d. Attitudes did not change significantly until the modern era
   2. Classical era (Greco-Roman)
      a. Certain attitudes changed toward mental illness
      b. Early scientific interest led to various descriptive or classification systems
      c. The idea of divine possession was rejected in favor of the concept of humors
      d. Humors were thought to be basic internal fluids capable of controlling behavior
      e. The terms melancholia and hysteria are derived from these ancient beliefs
   3. The Middle Ages
      a. Return to the idea of divine possession and spiritual explanations of mental illness
      b. The mentally ill person was often mistreated by incarceration

Historic Highlights

Eighteenth century

Phillipe Pinel (1745-1826, France): freed mentally ill persons from chains

Benjamin Rush (1746-1813, United States): founded Pennsylvania Hospital; the Father of American Psychiatry

Nineteenth century

Florence Nightingale (1860, England): founder of modern nursing

Dorthea Dix (1802-1887, United States): promoted legislation to establish mental hospitals

Linda Richards (1873, United States): first psychiatric nurse

Daniel Tuke (1827-1895, England): founded York Retreat based on Quaker principles

Twentieth century

Clifford Beers (1876-1943, United States): wrote the book, *The Mind that Found Itself*, generating public concern for the treatment of mentally ill persons

Adolf Meyer (1866-1950, United States): Director of the Johns Hopkins Clinic; founder of the mental hygiene movement

Emil Kraepelin (1856-1926, Germany): classified mental disorders

Eugene Bleuler (1857-1939, Switzerland): coined the word *schizophrenia* and classified it into types

Sigmund Freud (1856-1939, Austria): developed psychoanalytic theory; revolutionized psychiatry

Carl Jung (1875-1961, Switzerland): developed a personality theory that included the concepts of introversion and extroversion

Karen Horney (1885-1952, United States): theorized that culture had a great influence on mental illness

4. Modern era: numerous reforms were instituted (see the box above)
5. Later modern developments include
   a. Discovery of tranquilizing drugs: late 1950s
   b. Community mental health: 1960s; still in use today; aim is to provide care of mentally ill persons in their own communities rather than in large institutions: a primary goal of the community mental health concept is to return patients to their homes as quickly as possible and to foster the development of support systems in the community
   c. Patients released from large hospitals: late 1970s; large numbers of mentally ill persons were released into communities where they often did not receive treatment either because they did not seek it out or because adequate types of services were not available; this process is called deinstitutionalization; some believe that there is an increase of "street people" as a result of the process

THE NURSING ROLE

A. The nursing process
   1. Assessment: in assessing the mentally ill patient, the nurse must seek data in the following areas

   a. Physical appearance: posture, skin color, scars, abrasions, rashes, facial expression, dress and grooming, smoking, alcohol on breath, other evidence of drug use, apparent developmental level and age, height, and weight; question allergies, diet, sleep, elimination, previous illnesses, and impairments
   b. Psychologic state (mental state): alertness; orientation to time, place, and person; stated feelings (glad, sad, mad, scared); intellect; speech pattern (slow, loose, hesitant, pressured); potential for harm to self or others
   c. Relationships; married, single, living with whom, siblings, children, child care arrangements, parents, other care takers
   d. Sociocultural: race, religion, national origin, type of work, social activity, hobbies, education level
2. Diagnosing: nurses diagnose and treat human responses to illness; the nursing diagnosis is formulated by the registered professional nurse; the LP/VN contributes by recognizing and assisting with the collection of patient data. Sample nursing diagnoses used in mental health nursing include the following
   a. Use of disordered communication related to fear of intimate human contact
   b. Avoidance of heterosexual relationships related to sexual ambivalence
   c. Panic attacks, related to threat of abandonment, as manifested by dizziness, tremulousness, dyspnea, and sweating
   d. Feigned psychotic behavior related to preference for hospitalization over incarceration
   e. Negative self-concept related to overly high ego ideal
3. Planning: the plan of care is based on observations in the initial assessment; specific nursing interventions are devised to attain specifically stated goals; when possible, goals should be developed jointly with the patient and cooperation enlisted; goals may be short term or long term; all goals should be prioritized, emphasizing those that eliminate hazards to the patient or others in the environment; goals usually include the anticipated length of time for accomplishment and the standard for judging whether the goal has been met
4. Implementation: the specific treatment of the patient (psychotherapy or counseling), health teaching, activities of daily living, other prescribed treatments, and medications; this is an ongoing phase, and reactions to treatment are observed so that the care plan may be modified periodically as goals are met
5. Evaluation: usually done informally (formal evaluation is usually conducted by a designated committee) and determines how well each care plan is working; patients and their families may be involved in the process; this phase is also used to identify new problems, which are then included in the care plan

B. Principles of mental health nursing
   1. Understand your inner needs, thoughts, and feelings and be aware of how these affect patients
   2. Be aware of your own resources and limitations to function effectively in mental health nursing

3. Respect the patient as a person; take time to listen to what is said
4. Be aware of the patient's dignity; show patience and understanding
5. Be nonjudgmental and nonthreatening; patients must be accepted as they are
6. Be honest
7. Reassure patients by being available and allaying fears
8. Explain routine, rules, and regulations when appropriate
9. Maintain a calm, hopeful attitude
10. Encourage reality testing and avoid entering into patient's unrealistic thinking
11. Emphasize strengths that the patient displays by praising healthy behavior; offer warm understanding but do not encourage overdependency or intimacy
12. Remember that all staff members are role models and are often viewed as authority figures by patients
13. Help reduce anxiety by making as few demands as possible on patients
14. Explain what is happening to the patient in simple, understandable language
15. Remain objective but do not display aloofness or distance; maintain your awareness of the patient's humanity and dignity
16. Maintain a nurse/patient relationship that is always realistic and professional
17. Remember that there is a reason for all behavior
18. Note that behavior is changed through emotional experience rather than through rational means
19. Allow patients to exercise all of their basic human rights
20. Use the least restrictive method(s) of controlling behavior, such as communication
21. Respect the confidentiality of the patient

C. Communications in mental health nursing
   1. Communication: a complex activity consisting of a series of events, each interdependent on the other, which results in a negotiated understanding between two or more people in a given situation
      a. Communication is not merely the exchange of information
      b. Each message (input) generates an extremely complex reaction that eventually leads to a selective response (output), which in turn becomes a new input for the communicators
   2. Modes of communication
      a. The most apparent form is verbal (written or spoken language); spoken is the more important in mental health nursing
      b. Spoken communication is always accompanied by at least one of the following additional communication forms
         (1) Paralanguage: voice quality, tones, grunts, and other nonword vocalizations
         (2) Kinesis: facial expression, gestures, and eye and body movements
         (3) Proxemics: the spatial relationship between persons
         (4) Touch and messages to other sensory organs: aromas and cultural artifacts (jewelry, clothing, hair style)

   c. Effective communications are
      (1) Efficient: messages are simple, clear, and timed correctly
      (2) Appropriate: relevant to the situation
      (3) Flexible: open to alteration based on perceived response
      (4) Receptive: allow feedback (checking and correcting by either or both parties)
3. Therapeutic communication in mental health nursing involves
   a. Listening: deliberate use of nonverbal communication to indicate attention
   b. Silence: adds importance to the other person's communication and allows time to formulate responses
   c. Reflection: encourages continuation of the previous communication; for example, patient states, "I feel sad." Nurse responds, "You feel sad?"
   d. Encouraging comments: for example, "Go on."
   e. Open-ended statements: e.g., "Say more . . . "
   f. Questioning: may block communication and should be used carefully
   g. Accepting: permitting patient to speak freely without fear of judgment, threats, or put-downs
   h. Giving recognition: calling by name, responding nonverbally such as leaning forward, nodding, and so on
   i. Placing events in sequence: helps patient to sort out confusing ideas
   j. Making observations: for example, "You look sad as you say that."
   k. Encouraging comparison: for example, "Was that how you were treated as a child?"
   l. Restating: rearranging the patient's words to gain greater understanding
   m. Focusing: helping patient to keep to the subject
   n. Exploring: helping to make logical connections
   o. Giving information: concrete information, not advice
   p. Seeking clarification: for example, "Do you mean . . . ?"
   q. Presenting reality: for example, "I know you believe that, but . . . "
   r. Attempting to translate feelings: for example, "Are you feeling angry?"
   s. Summarizing: concisely stating the overall meaning of the conversation

NOTE: The nurse should always try to identify the underlying feelings associated with behavior (anger, fear, etc.) by using these therapeutic communication techniques.
4. Blocks to communication
   a. Excessive questioning or probing
   b. Using cliches that minimize patient's individuality
   c. Giving advice
   d. Avoiding emotionally charged topics (changing the subject)
   e. Missing important clues: verbal or nonverbal
   f. Rejecting: any open rejection will block communication
   g. Agreeing or disagreeing: adding your values about what is being said

h. Testing, challenging: for example, "How could you prove that..."

i. Defending: logically arguing your position

j. Requesting explanations: patients usually do not have reasons for their behavior; reasons are not useful in their understanding of their behaviors

D. Nurse-patient relationship

1. A one-to-one relationship between the nurse and a patient with a therapeutic goal or projected outcome

2. The goal or outcome is based on the relief of symptoms or modification of the patient's behavior

3. The relationship comprises three phases

a. Orientation: initial mutual expectations are outlined

b. Working phase: the nurse and the patient work toward agreed-on goal (e.g., activities of daily living)

c. Termination phase: the nurse and patient end the relationship in a satisfactory manner

E. Applications of mental health nursing

1. Community mental health center

2. Partial hospitalization setting: day or night hospitals

3. Mental health clinic

4. Liaison: use of mental health workers in general hospital setting

5. Alcohol and drug-abuse facilities and clinics

6. Inpatient units

PERSONALITY DEVELOPMENT

A. Definition: a consistent set of behaviors peculiar to a specific individual; the sum of thoughts, feelings, physical characteristics, and sociocultural biases on which all behavior is built

B. Heredity

1. Personality is influenced by inherited characteristics, both physical and psychologic

2. Controversy exists over the extent of genetic influence on specific human behaviors

C. Environment

1. The environment is a strong determining factor in the individual's development

2. Environment includes the intrauterine environment as well as all the external factors that influence the individual after birth

D. Physical basis: personality develops normally if the necessary physical basis is present

1. The brain is the major organ of thought and is necessary to development of personality

2. Other influential factors include a normally functioning endocrine system, which strongly influences behavior

E. Major theorists (Table 7-1)

F. Elements of personality

1. Levels of consciousness

a. The unconscious: always outside the awareness of the individual; influences actions in ways the individual may not understand; thought to include dreams

b. The preconscious: usually outside awareness; available to conscious mind in special circumstances such as under hypnosis or during therapy

c. The conscious: ordinary awareness

2. Structures: some theorists refer to personality structures

a. Freud: ego, id, superego

b. Berne: child, adult, parent

3. Functions: each structure is thought to perform specific functions

a. Id/child: basic, innate psychic energy; emotional

b. Ego/adult: mediates between person's perception and objective reality; always rational

c. Superego/parent: incorporates societal values; judgmental and critical

G. Developmental levels: various theorists describe levels of development

1. Freud: oral, anal, phallic, latency, genital

2. Erikson: basic trust vs. mistrust: autonomy vs. shame and doubt; initiative vs. guilt; industry vs. inferiority; identity vs. role diffusion; intimacy vs. isolation; generativity vs. stagnation; ego integrity vs. despair

H. Development of the self-concept

1. A family provides the basis of self-concept by offering

a. Feelings of adequacy or inadequacy

b. Feelings of acceptance or rejection

c. Opportunities for identification

d. Expectations of values, goals, and behaviors

2. Self-concept consists of

a. Body image: one's perception of one's body

b. Self-ideal: one's idea of what is "good" behavior

c. Self-esteem: personal judgment of one's own worth

d. Role: one's perception of how one fits into the society

e. Identity: the combination of all of the above into a unified whole

ADJUSTMENT MECHANISMS

Adjustment mechanisms are basic psychologic tools that individuals use at various times to manage life's crises. They may also be referred to as ego defenses, defense mechanisms, or protective mechanisms. As such, they defend the ego or self from untoward anxiety, help resolve conflicts, and return the individual to a point of psychologic homeostasis or comfort. They are usually outside conscious awareness and are not considered pathologic in and of themselves. They should not be removed or challenged until the individual is ready and has adequate strength to tolerate the stressful situation.

A. Common defenses

1. Repression (dissociation): feelings that are painful or unacceptable are unconsciously blocked from awareness; for example, painful events of childhood are not remembered

2. Suppression: similar to repression but on a conscious level; for example, painful thoughts or feelings are pushed out of the mind

3. Reaction formation: uses repression, in part, to dispose of unacceptable feelings while consciously expressing the opposite feeling; for example, being overly nice to someone you really dislike

4. Projection: assigning unacceptable feelings or acts to others; for example, a woman who wants to cheat on her husband accuses him of cheating on her

5. Rationalization: explaining away unacceptable thoughts, feelings, or acts by logical construction; e.g., a man who isn't hired for a job finds numerous reasons why the job wasn't very good anyway

Table 7-1. A comparison of the development stages postulated by Freud, Sullivan, Erickson, and Piaget

Freud	Sullivan	Erikson	Piaget

I) Oral stage (0-18 mo)
a) The mouth is a source of satisfaction
b) Two phases
  1) Passive
    Only interests are satisfying hunger and *sucking.*
    Completely helpless, *security* is the greatest need.
    Narcissistic and egocentric, operates on *pleasure principle.*
    Omnipotent feelings are prevalent
  2) Active
    Biting is a mode of pleasure.
    Continuous experimentation and associations.
    Sensory discriminations.
    Differentiation between mental images and reality.
    Differentiation of others and discovery of self
	I) Infancy (0-18 mo)
	a) The mouth is a source of satisfaction
	b) Mouth—takes in (sucking), cuts off (biting), and pushes out (spitting) objects introduced by others
	c) Crying, babbling, and cooing are modes of communication used by the infant to call attention of adults to self
	d) *Satisfaction response (pleasure principle).* Infant's biologic needs are met and a mutual feeling of comfort and fulfillment is experienced by mother and infant. (Mother gives and infant takes)
	e) *Empathic observation.* Capacity to perceive feelings of others as his or her own immediate feelings in the situation
	f) *Autistic invention.* State of symbolic activity in which the infant feels he or she is master of all he or she surveys
	g) Experimentation, exploration, and manipulation are methods used to acquaint self with environment
		I) Oral-sensory stage (0-12 mo)
		a) The mouth is a source of satisfaction and a means of dealing with anxiety-producing situations
		b) Focus is on the development of the basic attitudes of *trust* vs. *mistrust*
		c) Attitudes are formed through mother's reaction to infant needs
			I) Sensorimotor stage (0-12 mo)
			a) Emphasis is on preverbal intellectual development
			b) Learns relationships with external objects
			c) Focus is on physical development with gradual increase in ability to think and use language

II) Anal stage (1½-3 yr) a) Primary activity is on learning muscular control association with urination and defecation *(toilet training period)* b) Exhibits more self-control; walks, talks, dresses, and undresses c) *Negativism*—assertion of independence d) Introduction of *reality principle,* ego development e) Superego begins to develop f) Engages in *parallel* play	II) Childhood (1½-6 yr) a) Begins with the capacity for communicating through speech and ends with a beginning need for association with peers b) Uses language as a tool to communicate wishes and needs c) Anus is power tool used to give or withhold a part of self to control significant people in his environment d) Emergence and integration of *self-concept* and *reflected appraisal* of *significant persons* e) Awareness that postponing or delaying gratification of own wishes may bring satisfaction f) Begins to find limits in experimentation, exploration, and manipulation g) More aggressive h) Uses parallel play and curiosity to explore environment i) Uses exhibitionism and mastubatory activity to become acquainted with self and others j) Demonstrates a beginning ability to think abstractly	II) Anal-muscular stage (1-3 yr) a) Learns the extent to which the *environment* can be influenced by direct manipulation b) Focuses on the development of the basic attitudes of *autonomy* vs. *shame and doubt* c) Exerts self-control and will power	II) Preoperational stage (2-7 yr) a) Learns to use symbols and language b) Learns to imitate and play c) Displays egocentricity d) Engages in *animistic thinking*—endowment of objects with power and ability

Table 7-1. A comparison of the development stages postulated by Freud, Sullivan, Erickson, and Piaget—cont'd

Freud	Sullivan	Erikson	Piaget

III) Phallic stage (3-6 yr)
  a) *Libidinal energy* focus on the genitals
  b) Learns *sexual identity*
  c) *Superego* becomes internalized
  d) Sibling rivalry and manipulation of parents occurs
  e) Intellectual and motor facilities are refined
  f) Increased socialization and *associative play*
		III) Genital-locomotor stage (3-6 yr)
		  a) Learns the extent to which being *assertive* will influence the environment
		  b) Focus is on the development of the *basic attitudes* of *initiative* vs. *guilt*
		  c) Explores the world with senses, thoughts and imagination
		  d) Activities demonstrate direction and purpose
		  e) Engages in first real social contacts through *cooperative play*
		  f) Develops conscience	

IV) Latency (6-12 yr)
  a) *Quiet* stage in which sexual development lies dormant, emotional tension eases
  b) *Normal homosexual phase* For boys, gangs For girls, cliques
  c) Increased intellectual capacity
  d) Starts school
  e) Identifies with teachers and peers
  f) Weakening of home ties
  g) Recognizes authority figures outside home, age of *hero worship*
	III) Juvenile stage (6-9 yr)
	  a) Learns to form satisfactory relationship with peers
	  b) *Peer norms* prevail over family norms
	  c) Engages in *competition,* experimentation, exploration, and manipulation
	  d) Able to cooperate and compromise
	  e) Demonstrates capacity to love
	  f) Distinguishes fantasy from reality
	  g) Exerts internal control over behavior
	IV) Preadolescence (9-12 yr)
	  a) Learns to relate to a friend of the same sex—*chum relationship*
	  b) Concerned with group success and derives satisfaction from group accomplishment
	  c) Shows signs of *rebellion*—restlessness, hostility, irritability
	  d) Assumes less responsibility for own actions
	  e) Moves from egocentricity to a more full social state
	  f) Uses experimentation, exploration, manipulation
	  g) Seeks *consensual validation* from peers
		IV) Latency (6-12 yr)
		  a) Learns to use energy to create, develop and manipulate
		  b) Focus is on the development of basic attitudes of *industry* vs. *inferiority*
		  c) Able to initiate and complete tasks
		  d) Understands rules and regulations
		  e) Displays competence and productivity
			III) Concrete operations stage (7-11 yr)
			  a) Deals with visible concrete objects and relationships
			  b) Increased intellectual and conceptual development—uses logic and reasoning
			  c) More socialized and rule conscious

V) Genital stage (12 yr—early adulthood)
  a) Appearance of secondary sex characteristics, reawakening of sex drives
  b) Increased concern over physical appearance
  c) Strives toward independence
  d) Development of sexual maturity
  e) Identity crisis
  f) Identification of love object of opposite sex
  g) Intellectual maturity
  h) Plans future
	V) Early adolescence (12-14 yr)
	  a) Experience physiologic changes
	  b) Uses rebellion to gain independence
	  c) Fantasizes, overidentifies with heroes
	  d) Discovers and begins relationships with opposite sex
	  e) Demonstrates heightened levels of anxiety in most interpersonal relationships
		V) Puberty and adolescence (12-18 yr)
		  a) Demonstrates an ability to integrate life experiences
		  b) Focus is on the development of the basic attitudes of *identity* vs. *role diffusion*
		  c) Seeks partner of the opposite sex
		  d) Begins to establish identity and place in society
			IV) Formal operations stage (11-15 yr)
			  a) Develops true abstract thought
			  b) Formulates hypothesis and applies logical tests
			  c) Conceptual independence

Continued.

Table 7-1. A comparison of the development stages postulated by Freud, Sullivan, Erickson, and Piaget—cont'd

Freud	Sullivan	Erikson	Piaget

	VI) Late adolescence (14-21 yr)
	  a) Establishes an enduring intimate relationship with one member of the opposite sex
	  b) Self-concept becomes stabilized
	  c) Attains physical maturity
	  d) Develops ability to use logic and abstract concepts
	VII) Adulthood (21 yr and older)
	  a) Assumes responsibility relevant to station in life
	  b) Maintains balance and involvement between self, family, and community
	  c) Further develops creativity
	  d) Reaffirms values in life
		VI) Young adulthood (18-25 yr)
		  a) Primarily concerned with developing an intimate relationship with another adult
		  b) Focus is on the development of the basic attitudes of *intimacy and solidarity* vs. *isolation*
		VII) Adulthood (25-45 yr)
		  a) Primarily concerned with establishing and maintaining a family
		  b) Focus is on the development of the basic attitudes of *generativity* vs. *stagnation*
		  c) Displays a marked degree of creativity
		  d) Adjusts to circumstances of middle age
		  e) Reevaluates life's accomplishments and goals
		VIII) Maturity (older than 45 yr)
		  a) Acceptance of lifestyle as meaningful and fulfilling
		  b) Focus is on the development of basic attitudes of *ego integrity* vs. *despair*
		  c) Remains optimistic and continues to grow
		  d) Adjusts to limitations
		  e) Adjusts to retirement
		  f) Adjusts to reorganized family patterns
		  g) Adjusts to losses
		  h) Accepts death with serenity	

Modified from Kreigh H, Perko J: *Psychiatric and mental health nursing: commitment to care and concern,* Reston, 1979, Reston Publishing, pp 126-133.

6. Displacement: use of more socially acceptable substitutes for the expression of feelings; for example, a man yells at his wife when he is angry at his boss

7. Sublimation: more socially acceptable behavior is substituted for an unacceptable drive or wish; for example, a man who wishes to gamble becomes a charity organizer for "casino nights" at his church

8. Identification: unconsciously assuming the characteristics of another person; for example, a little boy plays at shaving like his father

9. Conversion (conversion reaction): unconscious expression of psychologic problems by converting them to specific physical symptoms; for example, a person becomes deaf after hearing bad news; this is not the same as psychosomatic illness, which is discussed elsewhere

10. Regression: returning to an earlier mode of behavior that is more comfortable to avoid current pain; for example, a toilet-trained child begins bed-wetting after the birth of a new sibling

11. Fantasy: the use of wishful imagination when real satisfaction is unavailable; for example, daydreaming about finishing a school program

12. Intellectualization: use of thinking or logic to avoid feelings; for example, a woman scheduled for hysterectomy studies the anatomy in detail but avoids all expression of feelings

13. Introjection: complete acceptance of another's values as one's own; for example, a teenage gang member accepts the values of the gang leader

B. Emotions: basic feelings that occur within the individual
   1. Happiness

2. Anger
3. Sadness
4. Fear

C. Thoughts: rational processes that occur within the individual; thoughts occur continuously as the individual processes sensory data and internal responses (including emotional responses) and correlates these with past experiences and possible future actions

ALTERNATIVE LIFE-STYLES

Today there are numerous modes of living that are not considered pathologic. Most mental health workers do not consider nonmarital living arrangements, homosexuality, or other differences as problems needing therapy. In general, unless there is specific symptomatology, these differences are not treated. Homosexuality was once considered a diagnosis but has been removed from that category in recent years.

HUMAN SEXUALITY

People have sexual needs throughout their lives. Sexuality is basic to human happiness and often is the cause of many problems. "Normal" sexuality varies with the time, place, and cultural setting. Minor sexual dysfunction is amenable to short-term, often behavioristic approaches, whereas sexual deviation requires intensive treatment.

A. Minor dysfunctions include premature ejaculation in men and lack of orgasm in women
B. Deviations include rape and child molestation, both of which are primarily acts of violence rather than sexual in nature; in these cases both the victim and the perpetrator require intensive therapy

MENTAL DISTURBANCES AND RESOURCES

Anxiety

A. Definition: a state of alertness or apprehension, tension or uneasiness; a major component of all mental disturbances. Anxiety is an internal state experienced by the individual when there is a perceived threat to the physical body or to the psychologic integrity of the person. It interferes with concentration, focusing attention on the perceived threat. In its mild form anxiety serves to alert the person to danger and to prepare the body to react to danger; in its severe form it is debilitating and may immobilize the person and interfere with activities. Anxiety is usually described in degrees or levels.

B. Degrees of anxiety
   1. Alertness level: awareness of danger; ready for action
   2. Apprehension level: individual feels uncomfortable and prepares to face imminent danger
   3. Free-floating: generalized sensation of discomfort; a feeling of impending danger or disaster
   4. Panic level: a total uncontrolled response dominates perceptions and distorts reality; great discomfort

C. Signs of anxiety
   1. Vocal changes
   2. Restlessness
   3. Rapid speech
   4. Fatigue
   5. Palpitations
   6. Perspiration
   7. Nausea
   8. Frequent urination
   9. Diarrhea
   10. Vomiting (occasionally)

Motivation

Motivation is the gathering of personal resources to perform a task or reach a goal; may be derived from perceived reward or perceived threat of punishment; important in treating mental disturbances.

Frustration

Anything that interferes with goal-directed activity results in frustration. Frustration is commonplace in a complex society, and it is necessary to understand the individual's response to it. Some people adapt better than others. When adaptation fails, their anxiety, use of defense mechanisms, and hostility may increase.

Stress

Hans Selye (1956) defined stress as "wear and tear on the body." All people are continuously exposed to varieties of stress: physical, chemical, psychologic, and emotional. Almost any situation, pleasant or unpleasant, that requires change leads to some level of stress. Stress produces a clearly identifiable response called the general adaptation syndrome. It is associated with concomitant physical and chemical changes that commonly occur in the body.

Conflict

Like frustration, conflict is commonplace in a complex society. Everyone experiences conflict when two drives are present at the same time; for example, the wish to sleep and the wish to finish homework. Conflicts of this nature are usually resolved easily; more complicated conflicts, particularly emotional conflicts, may increase anxiety and over time cause the development of pathologic strategies to reduce anxiety and frustration or to resolve the conflict.

Special Terms

A. Hallucination: a sensation without an external stimulus; may be:
   1. Auditory
   2. Olfactory
   3. Visual
   4. Tactile
   5. Gustatory

B. Delusion: a false belief, not based on fact, that cannot be changed by reasoning
   1. Delusions of grandeur: feeling of greatness
   2. Delusions of persecution: feelings of being mistreated
   3. Delusions of sin or guilt: feelings of deserving punishment
   4. Flight of ideas: extreme distractibility
   5. Anxiety: see above
   6. Depression: feeling of dejection or hopelessness

Thought Disorders

Schizophrenia is considered the psychiatric manifestation of thought disorder; this group of illnesses represents the largest number of mentally ill persons.

A. Types of schizophrenia
1. Disorganized: includes frequent incoherence, non-systematized delusions, and inappropriate affect
2. Catatonic: includes stupor, negativity, rigidity, excitement, and posturing
3. Paranoid: includes persecutory delusions, grandiosity, delusional jealousy, and hallucinations
4. Undifferentiated: does not fit criteria of other categories or combines them
5. Residual: presence of residual symptoms (e.g., marked social isolation, inappropriate affect, odd beliefs) without delusions, hallucinations, or gross disorganization
B. Characteristics during the acute phase
1. Delusions of being controlled
2. Somatic delusions (grandiosity, religious, or nihilistic)
3. Persecutory delusions accompanied by hallucination
4. Auditory hallucinations of a running commentary on behavior or thought
5. Auditory hallucination on several occasions with content of more than one word
6. Incoherence, looseness of association, illogical thinking with a deterioration in function
7. Continuation of symptoms for 6 months or more, occurring before 45 years of age

Affective Disorders

Disturbances in feeling or affective disorders, are classified as follows

Depressive Disorders

A. According to the *Diagnostic and Statistical Manual of Mental Disorders (DSM-III-R)*, major depression is the predominant mental illness in the United States and Canada with ranges from 5% to 12% in the male population and 9% to 26% in the female population
B. Common signs of depression as it deepens from mild to severe are
1. Irritation
2. Loss of interest in some or all usual activities
3. Change in appetite: usually decreased
4. Changes in weight: usually loss in weight
5. Sleep disturbances: usually insomnia, but may be increased hours of sleep per day
6. Withdrawal from family and friends
7. Hopelessness and helplessness may become profound and may lead to delusions or fantasies of "ending it all"
8. If left in this pattern, the patient eventually could justify how nonexistence may solve the problems
9. The patient may start to dwell on death, and to devise a plan of self-destruction
10. Self-destruction becomes the goal; this is suicidal ideation
C. See later sections on Suicide Prevention and Suicide Intervention

Bipolar Disorders

A. Category used when one or more manic episodes are noted whether or not a depressive episode is/has been experienced
B. Mania characterized by unstable mood, pressured speech, and increased motor activity
C. Clinically, it is more common to see depression in its pure form than to see mania in its pure form

Personality Disorders

A. Paranoid personality: characterized by suspicion, rigidity, secretiveness, oversensitivity and alertness, distortions of reality, and the use of projection as a major defense mechanism
B. Borderline personality: at times moderately neurotic and at other times, overtly psychotic; extremely difficult to treat and often unstable after numerous treatment attempts; symptoms include
1. Combined anger and depression
2. Anhedonia
3. Social isolation
4. Poor impulse control
5. Dependency
6. Substance abuse
7. Sexual promiscuity
C. Codependency: meeting goals successfully by relying on another person for the answers. Characteristics of the codependent person include
1. Partners are dependent on each other to make a whole relationship
2. One of the partners in this relationship assumes a passive role
3. One or both may have low self-esteem
4. One or both may have low self-image
5. One or both may have an addictive disorder (alcohol, drugs, etc.)
6. They tend to be manipulative—there is a constant conflict either between them or within the family
7. They tend to operate in a series of delusions
8. Because of delusions, they tend to promote their version of any story as the absolute truth
9. They exhibit poor boundaries in relationships
10. They are somewhat to totally insensitive to others' emotions and feelings
11. If the codependency exists within family boundaries, it is highly likely that a dysfunctional family unit will emerge and the children will become a part of the codependency
12. Codependency may be intergenerational, and therefore cyclical
The treatment of codependent persons is designed by identifying the underlying emotions that are fostering the codependency
D. Substance abuse disorders: a pattern of pathologic use of substances that entails such things as need for daily use, loss of control, efforts to control use, overdoses, impairment of social functioning, family disruptions, legal problems, and so on; abuse is distinguished from dependency by tolerance of the substance (increasing use requires increasing doses to achieve the same effect) and the presence or absence of a withdrawal syndrome.
1. Alcoholism
a. Abuse is distinguished from recreational use by such features as daily drinking, frequent need for the chemical, blackouts, social impairment, and decreased ability to function, such as job loss, driving while intoxicated, arrests, and so forth

b. Acute alcohol ingestion may result in a condition formerly known as delirium tremens (DTs), now known as acute alcohol withdrawal syndrome; key features are hallucinations, extreme agitation, and disorientation; treatment includes anxiolytics (benzodiazepines), anticonvulsants, and hydration

c. Long-term use may lead to peripheral neuropathy, Wernicke's syndrome (confusion, ataxia, and abnormal eye movements), or Korsakoff's syndrome (alcoholic amnesia syndrome), which is manifested by memory loss and confabulation. These effects are largely caused by deficiency of thiamine and may be partially reversed by the provision of thiamine. Usually Korsakoff's syndrome is irreversible but may be arrested by thiamine replacement therapy and cessation of alcohol abuse

2. Barbiturate and sedative abuse (barbiturates, minor tranquilizers such as diazepam, benzodiazepines, etc.)
   a. Cross tolerant with alcohol
   b. May be used by "street addicts" when unable to obtain opiates
   c. Second most abused substance after alcohol in the United States
   d. Legally obtained drugs are often used by middle-class women who overuse tranquilizers
   e. Intoxication similar to alcohol
   f. There is a withdrawal syndrome similar to alcohol withdrawal

3. Opiates (heroin, morphine, etc.)
   a. Includes street addicts using IV heroin as well as "medical addicts" using various prescribed substances such as codeine
   b. IV drug users are at a high risk for AIDS
   c. Intoxication: pupil constriction, poor attention span, apathy, slurred speech, euphoria, and psychomotor retardation
   d. There is a physical withdrawal syndrome

4. Cocaine
   a. Stimulant
   b. Increasing use among the middle class
   c. Considered a social drug; many believe that it is not addictive
   d. May be snorted or smoked as a "free-base" or as crack
   e. Intoxication: poor judgment, poor impulse control, feeling of confidence, euphoria, talkative, rapid speech, pacing, elevated heart rate and blood pressure, dilated pupils, nausea, and sweating
   f. May lead to hallucinations with prolonged use; severe depression occurs after the substance use is stopped, leading to strong psychologic craving
   g. There does not appear to be a true withdrawal syndrome

5. Amphetamines
   a. Abuse may begin in an effort to control weight
   b. May be used IV by street addicts for a "rush"; may be combined with other drugs such as heroin or barbiturates

   c. Intoxication: elevated heart rate and blood pressure, dilated pupils, chills, perspiration, nausea, and vomiting

6. Hallucinogens (LSD, mescaline, etc.)
   a. Used much less than in the early 1970s
   b. Use leads to altered perceptions and hallucinations; distorted perception of colors; illusions and delusions; unpredictable effects
   c. Intoxication: perceptual changes; dilated pupils; increased pulse, sweating, anxiety, tremors; feelings of paranoia; and poor judgment

7. Cannabis (marijuana, hashish, etc.)
   a. Widely used by various groups, usually smoked or eaten
   b. Intoxication: increased pulse rate, bloodshot eyes, increased appetite, dry mouth, distorted perception of time, euphoria, and apathy
   c. May precipitate panic attacks

Physically Based Mental Disorders

A. Organic brain syndrome may result from vascular disorders of the brain, brain infections, trauma, altered metabolism, poisoning, endocrine disorders, and deficiencies
   1. Global involvement: confusion, delirium, and dementia
   2. Selective involvement: may be limited to portions of the personality (e.g., amnesia, hallucinations, and psychosomatic disorders)
   3. Functional impairment: has the features of psychosis (e.g., paranoia, depression, and mania)

B. Mental retardation: subaverage intelligence; there are numerous causes including inherited defects in metabolism, genetic defects, birth injuries, and developmental anomalies

C. Other somatic manifestations of mental disturbance: several conditions have defined or suggested psychologic bases
   1. Ulcers
   2. Bowel disorders
   3. Cardiovascular disorders
   4. Asthma
   5. Allergies
   6. Eating disorders: anorexia, bulimia
   7. Headache
   8. Certain endocrine disorders

Anxiety Disorders

A. Panic disorder: recurrent panic attacks at unpredictable times; symptoms include shortness of breath, choking, palpitations, chest pains, and sweating

B. Agoraphobia (literal meaning, "fear of the marketplace"), without panic attacks: fear of being away from a safe environment or person

C. Social phobia: irrational fear of exposure to the scrutiny of others

D. Simple phobia: a disabling fear of some specific object or situation, such as the fear of animals or of being in a high place

E. Obsessive-compulsive disorder: incessant preoccupation with impulses and anxieties that the person believes are groundless

F. Posttraumatic stress disorder: characteristic symptoms after a psychologically traumatic event; these include numbness of responses, frequently reliving the event, dreams, depression, and anxiety

Eating Disorders

A. Obesity/compulsive overeating: consuming greater than required number of calories, which results in weight gain, usually considered more than 20% greater than the recommended weight for one's height

B. Anorexia nervosa: compulsive refusal to eat; person believes that he or she is overweight, regardless of his or her actual weight

C. Bulimia: an eating disorder characterized by episodes of binging and then purging; person may not appear overweight or underweight. Bulimia leads to other symptoms such as menstrual irregularities, gastric dilation, aspiration pneumonia, dental caries (caused by frequent vomiting), and esophagitis

PATIENT'S RIGHTS MOVEMENT

A. Although patients in psychiatric settings are ill, they retain their civil rights and are often specifically protected under special sections of the law

B. In most places, "commitment" only removes the patient's right to leave the hospital or terminate treatment

C. Recent legal decisions indicate that patients may expect treatment and may not simply be detained in hospitals where there is no active treatment available

D. In recent years, patient and former-patient groups have formed and demanded access to records of treatment rationales

CARE AND TREATMENT OF PATIENTS

A. Basic needs: the basic needs of patients in psychiatric settings are similar to those of other patients; usually, psychiatric patients do not have the accompanying impairments of the physically ill patient
   1. Most patients are ambulatory
   2. The nurse's role is to guide, encourage, and teach by example
   3. Patients may be socially deteriorated and require assistance in activities of daily living such as how to arrange time to complete their own care
   4. Reward such as praise is helpful in guiding patients in these activities

B. Specific interventions: the following are grouped by type of patient, but should be viewed as broad strategies useful in various settings and with various patients
   1. Thought disorders
      a. Do not enter into patient's delusions; maintain your own view of reality without demeaning the patient's view of reality
      b. Do not argue with hallucinations: the patient views these as real
      c. Offer reassurance: most patients are experiencing pain from their symptoms
      d. Touch only with permission; the thought-disordered patient may have a distorted sense of his or her own person
      e. If you are afraid, be aware that the patient will sense this; be sure you have sufficient backup for your own safety and comfort

f. Maintain patient safety
   2. Affective disorders
      a. Demonstrate sincere interest
      b. Accept patient's feelings; anger may be directed to the nearest safe object: often the nurse
      c. Allow patient to express feelings; for example, crying in a dignified environment
      d. Only encourage the expression of feelings that you feel capable of handling; for example, do not encourage ventilation of feelings and then go on your lunch hour
      e. If patient is overactive, limit setting or reduction of stimuli may be necessary
      f. Avoid power struggles: use force only if necessary to protect patient or others in the environment
   3. Personality disorders
      a. Be honest with patients
      b. These patients are often manipulative and attention seeking
      c. They tend to view people or situations as all good or all bad
      d. Patients need to begin developing meaningful relationships in which they can begin to trust
      e. Consistency is important; patients may split the staff to play one staff member against another
   4. Substance abuse
      a. Severe denial is a common defense mechanism
      b. Keep the patient focused on the purpose of treatment
      c. Manipulation may be used to obtain a substance for abuse
      d. The nurse must remain nonjudgmental
      e. These patients may require repeated attempts at treatment before they can conquer their addiction
      f. Adequate diet, rest, and vitamin supplements are helpful
      g. Long-term success is often achieved through a lifelong affiliation with abstinence programs such as Alcoholics Anonymous (AA) and Narcotics Anonymous
      h. Alcoholism is usually treated in several steps, the first being detoxification. In detoxification, the alcoholic is withdrawn from the chemical through the use of a cross-tolerant substance, usually a benzodiazepine, which is administered for 3 to 5 days in decreasing doses. Frequently, alcoholics are referred to Alcoholics Anonymous
         (1) Detoxification should occur in a controlled (monitored) setting because detoxification may become life threatening
         (2) After the acute detoxification period of 3 to 5 days, intense counseling occurs
         (3) The patient may find it beneficial to continue in a peer group setting on a regular full- or part-time schedule
         (4) In some cases, additional treatment may be suggested in the form of halfway houses, which may offer up to 6 months to 1 year of treatment
      i. Other forms of substance abuse are treated similarly, with combinations of detoxification, if

needed, and supportive long-term treatment settings; opiate abusers may also be treated with methadone maintenance in attempts to prevent heroin use and allow the addict to return to more socially acceptable behavior patterns

5. Mental retardation: classified as follows with interventions geared accordingly
   a. Profoundly retarded: needs total nursing care in early stages; later may develop rudimentary ability to care for self; always requires some care
   b. Severely retarded: may be able to care for self in protected environment; requires monitoring
   c. Moderately retarded: usually capable of self-care but requires supervision when under stress
   d. Mildly retarded: usually self-supporting; may require support of family or others when under stress

6. Special needs of children and adolescents: there are many similarities and some differences in therapeutics for children and adolescents
   a. Services in hospitals are usually short and aimed at assessment and evaluation
   b. Most ongoing treatment is on an outpatient basis
   c. Treatment is action oriented, using such modalities as play therapy
   d. There are many issues of trust vs. mistrust
   e. There are issues of self-image, limit testing, and developmentally specific concerns

7. Special needs of the elderly: special consideration is given to the role of declining physical attributes
   a. There may be prejudices regarding the elderly
   b. Most elderly persons do not suffer from senility
   c. Apparent senility may be depression or other forms of illness (e.g., alcoholism)
   d. The reaction to drugs of all types may be idiosyncratic among the elderly
   e. Special techniques
      (1) Life review
      (2) Group work aimed at socialization such as remotivation
      (3) Touch: many elderly are deprived of touch in the usual manner because of relational losses

8. Death and dying: Nursing intervention is aimed at ensuring the transition of the patient through each of the stages listed below. It is important to be aware of your own attitude about death and to ensure that you are meeting the patient's needs and not your own. Being nonjudgmental and allowing the expression of emotions by the patient are essential. Patient defenses are necessary in accepting his or her own death and should not be challenged. Elizabeth Kübler-Ross describes dying as a process that proceeds through the following stages
   a. Shock and denial: the patient cannot actually accept or believe that he or she is going to die; may repress information, seek to escape the truth by seeking other opinions, and be unable to hear the real message
   b. Anger and rage: a stage in which the patient becomes angry with the terrible truth of impending death; may be hypercritical of others, demanding, and resentful. Health care workers often bear the brunt of a patient's rage as they represent cure for others but not for him or her
   c. Bargaining: in this stage, acceptance has begun, and the patient begins to bargain for more time or for some specific request; during this stage, wills may be finalized and legacies of various kinds bestowed. If possible, requests should be granted because they bring comfort to the dying person
   d. Depression: after acceptance of the inevitable has begun, the person feels sad and alone. He or she may speak little, and cry often. Quiet acceptance is often the most helpful kind of intervention in this stage
   e. Acceptance: once this occurs, the person is often seen as tranquil and at peace with himself. Again, the patient may speak little, since most of what he or she has to say to others has been said; although still sad, the patient has made his or her peace with death and has accepted the inevitable. This phase may last for months or longer

9. Grieving: George Engel (1964) defined grieving as a process of sequential steps similar to those in the dying process
   a. Shock and disbelief: the person refuses to accept the loss, may feel stunned or numbed; similar to the first stage of dying
   b. Developing awareness: the person may experience varying degrees of physical symptoms such as nausea, vomiting, and loss of appetite. Crying is common, anger may be felt and expressed toward the lost person for the act of desertion. Anger may be self-directed and recriminations made
   c. Restitution (resolution): acceptance occurs and is aided by the culturally approved modes of grieving such as funerals and wearing black
   d. The process of grieving may take more than 1 year; all stages must be experienced for grief to be successfully completed. If grieving is not successful, it may lead to one of the following
      (1) Delayed reaction: a later reaction to the loss; delay is caused by repressing reality; it may result in more painful experiences than the normal immediate reaction
      (2) Distorted reactions: may include the development of symptoms similar to the lost person's: medical illnesses, social isolation, agitated depression, increased use of alcohol or other drugs

CRISIS INTERVENTION

Generally, there are common components in all crisis situations. With this knowledge, strategies are developed to assist people through a crisis and minimize its detrimental effects.

A. Crisis: an event that disturbs the equilibrium of the individual or family
B. The disturbance leads to development of certain symptoms, most notably, anxiety and depression
C. These feelings continue until a need is felt to reduce or alleviate them

D. If the person or family has adequate coping mechanisms, the problem will be resolved and balance restored

E. Without coping mechanisms, anxiety and depression increase to intolerable levels

F. Interventions are aimed at providing short-term therapy to increase coping behaviors

G. Most crises are resolved within 6 to 8 weeks

H. Intervention entails
   1. A thorough assessment of the situation
   2. Planned strategies that do not attempt to rearrange a person's life
   3. Strategies that increase intellectual understanding, explore current feelings, offer coping mechanisms, and support existing ties and helpful relationships

CRISIS OF RAPE OR INCEST

Assisting survivors of these violent acts requires substantial time. This intervention begins when the victim calls for help in any form or seeks treatment. There are two possible phases to this violence. One is the acute or immediate phase wherein the victim exhibits fear, confusion, disorganization, and restlessness. The second phase is a long-term process of reorganization and usually begins weeks after the attack.

A. Early relevant feelings include
   1. Physical pain
   2. Anger
   3. Fear of reattack
   4. Outrage at the perpetrator
   5. Total violation of (emotional) space
   6. Fear of involvement with anyone of the same sex as the perpetrator
   7. Emotionally drained
   8. Helplessness
   9. Fear of pregnancy

B. If these immediate feelings are not externalized and dealt with, the result may be permanent psychologic damage including but not limited to the following psychosexual dysfunctions
   1. Sexual arousal disorders
   2. Sexual deviations (several varieties)
   3. Sexual aversions
   4. Delusions of violent sexual behavior, which could be incorporated in the patient's life-style

C. Interventions include
   1. Assess the victim's safety: Are you in a safe place?; Is there help for you?
   2. Listen: accept what is said
   3. Respond as appropriate
   4. Refer patient to appropriate agency

SUICIDE PREVENTION

Suicide ranks as a leading cause of death in the United States. There are specific indicators that assist in assessing suicidal risk. Risk factors include

A. Age and sex: more women attempt suicide; more men are successful

B. Men over 35 are at higher risk; most suicides occur in men between the ages of 35 and 50 years

C. Anxiety and depression: many potential suicide victims report increasing anxiety and depression; most significant is a recent change in these feelings

D. Past coping pattern: not working in the current situation

E. Past suicide attempt is always considered a high-risk factor

F. Alcohol or drug abuse: many suicides are committed by alcoholics

G. Concrete plan: if there is a plan, considerations are
   1. Is it set in a current time frame
   2. Is it lethal
   3. Does the potential victim have the necessary resources to carry out the plan

H. Significant others: often a suicide is committed to communicate with others

I. Interventions include
   1. Focus on clear and present danger
   2. Reduce present hazards
   3. Give clear directions for victim to follow
   4. Assign to constant monitoring in a hospital
   5. Mobilize significant others when possible
   6. Mobilize past coping mechanisms
   7. Assign concrete specific tasks
   8. Explore positive alternatives to suicide
   9. Teach problem-solving techniques

SUICIDE INTERVENTION

Intervention becomes critical at the point of suicidal ideation. If intervention does not occur, suicide is highly likely. The patient may be having underlying feelings of hopelessness, helplessness, and impending doom. Frequently the patient will verbalize the need to "end it all."

A. Always ask
   1. Do I understand that you want to hurt yourself? (confirming suicide ideation)
   2. Do you have a plan or how will you hurt yourself? Will you share your plan with me? (suicidal gesturing may be evident)
   3. If the specific plan calls for using an enabling device or instrument: May I have the _____ that is included in the plan? (specify item: knife, razor, rope, etc.)

B. Ordinarily a loud cry for help can be heard before the suicide occurs if others are perceptive enough to hear it

NOTE: severely depressed patients are so physically impaired that they rarely have the energy to commit suicide. As the depression begins to lift, the potential to commit suicide increases, that is, especially if they have communicated that need to "end it all."

TREATMENT MODALITIES
Psychotherapy

A. Individual psychotherapy: one-to-one relationship between a therapist (physician, psychologist, social worker, nurse clinician) and a patient; sessions of 45 to 50 minutes are usually held weekly or more often; the aim is to improve the functioning of the person; it is most effective with the neuroses and in patients who have good verbal skills and high intelligence

B. Family group therapy: a family is seen as a group by a therapist, based on the premise that disturbance arises as a function of family interactions and that treatment must be aimed at the family as a whole

C. Group therapy: treatment provided to a group of persons related by age, symptom, or other commonality; treatment occurs on a weekly or biweekly basis and may include more than one therapist

D. Behavior modification: techniques based on conditioning; undesired behaviors are ignored and desired behaviors are rewarded

Milieu Therapy

Milieu therapy is the use of a controlled environment to influence the treatment of a patient

A. Interactions between patient and staff, as well as interpatient relationships, are used as a basis for treatment

B. Therapeutic communications: behavior modeling and some behavior modification techniques are often used

Therapeutic Community

Therapeutic community (Maxwell Jones, 1968) is a method of establishing a milieu for treatment wherein all members, staff as well as patients, have assigned responsibilities in the community and defined roles. The reasoning is that this type of democratic environment prepares the patient for release into the larger community.

Electroconvulsive Therapy

Electroconvulsive therapy (shock therapy) is an older treatment in controversial use in some settings. It is the application of an electrical current through the brain resulting in a grand mal seizure. Some patients suffer a short-term memory loss as a result of the treatment.

Psychopharmacologic Therapy

Psychopharmacologic agents are used in the treatment of mental health disorders.

NOTE: when administering medication to the mental health patient, remember to use a tongue blade to examine the interior of the mouth if you suspect the patient is "cheeking" the medication.

A. Anti-EPS (extrapyramidal symptoms): EPS, known locally as "pretzeling," is unusual muscle movement that involves the fine muscles of the body; these symptoms are acute and chronic dystonic reactions to the antipsychotic medication.

    1. Frequently EPS appears in the tongue or in the muscles of the upper chest, neck, and shoulders.

    2. Anti-EPS medications used to reverse the muscular effects of the antipsychotics are diphenhydramine hydrochloride (Benadryl) and benztropine mesylate (Cogentin)

b. Refer to Chapter 4 (Pharmacology) for greater detail regarding drugs that are commonly used to treat mental illness.

Adjunctive Therapies

A. Occupational therapy: the use of vocational tasks to allow patients to express various underlying feelings

B. Recreational therapy: the use of recreational activities to allow patients to express feelings

C. Art therapy: the use of the plastic and graphic arts to express feeling

D. Other therapies may include vocational counseling, bibliotherapy (writing or reading), and dance therapy

ETHICAL CONSIDERATIONS IN PATIENT CARE

A. In most places, patients may sue institutions under habeas corpus proceedings for their release from treatment

B. Laws guarantee rights to patients

C. Nurses and other staff members may be sued for assault and battery for forcing treatments on patients

D. Wrongful death suits have been brought in circumstances where a patient has died

E. There is a narrow line between treatment and abuse

F. Local laws vary in different parts of the country, and nurses should be aware of local statutes

G. Confidentiality is essential in mental health nursing

H. Communications between a patient and a nurse may be considered "privileged," whereas most medical records are open to subpoena

I. Documents should contain only factual material, not conjecture

J. If a patient threatens bodily harm to others, such information is no longer considered privileged and is required to be reported to the authorities

K. Oppressive mental institutions may infringe on a patient's rights, and nurses should be aware of their responsibilities in such situations

Suggested Reading List

Diagnostic and statistical manual of mental disorders, ed 3, rev, Washington, DC, 1987, American Psychiatric Association.

Kübler-Ross E: On death and dying, New York, 1969, Macmillan.

Lofstedt CR: *Mereness' essentials of psychiatric nursing learning and activity guide,* ed 3, St Louis, 1990, Mosby.

Pasquali EA, Arnold HM, DeBasio N: *Mental-health nursing: a holistic approach,* ed 3, St Louis, 1989, Mosby.

Physicians' desk reference, Montvale, NJ, Medical Economics (published annually).

Saxton DF, Haring PW: *Care of patients with emotional problems,* ed 4, St Louis, 1985, Mosby.

Stuart GW, Sundeen SJ: *Principles and practice of psychiatric nursing,* ed 4, St Louis, Mosby.

Taylor CM: *Mereness' essentials of psychiatric nursing,* ed 13, St Louis, 1990, Mosby.

Mental Health Nursing Review Questions

Answers and rationales begin on p. 436.

1. John is angry with and actually hates his boss, but to his co-workers he appears to be the boss's favorite employee. This is an example of:
   ① Repression
   ② Projection
   ③ Reaction formation
   ④ Rationalization

2. On the day before finals a student has sweaty palms and "butterflies" in the stomach. The anxiety level is most probably:
   ① Panic level
   ② Free floating
   ③ Apprehension level
   ④ Alertness level

3. A nursing diagnosis in psychiatric nursing is:
   ① A behavior or problem related to its probable cause
   ② Not used, because nurses do not diagnose
   ③ Based on the medical condition of the patient
   ④ Useful only in general hospital settings

4. Suicide is most likely to occur:
   ① On admission
   ② On discharge
   ③ As the depression deepens
   ④ As the depression lifts

5. You are attempting to communicate with your patient. The patient says, "My car is red, your hair is short, my socks are gold, DeWayne, Jewish, my wife's cooking is awful, she burns." This is called:
   ① Word salad
   ② Ambivalence
   ③ Confabulation
   ④ Flight of ideas

6. Anxiety can be expressed through emotional feelings. Which of the following signs is *least likely* to be observed in the anxious patient?
   ① Fear
   ② Phobias
   ③ Hostility
   ④ Depression

Situation: Mary, admitted 3 days ago to the inpatient unit, says that the television set is cursing her and that there are electrodes in her head that make her arms and legs burn. She has been increasingly disheveled and had not bathed for 4 weeks before admission.

7. The idea of the television cursing Mary is an example of:
   ① Persecutory delusion
   ② Visual hallucination
   ③ Incoherence
   ④ Flight of ideas

8. When Mary experienced the "burning" of her arms and legs, the nurse might respond:
   ① "That's silly, your legs are okay."
   ② "Does the fire travel from one leg to the other?"
   ③ "If your legs were burning, I would see it."
   ④ "I understand you feel the fire. How can you stop it?"

9. To help Mary in her activities of daily living, the nurse should:
   ① Insist that she bathe before she may have recreational privileges
   ② State in a manner-of-fact way that Mary is expected to bathe each morning at 8 AM, stay with her, and assist her with this task
   ③ Postpone Mary's bath until her symptoms subside as it is not the major concern now
   ④ Tell Mary she will be excluded from social groups because she is untidy

10. Thorazine is one of the oldest and most widely prescribed antipsychotic medications. The correct generic name for Thorazine is:
    ① Fluphenazine
    ② Mesoridazine
    ③ Chlorpromazine
    ④ Compazine

11. Paranoid thinking is characterized by feelings of:
    ① Anger and aggression
    ② Suspicion and jealousy
    ③ Self-pity and self-centeredness
    ④ Simultaneous hero worship and hero hating

12. The two outstanding examples of paranoia include:
    ① Grandiosity and poverty
    ② Poverty and persecution
    ③ Persecution and poisoning
    ④ Grandiosity and persecution

13. Patients who abuse alcohol may become tremulous and have hallucinations when they stop drinking. This is called:
    ① Tolerance
    ② Abstinence
    ③ Withdrawal
    ④ Dementia

14. Monoamine oxidase inhibitors are dangerous when used with certain foods. The substance in these foods is called:
    ① Histamine
    ② Phenylalanine
    ③ Lysine
    ④ Tyramine

15. Which of the following nursing measures is *most often* recommended when caring for a patient who is aggressive and hyperactive?
    ① Physically restraining the patient
    ② Secluding the patient
    ③ Providing safe, diversional activity
    ④ Explain that "this behavior is unacceptable" so the patient can control it

16. The chief defense mechanism used by the alcoholic (addict) is:
    ① Denial
    ② Compensation
    ③ Reaction formation
    ④ Sublimation

17. The medication most frequently given to the bipolar (manic depressive) patient is:
    ① Chlorpromazine (Thorazine)
    ② Perphenazine (Trilafon)
    ③ Imipramine (Tofranil)
    ④ Lithium (Lithane)
18. A patient rushes up to you and says, "They're after me. They want to torture me and kill me." Which of the following is the most appropriate response?
    ① "Tell me who they are?"
    ② "There's no one here except you and me."
    ③ "I need to go look for myself."
    ④ "You are safe here. Can you tell me more?"

Situation: Gwen, admitted for attempted suicide by superficially cutting her wrist, is sullen and angry. She has worked as a prostitute and recently her "man" told her she wasn't needed. She has a history of minor drug abuse. She states that she's bored with life and doesn't enjoy anything.

19. Gwen is probably best described as:
    ① Schizophrenic
    ② Ambivalent
    ③ Borderline personality
    ④ Psychotic
20. Gwen's attempted suicide is an example of:
    ① Poor impulse control
    ② Regressive behavior
    ③ Manipulation
    ④ Depression
21. One nursing goal for Gwen while she is hospitalized may be to:
    ① Show Gwen that her life of prostitution is immoral
    ② Eliminate self-destructive manipulative behavior
    ③ Get Gwen to settle down with a husband
    ④ Convince Gwen to have a tubal ligation to avoid pregnancy
22. Gwen needs to begin trusting relationships. One way to foster beginning trust is to:
    ① Show Gwen you are available regardless of her behavior
    ② Let Gwen know you care for her but may not always approve of her behavior
    ③ Avoid trust in the relationship, since Gwen will not be able to tolerate separation on discharge
    ④ Let Gwen know she can call you day or night

23. During the early phase of detoxification, an assessment for physical signs should be made when the patient:
    ① Asks for medication to stop the "shaking"
    ② Vomits
    ③ Complains of a sore throat
    ④ Asks to leave the hospital
24. A key feature of a patient with borderline personality disorder is they:
    ① Are able to cope successfully in society
    ② Learn from previous mistakes
    ③ Are driven by intense hallucinations
    ④ Manipulate everyone they can

25. A patient approaches you and says, "With all my troubles I feel worthless. I would like to end all this misery. Everyone would be better off if I were gone." Your most appropriate response to this statement would be:
    ① "Tell me more."
    ② "Are you thinking of killing yourself?"
    ③ "I can see that you are very upset."
    ④ "I have to take blood pressures right now, then we can talk."
26. During a group therapy session, a patient asks you what the difference is between a psychosis and neurosis. Your most correct reply to this question is:
    ① Psychotics can't think; neurotics can think
    ② Psychotics are always depressed; neurotics are not depressed
    ③ Psychotics have disorganized thinking; neurotics' thoughts are organized
    ④ Psychotics are always in touch with reality; neurotics are not in touch with reality
27. A patient complains of trouble with control of her or his tongue. Also, the neck muscles are beginning to tighten and the patient is having difficulty keeping her or his head in an upright position. Your first response would be:
    ① Check the medication administration record
    ② Call the physician
    ③ Draw blood per standing order
    ④ Fill out an incident report
28. Crisis intervention theory is based on which of the following assumptions:
    ① Crises lead to long-term damage
    ② Crises have common elements that are useful to know for intervention
    ③ A crisis is abnormal and occurs as a sign of deeper trouble
    ④ A crisis may take years to resolve
29. In a crisis the aim of intervention is to:
    ① Rearrange life elements of the people involved
    ② Provide treatment for as long as possible
    ③ Offer support and explore alternatives
    ④ Avoid old ties because these led up to the crisis

Situation: Sylvia, 46 years old, is admitted because of an increasingly depressed mood. She is unable to care for her house, and her husband reports that she has been up late at night and has difficulty getting up in the morning. In her interview, Sylvia reports she has abdominal pain, which she says is punishment for her sins.

30. Sylvia's symptoms are characteristic of:
    ① Alcoholic psychosis
    ② Affective disorder
    ③ Schizophrenia
    ④ Bipolar illness
31. Sylvia's inability to arise in the morning might be described as:
    ① Loose associations
    ② Difficulty in thinking
    ③ Psychomotor retardation
    ④ Mental retardation

32. After a few weeks of treatment you observe that Sylvia has started putting on large amounts of makeup, has become seductive with male patients, and stays up very late pacing the floor. You might conclude that Sylvia:
    ① Was initially diagnosed incorrectly
    ② May be having a manic episode as part of her illness
    ③ Is showing signs of recovery
    ④ May be having side effects of the medication

33. Four of the major features that clearly distinguish schizophrenia from other mental illness are:
    ① Low self-esteem, low morals, worthlessness, and poverty
    ② Fantasy, hallucinations, delusions, and personality flaws
    ③ Inappropriate affect, autistic behavior, ambivalence, and inability to associate thinking and reality
    ④ Ambivalence, autism, apathy, and associative looseness

34. Extreme mood swings ranging from deep depression to high activity levels is most often seen in:
    ① Paranoid disorders
    ② Bipolar disorders
    ③ Schizophrenia
    ④ Eating disorders

35. When dealing with a patient having somatic delusions, it is important to remember that:
    ① The patient really doesn't feel the delusional sensation
    ② Touching such a patient may be nontherapeutic, because they may have disturbed personal borders
    ③ Agreeing with the patient is helpful
    ④ Placebos can be used to alleviate somatic complaints

36. A patient on suicide precautions reports a recent change in mood. The nurse knows:
    ① This is a high-risk factor
    ② The crisis has probably passed
    ③ The patient may be manic-depressive
    ④ The patient is responding to the added attention of the precautions

37. In assessing suicidal risk, which of the following is a high-risk factor:
    ① Long psychotherapeutic treatment
    ② A concrete plan that is relatively lethal
    ③ Past attempts, because these usually mean the person is now able to cope better with stresses
    ④ Deviance in the person's background

38. If you were to select a single identifying characteristic of the obsessive-compulsive patient, it would be:
    ① Seclusiveness
    ② Aggression
    ③ Orderliness
    ④ Instant gratification

39. A teenager admits to you that he or she is smoking marijuana on a fairly regular basis. You would know that marijuana is considered a(n):
    ① Highly addictive substance
    ② Amphetamine
    ③ Hallucinogen
    ④ Cannabinol

40. Which of the following statements is most true about the difference between a delusion and a hallucination?
    ① Delusions are false beliefs; hallucinations are projections
    ② Delusions are systems; hallucinations are beliefs
    ③ Delusions are always true; hallucinations are always false
    ④ Delusions are based in fact; hallucinations are based in belief

41. Which of the following statements about suicide is most correct?
    ① Suicide is 100% preventable
    ② Suicide is only inherited
    ③ Suicide occurs without any prior warning
    ④ Suicide lethality increases in proportion to the details of the plan

42. Your patient tells you that he or she is depressed over the recent death of a parent. Which response would be the best communication intervention for this patient?
    ① Say nothing
    ② Wouldn't you rather talk about something else?
    ③ I have some time. Would you like to tell me more about your feelings?
    ④ I don't have time for sad people

43. You enter a patient's room and stand just inside the door. The patient is obviously agitated and is escalating to the point that physical harm may occur. What is your best action?
    ① Take the patient to the seclusion room
    ② Talk to the patient and try to identify why he or she is so agitated
    ③ Go to the nurses' station and report the patient's behavior
    ④ Call the physician

44. A patient who has just been admitted for polysubstance abuse is demanding to leave. Which of the following is the best nursing action?
    ① Ask the patient why he or she wants to leave so soon
    ② Inform the patient that no one is allowed to leave once he or she is admitted
    ③ Take the patient to the seclusion room
    ④ Respond, "I would like you to tell me how you feel. Can you do that?"

45. In working with mental health patients you would know that *all* records are confidential, which means:
    ① Everyone who asks may see the patient's records
    ② Only the medical and nursing staffs may view the records
    ③ Only nurses are allowed to make entries in the records
    ④ The patient may view her or his record on request

46. You are caring for a patient with major depression. When planning activities, you would know that the patient needs:
    ① Frequent changes in activities
    ② Constant redirection into numerous activities
    ③ Behavior modification that restructures feelings
    ④ Well-defined, structured interactions at the beginning of treatment

47. The dominant feeling that the patient with major depression is most likely to display is:
    ① Agitation
    ② Ambivalence
    ③ Anxiety
    ④ Hopelessness

48. The drug that cannot be given if the patient has consumed alcohol within the past 24 hours is:
    ① Chlorpromazine (Thorazine)
    ② Loxapine succinate (Loxitane)
    ③ Disulfiram (Antabuse)
    ④ Trifluoperazine (Stelazine)

49. To foster feelings that bolster a patient's self-esteem, it is important that the nurse:
    ① Constantly criticize the patient's behavior
    ② Accept and give positive reinforcement for appropriate behavior
    ③ Enforce behavior modification, including ignoring all previous unacceptable behavior
    ④ Remain very strict with unacceptable behavior and structure precise expectations for the patient

50. You have answered a phone call. The caller tells you that he or she is going to commit suicide. What would be your initial response?
    ① "People who talk about it, never do it."
    ② "Do you have a plan?"
    ③ "Why would you want to do a thing like that?"
    ④ "Could you tell me your phone number?"

CHAPTER 8

Obstetric Nursing

The aim of obstetrics is to offer health services to the childbearing mother, her baby, and her family that will ensure a normal pregnancy and a safe prenatal and postnatal experience. This chapter reviews components of the nursing process. Each topic presents pertinent information helpful in planning the nursing assessment and in analyzing the nursing needs. Nursing management is outlined, giving options for selecting appropriate plans for action. The evaluation of whether outcomes and goals of obstetrics have been met completes the nursing process. The information presented in this review will assist the nurse in understanding how to

- *Plan, implement, and evalute the nursing process as it relates to the maternity patient, her baby, and her family.*
- *Integrate selected theoretic information into the nursing process to effectively meet the basic aims of maternity nursing.*

BRIEF HISTORY

A. Primitive society
   1. Practiced infanticide
   2. Treated mothers with indifference and brutality
   3. Superstitions, incantations, taboos
B. Ancient civilizations
   1. Egypt: first to describe podalic version; first to practice cesarean section, as Egyptian law forbade burial of pregnant mother with infant
   2. China: published manual on obstetrics describing treatment of mother
   3. Greco-Roman: obstetric writings of Soranus of Ephesus (Father of Obstetrics); also wrote on midwifery (AD 200)
C. Evolution of modern obstetrics
   1. Middle Ages and early Christianity: pain of childbirth believed to be a means of expiation for sins
   2. Judaism: contributed to public health through its kosher dietary laws and to hygiene through its ritual of circumcision
   3. Renaissance: Leonardo da Vinci (Italy, 1452-1519): contributed to understanding human anatomy through his anatomic drawings
   4. Western European influence
      a. Abroise Paré (France, 1510-1590): started trend of doctors' replacing midwives
      b. Peter Chamberlen (England and Holland, 1560-1631): introduced forceps, paving the way for mechanical devices to assist in difficult deliveries
      c. William Smellie (England, 1697-1763): published book on midwifery in 1752 and wrote rules for the use of forceps during a delivery
      d. William Hunter (England, 1718-1783): described placental anatomy

   e. Jean Louis Baudelocque (France, 1746-1810): described positions, presentations, and pelvic measurements
   f. Ignaz Philipp Semmelweiss (Austria, 1818-1865): a pioneer in obstetric asepsis, Semmelweis found that handwashing before attending mothers greatly reduced the incidence of puerperal (child-bed) fever
   g. Louis Pasteur (France, 1822-1895): discovered *Streptococcus* as the causative organism in puerperal fever (1860)
   5. Contributors in the United States
      a. Anne Hutchinson (1634): midwife who delivered many babies of early settlers
      b. William Shippen: established first lying-in hospital and midwifery school in the United States in 1762
      c. Olive Wendell Holmes (1809-1894): stressed cleanliness and handwashing before caring for new mothers
      d. Margaret Sanger Research Bureau (1923): first organization to address question of contraception and planned parenthood
   6. United States legislation affecting mothers and children
      a. 1921: Sheppard Towner Act: promoted health and welfare for mothers and children
      b. 1936: Social Security benefits begun; later to include entitlement benefits for mothers and their dependent children
      c. 1943: Emergency Maternal and Infant Care Act to assist families of soldiers during World War II
      d. 1973: Supreme Court legalizes abortion
      e. 1974: WIC: federally funded nutritional program

providing supplementary food to eligible pregnant, lactating, or postpartum women, their infants, and children under 5 years of age

DEFINITIONS COMMONLY USED IN OBSTETRICS
Statistics

birth rates number of live births per 1000 population
fetal death (stillborn) infant of 20 weeks or more gestational age who dies in utero prior to birth
infant mortality rate number of deaths before the first birthday per 1000 live births
maternal mortality rate number of mothers dying in or because of childbearing per 100,000 live births
neonatal death death within first 4 weeks of life
neonatal death rate number of deaths within the first 4 weeks of life per 1000 live births

Abbreviations (Limited Listing)

ARM artificial rupture of membranes
BOW bag of waters; amniotic sac
CPD cephalopelvic disproportion
C/S cesarean section
DIC disseminated intravascular coagulation
EDC estimated date of confinement; due date for birth
FHR fetal heart rate
FHT fetal heart tone
G gravida; number of pregnancies
GTPAL gravida, term, premature, abortions, living children; identification of pregnancy status
HCG human chorionic gonadotropin
HELLP hemolysis, elevated liver enzymes, low platelet count; extention of pathology related to severe preeclampsia
HIV human immunodeficiency virus
LGA large for gestational age
LMP last menstrual period
P para; number of viable births
PIH pregnancy-induced hypertension
PROM premature rupture of membranes
Q quadrant; one of four equal parts into which the abdomen is divided to designate position of fetus in uterus
RhoGAM Antibody against Rh factor given early prenatally or within 72 hours postpartum to mother
SGA small for gestational age

Common Obstetric Terminology

Apgar score method of evaluating infant immediately after delivery; usually at 1 minute and at 5 minutes
Braxton Hicks contractions painless uterine contractions felt throughout pregnancy, becoming stronger and more noticeable during second and third trimester
caput head; cephalic portion of infant
cyesis pregnancy
dystocia long, painful labor and delivery
elderly primipara pregnant woman over 35 years of age giving birth to her first child
gestation developmental time of embryo, fetus, in utero
grand multipara more than five children
high risk pregnant woman with preexisting problems that could jeopardize the pregnancy, the fetus, or herself; under 18 years of age or over 35 years of age with no prenatal care (any one or more of these conditions)
lightening dropping of the uterus as the fetal head enters the pelvis during the last 2 weeks before EDC (usually just before labor in multiparas)
low risk pregnant woman with normal history, between ages 18 and 34, with no medical, psychologic, or other preexisting problems, and under good prenatal care

meconium first bowel movement of the newborn—thick, tarlike, greenish black substance
multigravida pregnant more than one time
multipara given birth to more than one child
postmature infant one born after 42 weeks' gestation
premature infant one born anytime before 37 weeks' gestation
primigravida pregnant for the first time
primipara giving birth to first child
pseudocyesis false pregnancy
quickening first movements of the fetus felt by the mother (16 to 18 weeks' gestation)
secundines afterbirth or placenta and membranes
term infant one born between 38 and 42 weeks' gestation
vernix caseosa cheesy material covering the fetus and newborn that acts as a protection to the skin
vis a tergo external pressure on the fundus to assist in the delivery of the infant
viable ability to live outside uterus; living

TRENDS

A. Prepared childbirth experience: mother and father (or alternate) jointly attend childbirth education classes to prepare for the child and for the childbearing and childbirth experience
B. Alternate birth settings
  1. Birthing centers outside of hospital; ABC (alternate birth centers)
  2. Individual's home
  3. Use of the birthing chair instead of traditional table
  4. Birthing room: labor, delivery, and postpartum hospital stay incorporated into one cheerful, homelike room set up with necessary labor and delivery equipment
C. Variety of positions used to assist labor and delivery (squat, side position, etc.)
D. Showering during first or second stage of labor
E. Inclusion of father or alternate: support person stays in labor and delivery area for both vaginal and cesarean section deliveries
F. Rooming in: allows newborn in room with mother for the day; fathers (properly gowned) allowed unlimited visiting time
G. Early discharge: may be discharged home within 12 to 24 hours (uncomplicated labor and delivery)
H. Sibling visits: designated hours that children may visit with mother and see baby (from nursery window)
I. Use of midwives: many hospitals and birthing centers throughout the United States now have nurse-midwives as the primary care person conducting prenatal, labor, delivery, and follow-up care
J. Cesarean sections: more frequent now because of sophisticated fetal monitoring; controversial because of high numbers of sections in recent years
K. Breast-feeding: accepted and encouraged; societies such as La Leche League and popularity of "natural" foods encourage breast feeding
L. Genetic counseling: increasingly accurate, safe amniocentesis and advances in genetics encourage counselors to advise couples with genetic problems
M. In vitro method of fertilization to assist pregnancy/fetal development: usually chosen by couples with fertility problems after exploring various methods, including fertility drugs and other insemination practices

PROCEDURES TO DETERMINE MATERNAL/FETAL PROBLEMS

A. Alpha fetoprotein (AFP) test
1. Screening procedure, not diagnostic
2. Serum from maternal blood sample is tested; best results if sample is taken 16 to 18 weeks gestation; identifies unrecognized high-risk pregnancies
3. Elevated levels of maternal serum indicate 5% to 10% open neural tube defect (spina bifida) in developing fetus
4. Recommend two samples of test followed by ultrasound and amniocentesis to confirm findings; genetic counseling availability if confirmed
5. Other causes of elevated AFP levels: multiple gestation, missed calculations, missed abortions, other abnormalities

B. Amniocentesis: invasive procedure during which a needle is inserted through abdomen and uterus to withdraw amniotic fluid; usually done after 14th week
1. Used for determination of sex, defects in fetus (e.g., Down's syndrome); fetal status (Rh isoimmunal problem, fetal maturity, other tests as listed below)
2. Lecithin/sphingomyelin ratio (L/S ratio): used to determine fetal maturity by testing surfactant by 35th week of pregnancy; lecithin level two times greater than sphingomyelin level indicates that lungs are mature
3. Creatinine level: used to test fetal muscle mass and fetal renal function; 0.2 mg/100 ml amniotic fluid at 36 weeks is normal level; large amount may also indicate large fetus, such as fetus of diabetic mother
4. Bilirubin level: used for determination of fetal liver maturity; should decrease as term progresses; 450 μm is optimal density
5. Cytologic testing: determines percentage of lipid globules present in amniotic fluid; indicates fetal age

C. Chorionic villi test
1. Permits first-trimester testing for biochemical and chromosomal defects; invasive and high-risk procedure during which a plastic catheter is inserted vaginally into the uterus; ultrasound guides catheter to chorionic frondosum
2. Can be done 8 to 10 weeks after LMP
3. Done earlier than amniocentesis; recent evidence shows that test may increase risk of babies born with missing toes and fingers or shortened digits (Burton, 1992)

D. Fetoscopy: invasive procedure using transabdominal insertion of metal cannula into abdomen; visualization of fetus and placenta for developing abnormalities
1. High-risk procedure; complications include spontaneous abortion and premature labor
2. Has limited usage, only if defect cannot be detected otherwise

E. Estriol level study: 24-hour urinalysis of urine from mother; determines estriol level to ascertain fetal well-being and placental functioning
1. Done at third trimester (32 weeks)
2. 12 mg in 24 hours is good; below 12 mg indicates that infant is in jeopardy

F. Heterozygote testing (mother's blood): done to detect clinically normal carriers of mutant genes
1. Tay-Sachs disease: common fatal genetic disease affecting children of Ashkenazi Jews (Eastern Europe)
2. Sickle cell anemia: common disorder among black Americans of African descent; 1 in 10 American blacks is a carrier
3. Cooley's anemia (beta thalassemia): genetic disorder frequent among Mediterranean ethnic groups: Italians, Sicilians, Greeks, Turks, Middle Eastern Arabs, Asian Indians, Pakistanis

G. Oxytocin challenge test (OCT) or (stress test): late trimester test to measure placental insufficiency and measure fetal reaction to uterine contractions
1. Usually done after estimated date of confinement (EDC) has passed
2. Invasive procedure during which IV oxytocin is administered, baseline recorded on monitor; takes 20 minutes to 1 hour
3. Results: late decelerations during contraction for at least three contractions indicate a positive test; no decelerations during three successive contractions within 10 minutes indicate a negative test; occasionally inconsistent decelerations indicate suspicious conditions

H. Nonstress test (NST): assesses and evaluates fetal heart tone (FHT) response to uterine movement or increased fetal activity

I. Umbilical cord technique: evaluates condition of fetus
1. Superior technique because fetal blood can be analyzed as early as 18th week of gestation
2. Can evaluate blood count, liver function, blood gases, acid-base status
3. Invasive procedure

J. Ultrasound procedure: use of high-frequency sound waves to determine fetal size, estimate amniotic fluid volume, neural tube defects, limb abnormalities, and so forth
1. Usually a second-trimester procedure
2. Risks still under investigation

ANATOMY AND PHYSIOLOGY OF REPRODUCTION
Obstetric Pelvis

A. Types (Fig. 8-1)
1. Gynecoid: "true" female pelvis
2. Anthropoid: resembles pelvis of anthropoid apes
3. Android: male pelvis
4. Platyploid: flat pelvis

B. Components
1. Ilium: flat or lateral, flaring part of pelvis or hip; iliac crest is top part of ilium
2. Ischium: inferior dorsal or lower part of hip bone; the ischial spines, sharp projections of the ischium, are important in obstetrics because they are landmarks to measure progress of presenting part of fetus
3. Sacrum: triangular bone between the two hip bones; flat part of the lower back (spine)
4. Coccyx: two to five rudimentary vertebrae that are fused and attached to lower part of sacrum (tail bone)

C. Measurements
1. Diagonal conjugate: measured through vagina from lower border of symphysis pubis to promontory of sacrum (12.5 to 13 cm)

PURE TYPES

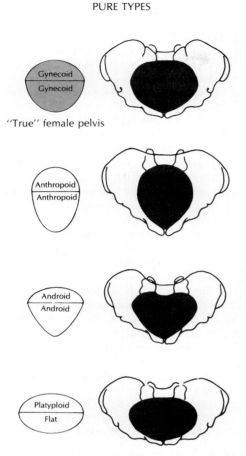

"True" female pelvis

FIG. 8-1. Female pelves: pure types. (From Bobak IM, Jensen MD: *Essentials of maternity nursing,* ed 2, St Louis, 1987, Mosby.)

2. Conjugate vera (true conjugate): measured from upper margin of symphysis pubis to promontory of sacrum by x-ray examination or sonogram (11 cm)
3. Transverse diameter: distance between inner surfaces of the tuberosities of ischium (13 to 13.5 cm)
4. Obstetric conjugate: measured by x-ray examination or sonogram or by subtracting 1.5 to 2 cm from diagonal conjugate (9.5 to 11.5 cm)

Fertilization and Implantation

A. Definitions
1. Fertilization: occurs when the sperm and ovum join, usually at the distal end of the fallopian tube within 12 to 48 hours after intercourse
2. Zygote: product of the union of a sperm and ovum
3. Implantation: occurs when zygote burrows into the endometrium of the uterus, approximately 7 days after fertilization
4. Nidation: completion of implantation
B. Processes
1. Mitosis: rapid cell division
2. Blastoderm: first division of the zygote
3. Morula: ball-like structure of the blastoderm; sometimes referred to as mulberry-like

4. Blastocyst: as morula enters uterus
5. Trophoblast: as blastocyst implants in the uterus, the wall becomes the trophoblast
6. Chorionic villi: trophoblasts develop villi that become fetal portion of the placenta
7. Decidua: endometrium undergoes a change when pregnancy occurs
8. Decidua vera: that portion of the decidua that becomes the lining of the uterus except for around implantation site
9. Decidua basalis: where implantation occurs and where chorionic villi become frondosum or the beginning of the placental formation
10. Decidua capsularis: covers blastocyst and fuses to form fetal membranes
11. Amnion: inner membrane, which comes from the zygote and blends with the cord
12. Chorion: outer membrane, which comes from the zygote and blends with the fetal portion of the placenta

Development of Human Organism

A. Ovum stage: preembryonic stage from conception until the primary villi appear (first 14 days)
B. Embryo: end of ovum stage to 8 weeks from LMP; period of rapid cellular development: disruption will cause developmental abnormality
C. Fetus: from end of embryonic stage (8 weeks) to term
D. Placenta: membrane weighing about 450g (1 lb); develops cotyledons that act as areas for nourishing fetus; maternal surface is beefy and red; fetal surface is shiny and gray
E. Amnionic cavity: fills with fluid (1000 ml) that is replaced every 3 hours; shelters fetus

Sex Determination

A. Normal sperm; carries 22 autosomes and 1 sex chromosome (either an X or a Y chromosome)
B. Normal ovum: carries 22 autosomes and 1 sex chromosome (always an X chromosome)
C. Combined number of chromosomes: 44 autosomes and 2 sex chromosomes (at conception)
D. Genetic component of sperm determines sex of child (see the example below)
E. Chromosome carries genes plus DNA and proteins
F. Genes: factors in chromosomes carrying hereditary characteristics

---

EXAMPLE

Sperm supplies 22 autosomes and an X sex chromosome
Ovum supplies 22 autosomes and an X sex chromosome
Result: 44 autosomes and XX = female

Sperm supplies 22 autosomes and a Y sex chromosome
Ovum supplies 22 autosomes and an X sex chromosome
Result: 44 autosomes and an XY = male

PHYSIOLOGY OF FETUS

A. Membranes and amniotic fluid
   1. Protect from blows and bumps mother may experience
   2. Maintain even heat to fetus
   3. Act as an excretory system
   4. Supply oral fluid for fetus
   5. Allow free movement of fetus
B. Placenta
   1. Transport organ: passes nutrients from mother to fetus and relays excretory material from fetus to mother
   2. Formation completed by 3 months
   3. Functions: kidney, lungs, stomach, and intestines
   4. Requirement: adequate oxygen from mother to function well
C. Monthly development
   1. Embryonic stage (1st to 8th week)
      a. Beginning: pulsating heart, spinal canal formation: no eyes or ears; buds for arms and legs
      b. By end: little over 1 inch (2.5 cm) long; eyelids fused; distinct divisions of arms, legs; cord formed; tail disappears
   2. Fetal stage (9th week to term)
      a. 3 months: 3 inches (7.5 cm) long; weighs 1 oz (28 g); fully formed arms, legs, fingers; distinguishable sex organs
      b. 4 months: development of muscles, movement; mother feels quickening; 6 to 7 inches (15 to 17.5 cm) long; weighs 4 oz (112 g); lanugo over body; head large
      c. 5 months: 10 to 12 inches (25 to 30 cm) long; weighs ½ to 1 lb (225 to 450 g); internal organs maturing; lungs immature; FHT heard on examination; eyes fused; rarely survives more than several hours
      d. 6 months: 11 to 14 inches (27.5 to 35 cm) long; weighs 1 to 1½ lb (450 to 675 g); wrinkled "old man" appearance; vernix caseosa covers body; eyelids separated; eyelashes and fingernails formed
      e. 7 months: begins to store fat and minerals; 16 inches (40 cm) long; may survive with excellent care
      f. 8 months: beginning of month weighs 2 to 3 lb (900 to 1350 g); by end of month, 4 to 5 lb (1800 to 2250 g); continues to develop; loses wrinkled appearance
      g. 9 months: 19 inches (47.5 cm) long; weighs 7 lb (3200 g) (girl) 7½ lb (3400 g) (boy); more fat under skin; vernix caseosa; has stored vitamins, minerals, and antibodies; fully developed
D. Fetal circulation
   1. Special structures
      a. Ductus venosus: passes through liver; connects umbilical vein to inferior vena cava; closes at birth
      b. Ductus arteriosus: shunts blood from pulmonary artery to descending aorta; closes almost immediately after birth
      c. Foramen ovale: valve opening that allows blood to flow from right atrium to left atrium; functionally closes at birth; all three fetal structures listed above allow blood to bypass the fetal lungs and liver
      d. Umbilical arteries: transport blood from the hypogastric artery to the placenta; functionally closes at birth
      e. Umbilical vein: transports oxygenated blood from placenta to ductus venosus and liver, then to the inferior vena cava (IVC); closes at birth
   2. Fetal circulation (Fig. 8-2)
      a. Oxygenated blood from placenta goes through umbilical vein, bypassing portal system of the liver by way of the ductus venosus
      b. From the ductus venosus blood goes to the ascending vena cava (inferior) to the heart, right auricle
      c. From the right auricle through the foramen ovale
      d. To the left auricle, then to the left ventricle
      e. Leaves the heart through the aorta to the arms and head
      f. The blood then returns to the heart, passing through the descending vena cava (superior)
      g. To the right auricle, then to the right ventricle
      h. Blood leaves the heart through the pulmonary arteries, bypassing the lungs
      i. Blood goes through the ductus arteriosus to the aorta and down to the trunk and lower extremities
      j. It then goes through the hypogastric arteries to the umbilical arteries on to the placenta, carrying carbon dioxide and waste materials

NORMAL ANTEPARTUM (PRENATAL)
Physiologic Changes During Pregnancy

A. Reproductive system
   1. External changes
      a. Perineum: increased vasculature; enlarges
      b. Labia majora: change especially in parous woman; separate and stretch
      c. Anal and vulvar varices: caused by increased pelvic congestion
   2. Internal changes
      a. Uterus: enlarges to accommodate growing fetus; walls thicken first trimester; *Hegar's* sign (soft, lower lip of uterus)
      b. Cervix: *Goodell's* sign (thickens, softens) 6 weeks from LMP because of vascular changes
      c. Vagina: *Chadwick's* sign (bluish violet color); mucosal changes about 8 weeks from LMP; estrogen activity may cause thick vaginal discharge
B. Other body system changes
   1. Breasts
      a. Increased size, tingling sensations, heavy
      b. Increased pigmentation, darkened areolae
      c. Montgomery's tubercles on areolae
   2. Cardiovascular changes
      a. Slight enlargement of heart resulting from increased blood volume
      b. Increased circulation (47%)
      c. Cardiac output increased 30% first and second trimester, then levels off until term; during labor and delivery increases; and about 13% above normal during postpartum period

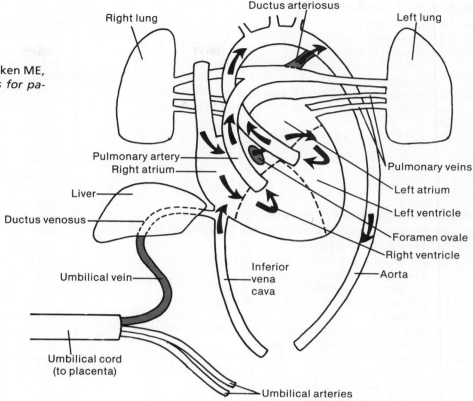

FIG. 8-2. Fetal circulation. (From Milliken ME, Campbell G: *Essential competencies for patient care,* St Louis, 1985, Mosby.)

Labels on figure: Right lung · Ductus arteriosus · Left lung · Pulmonary artery · Right atrium · Liver · Ductus venosus · Umbilical vein · Umbilical cord (to placenta) · Umbilical arteries · Inferior vena cava · Pulmonary veins · Left atrium · Left ventricle · Foramen ovale · Right ventricle · Aorta

3. Hematologic changes
   a. Increased RBC count; decreased hemoglobin level
   b. Increased tendency for blood to coagulate during pregnancy
   c. Coagulation factors return to normal during postpartum, increasing likelihood of thromboembolism
4. Respiratory/pulmonary changes: enlarging uterus presses on diaphragm, causing difficulty breathing
5. Skin: increased pigmentation
   a. Linea nigra: darkening line from below breast bone (sternum) over abdomen to symphysis pubis
   b. Chloasma gravidarum (mask of pregnancy): dark, frecklelike pigmentation over nose and cheeks; disappears after delivery
   c. Striae gravidarum: stretching of skin with silvery to reddish, bluish stretch marks on breasts, abdomen, thighs; never disappears completely; lotion, cocoa butter lubricants may help
6. Urinary system changes
   a. Traces of sugar in urine resulting from activity of lactiferous ducts
   b. Transitory albumin: may be indication of pending toxemia
   c. Cystitis: frequent because ureters lose some compliance or elasticity
7. Nervous system changes
   a. Nervous system may be affected in emotionally unstable women
   b. Prepregnancy psychosocial problems may be aggravated
8. Digestive system
   a. Morning sickness: nausea and vomiting common during first trimester
   b. Increased appetite after first trimester
   c. Indigestion (heartburn): caused by increasing upward pressure of enlarging uterus or by relaxin hormone, which slows metabolism and keeps food in stomach longer in pregnant women
   d. Constipation: caused by changes in organ positions; pressure of growing uterus on sigmoid colon
9. Weight gain: total weight gain varies from 25 to 30 lb (12 to 13.5 kg) (Table 8-1)

Table 8-1. Distribution of weight gain during pregnancy

Distribution	Pounds	Grams
Fetus	7½	3400
Placenta	1	450
Amniotic fluid	2	900
Uterus	2½	1125
Increased blood volume	3-4	1350-1800
Breasts	2-3	900-1350
Mother's gain (fat, tissue, etc.)	4-8	1800-3600
Total weight gain	21-28 lb	9.5-12.7 kg

Duration of Pregnancy

A. Length in terms of time
   1. 9 calendar months
   2. 10 lunar months
   3. 280 days (266 days from time of ovulation)
   4. 40 weeks
B. Nägele's rule: to calculate EDC count back 3 months from the month of the LMP and add 7 days to the first day of LMP

   EXAMPLE: first day of LMP was July 17

7 (July)	17
−3 months	+7
4th month	24 = EDC April 24

Signs and Symptoms of Pregnancy

A. Presumptive signs (subjective: mother usually notices)
   1. Missed menstrual period
   2. Breast changes: nipples tingle, fuller, darker areola in about 6 weeks
   3. Frequency of urination in about 6 weeks
   4. Morning sickness: nausea and vomiting in 4 to 6 weeks
   5. Skin changes: chloasma, linea nigra, striae (some authors call this "probable" sign)
B. Probable signs (objective: examiner usually notices)
   1. Uterus: enlarges; shape changes at 12 to 16 weeks; Hegar's sign: 8 weeks
   2. Cervix: Goodell's sign
   3. Vagina: Chadwick's sign
   4. Implantation site: softens, enlarges (von Fernwald's sign) 6 to 7 weeks
   5. Laboratory tests:
      a. Biologic: used before 1960; laboratory animals: Aschheim-Zondek (AZ) test and Friedman's test
      b. Immunologic: widely used today; faster, 90% accurate; beta subunit of HCG can be used even before missed period; home pregnancy tests can be used 9 days after missed period (for names of tests see Prenatal Care)
C. Positive signs (by examiner)
   1. Palpate: can feel fetal parts
   2. Hearing: fetal heart tone
      a. Electronic Doptone scope (audible at 8 to 11 weeks)
      b. Electrocardiogram (can ascertain at 12 weeks)
      c. Auscultation (17 to 24 weeks) with fetoscope (headscope) or Leff stethoscope
   3. Roentgenographic (x-ray) examination: reveals skeletal form; procedure not recommended during first and second trimester; use caution anytime during gestation
   4. Ultrasonographic (echographic) evidence of pregnancy visualized on screen

Prenatal Care

A. Importance
   1. Regular assessment and monitoring detect early signs and symptoms disrupting normal, healthy pregnancy
   2. Early evaluation of problem permits development of an appropriate plan of action based on findings
B. Visits and examinations
   1. Initial visit: establish diagnosis of pregnancy
      a. Latex agglutination inhibition (LAD) test: results in 2 minutes; accurate 4 to 10 days after missed period (e.g., Pregnosticon)
      b. Hemagglutination inhibition (HAD) test: more sensitive; results in 1 to 2 hours; accurate 4 days after missed period
      c. Radioreceptor assay test: serum test; results in 1 hour; accurate at time of missed period (e.g., Biocept G)
      d. Radioimmunoassay (RIA): most sensitive; results can range from 1 to 48 hours (depends on the degree of sensitivity required); can detect pregnancy 2 days after implantation
      e. Commercially sold pregnancy test: an HAI in-home test; results in 4 minutes; should be confirmed by a physician (e.g., ept [early pregnancy test])

      NOTE: All tests use urine from the mother
   2. Complete medical history
      a. General personal health, habits, diseases, and medical or surgical problems
      b. History of communicable diseases, especially scarlet fever, measles, rubella, streptococcus infections, kidney conditions that might adversely affect pregnancy
      c. Previous pregnancies, miscarriages, abortions, blood transfusions, gynecologic problems
      d. Family health status: diabetes, tuberculosis, heart disease, cancer, epilepsy, allergies, mental problems, drug abuse, particularly coke (cocaine), which is detrimental to both mother and baby
   3. Complete physical examination
      a. Routine laboratory tests
         (1) Matching blood type and Rh factor
         (2) Antibody screen (rubella, sickle cell) if appropriate
         (3) Hemoglobin and hematocrit
         (4) Venereal Disease Research Laboratory (VDRL) test (for syphilis)
         (5) Herpes 1 and 2 tests
         (6) HIV testing for the AIDS virus
         (7) Hepatitis A and B tests
      b. Physical examination to include
         (1) Pelvic examination and measurements
         (2) Abdominal palpation
         (3) Examination of breasts, nipples
         (4) Vital signs: blood pressure, weight, temperature, respirations
         (5) Urinalysis for sugar and albumin
         (6) Smears (Papanicolaou's test) for cytology, gonorrhea, chlamydia
   4. Usual schedule for prenatal visits
      a. Every month for 28 weeks
      b. Every 2 weeks thereafter to 36th week
      c. Every week from 37th week to term
      d. Adjusted to individual needs
   5. Usual routine for prenatal visits:
      a. Urinalysis each visit for sugar, acetone, albumin
      b. Capillary blood testing on a glucose oxidase strip for gestational diabetes mellitus (GDM); fol-

lowed by plasma glucose testing at 12 weeks'
gestation on all high-risk pregnancies

   c. Check vital signs (especially blood pressure)

   d. Check weight gain every visit

     (1) First trimester: 3 to 4 lb (1.5 to 2 kg) total

     (2) Second trimester: 1 lb (0.5 kg) per week; 12 to 14 lb (6 to 7 kg) total

     (3) Third trimester: 1 lb (0.5 kg) per week; 8 to 10 lb (4 to 5 kg) total

   e. Measure height of fundus to evaluate growth of fetus (Fig. 8-3)

   f. Listen to FHT and FHR by Doptone or auscultation

   g. Ask about fetal activity, attitude of family; answer mother's questions, fears

   h. Recommend childbirth education classes

C. Promotion of positive health

   1. Nutritional counseling

     a. Fetus receives all nourishment from mother

     b. Teenage pregnant mother requires extensive counseling (nutritional pattern poor); focus on positive effect of good nutrition on teenager as well as on fetus

     c. Salt restrictions may be advised in presence of edema, retention of fluids, sudden change in blood pressure

     d. Direct relationship between maternal nutrition and mental development of the child

   2. Nutritional needs during pregnancy: Table 8-2

   3. General health teaching

     a. Daily baths for cleanliness; showers during last 6 weeks for safety's sake

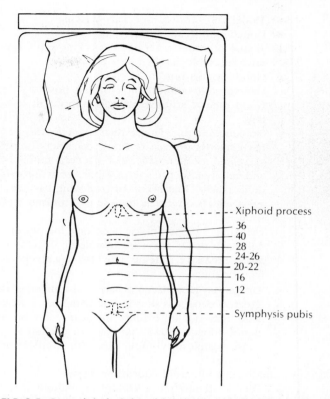

FIG. 8-3. Growth in height of fundus by weeks. (From Bobak IM, Jensen MD: *A modular study guide to maternity care*, St Louis, 1982, Mosby.)

Table 8-2. Nutritional needs during pregnancy

Nutrient	Nonpregnant woman (19-22 yr)	Pregnant woman	Usage	Food source

Protein	44 g	74-100 g; needs twice as much	Growth of fetus
			  Placental growth
			  During labor and delivery
			  During lactation
				Milk, cheese, eggs, meat, grains, legumes, nuts

Major minerals				

Calcium	800 mg	1200 mg; needs one and a half times as much	Fetal skeleton
			  Fetal teeth buds
			  Calcium metabolism in mother
				Milk, cheese, whole grains, leafy vegetables, egg yolk

Phosphorus	800 mg	1200 mg; needs one and a half times as much		Milk, cheese, lean meats
Iron (Fe)	18 mg	30-60 mg supplement; needs almost two to three times as much	Increased maternal blood volume Fetus stores iron in third trimester	Liver, meats, eggs, leafy vegetables, nuts, legumes, whole wheat
Vitamin C (not stored in body so pregnant mother should take at least 1 serving per day)	60 mg	80 mg	Tissue formation Increased iron absorption	Citrus fruits, berries, melon, tomatoes, green peppers, green leafy vegetables, broccoli

Vitamin D	5-10 µg*; 200-400 IU†	10-15 µg; 400-600 IU needs almost twice as much	Tooth buds
			  Mineralize bone tissue
			  Aid absorption of calcium and phosphorus
				Fortified milk
				Fortified margarine

*µg = microgram.
†IU = international units.

b. Moderate exercise, especially walking
c. Douching only on advice of physician
d. Sexual intercourse permissible as long as it is not uncomfortable and cervix is closed
e. Good support bra
f. Unrestrictive comfortable clothing, hose
g. Good mental attitude; discuss ambivalent feelings
h. Smoking: nicotine (more than six cigarettes per day) retards growth of fetus, constricts blood vessels in mother, decreases placental function, and may cause premature labor; growing evidence shows that secondary smoking has damaging effects on the mother, fetus, children, and spouses
i. Drinking: 5 oz of whisky, beer, or wine per day will have major adverse physiologic effects on fetus; excessive caffeine may also negatively affect the fetus
j. Drugs: May pass placental barrier and affect fetus; greatest danger is during first trimester, but effects may not be evident for years after birth; new evidence shows that crack or cocaine may cause significant complications for mother and newborn
4. Childbirth and parent education classes
a. Dick-Read method ("childbirth without fear") (1944): philosophy of relaxation coupled with abdominal and chest breathing and education
b. Lamaze method American Society for Prophylaxis in Obstetrics [ASPO]; psychoprophylactic method [PPM]) 1960: combines breathing techniques with preparation for childbirth by training mother to anticipate various stages of labor and meet each stage with practiced relaxation and breathing methods; coach to support mother and direct her if necessary
c. Bradley method, 1965: husband-coached childbirth, emphasizing quiet, darkened atmosphere, no stress
5. Teaching danger signs (those that must be reported to physician immediately)
a. Persistent, severe vomiting beyond first trimester
b. Epigastric or abdominal pain
c. Edema: face, fingers; especially in the morning
d. Visual disturbances: blurring, double vision, spots
e. Frequent or continuous headaches
f. Bleeding or "leakage of fluid" from vagina
g. Absence of fetal movements (after quickening)
h. Chills and fever (signs of infection)
i. Rapid weight gain (signs of possible preeclampsia)

Normal Discomforts of Pregnancy

Table 8-3

ABNORMAL ANTEPARTUM
Hypertensive States

A. Definition: a group of conditions that occur during pregnancy usually after 20 weeks' gestation: symptoms can range from high blood pressure (BP) to headaches, blurred vision, and convulsions with ensuing coma
1. Frequent in high-risk mothers
2. Greater likelihood during first pregnancies
3. Incidence: 5% to 7% of all pregnancies
B. Types
1. Pregnancy-induced hypertension (PIH): increase of blood pressure to or above 140/90 mm Hg
a. Increased BP only symptom
b. Disappears within 10 days following delivery
2. Preeclampsia: an acute hypertensive condition resulting in elevated BP and proteinurea; edema may also be present
a. Mild preeclampsia:
(1) BP 140/90
(2) Proteinurea 1+
(3) Rapid weight gain
b. Moderate-to-severe preeclampsia
(1) Hospitalize stat
(2) BP 160/110
(3) Albumin 2+ to 4+
(4) Persistent, severe headaches with visual disturbances
(5) Epigastric pain (late sign)
(6) Hyperactive: twitching musculature
3. Eclampsia
a. Definition: most severe form of the hypertensive states, characterized by hypertensive crisis, shock, or convulsions and possibly coma
b. Signs and symptoms
(1) Alarming weight gain
(2) Scanty urine (less than 30 ml/hour)
(3) Proteinurea 4+, red blood cells (RBCs) in urine
(4) BP 200/100 or higher
(5) Edema of retina; can cause blindness
(6) Severe epigastric pain
(7) Convulsions: tonic and clonic
NOTE: May start labor prematurely; infant may be severely compromised and die
C. Treatment and nursing management
1. According to classification and severity of symptoms; varies from home care precautions to absolute bed rest in a hospital with patient lying on left side
2. Reduce stimuli
3. Convulsion precautions
4. Selective antihypertensive and diuretic therapy may be ordered (e.g., hydalazine [Apresoline] hydrochloride, furosemide [Lasix], magnesium sulfate, mannitol); nurse should know effects and untoward symptoms
5. Monitor edema, BP, FHT, levels of consciousness, reflexes, impending labor signs

Hyperemesis Gravidarum

A. Definition: pernicious vomiting of pregnancy lasting into second trimester
B. Signs and symptoms
1. Excessive nausea and vomiting
2. Considerable weight loss
3. Severe dehydration
4. Depletion of essential electrolytes (sodium and potassium)

Table 8-3. Normal discomforts of pregnancy

Discomfort	Probable cause	Relief measures
First trimester		
Breasts: painful	Hypertrophy of glandular tissue Increased blood flow to area Hormonal effects	Firm, supportive bra; even a nursing bra
Urinary frequency	Pressure on bladder from expanding uterus reduces bladder capacity; increased vascular content	Pads if necessary
Yawning (tired, sleepy)	Whether result of relaxin hormone is questionable; possibly caused by sudden chemical changes in body	Frequent rest periods Balanced diet to prevent anemia
Nausea/vomiting	Hormonal changes Ambivalent feelings regarding pregnancy	Small, frequent meals Limited fluids Dry crackers with tea Avoid greasy fried foods
Second trimester		
Heartburn (acid taste in mouth)	Relaxin hormone effect Enlarging uterus displaces stomach upward	Avoid fatty foods Antacids: Milk of Magnesia, Gelusil, Maalox, Amphojel
Pigmentation (face)	Hormonal	Reassure mother that it is temporary and will disappear after delivery
Leg cramps	Calcium-phosphorus imbalance	Position relief Calf stretching Calcium supplements, milk
Constipation	Hormonal: slowing down of peristaltic movements Compression of colon by uterus and baby	Adequate fluids, fruits, foods with roughage Exercises Stool softener but no mineral oil
Third trimester		
Urinary incontinence	Lightening/dropping of fetus into pelvic cavity pushes presenting part on bladder	Pelvic floor exercise (Kegel): tighten perineal muscles, relax, then repeat
Hemorrhoids	Pressure from fetal presenting part Increased vascular activity	Knee-chest (elevate hips): Kegel exercises Comfort measures: frequent rest periods; sitting in warm tub; supporting legs with pillows
Low back pain	Increased pressure Fatigue Poor weight distribution	Pelvic exercises Pushing, stretching Comfort massaging Good posture
Insomnia	Increased fetal movements Muscular cramping Frequency Dyspnea	Adequate rest periods Warm milk at bedtime Relaxing shower Support with pillows Deep breathing
Varicosities (leg, vulva)	Hereditary disposition Pelvic vasocongestion Pull of gravity Pressure of uterus Forcing stool (constipation)	Support stockings Changing position frequently Abdominal support Keeping legs uncrossed
Edema (legs, feet)	Immobility (staying in one position for a prolonged time)	Periodic resting Moving around Support stockings Elevating legs Plenty of fluids (to serve as diuretic)
Dyspnea (shortness of breath)	Pressure on diaphragm from expanding uterus	Sitting erect Deep breathing Putting arms above head Keeping weight down
Leaking of colostrum	Increased blood supply Prominent nipples	Support bra Pads if necessary (keep clean and dry)
Supine hypotension syndrome (feel faint)	Pressure on ascending vena cava by uterus	Lying on left side with legs flexed or semi-sitting position
Vaginal discharge	Hormonal	No douching Keep area clean, dry (perineal care)

5. Vitamin, glucose, and protein deficiencies
6. Ketone bodies in urine: 1 + protein
7. Elevated hemoglobin level, RBC count, and hematocrit

C. Treatment and nursing management: untreated will lead to death of mother or child or both
   1. Hospitalize in well-ventilated, private, pleasant environment
   2. No visitors, not even husband first 48 hours
   3. Nothing by mouth (NPO) first 48 hours
   4. Record intake and output (I & O)
   5. Intravenous (IV) fluids to replace losses in nutrition
   6. Gradual serving of attractive, small portions of food on china dishes, starting with dry toast and tea
   7. Nonjudgmental nursing attitudes
   8. Refer for psychotherapy when appropriate

Hemorrhagic Conditions

A. Abortion (early pregnancy bleeding)
   1. Definition: the expulsion of uterine contents before term for medical reasons or spontaneously
   2. Types
      a. Induced abortion
         (1) Therapeutic: legal aborting of the fetus for medical or psychologic reasons by a licensed physician under controlled, aseptic conditions
         (2) Criminal: an abortion performed under illegal, unsafe conditions
      b. Spontaneous abortions
         (1) Definition: an abortion that occurs naturally (usually in the first trimester)
         (2) Possible causes: hormonal deficiencies, abnormalities of the fetus, incompetent cervix, abnormalities of the reproductive organs, emotional shock, physical injury, acute infections, growths, and so on
   3. Terminology of abortions
      a. Habitual abortion: three or more consecutive spontaneous abortions for unknown reasons
      b. Threatened abortion: minimal signs and symptoms of abortion such as bleeding and cramping but with no loss of uterine contents
      c. Imminent abortion: considerable blood loss, severe contractions, urge to push that without treatment will result in loss of uterine contents
      d. Inevitable abortion: bleeding, contractions, rupture of membranes, and cervical dilatation in which the uterine contents will be lost, so treatment will concentrate on the mother
      e. Incomplete abortion: part(s) of uterine contents retained, necessitating administration of oxytocins to accelerate expulsion of remaining contents, or dilatation and curettage (D & C; a minor surgical intervention) to prevent prolonged bleeding
      f. Complete abortion: entire uterine contents are expelled
   4. Signs and symptoms of abortion
      a. Vaginal bleeding: scant to profuse
      b. Abdominal cramping: slight to severe
      c. Contractions: intermittent, steady, mild, or severe

   5. Treatment and nursing management
      a. Prompt and immediate bed rest
      b. Hospitalization when appropriate
      c. Prevention of blood loss and shock
      d. Replacement blood treatment if necessary
      e. Checking vital signs and temperature for 24 hours
      f. Endocrine therapy when appropriate
      g. Surgical intervention when appropriate: Shirodkar operation (purse-string suturing) for known incompetent cervix
      h. Psychotherapy when appropriate
         (1) Prepare for grieving process
         (2) Provide assistance for burial regulations
         (3) Let mother vent feelings of love, loss, guilt
         (4) Quiet, supportive, compassionate nursing care

B. Ectopic pregnancy (early pregnancy bleeding)
   1. Definition: an extrauterine pregnancy in which the products of conception are implanted outside the uterine cavity; 90% occur in the fallopian tube (right tube more frequent); other sites include the abdomen or the ovary
   2. Signs and symptoms
      a. Abnormal or missed menstrual period
      b. Slight uterine bleeding or spotting
      c. Possible mass on affected side; pain, tenderness, rigid abdomen
      d. If tube ruptures, may be little bleeding externally, but massive internal hemorrhaging with accompanying severe shock
   3. Treatment and nursing management
      a. Hospitalization stat
      b. Treat shock, (warm, quiet, replacement therapy—IV fluids, oxygen, etc.)
      c. Cross match and other blood work: transfusion readiness
      d. Support mother who will be extremely frightened
      e. Prepare for stat surgery if appropriate
      f. Arrange for baptism of fetus when appropriate
      g. Postsurgical care with IV fluids, medications, other appropriate treatments (RhoGAM if necessary)
      h. Provide emotional support to mother and family; get assistance of clergy when requested

C. Hydatidiform mole (early pregnancy bleeding)
   1. Definition: rare degeneration of chorionic villi into a benign neoplasm in which the villi fill with clear viscous fluid and form grapelike clusters; the neoplasm fills the decidua and expands the uterus to larger than normal for gestational age
   2. Signs and symptoms
      a. Enlarging uterus, greater than for normal gestation
      b. Missed period; spotting to profuse bleeding
      c. Several shiny, tapioca-like "grape clusters" escape through vaginal tract
      d. Nausea and vomiting
      e. Signs of pregnancy-induced hypertension (PIH); usually before 20 weeks' gestation
      f. No FHT
      g. Ultrasound reveals no fetal structures

h. Laboratory findings: human chorionic gonado-tropin (HCG) titers up to 1 to 2 million (normally 350,000 to 400,000 at 8 weeks)

3. Treatment and nursing management
   a. Termination as soon as diagnosis confirmed
   b. Blood transfusion if indicated
   c. Assistance in grieving process of mother and family
   d. Follow-up very important
      (1) Contraceptive advice (no oral since that will distort HCG titers)
      (2) HCG titers for at least 6 months

D. Placenta previa (third-trimester bleeding)
   1. Definition: abnormal implantation of a normal placenta for unknown reasons, usually in the lower segment of the uterus; condition usually occurs in multiparas, and incidence appears to increase with age; may also be caused by fibroids
   2. Types (Fig. 8-4)
      a. Partial (incomplete): incomplete coverage of the uterine os
      b. Complete (total): entire uterine os completely covered
      c. Marginal (low lying): located in lower uterine segment but away from the os
   3. Signs and symptoms
      a. Painless uterine bleeding: may be intermittent or occur in gushes; scanty to severe; bright red
      b. Third-trimester occurrence
   4. Treatment and nursing management
      a. Diagnosis confirmed by ultrasound or x-ray examination
      b. Avoidance of vaginal examinations
      c. Hospitalization stat
      d. Quiet environment; fetus uncompromised; station high
      e. Fowler's position (head at 30-degree angle)
      f. Tocolytic therapy with use of magnesium sulfate to manage uterine irritability under certain circumstances

   g. Have double set-up ready so if vaginal examination is imperative, emergency cesarean section equipment is available and blood is ready for transfusion
   h. Foley catheter if condition is severe; shock care
   i. Count pads to determine amount, color, duration of bleeding
   j. Monitor vital signs, especially blood pressure
   k. Monitor FHT and FHR
   l. IV fluids
   m. Support patient and family; keep them informed

E. Abruptio placentae (third-trimester bleeding)
   1. Definition: premature separation of a normally implanted placenta before the birth of the fetus
   2. Causes
      a. Trauma
      b. Chronic maternal disease
      c. Grand multipara
      d. Unknown
   3. Types (Fig. 8-5)
      a. Complete: separation of the placenta from the uterine wall before birth of the fetus
      b. Partial: separation of a portion of the placenta from the wall of the uterus before the birth of the fetus
   4. Signs and symptoms
      a. Severe abdominal pain; sometimes called "exquisite"
      b. Patient is distressed, depressed, and exhibit signs of shock
      c. Painful bleeding: moderate to severe; internal or external; dark red, not clotted; amount varies
      d. Abdomen tense, boardlike; nurse unable to feel contractions; uterus irritable
      e. Hypovolemic shock can result in renal failure
      f. Sudden change in heart beat or bradycardia, or absence of FHT
   5. Treatment and nursing management
      a. Depends on stage and intensity of condition; for reasons not clearly understood, partial abruptio

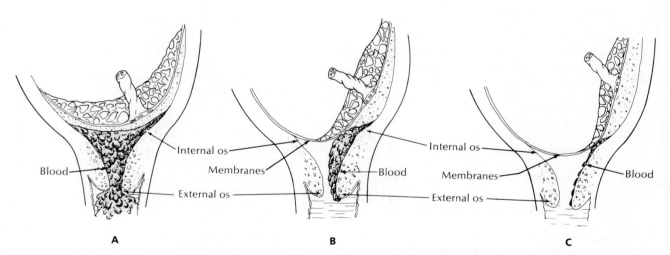

FIG. 8-4. Types of placenta previa after onset of labor. **A,** Complete, or total. **B,** Incomplete, or partial. **C,** Marginal, or low-lying. (From Bobak IM, Jensen MD: *Essentials of maternity nursing,* ed 2, St Louis, 1987, Mosby.)

ABRUPTIO PLACENTAE (Premature Separation)

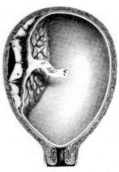
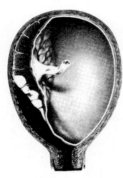
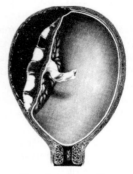

Partial Separation
(Concealed Hemorrhage)

Partial Separation
(Apparent Hemorrhage)

Complete Separation
(Concealed Hemorrhage)

FIG. 8-5. Abruptio placentae. (From Ross Laboratories Nursing Education Service, 1978. Reprinted with permission of Ross Laboratories, Columbus, Ohio.)

placentae may seal off bleeding spontaneously, and labor will proceed normally
   b. Check coagulation profile: fibrinogen/fibrin, platelets
   c. Prevent hypovolemic shock and fetal hypoxia
   d. Cross match, type, readiness for transfusions
   e. Monitor contractions, FHT, and vital signs
   f. Slight or moderate bleeding may indicate artificial rupture of membranes (ARM) to hasten delivery or seal off bleeding
   g. Severe bleeding (dark red) may indicate immediate cesarean section
   h. Support mother and family
   i. Continued bleeding after delivery may necessitate hysterectomy
F. Disseminated intravascular coagulation (DIC)
   1. Cause
      a. Unknown
      b. Coincidental with abruptio placentae, postabortal infection, amniotic fluid emboli
   2. Pathology: not clearly understood; massive clotting, depletion of coagulant factor
   3. Signs and symptoms: Excessive bleeding at placental site, incisional site, nose, mouth, gums
   4. Treatment and nursing management
      a. Halt or reverse DIC
      b. Eliminate cause
      c. Delivery stat
      d. Blood replacement
      e. IV fibrinogen/heparin

Medical and Infectious Conditions

A. Chickenpox (varicella)
   1. Causative agent: herpesvirus; varicella zoster virus (VZV)
   2. Effect on mother
      a. May manifest itself as herpes zoster (shingles)
      b. May be fatal if severe
      c. May cause abortion
   3. Effect on fetus

   a. May cause defects of skin, bones, hydrocephalus if contracted during first trimester
      b. Fetal death
B. German measles (rubella or 3-day measles)
   1. Causative agent: virus
   2. Effect on mother
      a. Rash, fever, photophobia
      b. Possible abortion
   3. Effect on fetus if infected during first trimester
      a. Rubella syndrome: heart defects, blindness, deafness, mental retardation
      b. Delayed effect on brain (15 to 20 years of age)
C. Genital herpes
   1. Causative agent: herpes simplex virus 2
   2. Effect on mother
      a. Vaginal discharge
      b. Genital blisters, ulcers
      c. Fever
      d. Painful inguinal lymph nodes
   3. Effect on fetus
      a. Abortion or premature birth
      b. Neonatal infections
      c. Survivors may have CNS symptoms
D. Group B streptococcus
   1. Causative agent: *Streptococcus* bacterium
   2. Effect on mother: septicemia
   3. Effect on fetus
      a. Neonatal death (stillborn)
      b. Blindness, deafness, mental retardation
E. Hepatitis A
   1. Causative agent: virus
   2. Effect on mother
      a. Abortion
      b. Liver failure
   3. Effect on fetus
      a. First-trimester infection: fetal anomalies
      b. Premature birth
      c. Neonatal hepatitis
F. Hepatitis B (serum hepatitis)
   1. Causative agent: virus (HBV)

2. Effect on mother
   a. Prolonged illness
   b. Destruction of liver cells
   c. Cirrhosis
3. Effect on fetus
   a. Preterm at birth
   b. May be asymptomatic at birth
   c. May exhibit signs of acute hepatitis
   d. Possible carrier
4. Vaccine available for high-risk women and health care workers

G. Influenza
   1. Causative agent: virus
   2. Effect on mother
      a. Pneumonia
      b. Abortion
      c. Premature labor
   3. Effect on fetus
      a. Abortion or premature birth
      b. Fetal death
   4. Vaccine for pregnant women available; live viral vaccine can infect fetus

H. Gonorrhea (clap)
   1. Causative agent: *Neisseria gonorrhoeae* bacterium
   2. Effect on mother
      a. Vaginal discharge
      b. Cervical tenderness
      c. Dysuria
      d. Affects ovaries, tubes, causing sterility
   3. Effect on fetus
      a. Ophthalmia neonatorum
      b. Conjunctivitis
      c. Mild-to-severe infections

I. Syphilis (lues)
   1. Causative agent: *Treponema pallidum* bacterium
   2. Effect on mother (if untreated)
      a. Primary chancre
      b. Secondary skin rash
      c. Latent or tertiary CNS problems
   3. Effect on fetus
      a. Rhagades of the corners of mouth and anus
      b. Snuffles
      c. Maceration of palms of hands and soles of feet
      d. Congenital syphilis (symptoms appearing later in life)
      e. Death (stillborn)

J. Cardiac disease
   1. Classification
      a. Class I: no limitation of activity
      b. Class II: slight limitation of activity
      c. Class III: considerable limitation of even ordinary activity
      d. Class IV: symptoms of cardiac insufficiency even at rest
   2. Treatment and nursing management
      a. Close medical and nursing supervision
      b. Watch for signs and symptoms of fatigue, dyspnea, coughing, palpitations, tachycardia
      c. Promote rest
      d. Hospitalize at end of second trimester
      e. Breast feeding contraindicated
      f. Contraceptive education (consider moral obligations)

g. Nutrition: offer foods high in iron and protein; avoid raw, deep green vegetables, because vitamin K counteracts effects of heparin
h. Prevent infections: report first signs of exposure
i. Teach comfortable positions: pillows, support, left side
j. During labor and delivery: saddle block; caudal block to minimize discomfort on bearing down
k. Watch for cardiac decompensation (pulse rate over 100 beats/min; respirations, 25+)
l. Vaginal delivery preferred
   (1) Episiotomy, low forceps
   (2) Oxygen to decrease pulmonary edema
   (3) Medication to regulate heart rate
   (4) Diuretic to reduce fluid retention
m. Postpartal care
   (1) Hospitalized at least 7 to 10 days to stabilize cardiac output
   (2) Application of abdominal binder (because of rapid change in intraabdominal pressure)
   (3) Bed rest with progressive bathroom privileges dependent on progress
   (4) Prevent overdistention of bladder
   (5) Encourage bonding; nurse should hold baby at eye level to allow mother to touch and talk to baby
   (6) Inform mother and family of progress

K. Diabetes mellitus
   1. Definition: inborn error in the transportation and metabolism of carbohydrates
   2. Classification
      a. Class A
         (1) Gestational diabetes mellitus (GDM) occurs with onset of pregnancy or later in pregnancy; caused by an intolerance to carbohydrates
         (2) Classified as *A* according to plasma glucose readings of 140 mg/dL after regular screening procedure
         (3) Return to normal after delivery (usually 6 weeks)
      b. Class B: frank diabetes; duration 9 years; unable to use oral hypoglycemics
      c. Class C: duration 10 to 19 years
      d. Class D
         (1) Duration 20 years or more
         (2) Vascular complications such as retinopathy and calcification of leg muscles
      e. Class E
         (1) Vascular complications
         (2) Calcification in pelvic area
      f. Class F; Same as class E plus retinopathy and kidney complications
   3. Effects of diabetes on pregnancy
      a. Difficult to control because of changing patterns of fetal growth and development and maternal demands
      b. Fluctuating insulin requirements
      c. Tendency to develop acidosis (diabetic coma) from lack of insulin
      d. Increased tendency to infection (urinary tract, vaginal tract), preeclampsia, and polyhydramnios

e. Increased incidence of premature labor
f. Oversized baby
g. Possibility of dystocia
h. Increased danger of placental deterioration causing hypoxia in fetus
i. Tendency to abruptio placentae
4. Changing insulin requirements during pregnancy
a. First trimester: insulin requirement decreased
b. Second trimester: insulin requirement increased
c. Third trimester: careful regulation (blood sugar); evaluation of placenta, oxytocin challenge test (OCT)
d. Intranatal: labor depletes glycogen
e. Postpartum: insulin reaction resulting from sudden drop in need
f. Watch for hypoglycemia, shock, infection, bleeding
g. No need for insulin 24 to 48 hours after delivery
h. Hospitalized until insulin balance restored
5. Early recognition of insulin reaction and diabetic coma
6. Treatment and nursing management
a. Weekly prenatal visits
b. Regulation of insulin dosage and dietary management
c. Mother taught to test urine/blood three or four times a day
d. Testing for placental adequacy: OCT (stress test) measures fetal response to uterine contractions; late deceleration indicates problem
e. Teach good nutrition
f. Help allay fears and anxieties
L. Addiction and pregnancy
1. Drug addiction
a. Effect on mother
(1) Abortion
(2) Premature birth
(3) Stillbirth
b. Effect on neonate: see Abnormal Newborn
2. Alcohol and pregnancy
a. Effect on mother
(1) Poor nutritional habits
(2) Poor hygiene
(3) Physical, psychosocial deterioration
b. Effect on neonate: see Abnormal Newborn
3. Treatment and nursing management
a. Supervised withdrawal
b. Substitute therapy

Acquired Immunodeficiency Syndrome (AIDS)

Pregnant women whose partners were drug users sharing common needles, high-risk category men—bisexual or homosexual—or men who were infected with the disease have been known to become infected. Transmission of the HIV virus to the unborn fetus has now been confirmed.
A. Confirmed avenues of transmission
1. Anal/vaginal intercourse
2. Drug addicts sharing needles of infected users
3. Contaminated blood transfusions
B. Statistics
1. Highest incidence of AIDS is in New York, then California, Florida, New Jersey, and Texas

2. In New York City, as of December 1987, 1 of every 61 newborns carried antibodies of the AIDS virus; 40% will eventually exhibit signs and symptoms of AIDS
C. Centers for Disease Control (CDC) guidelines for preventing transmission of the AIDS virus
1. Wear gloves when in contact with body fluids, mucous membranes and nonintact skin; wear gloves when performing venipuncture or when handling items soiled with blood or body fluids
2. Change gloves after caring for each patient; wash hands and most of your exposed surfaces with soap and water
3. Wear masks, gown, and apron (if available); protect mucous membranes of your mouth, nose, and eyes
4. Prevent injuries from needles, sharp instruments, toys, and other products; be alert when handling, cleaning, and disposing of instruments
5. Avoid needle pricks; all sharp items that have been used should be placed in puncture-resistant containers
6. To minimize need for emergency mouth-to-mouth resuscitation, keep resuscitation bags, mouthpieces, and ventilation devices in easily located areas
7. Refrain from direct patient care and do not handle patient care equipment if you have open lesions, weeping dermatitis, and so forth
8. Pregnant nurses should be especially careful, as an HIV infection could place the fetus at risk
D. Minimum precautions for invasive procedures
1. Wear gloves and surgical masks for all invasive procedures
a. Prevent skin and mucous membrane contact with blood and other body fluids by using appropriate barrier precautions
b. Wear protective eye wear or face shields, gowns, or aprons for procedures resulting in splashing of blood or other body fluids
2. Wear gloves and gowns when handling placenta or the infant until blood and amniotic fluid has been removed from the infant's skin and during postdelivery care of the umbilical cord
3. Put on new gloves as soon as patient safety permits should you tear a glove or be injured by a needlestick or other injury

Premature Labor

A. Definition: labor occurring before 37 to 38 weeks' gestation
B. Effect on family (focus on psychosocial problems)
1. Mother not ready for delivery: apprehensive and frightened; may feel guilty
2. Family plus professional staff: restrained, quiet, anticipating complications
C. Effect on fetus: see The Premature under Abnormal Newborn
D. Treatment and nursing management
1. Usually premature rupture of membranes precedes premature labor; test fluid with nitrazine paper: if alkaline, positive for amniotic fluid
2. If membranes intact and cervix undilated, halt labor if possible

3. Bed rest stat
4. Monitor maternal pulse and blood pressure
5. Know untoward effects of medications
6. Prevent infection
7. Offer constant emotional support to mother and family: inform, reassure, encourage mother and family

NORMAL INTRAPARTUM (LABOR AND DELIVERY)

A. Fetal head (passenger)
1. Two parietal bones: one each side of head
2. Two temporal bones: one each side of head near temple
3. Two frontal bones: one each side of forehead
4. One occipital bone: lower back of head
5. Sutures: membranous spaces between bones
   a. Sagittal suture: separates parietal bones and extends longitudinally back to front
   b. Frontal suture: between two frontal bones and is continuation of the sagittal suture
   c. Coronal suture: like a crown, separates frontal and parietal bones
   d. Lambdoidal suture: separates occipital bone from two parietal bones
6. Fontanels: formed by intersection of sutures; allow head bones to override and accommodate to birth passage
   a. Anterior fontanel: membranous, diamond-shaped space (bregma) formed by intersection of sagittal, frontal, and coronal sutures; called "soft spot"; closes within 12 to 18 months
   b. Posterior fontanel: small, membranous triangle-shaped space between occipital bone and two parietal bones; closes within 6 to 8 weeks
7. Principal measurements of the fetal head
B. Presentations, positions, station
1. Presentation
   a. Definition: refers to that part of the passenger (fetus) that enters the passage (true pelvis, uterine os, vaginal canal) first
   b. Types of presentations
      (1) Cephalic: head, vertex, occiput (93%)
      (2) Breech: buttocks, sacrum, leg(s), foot (feet) (3%)
      (3) Shoulder: scapula (3%)
2. Lie (Fig. 8-6)
   a. Definition: refers to the relationship between the long axis of the passenger to the long axis of the mother
   b. Types
      (1) Longitudinal (99%)
      (2) Transverse (sideways)
3. Position (Fig. 8-7)
   a. Definition: the way in which the presenting part of the fetus lies in relation to the four quadrants of the mother's pelvis and to her back (posterior) and her front (anterior)
   b. To determine position, fetal "reference points" are used, and they are
      (1) Occiput (back of fetal head): O
      (2) Chin (mentum): M
      (3) Brow (bregma): B
      (4) Buttocks (sacrum): S

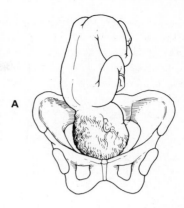

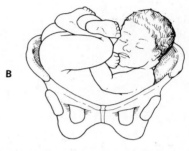

FIG. 8-6. **A,** Longitudinal lie. **B,** Transverse lie. (From Philips CR: *Family-centered maternity/newborn care: a basic text,* ed 2, St Louis, 1987, Mosby.)

      (5) Shoulder (scapula): Sc
      (6) Transversus
   c. Types of position with occiput presentations: LOA, LOT, LOP, ROA, ROT, ROP, (see Fig. 8-7)
4. Attitude
   a. Definition: relationship of the various fetal parts to one another, or the relationship of the fetal extremities to its body (trunk)
   b. Normal attitude: flexed; fetal head on sternum; arms folded against chest; knees bent, pressing abdomen; legs flexed so toes touch arm
5. Station
   a. Definition: degree to which presenting part is located in the true pelvis; points of reference are the ischial spines, which are designated as *0* (zero)
   b. Levels
      (1) Minus: as in -1, -2, -3 station, means that presenting part is above the ischial spines
      (2) Plus: as in $+1$, $+2$, $+3$ station, means that the presenting part is below the ischial spines
      (3) -5 = floating; $+5$ = presenting part on perineum; or -3 to -5 = floating; $+3$ to $+5$ = presenting part on perineum; check with agency for the numbers used
C. Mechanisms and stages of labor: labor cannot progress without power
1. Definition: the steps or maneuvers the fetus must undertake to accommodate to the passage and be delivered

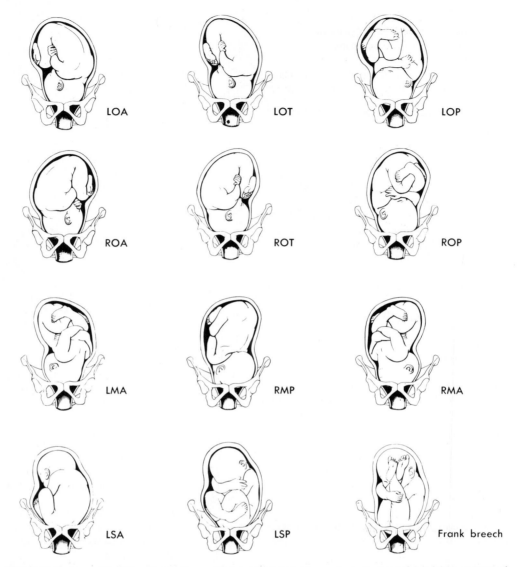

FIG. 8-7. Categories of presentations. (From Obstetrical presentation and position, Ross Laboratories Nursing Education Service, 1978. Reprinted with permission of Ross Laboratories, Columbus, Ohio.)

2. Process (mechanisms) (Fig. 8-8)
   a. Engagement: passage of the passenger into the pelvic inlet
   b. Descent: continuous slow progress of the fetus through the pelvis and the birth canal
   c. Flexion: head slowly adapts to birth canal by flexing chin
   d. Internal rotation: fetal head turns in corkscrew maneuver so the long diameter of the head is parallel to the longest diameter of the pelvic outlet
   e. Extension: the back of the fetal head goes under the pubic arch; the spine of the fetus extends to adapt itself to the curvature of the birth canal, and the head is delivered
   f. Restitution: as the head emerges, it rotates back 45 degrees to the position it was before internal rotation, which helps the shoulders accommodate to the outlet
   g. External rotation: the shoulders drop down and turn to the anteroposterior (AP) position, and the head slowly turns so both head and shoulders are aligned
   h. Expulsion: the posterior (underneath) shoulder is delivered by lateral flexion (upward motion); then the anterior upper shoulder will slide out (downward motion) from under the pubic arch, and the body slithers out easily

3. Stages of labor
   a. First stage: begins with the first true labor contraction; ends with complete dilatation and effacement of the cervix
   b. Second stage (expulsion): from complete effacement and dilatation to expulsion of the infant

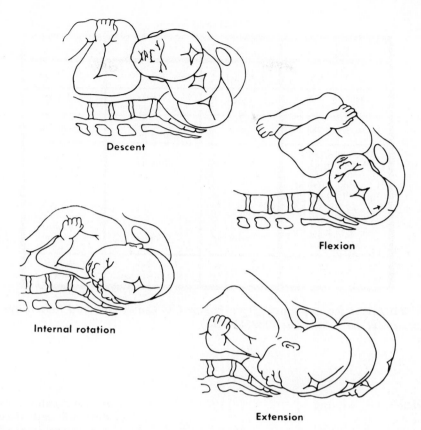

FIG. 8-8. Mechanisms of labor in left occiput anterior position. (From Hamilton PM: *Basic maternity nursing,* ed 6, St Louis, 1988, Mosby.)

c. Third stage (placental): from delivery of the infant to delivery of the placenta and membranes (5 to 20 minutes)

d. Fourth stage: from delivery of the secundines and repair of the perineum to 1 hour thereafter

D. Fetal evaluation during labor and delivery and immediately after

1. During labor

a. Fetal monitoring devices

(1) Phonotransducer: amplification of fetal heart activity

(2) Doppler transducer: ultrasonic device

b. Special stethoscopes for monitoring FHT

(1) Headscope (fetoscope): stethoscope on a head device; FHT conducted through monitor's frontal bone

(2) Leff stethoscope: stethoscope with large, heavy conductor

c. Direct fetal monitoring: an electrocardiogram (ECG) electrode is placed directly to the fetal head

2. Evaluation immediately after delivery

a. Establishment of patent airway

b. Apgar scoring (Fig. 8-9): system of evaluating newborn response 1 minute after birth and 5 minutes after birth

c. Observation for any visible anomalies

E. Nursing assessment

1. Premonitory (impending) signs and symptoms of labor

a. Lightening: descent of fetus down pelvic cavity

b. Braxton Hicks contractions: painless contractions more frequent, regular

c. Breathing easier; heartburn disappears; hungry

d. Weight loss (decrease in water retention)

e. Frequency (pressure on bladder by presenting part)

f. Bloody show (slight pinkish discharge with or without discharge of mucous plug)

g. Bag of waters (BOW) ruptures spontaneously without prior contractions

2. Differences between true and false labor

a. False labor

(1) Contractions irregular

(2) No progress in interval or duration of contractions

(3) Some abdominal discomfort

(4) No bloody show

(5) Relief by walking

(6) No cervical change

(7) Discomfort mostly in front (lower abdomen)

b. True labor

(1) Contractions regular and progressive

APGAR SCORING CHART

Sign	0	1	2
HEART RATE	Absent	Slow (below 100)	Over 100
RESPIRATORY EFFORT	Absent	Weak cry, hypoventilation	Good strong cry
MUSCLE TONE	Limp	Some flexion of extremities	Well flexed
REFLEX RESPONSE 1. Response to catheter in nostril (tested after oro-pharynx is clear)	No response	Grimace	Cough or sneeze
2. Tangential foot slap	No response	Grimace	Cry and withdrawal of foot
COLOR	Blue, pale	Body pink, extremities blue	Completely pink

FIG. 8-9. The Apgar scoring chart. (From Philips CR: *Family-centered maternity/newborn care: a basic text,* ed 2, St Louis, 1987, Mosby.)

(2) Not relieved by walking

(3) Cervical changes

(4) Progressive discomfort starting in back, going around lower abdomen, indentable fundus

3. Spontaneous rupture of membranes
   a. Note time, amount
   b. Prevent infection (handwashing, good hygienic practice)
   c. Observe for prolapsed cord (notify physician immediately)
   d. If leakage minimal, spontaneous resealing may occur
   e. If close to EDC, contractions may begin, usually within 4 to 16 hours

F. Nursing intervention
   1. Nursing management during first stage of labor
      a. Admit patient to labor room
      b. Establish rapport; ask pertinent questions regarding labor; observe reaction to labor process
      c. Offer bedpan frequently (keep bladder empty)
      d. Usually an IV is started to keep a vein open (KVO) (get equipment, solutions)
      e. Monitor contractions, FHR
         (1) Hook up to fetal monitoring device
         (2) Check every 30 to 60 minutes (dependent on progress)
      f. Keep mother, father informed on status and progress
         (1) Effacement, dilatation, station
         (2) Encourage father to follow monitor read-out
         (3) Encourage father to use comfort measures for mother
   2. Nursing management during second stage of labor
      a. Uterine muscles bring about effacement and di-

latation; abdominal muscles bring fetus down after dilatation and effacement are complete, and levator ani muscles assist in pushing and expelling fetus
      b. All monitoring equipment removed from mother
         (1) Transport to delivery room
         (2) Explain procedures
         (3) Clean perineal area according to hospital policy
         (4) Monitor FHR every 5 minutes with fetoscope; inform physician on rate, strength, position
         (5) Check blood pressure every 15 minutes as necessary
         (6) Prepare necessary equipment for delivery readiness and for reception of baby
         (7) Instruct mother to push with contractions when indicated
         (8) When infant delivered completely, note time
         (9) Establish patent airway
         (10) Encourage mother and father to see, touch, and speak to infant
         (11) Carefully place prophylactic drops in each eye
         (12) Follow proper identification routine
         (13) Transfer infant into warm crib to transport to nursery for further evaluation and care
   3. Nursing management during third stage (placental)
      a. Be sure cord blood specimen is taken
      b. Placenta delivered within 5 to 20 minutes from expulsion of infant
      c. Note time and which side of placenta delivered
         (1) Maternal side, raw and meaty: Duncan delivery
         (2) Fetal side, shiny and neat: Schultze delivery

d. Administer oxytocin immediately following delivery of placenta to contract uterus and prevent hemorrhage

e. Check blood pressure every 15 minutes

f. Check fundus for firmness; soft, boggy indicates possible hemorrhaging

g. Check and clean perineal area; apply sanitary napkin

h. Mother may experience knees shaking, teeth chattering

    (1) Sudden changes in abdominal pressure plus hormonal changes trigger these symptoms

    (2) Place several warm blankets over mother

    (3) Reassure mother and family that it is a normal physiologic phenomenon

i. Transfer mother to recovery area (if not in birthing room)

4. Nursing management during fourth stage of delivery

a. Critical hour after delivery; watch for complications, especially hemorrhaging

b. Perform fundal check every 5 minutes; massage gently if necessary

c. Check blood pressure and vital signs every 10 to 15 minutes until stable

d. Offer warm drink, toast or even meal tray if mother wishes and physician approves

e. Offer bedpan frequently to prevent bladder distention, which will impede involution

f. After 1 hour, when vital signs are stable, give sponge bath to refresh and clean body

g. Teach perineal care with peribottle

h. Transfer to postpartum room

i. Advise mother to request help the first time she wishes to use the bathroom

5. Commonly used medications during labor and delivery: prepared childbirth has greatly diminished use of analgesics and anesthetics during labor and delivery; patients who experience dystocia may need some medication for relief from exhaustion, fright, or prolonged pain

a. Amnesic

b. Tranquilizer

c. Analgesic

d. Regional anesthesia

    (1) Paracervical block: anesthetizes cervical area

    (2) Pudendal block: peripheral nerve block; may also block urge to push for 30 minutes

    (3) Caudal block (spinal): used during first and second stages; continuous or one dosage

    (4) Saddle block: third, fourth, or fifth lumbar interspace; anesthetizes saddle area (inner groin, perineal area)

    (5) Epidural: also administered into lumbar interspace: uses less anesthetic than caudal; blocks urge to push

e. Nursing management

    (1) Flat in bed after spinals

    (2) Observe for headache

    (3) Encourage urination

    (4) Force fluids

f. General anesthesia: rare

ABNORMAL INTRAPARTUM
Dystocia

A. Definition: prolonged, difficult, painful labor or delivery involving any one or more problems with the three *P*'s: passage, power, and passenger

B. Problems with passage

1. Inadequate pelvis

2. Soft tissue deviation

C. Problems with the power (uterine contractions)

1. Primary uterine inertia: inefficient contractions from the beginning

2. Secondary uterine inertia: well-established labor with good contractions at first; then progress suddenly or gradually slows and stops altogether

3. Hypotonic contractions (atonic uterus); most common; no progress in effacement or dilatation

4. Hypertonic uterine contractions

a. Intense, titanic

b. No interval between contractions

5. Dystonic contractions

a. Painful

b. Ineffective

c. Asymmetric (contractions in different segments of the uterus)

D. Problems with passenger (fetus)

1. Excessive size

2. Fetal anomaly

3. Fetal malposition or malpresentation

a. Occiput posterior (most common)

b. Breech

c. Transverse

d. Face

e. Soldier (military) presentation

4. Cephalopelvic disproportion (CPD)

a. Accommodation impossible

b. May note unusual contour of uterus or abdomen

E. Complications from dystocias

1. Premature rupture of membranes

2. Predisposition to infection

3. Trauma

4. Hemorrhage

5. Prolapse of cord

6. Hypoxia of fetus

7. Severe molding of fetal head: danger of intracranial hemorrhage

8. Extreme backache (posterior positions)

9. Flowering of anus early because of pressure of occiput on lower sacral region, with subsequent residual of hemorrhoids

10. Extreme fatigue

F. Treatment and nursing management

1. Electronic monitoring of fetus and mother

2. Frequent confirmation of cervical progress

3. Sterile techniques during vaginal examination

4. Check status of BOW

5. Check vital signs

6. Observe condition of mother

a. Need for pain relief

b. Sometimes after a medicated sleep or rest dystocia disappears

7. Support physical and psychologic needs

8. Watch for dehydration

9. Spontaneous rotation toward end of transition may occur in occiput posteriors

Supine Hypotensive Syndrome

A. Definition: condition caused by compression of vena cava by heavy uterus for a prolonged period; caused by mother's staying in one position for a long time
B. Signs and symptoms
   1. Pallor
   2. Light-headedness
   3. Dizziness
   4. Slight nausea
C. Treatment and nursing management: turn patient on left side to relieve pressure; advise frequent turning and changing of position

Ruptured Uterus

A. Causes
   1. Titanic, pauseless contractions for unexplainable reasons
   2. Stretching of uterine walls by extensive, rapid growth of hydatidiform mole
B. Treatment and nursing management
   1. Prepare for cesarean section (CS)
   2. Prepare for all anticipatory nursing responsibilities, surgical or medical

Prolapsed Cord

A. Definition: displacement of the cord below the presenting part and into the vaginal passage before delivery
B. Causes
   1. Spontaneous rupture of the membranes before engagement
   2. Breech presentations
   3. Prematurity
   4. Polyhydramnios
   5. Abnormal presentations
C. Signs and symptoms
   1. Cord may be seen, felt, or palpated
   2. Fetal heart pattern abnormal
D. Treatment and nursing management
   1. Do not compress cord; do not try to reposition it
   2. Sterile saline compress to keep cord moist and protected from infection
   3. Place mother in knee-chest position or in Trendelenburg's position so presenting part is pushed away from cord by gravity
   4. Preparation for cesarean section, blood cross-match, IV fluids, and so on
   5. Check FHR every 5 minutes
   6. Support frightened mother and family

Multiple Pregnancies

A. Definition: simultaneous gestation; twins, triplets, quadruplets, quintuplets, sextuplets, septuplets
B. Signs and symptoms
   1. Not always discernible
   2. History of twins (female lineage)
   3. Hearing two FHTs, each with own rate
   4. Disclosure of multiple limbs, heads, by palpation
   5. Larger than normal gestation uterus
   6. Weight gain increased more than in normal gestation
   7. Striae gravidarum more noticeable early on
   8. Confirmation by x-ray examination, sonogram
C. Types (Fig. 8-10)
   1. Single-ovum twins (monozygotic, identical)
      a. Union of one sperm with one ovum
      b. During mitosis divides into two embryos

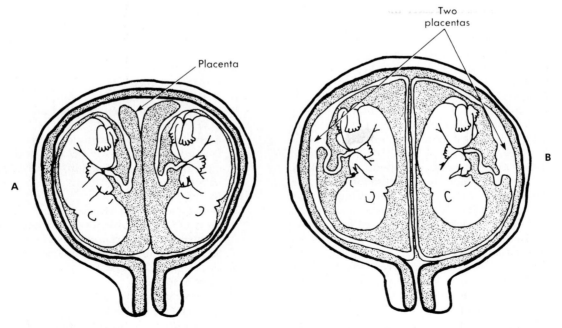

FIG. 8-10. Multiple pregnancy. **A,** Identical (monozygotic) twins: two sacs, one placenta. **B,** Fraternal (dizygotic) twins: two sacs, two placentas. (From Philips CR: *Family-centered maternity/newborn care: a basic text,* ed 2, St Louis, 1987, Mosby.)

c. One placenta, two amniotic sacs
d. Same sex
e. Heredity a factor
2. Fraternal twins (dizygotic, unidentical)
   a. Union of two sperm with two separate ova
   b. Two amniotic sacs
   c. Separate or fused placenta
   d. Same or different sex
   e. Do not look alike
   f. Age of mother a factor; older women tend to release more than one ovum
3. Formation of triplets and so on is varied

D. Treatment and nursing management
1. Prenatal care
   a. Visits increased
   b. Observe for signs and symptoms of preeclampsia
   c. Premature labor common
   d. Backaches common: support girdle, longer rest periods
   e. Varicosities common
   f. Watch for complications resulting from position, presentation, lie of fetuses
   g. Size of fetuses may cause problems
   h. Be alert for possible cesarean section
2. Natal care
   a. Be prepared for premature labor and premature babies
   b. High-risk second stage
3. Third and fourth stages
   a. Possibility of hemorrhage because of oversized uterus
   b. Blood loss greater than for single births
   c. Oxytocin not administered to mother until all babies delivered
   d. Risk of infection greater than in normal single births
   e. Perinatal mortality greater than in single deliveries

Induction of Labor

A. Definition: the use of medication (oxytocin) to stimulate contractions
B. Indications
1. Overdue fetus (over 42 weeks' gestation)
2. Fetal death/uterine death
3. Uterine inertia, primary or secondary
4. Atonic or hypotonic uterine contractions (may be enhanced by a boost of oxytocin)
5. Prolonged rupture of membranes (over 24 hours) if uterine contractions have not begun
6. Diabetic mother
7. Severe preeclampsia (exercise extreme caution)
8. Steeply rising Rh titer
C. Contraindications
1. Cephalopelvic disproportion (CPD)
2. Fetal distress
3. Previous cesarean section
4. Multiple births
5. Heart conditions
6. Prematurity
7. Unengaged presenting part
D. Treatment and nursing management

1. Monitor contractions carefully
2. If there are no intervals between contractions, stop medication drip and call physician immediately
3. Monitor FHR and report any changes stat
4. Check blood pressure: gradual elevation warrants immediate discontinuation of medication and prompt notification of doctor
5. Keep family and mother informed of progress and procedure

Operative Obstetrics

A. Episiotomy
1. Definition: surgical incision of the perineum during delivery to enlarge the vaginal outlet
2. Types (Fig. 8-11)
3. Indications
   a. To avoid tearing
   b. To shorten second stage of labor
   c. Fetus or mother is in jeopardy
4. Treatment and nursing management
   a. Comfort measures (promote healing)
   b. Encourage Kegel exercises, lessen pain and promote healing
   c. Apply witch hazel pads to perineal area (decrease swelling, promote healing)
B. Forceps deliveries
1. Definition: an operative procedure using various instruments to deliver the presenting part
2. Indications for use
   a. To shorten second stage
   b. Assist in descent of presenting part when there has been poor progress
   c. Maternal exhaustion
   d. When rotation (of head) is necessary, e.g., left occiput posterior (LOP) to occiput anterior (OA)
   e. To save fetus in jeopardy
3. Requirements for application
   a. No cephalopelvic disproportion
   b. Presenting part engaged and below ischial spines
   c. Full dilatation and effacement
   d. Ruptured membranes
   e. Empty bladder
   f. FHR checked before and after application
4. Complications
   a. Lacerations and tears
   b. Hemorrhage
   c. Rupture of uterus
   d. Facial marks or facial paralysis of fetus
   e. Intracranial hemorrhage or brain damage to fetus
C. Cesarean section
1. Definition: an operative procedure to deliver the fetus through a surgical incision made through the abdominal and uterine walls
2. Indications
   a. Cephalopelvic disproportion
   b. Fetal distress
   c. Prematurity
   d. Dystocia
   e. Prolapsed cord
   f. Oversized infant
   g. Positions and presentations undeliverable through the vagina

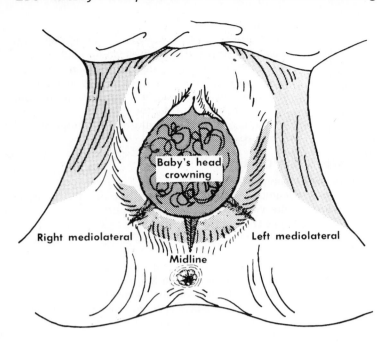

FIG. 8-11. Three types of episiotomies. (From Hamilton PM: *Basic maternity nursing,* ed 6, St Louis, 1988, Mosby.)

h. Some hypertensive states, placenta previa, abruptio placentae, prolapsed cord abnormalities
i. Maternal exhaustion
3. Types
  a. Elective
    (1) Anticipated difficulties: for example, inadequate pelvis or vaginal deliveries inadvisable because mother has AIDS or herpes
    (2) Previous cesarean sections (selective)
  b. Emergency
    (1) Sudden fetal distress
    (2) Accident
4. Treatment and nursing management
  a. Routine surgical preoperative and postoperative care plus normal postpartum care
  b. Promote involution
  c. Perineal care
  d. Lochia; color amount same as for vaginal delivery
  e. Support mother and family; allay fears
  f. Watch for signs and symptoms of infection (chills, fever)
5. Care of cesarean section newborn
  a. Place in incubator or Isolette for 24 hours
  b. Section babies prone to respiratory distress
  c. Controlled humidity to assist absorption of fluid in lungs
6. Vaginal birth after cesarean (VBAC): vaginal delivery after a cesarean section may be encouraged; depends on reason for cesarean section

NORMAL POSTPARTUM

A. Definition: period from end of fourth stage of labor to 6 weeks after day of delivery
B. Immediate care following delivery
  1. Continue checking of vital signs
  2. Encourage urination

    a. Full bladder impedes involution
    b. Full bladder may cause excessive bleeding
  3. Offer food: if policy permits, offer food and drink to mother after vital signs are stable
  4. Care of fundus
    a. Check for firmness
    b. Lochia checked for color, amount, and presence of clots
  5. Provide perineal care and care of breasts
  6. General hygiene: shower may be permissible to clean, refresh mother after vital signs are stable (policies vary)
  7. Encourage putting infant to breast for feeding and bonding
C. Physiologic changes during puerperium
  1. Reproductive organs
    a. Uterus: involution (return of uterus to normal size and function)
      (1) Walls of uterus return to normal in 3 to 4 weeks
      (2) Menstruation may return in 3 to 4 weeks
      (3) Nursing mothers: menstruation may be delayed several months
      (4) Fundus involutes 1 finger width every day if umbilicus is used as point of reference (Fig. 8-12)
    b. Vagina
      (1) Returns to normal within 3 to 6 weeks after delivery, depending on type of delivery, length of labor, lacerations, healing process, and so on
      (2) Cesarean sections: vaginal recovery rapid
    c. Perineal area
      (1) Should be intact and clean
      (2) Complete healing should take 5 to 7 days

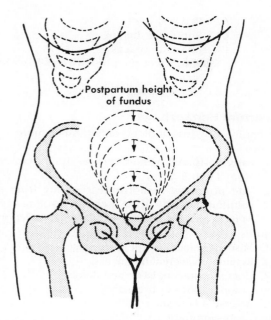

FIG. 8-12. Involution. Height of fundus as it descends to prepregnant levels postpartum. (From Hamilton PM: *Basic maternity nursing,* ed 6, St Louis, 1988, Mosby.)

2. Return to normal of body system and functions
   a. Hormonal recovery begins immediately
   b. Lochia: vaginal discharge coming from decidual lining of uterus after delivery
      (1) Lochia rubra: dark red to bright red; occasional clots; flow lasts 2 to 3 days
      (2) Lochia serosa: pale pink to brownish lochia; lighter flow, dependent on ambulation; lasts 2 to 5 days
      (3) Lochia alba: yellowish, creamy discharge consisting of leukocytes and dead cells; lasts 5 to 10 days
      (4) Prolonged or recurring bleeding may indicate a medical problem
   c. Vascular system
      (1) Average loss of blood at delivery: 250 to 400 ml
      (2) Blood loss of 500 ml or more considered hemorrhage
   d. Urinary tract
      (1) Perineal soreness may temporarily reduce voiding reflexes
      (2) Marked diuresis 8 to 12 hours postpartum
D. Treatment and nursing management during postpartum
   1. Objectives for daily care
      a. Assist in normal process of involution
      b. Prevent infection
      c. Promote infant bonding with mother and family
   2. Nursing techniques for postpartum care
      a. Vital signs: watch for symptoms of hypovolemic shock and hemorrhage (fainting); stay with mother who is out of bed (OOB) for the first time since delivery
   b. Check breasts
      (1) Should be soft until milk comes in
      (2) Daily cleansing in shower
      (3) Daily breast examination to note any complications; nodules may be felt second or third day as milk production begins; teach breast self-examination; report any abnormalities
   c. Engorgement
      (1) Nursing usually prevents this; breast pump; nipple shield
      (2) Nonnursing mother
         (a) Cold compresses or ice bag on breasts
         (b) Tight binder for 1 to 2 days
         (c) Restrict fluids for 1 to 2 days
         (d) Follow steps *a, b, c* only if requested
   d. Infections
      (1) Redness, warmth, pain, elevated temperature
      (2) May require minor surgical intervention to release drainage
   e. Check fundus
      (1) Height and firmness for proper involution
      (2) Relaxed fundus may indicate problem (hemorrhage or infection)
   f. Check lochia: color, amount, odor
   g. Check perineal area: healing and cleanliness
   h. Check legs: pain, tenderness, swelling (thrombi); check for Homans' sign
   i. Check urination: overdistention (subinvolution)
   j. Bowels: keep open (force fluids with balanced diet): administer stool softener (e.g., docusate sodium sulfosuccinate [Colace])
   k. Afterpains: involution
   l. Postpartum blues (baby blues): possible hormonal transitory depression
3. Teaching: important component of postpartum nursing management
   a. Personal hygiene
   b. Weight loss
      (1) Immediately after delivery, 7- to 10-lb weight loss
      (2) Total weight loss of pregnancy may take 6 weeks to 6 months or more to achieve
   c. PKU tests: requirement by law to test for inborn error of metabolism involving proteins and amino acids
   d. Capacity of newborn and infant stomach:
      (1) At birth can take 1 to 2 oz (30 to 60 ml) per feeding
      (2) By 1 to 2 weeks, can nurse 4 oz (120 ml) per feeding
      (3) Gradual increase to 6 to 8 oz (180 to 240 ml) per feeding in 1 month
   e. Discuss with mother and father
      (1) Importance of bonding
      (2) Readiness for parenthood
   f. Postpartum exercises
   g. Review methods of holding, bubbling, or burping baby

ABNORMAL POSTPARTUM
Postpartum Infection

A. Definition: any infection in the reproductive organs during labor, delivery, or up to 1 month postpartum
B. Signs and symptoms
  1. Chills, fever, localized back pain (kidney involvement)
  2. Malaise
  3. Lower abdominal tenderness, lower back pains
  4. Foul-smelling lochia (retained placental infection)
  5. Fundal height changes abnormal
C. Treatment and nursing management in general
  1. Administration of appropriate antibiotics on time and as directed
  2. Comfort measures appropriate to discomfort
  3. Check vital signs q4h
D. Specific infections
  1. Urinary tract infection (cystitis, pyelitis)
    a. Cause: trauma (stretching or tearing) or by an organism
    b. Signs and symptoms
      (1) 3 days postpartum
      (2) Low back pain
      (3) Localized pain (pyelitis)
      (4) Chills, high fever, apprehension
      (5) Frequency and burning urination (cystitis)
      (6) Discomfort
    c. Treatment and nursing management
      (1) Bed rest until symptoms subside (1 day)
      (2) Drugs (antibiotics)
      (3) Force fluids
      (4) Careful handwashing by mother and nursing staff
  2. Mastitis
    a. Definition: inflammation of the glands in the breast(s)
    b. Cause
      (1) Staphylococcus infection
      (2) Stasis of milk
      (3) Bruising of breast tissue
      (4) Open cuts in nipple or areola
    c. Signs and symptoms
      (1) High fever (103° F; 39.5° C)
      (2) Chills
      (3) Red, tender, painful, hard
    d. Treatment and nursing management: if untreated, abscess complications
      (1) Support bra
      (2) Antibiotic therapy
      (3) Check incision for drainage
      (4) Reassurance of mother
      (5) Discontinuing of breast-feeding varies
  3. Thrombophlebitis
    a. Definition: infection or clot occurring in the deep pelvic veins when placental site becomes infected
    b. Signs and symptoms
      (1) Local tenderness: femoral vein
      (2) 1 to 2 weeks postpartum
      (3) Swelling, chills, fever
    c. Treatment and nursing management
      (1) Administration of anticoagulant

      (2) Bed rest
      (3) Antibiotic therapy
      (4) Elevation of legs
      (5) Warm, wet compresses every 15 to 30 minutes
      (6) Never massage

Postpartum Hemorrhage

A. Definition: any loss of blood of 500 ml or more
B. Types
  1. Early postpartal hemorrhage resulting from uterine atony (1 to 3 days)
  2. Late postpartal hemorrhage resulting from subinvolution (inability of the uterus to involute or return to its prepregnant state) or placental infection
C. Causes
  1. Mismanagement of the third stage
  2. Retained placental fragments
  3. Complications of labor and delivery
  4. Complications of pregnancy
  5. Inversion (uterine)
D. Signs and symptoms
  1. Visible blood loss
  2. Shocklike symptoms: pale, clammy, hypotensive, apprehensive
E. Treatment and nursing management
  1. Warm drink, warm covers
  2. IV fluids
  3. Replacement transfusion if appropriate
  4. Quiet assurance; support to family and mother
  5. Medical management of cause

Hematomas

A. Definition: local accumulation of blood caused by
  1. Undue pressure of heavy gravid uterus
  2. Bearing down inappropriately
  3. Long second stage
  4. Primigravida's prolonged pushing
B. Signs and symptoms
  1. Visible vaginal hematoma
  2. Vulvular hematoma
  3. Large blood-filled sac visible
C. Treatment and nursing management
  1. Ice to area for 24 hours
  2. Analgesics if ordered
  3. Incision or ligation if necessary
  4. Comfort measures similar to episiotomy care, that is, sitz bath

Subinvolution

A. Definition: inability of the uterus to return to its normal size after delivery
B. Cause
  1. Retention of placental pieces
  2. Infection (endometrium)
C. Signs and symptoms
  1. Involution process abnormal
  2. Boggy uterus (not firm); foul odor
  3. Intermittent or constant lochia rubra after cycle has passed
D. Treatment and nursing management
  1. Surgical intervention (D & C)
  2. Support and reassurance to mother and family

NORMAL NEWBORN

A. Immediate care following delivery
1. Maintain patent airway
2. Apply cord clamp, check for bleeding, follow procedure for daily cord care and teach it to mothers
3. Maintain warmth
   a. Wrap in prewarmed receiving blankets
   b. Place in preheated crib
4. Preventative care
   a. Instill prophylactic eye drops to each eye as required by law to prevent ophthalmia neonatorum
   b. Commonly used prophylactic drugs: silver nitrate, erythromycin, penicillin ointments/drops
   c. Administer intramuscular (IM) injection of vitamin K to reduce likelihood of hemorrhage (optional)
5. Identification procedures
   a. Complete identification bands as required
   b. Record footprints of baby and pointer fingerprint of mother
6. Apgar scoring
7. Initial observation of newborn
   a. Is the primary responsibility of physician/pediatrician
   b. Nurse should wear gloves when handling newborn during immediate care and until initial bath; regulations differ for daily routines
   c. Nurse also makes quick observation, checking for visible anomalies such as cleft lip, cleft palate, extra digits, spinal column, limbs, skin, head
   d. Reflexes that nurse may check include Moro's, sucking, rooting, blinking, grasping
8. Encourage bonding
   a. After initial delivery room care, wipe off excess blood and debris from baby; wrap securely in clean, warm receiving blanket and let parents hold baby
   b. Allow time for mother and father to look, touch, and hold infant

B. Normal physiology of newborn
1. Vital signs
   a. Temperature: 96° to 99° F (35.5° to 37° C); baby loses body heat in delivery room and during transit
   b. Pulse rate: 120 to 160 beats/min
      (1) Apical pulse rate
      (2) Irregular in rate and cadence (normal)
   c. Respirations: abdominal and irregular, 32 to 40 per minute
2. Measurements
   a. Weight
      (1) Girls 7 lb (3100 g)
      (2) Boys 7½ lb (3300 g)
      (3) 5 to 8 lb (2500 to 4000 g) considered normal
      (4) 5% to 10% weight loss in first 2 to 3 days
      (5) Regains birth weight in 5 to 7 days
   b. Length: 18 to 22 inches (45 to 55 cm) long
   c. Head circumference: 13 to 14 inches (33 to 35 cm)
   d. Chest circumference: 12 to 13 inches (30 to 33 cm)

3. Skin
   a. Milia: small, white sebaceous glands visible about nose, forehead, chin
   b. "Stork bites": telangiectasis or capillary hemangiomas
   c. Red nevi: discoloration, circumscribed, blanch on touch, prominent during crying, disappear in 6 months to a year
   d. Mongolian spots: bluish, bruiselike spots on buttocks, back, shoulders; disappear by toddler or preschool age and found in babies of Hispanic, black, Slavic, or oriental background
   e. Erythema toxicum neonatorum (newborn rash): appears as scratches and pimples; may be nosocomial infection
   f. Nevi vasculosus (strawberry mark): bright red or dark capillary hemangiomas with raised, rough surfaces; usually disappear by school age
   g. Nevi flammeus (port-wine stain): reddish purple raised capillary hemangiomas; do not blanch on pressure and may not disappear
   h. Lanugo: soft, downy hair on top of skin on ears, forehead, neck, shoulders; disappears in weeks
   i. Vernix caseosa: cheeselike protective material coating fetus, especially under arms, beneath knees, and in folds of thighs
   j. Acrocyanosis: extremities are bluish for several hours after delivery
4. Elimination
   a. Urine: 3 to 4 times a day for first few days; usually urinates after every feeding
   b. Bowel movement: 5 to 6 times a day for first week
      (1) Meconium: expelled within 2 to 12 hours; black, tarry, thick unformed stool
      (2) Transient stool: blackish or greenish stool expelled after first few feedings
   c. Breast-fed stool: yellow, odorless, slightly runny
   d. Bottle-fed stool: formed, brownish yellow, distinct odor
   e. Each infant establishes own pattern of stool movement
5. Hyperestrogenism and its effect on the newborn
   a. Swelling of the breasts in male or female infant because of hormones from mother; the ensuing discharge is called "witches milk"
   b. Swelling of the male scrotum: large, with rugae; disappears within days
6. Reproductive organs of the male newborn
   a. Cryptorchidism: testes have not descended into scrotum; often present in premature infants
   b. Occasionally testes are in inguinal sac at birth but will descend within hours or more; if undescended after 1 month, pediatrician should evaluate
   c. Prepuce (foreskin) should be carefully retracted daily during bath time if newborn is uncircumcised; some prepuces will not retract for months or years
7. Circulatory system: pulmonary circulation established within minutes of birth
8. Digestive system: immature at birth but can metabolize nutrients except fats

9. Visual capabilities: immature coordination and muscle control
10. Hearing capabilities: acute hearing within 2 minutes of birth
11. Taste perception: can distinguish sweet and sour in 1 to 3 days
12. Smelling perception: can distinguish smell of mother at 5 days
13. Sleep patterns
    a. Unstable for 6 to 8 hours after birth
    b. Has regular and irregular sleep cycles
14. Newborn reflexes
    a. Sucking, rooting, swallowing, extrusion reflexes
    b. Tonic neck (fencing) should disappear in 3 to 4 months
    c. Grasping (palmar) lessens in 3 to 4 months
    d. Moro's (startle) disappears in 2 months
    e. Dancing (stepping, walking) disappears in 3 to 4 weeks
    f. Babinski's (plantar): absence indicates CNS damage
    g. Blinking, sneezing
15. Immunity in the newborn
    a. Has 3-month supply from mother if baby is term
    b. Begins own synthesis by 3 months of age
C. Daily observation and nursing care
    1. Newborn nursery care and observation
       a. Constant, careful observation
       b. After transferring infant from delivery room, place in warmer until vital signs are stable
       c. Check temperature; follow agency policy (rectal, axilla, etc.)
          (1) Drops 3° first hour after delivery
          (2) Heat production normal in 2 to 3 days
          (3) Newborn loses heat through convection, conduction, radiation, and evaporation
       d. Check respirations
       e. Place infant on right side to promote expansion of lungs and drain excess mucus
       f. Observe for signs and symptoms of respiratory distress syndrome (RDS)
       g. Check for bleeding
       h. Cord
          (1) Removal of cord clamp within 8 to 24 hours
          (2) Daily application of antigermicidal agent to prevent infections
       i. Check eyes and ears for abnormal drainage
    2. Daily nursery routine
       a. Daily weight and vital signs, especially temperature
       b. Observation and recording condition of skin, cord, eyes, elimination
       c. Daily care and changing of crib linen
          (1) Daily cord care
          (2) General observation
       d. During feeding routine observe infant-mother bonding
    3. Teaching mothers care of newborn: mothers' classes should incorporate the care, handling, and dressing of the newborn in addition to procedures and demonstrations in sponge baths, tub baths, and cord care

4. Daily bath routine
   a. Purpose
      (1) Cleansing
      (2) Exercise time
      (3) Play, social time with mother (bonding time)
   b. Prepare environment: select safe, convenient, warm area
   c. Select and prepare equipment
      (1) Utensils for sponge or tub bath
      (2) Necessary articles for procedure
      (3) Clean clothing
   d. Sponge baths: recommended for babies with cord intact
   e. Tub baths: recommended for babies whose cord has fallen off
5. Cord care
   a. Wipe base of cord with alcohol or designated antiseptic every time diapers are changed and during bath time
   b. After cord falls off
      (1) Wipe with alcohol as instructed after daily bath routine for first day or two
      (2) If drainage persists, cleanse with alcohol and notify pediatrician
6. Diaper rash
   a. Change diapers frequently
   b. Wash area with warm tap water
   c. Apply A and D ointment as a preventative and protective
   d. Expose to air if possible
      (1) Lay infant on abdomen and expose buttocks to air
      (2) Apply Desitin or Balmex if A and D ointment does not help
7. Circumcision
   a. Definition: the surgical cutting and removal of foreskin; usually done 1 to 3 days after birth
   b. Treatment and nursing management
      (1) Observe for bleeding
      (2) Petrolatum (Vaseline) gauze for 3 days
      (3) Check and record first voiding after procedure
      (4) Complications: rare
8. Facts about feeding the newborn
   a. Newborn metabolic rate twice that of adult
   b. Carbohydrates needed for brain growth and as source of energy
   c. Protein needed for building tissue; inadequacy results in infection, slow growth, flabby muscles
   d. Fat difficult to digest and metabolize but needed to maintain integrity of skin
   e. Iron: continuous supply needed for growth and development; storage from mother depleted in 4 to 6 months
9. Facts about breast milk
   a. Less protein than cow's milk; easier to digest
   b. More lactose than cow's milk, which facilitates metabolism and is good for bones
   c. Lactoferrin decreases dangers to infection
   d. Sucking stimulates posterior pituitary of mother to trigger let-down reflex, which allows milk to flow

10. Guidelines for breast-feeding
    a. A general rule of thumb is to nurse until breasts are soft
    b. To ensure a good supply of breast milk, the mother should
       (1) Have adequate rest
       (2) Drink sufficient fluids
       (3) Eat a balanced, nutritious diet
       (4) Maintain psychologic equilibrium
11. Suggested time limits for breast feeding: time limits are flexible, dependent upon condition of nipple
    a. First day: 2 to 3 minutes each breast
    b. Second day: 3 to 5 minutes each breast
    c. Third day: 5 to 7 minutes each breast

ABNORMAL NEWBORN
The Premature

A. Definition: a baby born before 37 weeks' gestation and weighing less than 5½ lb (2500 g)
B. Statistics
   1. Of all live births 8% are premature
   2. Prematurity is leading cause of death in infants in the United States
C. Cause
   1. Young, adolescent mothers
   2. Elderly primigravidas
   3. Multiple births
   4. Poor prenatal care
   5. Congenital anomalies
   6. Diseases or conditions that compromise fetus
      a. Toxemia
      b. Diabetes
      c. Heart disease
      d. Nutritional deficits
      e. Neglect
      f. Drug or alcohol addictions
D. Characteristics of a premature infant
   1. Central nervous system
      a. Poor muscle tone
      b. Poor reflexes
      c. Limp
      d. Assumes froglike position
      e. Weak, feeble cry
      f. Unstable heating mechanism: temperature fluctuates from 94° to 96° F (34° to 36° C)
      g. Poor sucking reflexes
      h. Weak gagging and swallowing reflexes
   2. Respiratory system
      a. Insufficient surfactant
      b. Immature lungs, rib cage, muscles
      c. Prone to respiratory distress syndrome (RDS)
      d. Poor oxygenation
   3. Digestive system: immature gastric system
   4. Integumentary system
      a. Harlequin pattern observed
      b. Veins and capillaries visible
      c. Lanugo prominent
      d. Vernix prominent
      e. No subcutaneous fat
      f. Skin tight, shiny, taut
   5. Circulatory system
      a. Fragile capillaries
      b. Susceptible to hemorrhages (intracranial)
   6. Renal system
      a. Inability to urinate properly
      b. Easily dehydrated
      c. Fragile electrolyte balance
   7. Immune system
      a. Too young to have obtained any immunity from mother
      b. Vulnerable to infection
   8. Head
      a. Fontanels large
      b. Suture lines prominent
      c. Old looking in appearance
E. Treatment and nursing management
   1. Maintain patent airway
   2. Frequently monitor blood gases to determine oxygen need
   3. Maintain body temperature by placing in Isolette
   4. Conserve energy: basic care only
   5. Provide adequate nutrition
      a. Nasogastric feedings
      b. Special soft nipples
      c. Parenteral fluids
   6. Prevent infection
      a. Prevent skin breakdown: change positions
      b. Keep dry and clean
   7. Length of hospitalization: until a weight of 5½ lb (2500 g) is reached
   8. Mothering stimulation taught and practiced
      a. Encourage parents to stroke, cuddle, talk
      b. Feed, diaper infants
      c. Play soft music
      d. Encourage tapping on Isolette and talking
   9. Listen to concerns of mothers and fathers

Dysmature Infant (Immature)

A. Definition
   1. Small for gestational age
   2. Intrauterine growth retardation
B. Causes
   1. Defective development
   2. Maternal factors: smoking, malnutrition
   3. Placental insufficiency
C. Nursing management
   1. Same as for premature infants
   2. Common complication: hypoglycemia

Postmature Infant

A. Definition: over 43 weeks' gestation
B. Cause: unknown
C. Characteristics of postmature infant
   1. Old looking
   2. No vernix; no lanugo
   3. Color: yellow-green or meconium stained
   4. Desquamation of hands (palms) and feet (soles)
   5. May have respiratory problems
D. Nursing management
   1. Observe for hypoglycemia
   2. Observe for RDS
   3. Look for birth injuries
   4. Symptomatic nursing care

Neonatal Respiratory Distress Syndrome

A. Definition
1. A series of symptoms signifying respiratory distress
2. Synonyms: RDS, hyaline membrane disease (HMD)

B. Statistics
1. Common in premature babies
2. Leading cause of death in infants in the United States

C. Cause
1. Lack or loss of surfactant in lungs
2. Immaturity
3. Hypoxia
4. Hypothermia

D. Signs and symptoms
1. Appears within minutes to hours after birth
2. Grunting, rib retraction, nasal flaring (RDS symptoms)
3. Inadequate oxygen: 60 or more respirations per minute

E. Diagnosis: x-ray examination shows collapsed portions of lung

F. Treatment and nursing management
1. Transfer to intensive care unit and Isolette care
2. Initiate oxygen therapy: 60%; hood is best
   a. IPPB (intermittent positive pressure breathing)
   b. CPAP (continuous positive airway pressure)
   c. Monitor blood gases
3. Endotracheal tube if necessary
4. IV hydration and nutrition and antibiotic therapy
5. Place in modified Trendelenburg's position

G. Complication
1. Retrolental fibroplasia
2. Causes
   a. High arterial oxygen levels
   b. Retinal vascular immaturity

Birth Injuries

A. Normal deviations of the head
1. Caput succedaneum
   a. Definition: edema (water) under the scalp
   b. Cause: continuous pressure of the fetal head on cervix
   c. Signs and symptoms
      (1) Crosses suture lines
      (2) Appears at birth
      (3) Disappears in 3 to 4 days
   d. Treatment: none
2. Cephalhematoma (Fig. 8-13)
   a. Definition: blood between the periosteum and bone
   b. Cause: pressure during delivery (forceps)
   c. Signs and symptoms
      (1) Never crosses suture lines
      (2) Appears several hours to several days after birth
      (3) Disappears within 3 to 6 weeks
   d. Treatment: none
3. Molding (Fig. 8-14)
   a. Definition: changes in the shape of the head
   b. Cause: accommodation of fetal bones to birth canal during labor and delivery
   c. Signs and symptoms: visual
   d. Treatment: disappears without treatment in 3 days

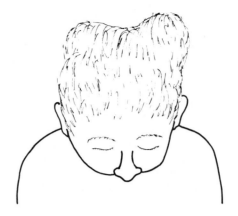

FIG. 8-13. Cephalhematoma. (From Philips CR: *Family-centered maternity/newborn care: a basic text,* ed 2, St Louis, 1987, Mosby.)

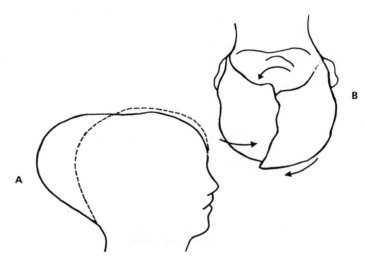

FIG. 8-14. A, Various types of molding. **B,** Bones overlapping during molding. (From Hamilton PM: *Basic maternity nursing,* ed 6, St Louis, 1988, Mosby.)

4. Soft tissue injuries (subcutaneous fat necrosis)
   a. Definition: pressure necrosis
   b. Signs and symptoms: purplish, movable mass
   c. Treatment: resolves spontaneously

B. Subconjunctival hemorrhage (scleral or retinal)
1. Definition: rupture of small capillaries in eye
2. Cause: increased intracranial pressure of birth
3. Signs and symptoms: small, red pin dots in white of sclera, or hemorrhaging in retina
4. Treatment: resolves without treatment in 5 days

C. Ecchymosis, petechiae, edema
1. Definition: blood within tissues; does not blanch with pressure
2. Cause: forceps, manipulation, pressure
3. Signs and symptoms: visual in affected areas
4. Treatment: resolves without treatment in 2 days

D. Skeletal injuries
1. Skull fracture: rare, and unless blood vessels are involved, heals without treatment

2. Fracture of the clavicle: most common fracture; usually caused by shoulder impaction
   a. Treatment: handle infant with care
   b. Prognosis: good
3. Fracture of the humerus or femur: rare
   a. Cause: dystocia and difficult delivery
   b. Treatment
      (1) Immobilize
      (2) Heals rapidly
   c. Complications: rare
E. Neurologic injuries
   1. Brachial paralysis of upper arm: Erb-Duchenne
      a. Definition: nerves of the brachial plexus are crushed or severed
      b. Cause
         (1) Difficult labor
         (2) Shoulder impaction
         (3) Malposition of forceps
      c. Treatment: immobilize with brace or splint
      d. Nursing management
         (1) Skin care as necessary
         (2) Gentle range-of-motion exercises after healing
   2. Brachial paralysis of lower arm: Klumpke's
      a. Definition: nerves of hand and wrist crushed or severed
      b. Treatment
         (1) Pad wrist and fingers
         (2) Corrective surgery
         (3) Gentle massage after surgery
         (4) Range-of-motion exercises when appropriate
      c. Prognosis: good
   3. Facial paralysis
      a. Definition: crushed or severed nerves of face that cause grimacing and distortion, especially when crying; asymmetric paralysis
      b. Cause: misapplication of forceps
      c. Treatment: condition transitory; reassure parents
F. Central nervous system injuries
   1. Definition: injuries causing intracranial hemorrhaging
   2. Cause
      a. Prematurity
      b. Large full-term babies
      c. Dystocia
      d. Hypoxia
      e. Hypovolemia
   3. Types
      a. In brain itself
      b. Subdural hematoma
   4. Signs and symptoms
      a. Suture line separation
      b. Bulging anterior fontanel
      c. High-pitched cry
      d. Abnormal respirations
      e. Cyanosis
      f. Irritability or lethargy
      g. Twitching; convulsions
   5. Treatment and nursing management
      a. Head higher than hips
      b. Warmth
      c. Oxygen

d. IV therapy
e. Minimal handling
f. Surgical aspiration (if appropriate)
g. Measurement of head size weekly
h. Convulsion precautions

Infections of the Newborn

A. Causes
   1. Dystocia
   2. Premature rupture of the membranes of 24 hours or more
   3. Aspiration of fluid by the fetus in utero
   4. Maternal infection
   5. Nosocomial infection (hospital-based infection; usually staph)
   6. *Monilia* or yeast infection in mother's vagina
B. Signs and symptoms
   1. Appears within first 48 hours
   2. Vague symptoms
   3. Lethargy, irritability, lack of appetite
   4. Low-grade temperature
   5. Diarrhea
   6. Jaundice
C. Treatment and nursing management
   1. Take cultures of blood, urine, throat
   2. Administer antibiotic therapy
   3. Keep warm
   4. Administer oxygen therapy if necessary
   5. Isolate if appropriate
   6. Weigh daily
   7. Watch for signs of jaundice
   8. Keep parents informed of progress

Congenital Malformations

A. Perinatal signs
   1. Polyhydramnios: excessive amniotic fluid
   2. Oligohydramnios: scant amniotic fluid; indicates urinary tract anomalies and renal disturbances
B. Postnatal congenital malformations
   1. Choanal atresia (gastrointestinal anomaly)
      a. Definition: postnares obstructed by bone or membrane; unilateral or bilateral condition
      b. Signs and symptoms
         (1) Cyanotic at rest
         (2) Color improves when crying
         (3) Snorts when feeding
      c. Treatment and nursing management
         (1) Physician may pierce obstruction with a probe if it is only a membrane
         (2) Minor surgical repair if bone involved; prognosis excellent
         (3) Feeding problems; positioning important
         (4) Gavage feeding may be necessary
         (5) Watch closely for aspiration
   2. Esophageal atresia: refer to Chapter 9, Pediatric Nursing
   3. Congenital laryngeal stridor
      a. Definition: abnormal condition around larynx that causes noisy respiration, especially a crowing sound on inspiration
      b. Cause:
         (1) Flabby epiglottis
         (2) Extraglotteal structures

(3) Relaxation of laryngeal wall
(4) Absence of tracheal rings
(5) Deformity of vocal cords
c. Signs and symptoms
(1) Noisy respirations on inspiration
(2) Most noticeable when crying
(3) Mild-to-severe intercostal or supraclavicular retractions
(4) Cyanosis
(5) Dyspnea
d. Treatment and nursing management
(1) Depends on cause
(2) Mild stridor may subside in 6 to 18 months
(3) Mother taught to position baby upright for feeding
(4) Feed slowly, pausing to let infant catch his breath
(5) Use small nipple
(6) Watch for aspiration of feedings
(7) Prevent respiratory complications
(8) Keep infant warm, dry, away from drafts
(9) Oxygen in readiness
(10) Tracheotomy preparedness
e. Prognosis: good
4. Cleft lip and cleft palate
a. Definition: bilateral or unilateral fissure or opening on the palate or the upper lips resulting from failure of the bony and soft tissue structures to unite
b. Cause: developmental failure during the embryonic stage because of heredity, age, and so on
c. Signs and symptoms
(1) Visual on lips
(2) Palate more difficult to notice sometimes
(3) Occurs more frequently in males
(4) Difficulty feeding
(5) Choking
(6) Drooling
(7) Milk may drain through nostrils
d. Treatment
(1) Cleft lips may have butterfly adhesive taping as initial treatment; may be helpful in feeding so milk does not continually drain through fissure
(2) Cleft lip may be surgically repaired at 1 to 2 weeks of age, or at 12 lb (5.5 kg)
(3) Cleft palate; first repair usually by 18 months
e. Nursing management
(1) Feeding precautions
(a) Use soft duck nipple, medicine dropper with rubber tip
(b) Place nipple away from cleft side
(c) Feed slowly
(d) Bubble frequently
(e) Rinse mouth after feedings
(f) Watch for aspiration, respiratory distress, gastrointestinal disturbances
(2) Mouth care: prevent cracks, fissures on lips
(3) Postoperative care for cleft lip
(a) Place infant on side
(b) Mouth care important because of Logan bar applied to prevent stretching of sutures

(c) Prevent crying
(d) Check swelling (tongue, nose, mouth)
(e) Watch for hemorrhage
(f) Apply elbow restraints
(g) Prevent crust formation
(h) Feed on opposite side of surgery
(i) Use rubber-tipped dropper (3 weeks)
5. Diaphragmatic hernia
a. Definition: herniation of abdominal viscera into the thoracic cavity as a result of incomplete development during embryonic stage, ranging from minimal to complete herniation
b. Signs and symptoms
(1) Constant respiratory distress
(2) Bowels distended
(3) Bowel sounds heard in chest
(4) Asymmetric chest contour
c. Treatment and nursing management
(1) Early recognition and prompt surgery
(2) Usual preoperative and postoperative management
d. Prognosis guarded, depending on severity
6. Omphalocele: see Chapter 9, Pediatric Nursing
7. Imperforate anus: see Chapter 9, Pediatric Nursing
C. Congenital anomalies of central nervous system
1. Spina bifida occulta
a. Definition: defect in vertebral column without protrusion of spinal cord and meninges; this is one of three types of spina bifida, which is a malformation of the spine, most common in the lumbosacral region, in which the posterior portion of the vertebrae fails to close
b. Signs and symptoms
(1) Dimple in lower lumbosacral skin
(2) Hair over area sometimes
(3) X-ray film confirmation
c. Treatment and nursing management: no treatment necessary unless neurologic symptoms occur
2. Meningocele (another form of spina bifida)
a. Definition: defect in spinal cord with protrusion of meninges through an opening in spinal canal
b. Surgical correction with excellent results
3. Meningomyelocele
a. Definition: both spinal cord and meninges protrude through defective bony rings in spinal cord; possible paralysis
b. Signs and symptoms
(1) Arnold-Chiari syndrome
(2) Observe for change in intracranial pressure
(3) Check head measurements
(4) Report signs and symptoms of CNS involvement
c. Preoperative management
(1) Flat on abdomen with sterile gauze, petroleum jelly (Vaseline), or Telfa pad
(2) No diapers
(3) Keep clean
(4) Use care to prevent sac from breaking
(5) Prevent infection: sterile technique
(6) Prevent deformity
(7) Prevent injury

d. Postoperative management
    (1) Vital signs
    (2) Symptoms of shock
    (3) Oxygen readiness
    (4) Head measurements
    (5) Cast care if necessary; sometimes casts applied to legs
    (6) Importance of good nutrition
    (7) Orthopedic and urologic habilitation
    (8) Encourage normal use of functions
    (9) Minimize disabilities
    (10) Paralysis (if present) may not be alleviated, but further damage could be prevented; aim of surgery is to give infant opportunity for optimal growth and development
    (11) "Crede" bladder to keep it empty and free from infection

4. Hydrocephalus: refer to Chapter 9, Pediatric Nursing
5. Congenital dislocation of the hip: refer to Chapter 9, Pediatric Nursing
6. Talipes equinovarus (clubfoot): refer to Chapter 9, Pediatric Nursing
7. Phocomelia
   a. Definition: developmental congenital anomaly in which only stubs or parts of arms and legs are present; involvement varies
   b. Cause: believed to be drug taken by mother during the first trimester to alleviate nausea
   c. Treatment and nursing management
    (1) Psychosocial problems for family and infant
    (2) Body surface limited, so heating mechanism overheats rest of body, causing diaphoresis
    (3) Personal hygiene: frequent baths
    (4) Special education imperative
8. Polydactyly
   a. Definition: supernumerary fingers or toes
   b. Cause: possibly hereditary
   c. Treatment and nursing management
    (1) Usually no bone or nerve involvement
    (2) Tie digit with silk suture in newborn nursery; it falls off
    (3) Surgical intervention necessary with bone involvement
9. Exstrophy of bladder
   a. Definition: anomaly of lower urinary tract in which bladder, mucosa, and ureters are exposed, sometimes without a ventral covering
   b. Signs and symptoms
    (1) Lining of posterior bladder exposed and red
    (2) Urine drips into abdominal wall from abnormal ureters
    (3) Ulceration of bladder mucosa from seepage
   c. Treatment and nursing management
    (1) Surgical corrective procedures dependent on extent of exstrophy
    (2) Adequate hydration to keep ureter patent
    (3) Avoid infections
    (4) Good skin care

    (5) Involvement of parents in problems, surgical procedures, nursing care, management, and prognosis
    (6) Long-term hospitalization and care
10. Hypospadias: refer to Chapter 9, Pediatric Nursing
11. Epispadias: refer to Chapter 9, Pediatric Nursing

Hemolytic Disease of Newborn

A. Hyperbilirubinemia (erythroblastosis fetalis)
  1. Definition: a congenital condition in which red blood cells are broken down by an antigen-antibody reaction
  2. Cause: an Rh-negative mother giving birth to an Rh-positive baby
  3. Pathophysiology: fetal Rh antigen enters the Rh-negative mother, who then produces anti-Rh antibodies, which return through placenta to the fetal circulation, attach to fetal red blood cells, and destroy (hemolyze) them
  4. Signs and symptoms
   a. Jaundice
   b. Anemia
   c. Enlarged liver and spleen
   d. Generalized edema
   e. If untreated, "yellow bodies" will travel to brain, causing brain damage, heart failure, kernicterus, and death
  5. Treatment and nursing management
   a. Blood types of mother and father important for anticipatory guidance
   b. Usually first babies do not present a problem
   c. If baby's bilirubin is above 10 or 12 mg/dl, phototherapy may be applied to reduce jaundice; exchange transfusions may be necessary
   d. After birth of Rh-positive baby, an unsensitized Rh-negative mother is given RhoGAM, a specific gamma globulin that will prevent the production of Rh antibodies; this must be given within 72 hours after delivery; the effect is the assurance that subsequent pregnancies will not be harmful to the baby
   e. Rh-antibody titers can be monitored throughout pregnancy (prenatal)
   f. Amniocentesis will reveal, by indirect Coombs' test, if mother has antibodies circulating in the maternal plasma or serum

B. ABO incompatibility
  1. Definition: an incompatibility of blood groups A and B because of the presence of antigens developed and passed on to the fetus by a type O mother
  2. Signs and symptoms
   a. Jaundice: mild, occurring during first day or two
   b. Slight enlargement of liver and spleen
  3. Treatment and nursing management
   a. Phototherapy
   b. If bilirubin is above 20 mg/dl, an exchange transfusion with group O and appropriate Rh type
   c. Observe for progressive lethargy
   d. Level of jaundice (visual and laboratory)
   e. Observe color of urine
   f. Observe for edema
   g. Observe for convulsions
   h. Symptomatic nursing care

Down's Syndrome (Trisomy 21)

Refer to Chapter 9, Pediatric Nursing

Drug Addiction in Newborns

A. Defined: secondary addiction, caused by drugs being ingested or injected by mother-addict; drugs cross placental barrier and create a drug-dependent newborn (immature liver unable to excrete drug rapidly during fetal life)
B. Signs and symptoms
  1. Low birth weight
  2. Premature
  3. Immature
  4. Withdrawal symptoms within 48 to 72 hours; watch for
    a. Sneezing
    b. Respiratory distress
    c. Excessive sweating
    d. Feeding problems
    e. Frantic sucking of fists
    f. High-pitched cry
    g. Irritable, hyperactive, tremors
    h. Fever
    i. Diarrhea
C. Treatment and nursing management
  1. Prevent infection
  2. Promote good nutrition
  3. Keep quiet (quiet, darkened environment)
  4. Offer loving, soothing, cuddling care
  5. Give medications on time
  6. Monitor vital signs
  7. Keep warm
  8. Protect from injury since child is hyperactive
  9. Good skin care because of excessive sweating and diarrhea
  10. Adequate fluids (prevent dehydration)
  11. Encourage mother to assist in care
    a. Teach holding, diapering, talking, bathing
    b. Encourage visits

Infants of Diabetic Mothers

A. Complications
  1. Delivery date may be recommended before EDC or about 36 to 37 weeks' gestation to prevent
    a. Oversized baby
    b. High-risk infant (diabetic babies have high infant mortality)
  2. Neonatal hypoglycemia common
  3. RDS complications
  4. Hyperbilirubinemia (severe jaundice)
  5. Intracranial hemorrhage
  6. Congestive heart failure
  7. Congenital anomalies in 5% of infants
  8. Hypocalcemia
B. Signs and symptoms
  1. Lethargic
  2. Plump, puffy face
  3. Long and heavy
  4. Respiratory problems evident
  5. Enlarged heart, liver, and spleen
  6. Symptoms of hypoglycemia
  7. Symptoms of hypocalcemia

C. Treatment and nursing management
  1. Medical management difficult because of rapid, changing growth patterns, nutritional demands, illness
  2. Urine must be tested several times a day; placing cotton balls in diaper and squeezing urine out is an easy method to teach parents
  3. Short-acting insulin best (easier to control)
  4. Treat hypoglycemia and hypocalcemia
  5. Oral feedings when tolerated and blood sugar levels stable

Cretinism (Congenital Hypothyroidism)

Refer to Chapter 9, Pediatric Nursing

FAMILY PLANNING

A. Trends
  1. Smaller families (except for the poor and disadvantaged)
  2. Delayed parenthood by choice
    a. Career women
    b. Desire for higher education
    c. Alternate living arrangements
  3. Single parents
    a. High divorce rate
    b. Expanding role of father as single parent since custody of children, traditionally awarded to mother, is now being awarded to fathers
    c. Lessening barriers for adoption by single men and women
    d. Cultural and ethnic acceptance of unmarried mothers
    e. Opportunities to continue education for pregnant teenager without pressure of forced marriage
B. Communes: labor and delivery in communal community homes
C. Early sexual encounters (teenage pregnancies)
  1. Need for referrals to family planning centers for guidance and counseling
    a. Teach use of condoms (controversial)
    b. Practice abstinence
  2. Problems originating from early sexual encounters
D. Surrogate mothers
  1. In vitro transplantation of embryo in the uterus of a woman who agrees to have a full-term pregnancy for another woman
  2. Moral and legal implications

Possible Influencing Factors

A. Sex education: incorporation of sex education in public and parochial schools at an early age
B. Freedom of choice
  1. Availability of over-the-counter pregnancy tests
  2. Availability of over-the-counter contraceptives
  3. Abortions mandated as legal by the United States Supreme Court, 1977
C. Postponement of family: using available contraceptive devices
D. Economic factor: high cost of medical care forces young people to consider waiting until affluent enough to "afford" a family

Common Methods of Birth Control (Contraception)

A. Natural
   1. Rhythm (calendar) method
      a. Based on the principle that ovulation occurs during midcycle of a menstrual period; that is, in a 28-day cycle, ovulation would occur on the 14th day
      b. Accordingly the most fertile days are considered to be 3 to 4 days before and 3 to 4 days after ovulation
   2. Basal metabolism method: daily monitoring of early morning temperature for a period of several months and entering it on a graph (Fig. 8-15) will establish an ovulation time; "safe" and "fertile" times can be determined, and mother advised on use of this method
B. Coitus interruptus
   1. Penis is withdrawn from vagina just before ejaculation
   2. Least effective of all methods
C. Condom (sheath, snake skin, rubbers): thin rubber or plastic sheath that fits over penis and acts as barrier, preventing sperm from entering the vagina
D. Diaphragm: mechanical barrier placed at mouth of cervix; used with contraceptive cream or jelly to be effective; may engage in intercourse immediately after placement; should be left in place for 6 hours after intercourse; spermicide must be added each time intercourse occurs
E. Chemical agents: foam, creams, jelly, vaginal suppositories, and the newest on the market, sponges, form a chemical barrier in the vagina and render the area unsafe for sperm
F. Intrauterine device (IUD)
   1. Devices come in various shapes made of memory plastic; inserted into the uterine cavity by a physician during or immediately following the woman's menstrual cycle
   2. Mode of action unclear: thought to interfere with implantation by creating peristaltic waves
   3. Disadvantages:
      a. Excessive bleeding during menstrual cycle
      b. Extremely controversial: Dalkon shield taken off the market—court cases pending on settlement of permanent sterility and multiple gynecologic problems
      c. Possible contamination from IUD string hanging in vaginal orifice
   4. Advantage: once IUD is inserted, only periodic checking to confirm that it is still intact
G. Oral contraceptives (birth control pill)
   1. Most widely used
   2. Considered 90% or more effective
   3. Prevent anterior pituitary from releasing follicle stimulating hormone (FSH); artificially raises estrogen and progesterone levels and prevents ovulation
   4. Stimulates endometrium, creating hostile environment for sperm

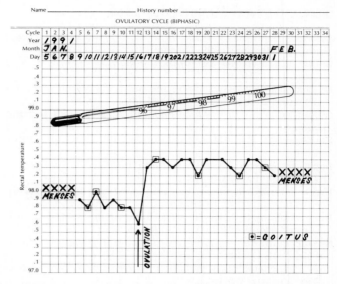

FIG. 8-15. Basal temperature record shows drop and sharp rise at time of ovulation. (From Bobak IM, Jensen MD: *Essentials of maternity nursing,* ed 3, St Louis, 1991, Mosby.)

   5. Minor side effects lasting few weeks to few months: nausea, weight gain, full breasts
   6. Major side effects: thrombophlebitis, hypertension, embolism, cardiovascular disturbances
H. Sterilization
   1. Surgical procedures for females are permanent
      a. Tubal ligation (cutting or tie) most commonly done
      b. Hysterectomy (removal of uterus)
      c. Oophorectomy (removal of ovaries)
   2. Surgical procedure for the male—vasectomy: tieing or ligating duct from each testicle so sperm cannot escape
   3. Careful consideration of these procedures because they are permanent
I. Newer methods
   1. Morning after pill: (diethylstilbestrol [DES]); must be taken orally within 72 hours after intercourse; prevents ovulation, alters endometrium, prevents implantation; not 100% effective; most commonly used in emergencies such as rape
   2. Contraceptive sponge: can be worn up to 24 hours; must be left in place for 6 hours after intercourse to be effective; danger of toxic shock syndrome (TTS)
   3. RU486: binds progesterone and appears to block its action; widely used in Europe
   4. Depo-Provera: injectable progesterone every 3 months
   5. Steroid implants: inhibits gonadotropins; not widely used
   6. Patches: time-released hormones; experimental

Suggested Reading List

Anderson B, Shapiro P: *Basic maternal and newborn nursing,* ed 5, Albany, NY, 1989, Delman.

Bobak IM, Jensen MD: *Essentials of maternity nursing,* ed 3, St Louis, 1991, Mosby.

Dulock DNS: Hypoglycemia in the newborn, March of Dimes BFD mod 2, ser 1, ed 2, White Plains, NY, 1990.

Guzzetta C et al: *Clinical assessment tools for use with nursing diagnoses,* St Louis, 1989, Mosby.

Hamilton PM: *Basic maternity nursing,* ed 6, St Louis, 1989, Mosby.

Ingalls JA, Salerno CM: *Maternal and child health nursing,* ed 7, St Louis, 1991, Mosby.

Karch A, Boyd E: *Handbook of drugs and the nursing process,* Philadelphia, 1989, JB Lippincott.

King J: Helping patients choose an appropriate method of birth control, *Matern Child Nurs* 17:91-95, March/April 1992.

Kosanek J: *Manual of labor and delivery nursing procedures,* 1990, ABC Decker.

Lone P: Silencing crack addiction, *Matern Child Nurs* 16:264-266, July/Aug 1991.

Long JW: *The essential guide to prescription drugs,* New York, 1990, Harper & Row.

Plovie B: Diabetes in pregnancy, prenatal care, March of Dimes BDF mod 10, ser 2, White Plains, NY, 1989.

Richardson J, Richardson LI: *The mathematics of drugs and solutions: with clinical applications,* ed 4, St Louis, 1990, Mosby.

Stringer M, Libizzi R, Weiner S: Establishing a prenatal genetic diagnosis: the nurse's role. *Matern Child Nurs* 16:152-156, May/June 1991.

Whaley L, Wong D: *Nursing care of infants and children,* ed 4, St Louis, 1991, Mosby.

Obstetric Nursing Review Questions

Answers and rationales begin on p. 439.

1. There are three categories of signs of pregnancy: presumptive signs, probable signs, and positive signs. Which of the following would be a positive sign of pregnancy?
   ① An immunologic pregnancy test
   ② Hegar's sign
   ③ Missed menstrual cycle
   ④ Echographic testing

2. Which of the following is considered the most effective method of birth control?
   ① Insertion of intrauterine device (IUD)
   ② Coitus interruptus
   ③ Use of condom
   ④ Oral contraceptives

3. Prenatal care is considered the primary deterrent to complications during pregnancy. Which complication would you consider as most affected by good prenatal care?
   ① Placenta previa
   ② Hyperemesis gravidarum
   ③ Pregnancy-induced hypertension (PIH)
   ④ Abortion

4. Pregnancy affects every major system in the body. Changes occur to the respiratory, skin, urinary, nervous, and digestive systems. Changes in the digestive system include:
   ① Aggravation of prepregnancy psychosocial problems
   ② Traces of sugar in the urine
   ③ Cholasma gravidarum
   ④ Increased appetite after the first trimester

5. Mothers are routinely screened during their first prenatal examination for a variety of conditions. One of the most important tests is the alpha-fetoprotein (AFP) test, which
   ① Determines fetal maturity
   ② Detects a neural tube defect such as spina bifida
   ③ Detects Tay-Sachs disease
   ④ Detects respiratory distress syndrome (RDS) in the newborn

6. Which female hormone is said to "hold" the pregnancy?
   ① Estrogen
   ② Luteinizing hormone
   ③ Progesterone
   ④ Human gonadotropic hormone

7. Which of the following statements is correct relative to a stress test and a nonstress test?
   ① A nonstress test is done by abdominal palpation by the physician
   ② A nonstress test is done early in pregnancy to determine sex of the infant
   ③ A stress test is usually done late in pregnancy to measure fetal response to uterine contractions
   ④ A stress test is done after the mother has been given orange juice to drink

8. You are to interview several pregnant women in the prenatal clinic. In today's psychosocial climate, which would be an *important* item to include in your initial interview?
   ① Economic and ethnic status
   ② Family and genetic history
   ③ Abuse of drugs or alcohol
   ④ Educational or schooling status

Situation: You are working on a unit caring for prenatal patients with problems. Miss Jay, 16 years old, is admitted with elevated blood pressure (BP), increased weight gain, and edema. Her diagnosis is preeclampsia. Orders include intake and output (I & O) every 4 hours, temperature, pulse, and respirations every 4 hours, BP and deep tendon reflexes (DTRs) every hour, and magnesium sulfate 1 g every hour intravenously.

9. Magnesium sulfate is a CNS depressant and should not be given if:
   ① BP is elevated
   ② DTRs are absent
   ③ DTRs are brisk
   ④ Should never be withheld for any reason

10. Miss Jay's magnesium sulfate in 100 ml D5W is due to run out in 1 hour. The administration set has 15 gtt/ml. How many drops per minute would you run the IV?
    ① 15 gtt/min
    ② 18 gtt/min
    ③ 25 gtt/min
    ④ 100 gtt/min

11. Miss Jay appears to be an impending eclamptic. She has complained of visual disturbance and severe epigastric pain. You would observe her closely for signs of:
    ① Seizure
    ② Elevated BP
    ③ Lowered BP
    ④ Labor

12. Because Miss Jay is 36 weeks' pregnant and in danger of becoming eclamptic, delivery is induced. She delivers a 5 lb 8 oz (2500 g) boy after just 6 hours of labor. She must continue to be watched for impending eclampsia for how long?
    ① 1 hour
    ② 2 hours
    ③ 24 hours
    ④ 72 hours

13. What is considered to be a major problem in teaching prenatal care to the pregnant teenager today?
    ① Inability to comprehend the psychosocial impact of her pregnancy on herself and on her unborn child
    ② Nutritional counseling
    ③ Physical immaturity
    ④ Dangers of HIV

14. Which would be the best source of calcium?
    ① Calcium tablets
    ② Milk
    ③ Greens
    ④ Multivitamin D

Situation: Elisabeth Tippens, age 29, is pregnant for the first time, has enrolled in a childbirth education class, and is eager to learn.

15. Elisabeth wants to know what substance in her urine specimen showed she was positive for pregnancy. As her instructor you would explain that a hormone presents itself at implantation and can be detected in the urine within 42 days after the LMP. It is called:
    ① Estrogen
    ② Progesterone
    ③ Relaxin hormone
    ④ Chorionic gonadotropin

16. Elisabeth has learned that the placenta is an all-purpose organ that nourishes the fetus, excretes waste materials, and acts as a respiratory organ. She is curious about the role of the umbilical cord. Your best answer would be:
    ① The cord is the staff of life and is surrounded by Wharton's jelly for protection of its contents
    ② It contains two veins and an artery that carry the vital life-sustaining products to the fetus
    ③ The umbilical cord contains the umbilical vein, which supplies oxygen and nutrients to the fetus while two arteries carry away the waste products
    ④ The oxygen flows from the umbilical vein to the liver through a fetal structure called the ductus venosus, then the arteries go through another fetal structure called the ductus arteriosus into the aorta and eventually back to the umbilical arteries

17. Elisabeth is curious to know when the fetal heart begins to function. You tell her it is usually:
    ① By the third or fourth week after LMP
    ② Within 6 weeks after implantation
    ③ By the first trimester
    ④ By the time the placenta is formed

18. Elisabeth is a chain-smoker, and as her prenatal nurse you have taught her the effect of nicotine and hazards of passive smoking. She does not drink, but you have taught her that fetal alcohol syndrome is a major concern today. In addressing the abuse of tobacco, you would stress that it:
    ① Is a dirty, nasty habit that yellows your teeth, can cause lung cancer, and can offend nonsmokers
    ② Is becoming socially unacceptable and has widespread negative effects on children as well as grown-ups
    ③ May cause adverse physiologic effects on the fetus
    ④ Retards fetal growth, constricts blood vessels in the mother, decreases placental function, and may cause premature labor

19. There are identical twins and fraternal twins. How would you distinguish the kind of twins Elisabeth has if she delivered a boy and a girl?
    ① Monozygotic or single-ovum twins: union of one sperm and one ovum, divides during mitosis into two embryos; one placenta, two amniotic sacs; heredity is a factor
    ② Dizygotic twins: union of two sperms with two ovas; two amniotic sacs; separate or fused placenta; same or different sex
    ③ They look exactly alike even though they are of a different sex; blood test will reveal if they are identical or fraternal
    ④ DNA will identify the type of twins they are

Situation: Mrs. Ketzler is a mother of a 5-year-old son. Her last menstrual period of 5 days began on May 18. Her first prenatal visit was on July 22. Her first pregnancy was normal in all respects.

20. As her pregnancy progresses, her urine specimen occasionally reveals traces of sugar. What is your assessment of this finding?
    ① She is eating a diet high in carbohydrates
    ② She is experiencing pregnancy-induced diabetes
    ③ This is probably the result of absorption of lactose from the breasts
    ④ Because she is a multipara, there is more absorption of lactose from the breasts

21. Mrs. Ketzler would be classified as:
    ① Gravida 1 para 1
    ② Gravida 2 para 2
    ③ Gravida 2 para 1
    ④ Gravida 2 nullipara

22. If a blood typing was Rh negative, there would be no complications to the new baby if:
    ① Mr. Ketzler was Rh negative
    ② Mr. Ketzler was Rh positive
    ③ Her son was Rh positive
    ④ She did not receive RhoGAM after the birth of her first son

23. The estimated date of confinement (EDC) would be:
    ① February 9
    ② February 11
    ③ February 18
    ④ February 25

24. In her third trimester Mrs. Ketzler suddenly notices that she is bleeding—at first the bleeding was scanty but has become heavier. She reports she has no pain. As her nurse in the prenatal clinic, you would suspect:
    ① Abruptio placentae
    ② Placenta previa
    ③ Ruptured uterus
    ④ Vasa previa

25. To relieve supine hypotensive syndrome in Mrs. Ketzler, you would:
    ① Massage her leg
    ② Instruct her to breathe deeply
    ③ Turn her on left side and advise frequent changing of position
    ④ Advise her to walk slowly and carefully

26. During this pregnancy Mrs. Ketzler is experiencing some leg cramps. Your nursing intervention would include:
    ① Advising hot compresses bid
    ② Instructing her to elevate her legs at least 15 minutes 3 times daily
    ③ Informing her of the cause (excessive phosphorus) and encouraging her to drink milk
    ④ Advising her to chew Tums for calcium

27. For relief of her low back pains, you might suggest:
    ① Sitz baths
    ② Heating pads to her back
    ③ Pelvic rocking or pelvic tilting exercises
    ④ Visits to the chiropractor

28. In looking over Mrs. Ketzler's chart you see that her hemoglobin is 7. What does this mean to you?
    ① That your patient is anemic and needs treatment stat
    ② That this is probably resulting from increased blood volume of pregnancy
    ③ That this must be her baseline
    ④ That you should give her Z-track iron dextran (Imferon)

29. Should Mrs. Ketzler have needed to confirm her pregnancy, how would you have instructed her regarding the required urine specimen?
    ① Give a voided specimen during her first visit
    ② Instruct her on how to give a sterile specimen in the office
    ③ Tell her to withhold fluid intake during the night and bring in the first voided specimen in the morning
    ④ A catheterized specimen will be required

30. After a review of prenatal care for Mrs. Ketzler, you would include an advisory that she notify the physician immediately:
    ① If she experiences abdominal pain, discharge of bright red blood, chills, and fever
    ② Blood-streaked mucus, Braxton Hicks contractions
    ③ Constipation, urgency, hemorrhoids
    ④ Quickening, varicosities, and discomfort

---

31. Estriol testing is a urine test taken at certain intervals to determine:
    ① Fetal age
    ② Lung surfactant of the fetus
    ③ Uterine nomenclature
    ④ Placental functioning

32. The communicable (childhood) disease most likely to affect pregnancy, with harmful effects to the fetus is:
    ① Chickenpox ③ Varicella
    ② Rubella ④ Rubeola

33. Orders for a patient on the maternity floor include notifying the physician immediately of any changes in status, no vaginal or rectal examinations, fetal monitoring, pad count, oxygen if necessary, and laboratory work (type and cross match, Hgh, Hct). These orders would alert the nurse to prepare for which of the following?
    ① Pending abortion
    ② Ectopic pregnancy
    ③ Third-trimester bleeding
    ④ Postpartum hemorrhage

Situation: Virginia Bauer has been admitted in active labor. Admission notes: Primipara, aged 33 years, excellent health. Lamaze mother, well prepared. Initial examination: 7 cm dilated, 75% effaced, 0 station, membranes intact. Contractions q 2 minutes, very strong, considerable bloody show. Tolerating contractions well. Routine hospital procedures completed.

34. Dr. Sono has just ruptured the membranes. Your primary responsibility as the attending nurse is to:
    ① Clean up after the procedure
    ② Note the time of the procedure, color, odor, other pertinent data
    ③ Chart the physician's name and the procedure done, sign your name in full
    ④ Hold patient's hand, reassure her, change the bed

35. As the labor-room nurse, you should encourage Mrs. Bauer to void and avoid a full bladder, because:
    ① A full bladder during labor may cause postpartum hemorrhage
    ② It may cause a rupture of the bladder during descent of the head
    ③ It may cause cystitis
    ④ It may impede the progress of labor

36. Nursing management during the first stage of labor includes which of the following?
    ① Admit patient to labor room, establish rapport, monitor FHT, keep patient and significant others apprised of progress
    ② Monitor FHT with fetoscope, monitor blood pressure (BP) q 15 minutes, give pushing instructions, maintain patent airway for newborn, follow proper identification routine
    ③ Be sure cord blood specimen is obtained, observe time and delivery of placenta, check perineal area, check fundus, administer oxytocin IV after placenta is delivered; check BP and fundus q 5 minutes
    ④ Watch for hemorrhaging, check fundus q 15 minutes, monitor BP q 15 minutes, offer warm food and fluid, offer bedpan for urination, teach perineal care, transfer patient to postpartum room when condition is stable

37. The greatest comfort you can give Mrs. Bauer or any woman in labor is to assure her that:
    ① Her progress is normal
    ② She will not be left alone
    ③ Her physician is in the building
    ④ She will be able to hold the baby after delivery

38. Why does a fetal position of left occiput posterior (LOP) create dystocia and severe back pain?
    ① The baby's face is descending, facing toward the spine
    ② The fetus is descending with its occipital bone against the mother's spine
    ③ The left shoulder is against the spine
    ④ The presenting part is pressing against the symphysis pubis

39. After the placenta is delivered and the suturing complete, you notice that Mrs. Bauer is beginning to shiver. You quickly get some warm blankets to cover her. The reason why she probably is shivering is:
    ① The sudden emptying of the uterine contents, plus the return of the body chemistry and hormones to the prepregnant state, causes a certain shock to the system
    ② Loss of blood, length of labor, and a certain tiredness cause the lowering of the body temperature; the warm blankets will help
    ③ Pitocin is given after the delivery of the placenta and may cause the body to respond by shivering
    ④ The shiver is a normal reaction, since she has been in a cold delivery room, swallowing ice chips, and only covered with a thin sheet

40. What Apgar score would you give a newborn who exhibited the following:
    Heart rate—below 100 beats/min
    Respiratory effort—weak cry
    Muscle tone—some flexion
    Reflex response—cough or sneeze
    Color—body pink; extremities blue
    ① 4   ③ 7
    ② 6   ④ 8

41. Of the following normal newborn conditions, which is *not* correct?
    ① Milia are small, white sebaceous glands found in the chin, forehead, nose, cheek, and upper lip
    ② Mongolian spots are noted as dark pigmented areas on the lower back and buttocks
    ③ Erb-Duchenne, brachial plexus
    ④ Cephalhematoma, molding, or caput succedaneum

Situation: Kathy and George Cone have attended private psychoprophylactic Lamaze classes. Both are looking forward to their first baby. Labor has started at home, and both Kathy and George have managed for 3 hours doing simple breathing. A sudden sharp pain made Kathy gasp for breath. She had beads of perspiration on her forehead, became almost ashen, cold, and clammy. George noticed also that Kathy's abdomen was rigid and boardlike. Frightened, he called the physician, who ordered them to go to the hospital immediately and added that he would be there waiting for them.

42. George and Kathy arrive at the hospital minutes later, and you are the admitting obstetric nurse. The most likely complication, judging from the symptoms described, would lead you to suspect:
    ① Low marginal placenta previa
    ② Appendicitis
    ③ Premature separation of the placenta
    ④ Rupture of the uterus

43. George tells you he cannot understand why Kathy looks so pale and weak when there is no significant bleeding. Your explanation would be:
    ① The bleeding is all internal; perhaps you should line up some blood donors
    ② In this condition, shock is out of proportion to blood loss, but we are watching her closely and will not leave her bedside
    ③ It is a good sign that you can't see much bleeding
    ④ As you can see we are doing everything to treat the shock; she should be coming out of it soon

44. The physician is checking Kathy's blood q 15 minutes in the room. Mr. Cone asks you what the physician is doing. Your best answer would be:
    ① "Ask the physician yourself."
    ② "Do you want me to ask the physician for you?"
    ③ "The physician is checking the fibrinogen level to determine the status of the clotting factor so he can plan what further action to take. We will keep you informed."
    ④ "The physician is finding out whether he should give her a blood transfusion or whether he should operate."

45. As the nurse responsible for obtaining equipment for the physician you would quickly prepare the delivery room for:
    ① A cesarean section
    ② A natural vaginal delivery
    ③ A double setup
    ④ A precipitate delivery

46. Kathy's pain has subsided as quickly as it started, and she is laughing and telling the physician she cannot believe what just happened. She progresses very well and delivers a baby girl; Apgar score is 9-10. Both mother and baby are fine. After the delivery, the physician wants to examine the placenta more thoroughly. Why?
    ① The placenta will reveal a tear where the original abruptio occurred
    ② The placenta will clearly show calcified areas that caused the problem
    ③ The placenta will be much heavier in weight than normal
    ④ The placenta will be sent to the laboratory for further analysis

Situation: Mrs. Downs, gravida II, para I, is brought to the emergency room by ambulance. Contractions are strong, she is pushing, and delivery is imminent.

47. With the next contraction Mrs. Downs delivers a 7 lb 8 oz (3400 g) baby girl spontaneously. You are still alone, so your first responsibility is to:
    ① Ascertain whether the fundus is likely to hemorrhage
    ② Establish an airway for the baby by milking the trachea and maintaining the head lower than the body
    ③ Quickly tie and cut the umbilical cord
    ④ Look for the uterus to rise, watch the perineum for a trickle of blood, and deliver the placenta

48. The physician arrives after the baby is delivered, examines the baby, then examines the mother. He has her wheeled into a delivery room, where he delivers the secundines intact. He reexamines the mother internally, orders oxytocin (Pitocin) IM, and starts an IV with a piggyback of an antibiotic. Because Mrs. Downs had a precipitous delivery, your nursing responsibility would be to:
    ① Watch for infiltration of the IV and observe for antibiotic reaction
    ② Watch for excessive bleeding or signs of hemorrhage
    ③ Anticipate Mrs. Downs' legs shaking and chills
    ④ Watch for sudden elevation of temperature as a forerunner of an infection or infectious process

49. The delivery is termed nonsterile birth (NSB), so your responsibilities as the emergency room nurse will include:
    ① Checking the cord, the Apgar score, making identification bands as for a normal delivery
    ② Informing the nursery of the baby's status so they will observe predesignated hospital precautions for deliveries performed outside the hospital
    ③ Ordering an antibiotic because of the circumstances of birth
    ④ Placing the baby in an Isolette for observation

50. After a particularly stormy labor, posterior presentation, severe back pains, nausea, and vomiting during transition and difficulty pushing, Mary Anderson delivered a 9 lb 14 oz baby boy. The placenta was not yet delivered when suddenly Mary started to hemorrhage profusely from the vaginal orifice. Within minutes you see blood trickling from her nose and mouth. What can you do to help in alleviating this condition the physician has labeled as disseminated intravascular coagulation (DIC)?
    ① Call the laboratory for blood replacement (fresh whole blood) and assist the physician to deliver the placenta as quickly as possible
    ② Prepare all necessary equipment for possible blood replacement, get extra IV poles for possible fibrinogen and heparin administration if ordered, get extra warm blankets for both fetus and mother, monitor blood pressure, and prepare dressings as necessary
    ③ Apply fundal pressure to help deliver the placenta stat
    ④ Hold patient's hand and reassure her

51. Mrs. Gwen Amora is a primipara. She has passed her due date by 2 weeks. She is apprehensive and does not know why she was instructed to come in for a test. She appears confused and bewildered. How can you help her?
    ① To ease her distress you could engage her in trivial conversation regarding the weather, current styles, and so forth
    ② Explain that she will be placed on a monitor for 20 minutes to an hour to see if her baby responds to her drinking water or to gentle external pressure by the nurse on her abdomen. The procedure is called a nonstress test
    ③ Tell Gwen she may have to have an oxytocin challenge test (OCT) at a later date but that it is invasive
    ④ Tell her many people are often past due, and she probably miscalculated her dates

52. As you watched the monitor during an OCT procedure on Gwen, you noted at least three late decelerations during at least three contractions. What would you do?
    ① This indicates a positive test; call the head nurse immediately
    ② This is not a positive test; wait until the pattern changed
    ③ Stop the oxytocin (Pitocin) and administer nasal oxygen
    ④ Wheel her into the delivery room for immediate delivery

53. At her age (over 35 years) Gwen would undoubtedly be classified as:
    ① A good candidate for a normal pregnancy and delivery
    ② A high-risk pregnant mother
    ③ A candidate for eclampsia
    ④ A granmultipara

54. You would explain to Gwen that the OCT test is an invasive test because medication is given in the veins and:
    ① Is uncomfortable for a short while
    ② Is not painful at all
    ③ Will take a few minutes to complete
    ④ Is a routine procedure for all pregnant women

55. If Gwen were truly overdue, her newborn baby may have:
    ① Polydactyly and jaundice
    ② Desquamated palms of hands and soles of the feet
    ③ Meconium-stained amniotic fluid
    ④ None of the above

56. Baby Joe C., 3 days old, vertex delivery, 10 lb 2 oz (4500 g), fourth baby of Mr. and Mrs. C., has a condition often described as pathologic jaundice. His sclera is yellow, his bilirubin index is 17, and he is not nursing well. If Baby Joe's bilirubin index continues to rise, you would:
    ① Tell the mother the baby will probably need an exchange transfusion and plan a teaching module of pros and cons
    ② Prepare unit for possible exchange transfusion procedure; obtain supplies, review procedure, wait for physician's orders
    ③ Place the baby under phototherapy light for longer periods of time; offer water every 2 hours until jaundice begins to fade
    ④ Suggest that the family all be tested for proper blood type

Situation: When admitted to the hospital, Mrs. Sweeney seemed alert and calm. She could not recall anything that had happened since noon. It is now 3PM. Mr. Sweeney said his wife, 38 weeks' pregnant, had been bothered by headaches and "blind spots" for about a week. She got up in the morning, complaining of severe pain in the upper abdomen, then had a convulsion about noon. Mr. Sweeney did not realize this until later; he then called the physician, who told him to take his wife to the hospital immediately.

Admitting record:

BP 190/112	Cervix effaced, dilatation 3 cm
Albumin 4+	Presenting part: station 0
FHT 140 strong	Membranes intact

57. As the admitting nurse in the maternity ward, apprised of the situation, you would place Mrs. Sweeney in:
    ① A semiprivate room with plenty of sunlight and air
    ② A semiprivate room, darkened and quiet; restricted visitors
    ③ A single, darkened room; no visitors, close to nurses' station
    ④ Single room, plenty of sunlight; no visitors, away from the nurses' station

58. The symptom experienced by Mrs. Sweeney that is often considered a warning sign of an impending convulsion in the toxic mother is:
    ① Headache
    ② Severe epigastric pain
    ③ Scotoma
    ④ Puffy face

Situation: Mrs G. delivered her first baby, a boy, several hours ago. She has been admitted to her postpartum room in stable condition. She is euphoric over her successful implementation of the Lamaze techniques. You find her uterus firm, slightly above the umbilicus. She has saturated one pad with red lochia. Her episiotomy appears clean, but her labia and perineal area are swollen and slightly black and blue.

59. Your first priority in nursing care would be:
    ① To apply an ice glove to the perineal area
    ② To massage her uterus so it will go down below the umbilicus
    ③ To administer a tranquilizer because she is so euphoric
    ④ To watch for hemorrhage because her lochia is so red

60. Mrs G. delivered a macrosomic infant, which means the infant is:
    ① Small for gestational age (SGA)
    ② Large, somewhat lethargic, weighing over 4500 g
    ③ Covered with newborn milia, which will disappear without treatment.
    ④ Definitely diabetic and will be insulin dependent

61. The most important precaution that the nurse should follow in working with AIDS or HIV-positive patients is to use:
    ① Frequent handwashing procedures
    ② The designated forms to notify the Centers for Disease Control and report the name of your patient(s)
    ③ Universal precaution protocol
    ④ Masks, gloves, and gowns at all times

62. As a rule, the nurse should schedule the high-risk pregnant mother to be screened for gestational diabetes mellitus (GDM) at:
    ① 12 weeks' gestation
    ② 20 to 24 weeks' gestation
    ③ 32 weeks' gestation
    ④ 40 weeks' gestation

63. Postpartum teaching of a pregnancy-induced diabetic would include which of the following?
    ① Her symptoms should disappear in about 6 weeks
    ② She must be careful because she may become insulin dependent
    ③ She should try not to gain over 25 lb
    ④ She should have her glucose level checked for 5 years

64. A major health concern in women is alcohol consumption. When should nurses ideally direct their efforts toward counseling to prevent fetal alcohol syndrome (FAS)?
    ① Before pregnancy
    ② By the first trimester
    ③ Aggressive counseling during the second trimester
    ④ During the third trimester

65. Cocaine is addictive to newborns because of:
    ① Inability of the newborn's immature liver to excrete the drug rapidly
    ② The mother's long-term use of drugs before conception
    ③ The mother's ingestion of several different drugs is doubly addictive to the newborn
    ④ The mother's impaired uterine growth resulting in newborn having respiratory distress syndrome (RDS) after birth

CHAPTER 9

Pediatric Nursing

Pediatric nursing includes the care of both well and sick children and covers both preventive health care and restorative nursing care. This chapter is divided into the following age groups: infancy, toddlerhood, preschool age, school age, and adolescence. The areas covered include normal growth and development, psychosocial development, health promotion, and health problems specific to each age group. Other topics discussed include the battered child syndrome, hospitalization and the child, and nursing care of the hospitalized child. The information provided in this chapter presents both the physical and psychologic aspects of care necessary in providing pediatric nursing care.

ASSESSMENT OF CHILD AND FAMILY

A. Functions and structure of family
1. The functions and structure of the family are vital to the normal growth and development of the child
2. Three primary functions of the family are
   a. Providing physical care such as food, clothing, shelter, safety, prevention of illness, and care during illness
   b. Education and training: language, values, morals, and formal education
   c. Protecting psychologic and emotional health
B. Physical assessment of child
1. Performing a health history, including the child's past history as well as current complaints or problems, is done by the nurse, physician, or nurse practitioner
2. Assessment of child's physical growth and development level is done by the physician or nurse practitioner
C. Concepts of child development (Table 9-1)
1. Freud's theory of development is based on the child's psychosexual development
2. Erikson's theory of development is based on psychosocial development as a series of developmental tasks
3. Piaget's theory of development is based on intellectual (cognitive) development: how the child learns and develops his or her intelligence

Infancy (Ages 4 Weeks to 1 Year)
NORMAL GROWTH AND DEVELOPMENT
Physical Development*

A. 1 month
1. Physical
   a. Weight: gains about 150 to 210 g (5 to 7 oz) weekly during the first 6 months of life

---

*From Saxton DF, Nugent PM, Pelikan PK: *Mosby's comprehensive review of nursing,* ed 13, St Louis, 1990, Mosby.

   b. Height: gains about 2.5 cm (1 inch) a month for the first 6 months of life
2. Motor
   a. May lift the head temporarily, but generally the head must be supported
   b. Holds the head parallel with the body when placed prone
   c. Can turn the head from side to side when prone or supine
   d. Asymmetric posture dominates, such as tonic neck reflex
   e. Primitive reflexes still present (grasp, Moro's, tonic neck)
3. Sensory
   a. Follows a light to midline
   b. Eye movements coordinated most of the time
   c. Visual acuity 20/100 to 20/50
4. Socialization and vocalization
   a. Smiles indiscriminately
   b. Utters small throaty sounds
B. 2 to 3 months
1. Physical: posterior fontanel closed
2. Motor
   a. Holds the head erect for a short time and can raise chest supported on the forearms
   b. Can carry hand or an object to the mouth at will
   c. Reaches for attractive objects but misjudges distances
   d. Grasp, tonic neck, and Moro's reflexes are fading
   e. Can sit when the back is supported; knees will be flexed and back rounded
   f. Step or dance reflex disappears
   g. Plays with fingers and hands
3. Sensory
   a. Follows a light to the periphery
   b. Has binocular coordination (vertical and horizontal vision)
   c. Listens to sounds

Table 9-1. Concepts of child development

Age	Developmental stage	Freud's theory	Erikson's theory	Piaget's theory
4 wk–1 yr	Infancy	Oral stage	Trust vs. mistrust	Sensorimotor phase
1–3 yr	Toddlerhood	Anal stage	Autonomy vs. shame and doubt	Preoperational phase
3–5 yr	Preschool age	Oedipal stage	Initiative vs. guilt	Preoperational phase continued
		Latency stage		
6–12 yr	School age	Latency stage continued	Industry vs. inferiority	Concrete operational phase
		Genital stage		Formal operational phase
13–18 yr	Adolescence	Genital stage continued	Identity vs. identity confusion	Formal operational phase continued

    4. Socialization and vocalization
       a. Smiles in response to a person or object
       b. Laughs aloud and shows pleasure in making sounds
       c. Cries less
C. 4 to 5 months
    1. Physical: drools because salivary glands are functioning, but the child does not have sufficient coordination to swallow saliva
    2. Motor
       a. Balances the head well in a sitting position
       b. Sits with little support; holds the back straight when pulled to a sitting position
       c. Symmetric body position predominates
       d. Can sustain a portion of own weight when held in a standing position
       e. Reaches for and grasps an object with the whole hand
       f. Can roll over from back to side
       g. Lifts the head and shoulders at a 90-degree angle when prone
       h. Primitive reflexes (e.g., grasp, tonic neck, and Moro's) have disappeared
    3. Sensory
       a. Recognizes familiar objects and people
       b. Has coupled eye movements; accommodation is developing
    4. Socialization and vocalization
       a. Coos and gurgles when talked to
       b. Definitely enjoys social interaction with people
       c. Vocalizes displeasure when an object is taken away
D. 6 to 7 months
    1. Physical
       a. Weight: gains about 90 to 150 g (3 to 5 oz) weekly during second 6 months of life
       b. Height: gains about 1.25 cm (½ inch) a month
       c. Teething may begin with eruption of two lower central incisors, followed by upper incisors (Fig. 9-1)
    2. Motor
       a. Can turn over equally well from stomach or back
       b. Sits fairly well unsupported, especially if placed in a forward-leaning position
       c. Hitches or moves backward when in a sitting position
       d. Can transfer a toy from one hand to the other
       e. Can approach a toy and grasp it with one hand

       f. Plays with feet and puts them in mouth
       g. When lying down, lifts head as if trying to sit up
       h. Transfers everything from hand to mouth
    3. Sensory
       a. Has taste preferences
       b. Will spit out disliked food
    4. Socialization and vocalization
       a. Begins to differentiate between strange and familiar faces and shows "stranger anxiety"
       b. Makes polysyllabic vowel sounds
       c. Vocalizes "m-m-m-m" when crying
       d. Cries easily on slightest provocation but laughs just as quickly
E. 8 to 9 months
    1. Motor
       a. Sits steadily alone
       b. Has good hand-to-mouth coordination
       c. Developing pincer grasp, with preference for use of one hand over the other
       d. Crawls and then creeps (creeping is more advanced because the abdomen is supported off the floor)
       e. Can raise self to a sitting position but may require help to pull self to feet
    2. Sensory
       a. Depth perception is beginning to develop
       b. Displays interest in small objects
    3. Socialization and vocalization
       a. Shows anxiety with strangers by turning or pushing away and crying
       b. Definite social attachment is evident: stretches out arms to loved ones
       c. Is voluntarily separating self from mother by desire to act on own
       d. Reacts to adult anger: cries when scolded
       e. Has imitative and repetitive speech, using vowels and consonants such as *Dadda*
       f. No true words as yet, but comprehends words such as *bye-bye*
F. 10 to 12 months
    1. Physical
       a. Has tripled birth weight
       b. Upper and lower lateral incisors usually have erupted for total of 6 to 8 teeth
       c. Head and chest circumferences are equal
    2. Motor
       a. Stands alone for short times
       b. Walks with help: moves around by holding onto furniture

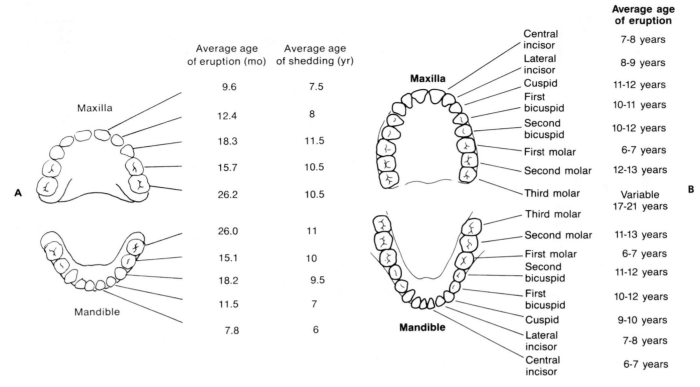

FIG. 9-1. Sequence of eruption and shedding of **A,** primary, and **B,** secondary, teeth. (From Whaley LF, Wong DL: *Nursing care of infants and children,* ed 4, St Louis, 1991, Mosby.)

c. Can sit down from a standing position without help

d. Can eat from a spoon and drink from a cup but needs help; prefers using fingers

e. Can play pat-a-cake and peek-a-boo

f. Can hold a crayon to make a mark on paper

g. Helps in dressing, such as putting arm through sleeve

3. Sensory
   a. Visual acuity 20/50+
   b. Amblyopia may develop with lack of binocularity
   c. Discriminates simple geometric forms

4. Socialization and vocalization
   a. Shows emotions such as jealousy, affection, anger
   b. Enjoys familiar surroundings and will explore away from mother
   c. Fearful in strange situation or with strangers; clings to mother
   d. May develop habit of "security" blanket
   e. Can say two words besides *Dadda* or *Mama*
   f. Understands simple verbal requests, such as "Give it to me"
   g. Knows own name

Psychosocial Development

A. Infants are in Erikson's stage of "trust vs. mistrust." Infants will develop a sense of trust or mistrust depending on how their needs are met by their parents (or other caregivers)

B. As infants grow older, they slowly realize that they are separate from their environment and that they influence their environment with their actions

C. Infants' early activities are mostly reflexes: crying, sucking, kicking, and so on. As the months progress, they learn to move in certain ways, follow with their eyes, and smile in response to a smile and soft words

HEALTH PROMOTION

A. Immunizations should be given on schedule; Table 9-2

B. Nutrition appropriate to the age and needs of the infant should be provided

   1. Introduction of strained foods may begin between 4 and 6 months of age, starting with strained fruits

   2. Solid foods should be introduced slowly, in small amounts, and one at a time, to determine the infant's likes and dislikes; this also helps detect possible allergies to certain foods

   3. Weaning from breast or bottle to a cup can begin between 5 and 6 months of age, although it is usually between 12 and 24 months of age before the infant can be weaned completely

   4. If breast-feeding must be stopped before the infant is 6 months of age, weaning should be to a bottle first to continue to provide for the infant's sucking needs

C. Safety and accident prevention includes a safe home environment, safe toys, use of car seats, and close attention to the infant who is crawling or walking

Table 9-2. Recommended schedule for immunization of healthy infants and children[a]

Recommended age[b]	Immunizations[c]	Comments
2 mo	DTP, HbCV,[d] OPV	DTP and OPV can be initiated as early as 4 wk after birth in areas of high endemicity or during epidemics
4 mo	DTP, HbCV,[d] OPV	2-mo interval (minimum of 6 wk) desired for OPV to avoid interference from previous dose
6 mo	DTP, HbCV[d]	Third dose of OPV is not indicated in the United States but is desirable in other geographic areas where polio is endemic
15 mo	MMR,[e] HbCV[f]	Tuberculin testing may be done at the same visit
15-18 mo	DTP,[g,h] OPV[i]	(See footnotes)
4-6 yr	DTP,[j] OPV	At or before school entry
11-12 yr	MMR	At entry to middle school or junior high school unless second dose previously given
14-16 yr	Td	Repeat every 10 yr throughout life

From American Academy of Pediatrics, *Red Book*, Elk Grove, Ill, 1991.

[a]For all products used, consult manufacturer's package insert for instructions for storage, handling, dosage, and administration. Biologics prepared by different manufacturers may vary, and package inserts of the same manufacturer may change from time to time. Therefore the physician should be aware of the contents of the current package insert.

[b]These recommended ages should not be construed as absolute. For example, 2 months can be 6 to 10 weeks. However, MMR usually should not be given to children younger than 12 months. (If measles vaccination is indicated, monovalent measles vaccine is recommended, and MMR should be given subsequently, at 15 months.)

[c]DTP, diphtheria and tetanus toxoids with pertussis vaccine; HbCV, *Haemophilus* b conjugate vaccine; OPV, oral poliovirus vaccine containing attenuated poliovirus types 1, 2, and 3; MMR, live measles, mumps, and rubella viruses in a combined vaccine; Td, adult tetanus toxoid (full dose) and diphtheria toxoid (reduced dose) for adult use.

[d]As of October 1990, only one HbCV (HbOC) is approved for use in children younger than 15 months.

[e]May be given at 12 months of age in areas with recurrent measles transmission.

[f]Any licensed *Haemophilus* b conjugate vaccine may be given.

[g]Should be given 6 to 12 months after the third dose.

[h]May be given simultaneously with MMR at 15 months.

[i]May be given simultaneously with MMR and HbCV at 15 months or at any time between 12 and 24 months; priority should be given to administering MMR at the recommended age.

[j]Can be given up to the 17th birthday.

HEALTH PROBLEMS
Failure to Thrive (FTT)

A. Definition: a state of inadequate growth resulting from inability to obtain and/or use calories; leads to malnutrition

B. Symptoms: below normal weight and height (below 5th percentile for age), listlessness, poor feeding habits, unresponsive to holding and attention, voluntary regurgitation, prolonged periods of sleep

C. Diagnosis
   1. Based on symptoms and a continued deviation from an established growth curve
   2. Three general categories of FTT
      a. Organic: result of a physical cause such as congenital defects of gastrointestinal (GI) system or heart
      b. Nonorganic: unrelated to a disease; usually caused by psychosocial factors
      c. Idiopathic: unexplained cause; may be grouped with nonorganic FTT

D. Treatment/nursing interventions (directed at correcting the malnutrition)
   1. Correction of organic causes, if possible
   2. Sensory stimulation
   3. Adequate food for weight gain; this may include nasogastric feedings as well as bottle feedings during early treatment
   4. Tender loving care; holding and cuddling, talking to the infant

   5. Teaching and encouragement of the mother regarding feeding and care of the infant
   6. Family counseling when needed

Respiratory Disorders
Upper Respiratory Infections (URIs)

A. Definition: viral or bacterial infection affecting the upper respiratory tract; nasopharyngitis or the "common cold" is particularly common in children of all ages

B. Symptoms: fever, sore throat, sneezing, nasal congestion, occasional cough, irritability, anorexia

C. Diagnosis: based on the symptoms

D. Treatment/nursing interventions
   1. Bed rest until free of fever for at least 1 day
   2. Encourage oral fluids
   3. Antipyretics for fever
   4. Nose drops to relieve nasal congestion
   5. Oral decongestants as ordered
   6. Adequate nutrition for age; high-calorie fluids and soft foods are better tolerated by infants and young children
   7. Cool air humidifier for moistened air (to assist in decreasing congestion)

Acute Otitis Media

A. Definition: middle ear infection; frequently caused by nasopharyngeal infections that travel through the infant's shortened, widened eustachian tubes

B. Symptoms: fever, irritability, restlessness, and pulling or rubbing of the ears

C. Diagnosis: based on the symptoms and history of recent URI
D. Treatment/nursing interventions
   1. Antibiotics as ordered for bacterial infections
   2. Ear drops as ordered
   3. Encourage oral fluids
   4. Promote rest
   5. Myringotomy and insertion of polyethylene tubes by the physician, to allow for drainage of fluid
   6. Observe for drainage
   7. Keep ears clean

Lower Respiratory Infections
Bronchiolitis

A. Definition: viral infection that causes the bronchioles to become plugged with a thick mucus; the mucus traps the air in the lungs, making it difficult for the infant to expel the air; respiratory syncytial virus (RSV) is responsible for over 50% of the cases of bronchiolitis
B. Symptoms: shallow respirations, dry cough, air hunger and cyanosis, retractions, rapid respirations (60 to 80 per minute), slight elevation in temperature
C. Diagnosis: based on the symptoms
D. Treatment/nursing interventions
   1. Elevate the head of the crib
   2. Croup tent for humidified oxygen inhalation (to relieve dyspnea and hypoxia)
   3. Monitor vital signs frequently
   4. Keep nose clear of mucus when possible
   5. Administer intravenous (IV) fluids if infant cannot take fluids by mouth (because of fatigue and tachypnea)
   6. Allow infant to rest as much as possible

Interstitial Pneumonia

A. Definition: localized acute inflammation of the lung, usually confined within the alveolar walls (interstitium)
B. Symptoms: fever, cough, rapid respiratory rate, and slight cyanosis
C. Diagnosis: based on the symptoms and results of chest x-ray films
D. Treatment/nursing interventions
   1. Elevate the head of the crib
   2. Croup tent for humidified oxygen inhalation
   3. Antibiotics as ordered (for bacterial pneumonia)
   4. Monitor vital signs frequently
   5. Encourage clear fluids by mouth
   6. Allow infant to rest to prevent dyspnea

Gastrointestinal Disorder: Gastroenteritis

A. Definition: diarrhea and vomiting that may be caused by malnutrition, allergies, and viral or bacterial infections
B. Symptoms: frequent, loose stools, irritability, vomiting, abdominal distention, dehydration, sunken fontanel, poor skin turgor, weak, rapid pulse
C. Diagnosis: based on the symptoms; specific bacterial cause can be isolated in a stool culture (most commonly *E. coli* or rotavirus in the infant)
D. Treatment/nursing interventions
   1. Give IV fluids with electrolytes as ordered
   2. Give infant nothing by mouth (NPO); resume oral feedings gradually as ordered (usually begins with glucose water, clear fluids, and skim milk), progressing to a "BRAT" diet: bananas, rice cereal, applesauce, toast/tea (in the older infant and toddler)
   3. Note amount, color, and consistency of stools and emesis
   4. Keep accurate intake and output record (if necessary, weigh diapers to measure urine output)
   5. Maintain proper isolation technique (enteric precautions)
   6. Provide good skin care to buttocks and perineum; cleanse well; leave area open to air when possible; apply ointments as ordered
   7. Provide time for stimulation, holding and cuddling

Nervous System Disorders
Febrile Seizures

A. Definition: seizures caused by high fever (102° to 105° F; 38.8° to 40.5° C); most often seen between 6 months and 3 years of age
B. Symptoms: seizures characterized by stiffening of the body, with jerking movements of the extremities and face, ending with a lapse of consciousness
C. Diagnosis: based on evidence of seizure activity preceded by high fever
   1. Simple febrile seizures are brief and generalized
   2. Complex febrile seizures are prolonged and may have focal features
D. Treatment/nursing interventions
   1. Anticonvulsant (phenobarbital) and antianxiety (diazepam) medications to control the seizures; antipyretics (acetaminophen) to control fever (see Chapter 4, Pharmacology)
   2. Padded side rails
   3. Airway and suction equipment at bedside
   4. During seizure, do not restrain the infant; turn his or her head to the side to allow saliva to drain out of the mouth; *do not* try to insert a seizure stick or airway in the infant's mouth during a seizure; observe the seizure and protect the infant from harm
   5. Documentation: note the kinds of movements, behavior before the seizure (if known), duration of the seizure, skin color and vital signs during and after the seizure, and medications given during the seizure, including the infant/toddler's reaction to the medications
   6. Parent teaching should include care of the infant during a seizure

Meningitis

A. Definition: infection of the spinal meninges and fluid; caused by several bacteria and viruses
B. Symptoms: elevated temperature, irritability, high-pitched cry, nuchal rigidity, seizures, bulging fontanel
C. Diagnosis: based on the symptoms and the presence of cloudy spinal fluid when lumbar puncture is performed (increased WBC count; decreased glucose level and increased protein level in the spinal fluid) (Fig. 9-2)
D. Treatment/nursing interventions
   1. Isolation from other children (for bacterial meningitis)

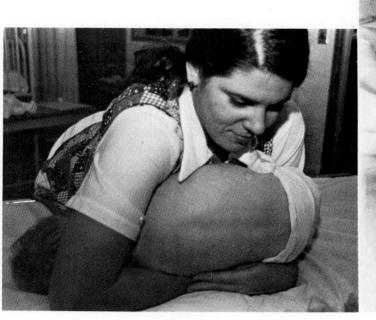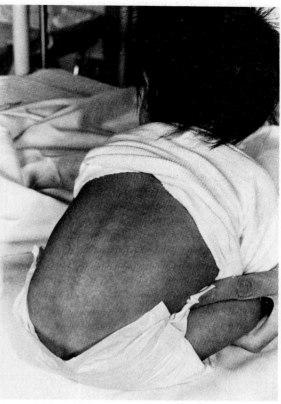

FIG. 9-2. Position for lumbar puncture. **A,** Older child. **B,** Infant. (From Whaley LF, Wong DL: *Nursing care of infants and children,* ed 4, St Louis, 1991, Mosby.)

2. IV antibiotics as ordered
3. Monitor vital signs and level of consciousness frequently
4. IV fluids as ordered
5. Diet: infant may be NPO at first, until liquids can be tolerated
6. Sponge with tepid water to reduce elevated temperature
7. Handle the infant as little as possible when the infant is irritable and uncomfortable

Integumentary Disorders
Infantile Eczema

A. Definition: atopic dermatitis caused by an allergic reaction to some irritant; usually begins between 2 and 6 months of age, and undergoes spontaneous remission around age 3
B. Symptoms: reddened, raised rash starting on cheeks and spreading to arms and legs; itching, oozing of vesicles
C. Diagnosis: based on the symptoms; the cause of the eczema (the allergen) must also be determined to control further episodes
D. Treatment/nursing interventions
   1. Good skin care; keep affected areas clean
   2. Tub baths with tepid water, baking soda, and corn starch to relieve the itching

3. Antihistamines and topical steroids as ordered to control itching
4. "Mittens" to prevent scratching
5. Elbow restraints to prevent scratching (only if necessary)
6. Provide for sensory stimulation, holding and cuddling at frequent intervals

Impetigo

A. Definition: infection of the skin caused by *Streptococcus* or *Staphylococcus* bacteria; occurs in nurseries when strict handwashing technique is not followed (impetigo neonatorum); also occurs in pre-school and school-age children
B. Symptoms: reddened, vesicular lesions (pustules)
C. Diagnosis: based on the symptoms; specific bacterial cause can be determined by culture of the draining lesions
D. Treatment/nursing interventions
   1. Isolation of infant (child)
   2. Strict handwashing technique by all persons coming in contact with the infant
   3. Antiseptic solution to wash lesions as ordered
   4. Antibiotic ointment to lesions as ordered
   5. Systemic antibiotics and corticosteroids may be ordered for infants/children with widespread lesions

Congenital Defects and Hereditary Disorders
Gastrointestinal System
Hypertrophic Pyloric Stenosis

A. Definition: hypertrophy of the pyloric muscle fibers and narrowing of the pylorus, which is at distal end of the stomach (Fig. 9-3)

B. Symptoms: usually appear between 3 and 8 weeks of age; projectile vomiting of formula and mucus, irritability, weight loss, and dehydration; the physician can often palpate the olive-size pyloric mass in the abdomen

C. Diagnosis: based on the symptoms, physical examination, and if necessary, upper gastrointestinal radiographic studies

D. Treatment/nursing interventions
   1. Preoperative
      a. IV fluids with electrolytes as ordered
      b. NPO unless ordered to feed
      c. Nasogastric (NG) tube is often inserted to remove excess stomach contents immediately before surgery
   2. Postoperative
      a. Position the infant on right side or abdomen or in infant seat to prevent aspiration
      b. NPO; first feeding begins about 4 to 6 hours after surgery (glucose water); amounts are increased slowly, with feedings every 2 hours as ordered, formula is started 24 hours postoperatively if clear fluids are retained
      c. General postoperative nursing care

Hirschsprung's Disease

A. Definition: distention of a portion of the lower colon caused by a congenital lack of nerve cells in the wall of the colon just below the distended section (Fig. 9-4)

B. Symptoms: constipation (including a lack of meconium stool in the newborn in the first 24 hours), abdominal distention, bile-stained mucus and emesis

C. Diagnosis: based on the symptoms, results of barium enema and rectal biopsy

D. Treatment/nursing interventions: based on the type of surgery done (bowel resection, sometimes with temporary colostomy); surgery done in two or three stages
   1. Preoperative
      a. Observation of stools: color, amount, and consistency
      b. Enemas/irrigations to clean out colon
   2. Postoperative
      a. NG tube to low-suction or gravity drainage
      b. General postoperative care
      c. Routine colostomy care as necessary (prn)
      d. Vital signs as ordered; axillary temperatures should be taken
      e. IV fluids as ordered
      f. NPO; resume diet as ordered
      g. Record intake and output (I&O) every shift
      h. Observe stools and record amount and characteristics
      i. Observe for rectal bleeding and abdominal distention

Omphalocele

A. Definition: the abdominal organs protrude through an abnormal opening in the abdominal wall and form a sac lying on the abdomen

B. Diagnosis: based on symptoms and physical examination

C. Treatment/nursing interventions
   1. Preoperative
      a. Keep the omphalocele covered with sterile gauze, moistened with normal saline until surgery can be performed
      b. Maintain sterile technique as much as possible in caring for the omphalocele
   2. Postoperative
      a. Surgery: the organs are returned to the abdom-

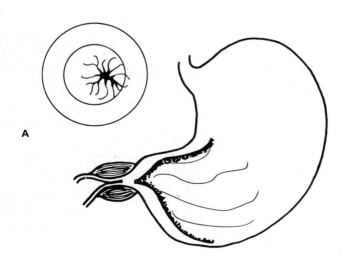

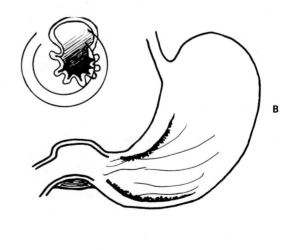

FIG. 9-3. Hypertrophic pyloric stenosis. **A,** Enlarged muscular tumor nearly obliterates pyloric channel. **B,** Longitudinal surgical division of muscle down to submucosa establishes adequate passageway. (From Whaley LF, Wong DL: *Nursing care of infants and children,* ed 4, St Louis, 1991, Mosby.)

inal cavity, and the abdominal wall is closed
   b. General postoperative care
   c. Observe stools and record amount and characteristics

Imperforate Anus

A. Definition: the rectal pouch ends blindly at a distance above the anus; sometimes there is no anal opening; there are various forms of this defect
B. Symptoms: no stools in the first 24 hours after birth; rectal thermometer cannot be inserted properly
C. Diagnosis: made by digital rectal examination, intestinal x-ray examination, and endoscopy
D. Treatment/nursing interventions
   1. Surgical procedure to reconnect the ends of the rectum and form an anal opening
   2. General postoperative nursing care

Esophageal Atresia

A. Definition: the upper end of the esophagus ends in a blind pouch; the lower end may also end in a blind pouch or may be connected to the trachea by fistula defect (tracheoesophageal fistula) (Fig. 9-5)
B. Symptoms: excessive salivation and drooling, coughing and choking during feedings, regurgitation of all feedings
C. Diagnosis: based on symptoms as well as passage of an NG tube or catheter down the esophagus to test for patency; exact anomaly is determined by x-ray studies
D. Treatment/nursing interventions
   1. NPO with administration of IV fluids as ordered
   2. Suctioning of nose and mouth as needed
   3. Insertion of an NG tube to drain mucus and fluid from the blind pouch
   4. Surgical repair to correct the defects and reconnect the ends of the esophagus

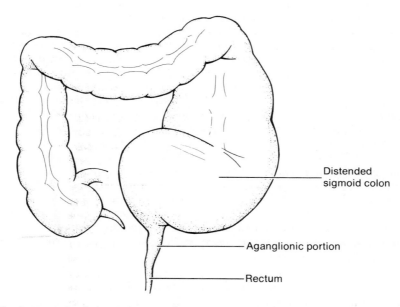

FIG. 9-4. Hirschsprung's disease. (From Whaley LF, Wong DL: *Nursing care of infants and children,* ed 4, St Louis, 1991, Mosby.)

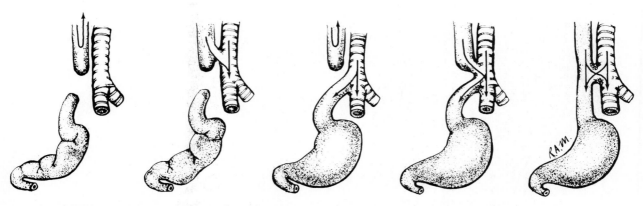

FIG. 9-5. The five most common types of esophageal atresia and tracheoesophageal fistula. (From Whaley LF, Wong DL: *Nursing care of infants and children,* ed 4, St Louis, 1991, Mosby.)

Intussusception

A. Definition: telescoping of one portion of the bowel into a distal portion; usually occurs between 3 and 12 months of age

B. Symptoms: appear suddenly; color pale; sharp, colicky pain causes infant to draw up legs and cry out (this occurs every 5 to 10 minutes); vomiting; stools with blood and mucus ("red currant jelly" stools); signs of shock

C. Diagnosis: based on symptoms; definitive diagnosis can be made radiographically with barium enema

D. Treatment/nursing interventions: this is an emergency that requires immediate treatment. The initial treatment of choice is hydrostatic reduction by barium enema; if this is not effective, surgery is necessary
   1. Preoperative
      a. Careful observation and recording of vital signs frequently
      b. IV fluids as ordered
      c. NPO
      d. NG tube to remove gastric contents
      e. Emotional support for parents; explain all procedures; answer questions
      f. Observe for passage of abnormal brown stool (indicates the intussusception has reduced itself); report to physician immediately
   2. Postoperative
      a. General postoperative care
      b. IV fluids as ordered; NPO
      c. Record intake and output
      d. Auscultate for return of bowel sounds
      e. Observe all stools and record
      f. Resume feedings slowly as ordered

Nervous System
Hydrocephalus

A. Definition: disorder caused by an obstruction of cerebrospinal fluid drainage; characterized by an excess of cerebrospinal fluid (CSF) within the cranial cavity, which causes an enlarged head and potential brain damage or retardation; it occurs in association with several other anomalies

B. Symptoms: bulging of the anterior fontanel, enlargement of the head, irritability, opisthotonos, "setting-sun" sign (sclera can be seen above the iris because of increased intracranial pressure)

C. Diagnosis: based on the symptoms, frequent measurements of head circumference, computerized tomography (CT), and magnetic resonance imaging (MRI)

D. Treatment/nursing interventions
   1. Surgical repair is necessary to relieve the obstruction or to shunt the CSF from the ventricles of the brain into the heart (ventriculoarterial shunt) or the abdomen (ventriculoperitoneal shunt) (Fig. 9-6)
   2. Postoperative care includes frequent position changes to prevent pressure on the head, care of the shunt, general postoperative care, and assessment for return of increased intracranial pressure

Down's Syndrome

A. Definition: an abnormality caused by extra chromosome 21 (trisomy 21). Children with Down's syndrome are born to women of all ages. Although there is a higher risk in women over age 35, the majority of infants with Down's syndrome are born to women under age 35

B. Symptoms: hypotonia; small, low-set ears; slanted eyes, protruding tongue; small, flattened nose; short, broad neck; single transverse palmar (simian) crease; dry, cracked skin; congenital heart defects; and mental retardation

C. Diagnosis: based on the physical defects; chromosomal studies are done to determine specific defects

D. Treatment/nursing interventions
   1. Emotional support for parents; they expected a "normal" infant without defects

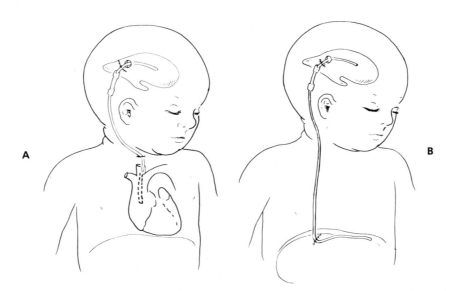

FIG. 9-6. A, Ventriculoarterial shunt. **B,** Ventriculoperitoneal shunt. (From Whaley LF, Wong DL: *Nursing care of infants and children,* ed 3, 1987, Mosby.)

2. Helping parents to set realistic goals for the child
3. Encourage activity and intellectual stimulation for the child
4. Genetic counseling for the parents

Genitourinary System
Epispadias and Hypospadias

A. Definition: congenital conditions in male infants where urethra ends on the under side (hypospadias) or the top side (epispadias) of the penis, rather than at the end
B. Symptoms: obvious physical defects evident on physical examination
C. Diagnosis: based on physical examination
D. Treatment/nursing interventions
    1. The surgery to extend the urethra to the end of the penis is usually done in several stages when the child is 6 to 18 months of age
    2. Postoperative care includes inspection of the operative site for bleeding, catheter care, and emotional support for the child and parents, as well as general postoperative care

Cryptorchidism

A. Definition: failure of one or both testes to descend into the scrotal sac; sterility may result if not treated
B. Symptoms: testes not palpable in the scrotal sac on physical examination
C. Diagnosis: based on symptoms
D. Treatment/nursing interventions
    1. The testes often descend during early childhood
    2. Hormonal therapy (human chorionic gonadotropin [HCG]) may be used at an early age to promote descent of the testes into the scrotum
    3. Surgical intervention (orchiopexy) is usually necessary to bring the testes down the inguinal canal and into the scrotum; routine postoperative care

Wilms' Tumor

A. Definition: tumor (nephroblastoma) in the kidney region
B. Symptoms: occasional hematuria and elevated blood pressure; swelling or mass in the abdomen
C. Diagnosis: the tumor is often palpable through the abdominal wall; it occurs most often in children under 2

years of age and is usually found before the child reaches the age of 3
D. Treatment/nursing interventions
    1. Surgery to remove the tumor is performed within 48 hours of diagnosis; routine postoperative care is given
    2. Radiation therapy is given postoperatively
    3. Chemotherapy as ordered (see Chapter 4, Pharmacology)
E. Prognosis is good with early diagnosis and treatment for children under 2 years of age

Musculoskeletal System
Congenital Clubfoot (Talipes Equinovarus)

A. Definition: defect in which the entire foot is inverted, heel is drawn up, and front of the foot is adducted; can affect one or both feet (Fig. 9-7)
B. Symptoms: obvious physical defect evident on physical examination
C. Diagnosis: based on the presence of the physical defect on examination
D. Treatment/nursing interventions
    1. The deformity is usually repaired in stages; the type of treatment depends on the severity of the defect
    2. Various methods of treatment include serial casting, splints (Denis Browne splint, Fig. 9-8), and surgery when necessary to repair the deformities; nursing care depends on method chosen

Congenital Dislocation of Hip (Developmental Dysplasia of the Hip [DDH])

A. Definition: congenital dislocation of the hip is caused by a defect in the acetabulum; it is usually bilateral
B. Symptoms: limited hip abduction, apparent shortening of femur, asymmetry of gluteal and thigh folds
C. Diagnosis: symptoms found on physical examination by the physician
D. Treatment/nursing interventions
    1. Treatment is started as soon as the defect is diagnosed; the hip is manipulated into proper position, and an abductor splint or hip spica cast is applied (Fig. 9-9); Bryant's traction, modified Bryant's, or modified Buck's extension may also be used

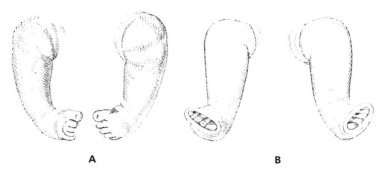

A   **B**

FIG. 9-7. Feet casted for correction of bilateral congenital talipes equinovarus. **A,** Before correction. **B,** Undergoing correction in plaster casts. (From Brashear HR Jr, Raney RB: *Shands' handbook of orthopaedic surgery,* ed 10, St Louis, 1986, Mosby, p 34.)

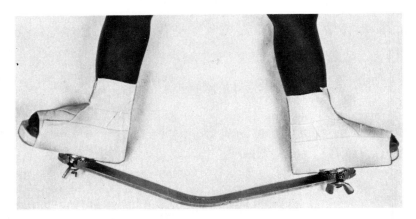

FIG. 9-8. Denis Browne splint for correction of clubfoot. Felt-padded plates are strapped to feet in corrected position with adhesive tape. Control of rotation, eversion, and dorsiflexion is adjustable. (From Brashear HR Jr, Raney RB: *Shands' handbook of orthopaedic surgery,* ed 10, St Louis, 1986, Mosby, p 35.)

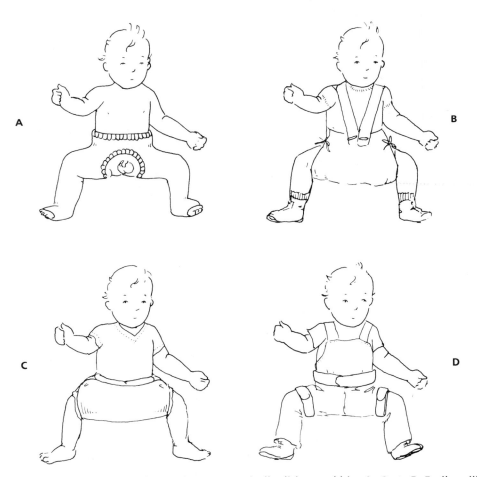

FIG. 9-9. Various devices used to reduce congenitally dislocated hip. **A,** Cast; **B,** Frejka pillow splint; **C,** abduction splint; **D,** brace. (From Whaley LF, Wong DL: *Nursing care of infants and children,* ed 4, St Louis, 1991, Mosby.)

2. When the defect is diagnosed in the newborn stage, abduction achieved by double diapering the child is often sufficient to keep the hip in proper position

3. Nursing care includes parent teaching regarding cast care, application of the splint, or double diapering

Cardiovascular System
Congenital Heart Defects

A. Atrial septal defect (ASD): abnormal opening in the septum between the two atria, or a patent foramen ovale, that causes left-to-right shunting of the blood

B. Ventricular septal defect (VSD): abnormal opening in the septum between the two ventricles that causes left-to-right shunting of the blood

C. Patent ductus arteriosus (PDA): the ductus arteriosus remains open after birth instead of closing off as normal, causing an overload of the left heart and a slight murmur

D. Coarctation of the aorta: constriction of the aortic arch, causing hypertension in the upper body and hypotension in the lower body

E. Tetralogy of Fallot: consists of four congenital defects: pulmonary stenosis, ventricular septal defect, overriding of the aorta, and right ventricular hypertrophy

F. Classic symptoms of congenital heart defects: dyspnea, difficulty with feeding, clubbing of fingers, cyanosis (in certain defects), heart murmurs, rapid pulse, and recurrent respiratory infections

G. Diagnosis: based on the symptoms, electrocardiograms, echocardiograms, cardiac catheterizations, and chest x-ray films

H. Treatment/nursing interventions
1. Most defects must be corrected by surgical intervention, often in stages; some symptoms can be treated with medications as ordered
2. Nursing care measures depend on the type of treatment or surgery; most often, immediate postoperative care is given in intensive care units

Sickle Cell Anemia

A. Definition: autosomal disease occurring mainly in blacks, but also occurs on occasion in whites of Mediterranean descent; causes breakdown of red blood cells carrying an abnormal hemoglobin S, which leads to a severe hemolytic anemia

B. Symptoms: appear only in children who inherit the trait from both parents; fatigue, anorexia, decreased hemoglobin; sickle cell crisis may occur, causing severe joint pain, abdominal pain, fever, and firm and distended abdomen

C. Diagnosis: based on the symptoms, family history of the disease, and specific blood tests including the sickle-cell slide preparation, sickle-turbidity test (Sickledex), and hemoglobin electrophoresis ("Fingerprinting")

D. Treatment/nursing interventions
1. IV fluids and fluids by mouth (PO) as ordered
2. Oxygen therapy, especially during sickle cell crisis
3. Bed rest
4. Electrolyte replacement
5. Analgesics for pain as ordered
6. Blood transfusions as ordered (packed red blood cells)
7. Antibiotic therapy as needed
8. Genetic counseling for parents

Endocrine System
Hypopituitarism (Dwarfism)

A. Definition: growth retardation due to deficiency of the growth hormone (GH)

B. Symptoms: short stature, well-nourished appearance, delayed physical development

C. Diagnosis: based on the family history, child's growth patterns, physical examination, x-ray studies, and endocrine studies

D. Treatment/nursing interventions
1. Replacement of the growth hormone by injections
2. Early diagnosis and treatment helps to prevent many physical and emotional problems that occur later in childhood
3. Provide emotional support for the child and parents during diagnostic procedures and early stages of treatment (even after growth hormone therapy is started, growth will be slower than normal)

Congenital Hypothyroidism (Cretinism)

A. Definition: lack of thyroid function resulting from a failure of the embryonic development of the thyroid gland

B. Symptoms: usually do not appear until 6 to 12 weeks of age in bottle-fed infants and after weaning in breast-fed infants; include feeding problems, inactivity, anemia, thick, dry, mottled skin, bradycardia, relaxation of the abdominal muscles, and delayed development of the nervous system, which leads to mental retardation

C. Diagnosis: based on the symptoms and tests of thyroid function, such as initial measurement of the newborn's T_4 (thyroxin) and thyroid stimulating hormone (TSH) level

D. Treatment/nursing interventions
1. Early diagnosis and treatment is essential in preventing retardation and other severe physiologic symptoms
2. Treatment is indefinite replacement therapy of the thyroid hormone
3. Parent teaching concerning administration of the thyroid hormone, including signs and symptoms of thyroid overdose

Disorder of Unknown Etiology
Sudden Infant Death Syndrome (SIDS)

A. Definition: sudden, unexplained death of an infant under 1 year of age who was healthy immediately before death; also known as crib death; 90% of SIDS cases occur by 6 months of age

B. Research: SIDS research has yet to determine a specific cause for the syndrome; it may be related to a brainstem abnormality in the regulation of cardiorespiratory control

C. Emotional support for the parents
1. Parents always feel guilty and must be reassured that SIDS is not their fault
2. Encourage them to allow an autopsy to try to determine a specific cause of death; this helps to allay their guilt and feelings that they could have prevented it
3. Allow parents to spend some time with the child to say good-bye
4. Refer the parents to the SIDS Foundation for counseling and support

Toddlerhood (Ages 1 to 3 Years)
NORMAL GROWTH AND DEVELOPMENT
Physical Development

A. Toddlerhood shows a decrease in the rate of growth but an increase in the rate of development

B. Toddlers gain approximately 5 to 10 lb (2 to 4.5 kg) each year, and add 3 inches (7.5 cm) in height per year

C. They have learned, and continue to learn, to walk between 1 and 2 years of age

D. Toddlers continue to learn to talk, learning new words and phrases; their favorite word is "no!"

Psychosocial Development

A. Behavior in the toddler is characterized by several things
   1. Negativism: toddlers say "no!" to almost everything; this is part of their becoming an individual person separate from their parents
   2. Ritualism: developing and following certain patterns of behavior to develop their own security
   3. Temper tantrums: toddlers like to do everything for themselves; when they can't, they are frustrated, and this frustration leads to temper tantrums; tantrums should be ignored as much as possible, and the child should be dealt with after the "storm" is over

B. Toddlers are in Erikson's stage of "autonomy vs. shame and doubt"; they need to develop a sense of autonomy and self-control; to do this, toddlers must be able to make some choices as well as learn to function within the limits set for them

C. Discipline and limit setting must be consistent to be effective; it is also important to remember to criticize the behavior, not the child

D. Toilet training is an important part of the socialization process in toddlers; they should be praised when they use the "potty chair" or toilet properly, rather than being punished for not using it; toilet training should only begin when the toddler is physically capable of controlling bowel and bladder (15 to 18 months)

HEALTH PROMOTION

A. Nutrition needs change because of change in growth rate; toddlers need less food, and their appetites decrease
   1. Teach parents that the decrease in food intake is normal
   2. The child is more autonomous now; should be allowed to feed himself or herself as much as possible; "finger foods" are ideal
   3. Snacks should be nutritious; cheese, fruits, and crackers are good choices
   4. Desserts should not be used as rewards; this gets the toddler into a habit of expecting something sweet whenever doing something good

B. Prevention of accidents is a major responsibility with toddlers; keep dangerous items (sharp objects, medications, cleaning supplies) out of their reach; toddlers should not be left unattended near a bathtub, swimming pool, whirlpool bath, or hot objects, such as pans on the stove or open flames

C. Teaching the toddler good oral hygiene habits is necessary to prevent early tooth decay and problems with gums

1. Brushing the teeth should begin between 18 to 24 months of age
2. Dental checkups with the dental hygienist or dentist should begin at about 2 years of age
3. Proper nutrition helps prevent a large amount of early dental caries

HEALTH PROBLEMS
Respiratory Disorders
Epiglottitis

A. Definition: one of the croup syndromes; a severely inflamed epiglottis; begins abruptly and progresses rapidly into severe respiratory distress; usually caused by *Haemophilus influenzae* bacteria

B. Symptoms: fever, sore throat, difficulty swallowing; child insists on sitting up, leaning forward with chin thrust out, mouth open, and tongue protruding; drooling is common

C. Diagnosis: based on the symptoms and visualization of enlarged reddened epiglottis on careful throat examination and enlarged epiglottis on lateral neck x-ray examination

D. Treatment/nursing interventions
   1. Do *not* examine throat unless immediate intubation can be performed if necessary
   2. Keep child as quiet as possible; allow child to sit up in bed or on lap of parent
   3. Keep emergency tracheostomy tray (and intubation tray) with patient at all times
   4. IV fluids and antibiotics as ordered
   5. Monitor child closely

Cystic Fibrosis

A. Definition: an autosomal recessive hereditary disease affecting the exocrine glands; the lungs, pancreas, and liver produce abnormal mucus secretions and become obstructed

B. Symptoms
   1. In newborns: meconium ileus, bile-stained emesis, distended abdomen, no stools, and salty "taste" to the skin resulting from increased sodium in the perspiration
   2. In infants and children: harsh, dry cough, frequent bronchial infections, malnutrition, distended abdomen, barrel chest, clubbed fingers, and bulky, greasy, foul-smelling stools (steatorrhea)

C. Diagnosis: based on family history, a history of FTT, the symptoms, lung changes revealed by chest x-ray films, an elevated sweat chloride level (increased sodium in the perspiration), and stool analysis for fat and enzymes

D. Treatment/nursing interventions
   1. Pancreatic enzymes are given as ordered with food to improve digestion of fats and proteins
   2. High-carbohydrate, high-protein, and low-fat diet
   3. Increased amounts of salt and water-soluble vitamins
   4. Inhalation therapy to break up mucus; nebulizer, humidifier, intermittent positive pressure breathing (IPPB) and bronchodilators (in an aerosol)
   5. Postural drainage and chest physiotherapy to help in expectoration of mucus
   6. Mucolytic drug as ordered; see Chapter 4
   7. Physical exercise to stimulate mucus secretion

8. Antibiotics for all pulmonary infections
9. Parent teaching regarding diet, medications, and inhalation therapy for proper home care after discharge
10. Referral to the Cystic Fibrosis Foundation for financial or emotional support
11. Genetic counseling for parents

Gastrointestinal Disorders
Celiac Disease (Gluten Enteropathy)

A. Definition: a defect of metabolism precipitated by the ingestion of wheat or rye gluten, leading to impaired fat absorption
B. Symptoms: usually appear between 9 and 12 months of age; chronic diarrhea with bulky, greasy, foul-smelling stools; malnutrition; anorexia; unhappy disposition; retardation of growth; distended abdomen; and muscle wasting especially of extremities and buttocks
C. Diagnosis: laboratory tests including stool analysis for fecal fat; blood studies for anemia, hypoproteinemia, and serum iron; definitive diagnosis is based on these tests, the symptoms, and a jejunal biopsy to demonstrate changes in the jejunal mucosa
D. Treatment/nursing interventions
   1. Gluten-free, low-fat diet; rice cereal for infants
   2. Parent teaching regarding diet and specific foods to avoid
   3. The child should be protected from respiratory infections, which may lead to exacerbations of the disease known as celiac crisis (characterized by severe vomiting and diarrhea, dehydration, and acidosis)

Neurosensory Disorders
Eye Disorders
Strabismus (Fig. 9-10)

A. Definition: failure of the eyes to direct and focus on the same object at the same time
B. Symptoms: deviation of one eye to the center (esotropia) or to the other corner (exotropia)
C. Diagnosis: based on the symptoms

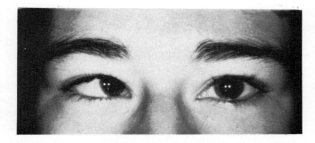

FIG. 9-10. Strabismus. Note the obvious malalignment of the eyes. The light reflections are centered in the left cornea and to the side of the right cornea. (From Havener WH et al: *Nursing care in eye, ear, nose, and throat disorders,* ed 4, St Louis, 1979, Mosby.)

D. Treatment/nursing interventions
   1. Patching of good eye to increase visual stimulation to weaker eye
   2. Glasses and exercises to help improve vision
   3. Surgery to correct the muscle defects is often necessary when conservative treatment is ineffective
   4. Preoperative and postoperative nursing care as indicated

Amblyopia ("Lazy Eye")

A. Definition: reduced visual acuity in one eye, usually caused by strabismus; the eyes are unable to focus and work together, and blindness may occur in the weaker eye if there is no treatment
B. Symptoms: blurred vision, double vision, development of a "blind spot"
C. Diagnosis: based on results of Snellen's eye test and the symptoms
D. Treatment/nursing interventions: patching of the good eye so that the child is forced to use and focus the weaker eye; the best time for treatment is during early childhood

Cerebral Palsy

A. Definition: a group of nonprogressive disorders caused by a malfunction of the motor centers of the brain; oxygen deprivation (anoxia) damages the brain's motor centers prenatally, during or immediately after delivery, or during childhood after an accident or disease
B. Symptoms: difficulty in controlling voluntary muscle movements, delays in development, hearing and vision impairment, seizures, and in some cases, mental retardation
C. Diagnosis: based on the mother's prenatal history, birth history, history of an accident or disease, presence of delays in growth and development, and abnormal neurologic examination
D. Types of cerebral palsy
   1. Spastic: hyperactive muscle and tendon reflexes, accompanied by continuous spasms and muscle contractures
   2. Dyskinetic (athetoid): the body muscles are in a constant state of motion and slow muscle contractions
   3. Ataxia: a lack of coordination and balance when walking
E. Treatment/nursing interventions
   1. Treatment and care are supportive to ensure optimal level of development for the child
   2. Physical and occupational therapy to help the child learn some control over muscle movements
   3. Braces as needed to hold extremities in correct positions of function
   4. Use of wheelchairs, walkers, and crutches as needed for ambulation/locomotion
   5. Speech therapy as needed
   6. Emotional support for the family and child; most often, cerebral palsy children are of normal intelligence and have only physical handicaps
   7. Encourage the child to live as normal a life as possible; refer the family to supportive groups such as the Easter Seal Society

Accidents

A. Accidents are the major cause of death in children between 1 and 4 years of age, chiefly because of their ability to walk and move about more freely than during infancy, along with their unawareness of danger within the environment

B. Accident prevention during toddlerhood is a major task requiring the involvement of both parents and other family members; following are several basic suggestions for accident prevention

    1. Supervise play, especially around dangerous areas such as cars, swimming pools, and open flames or hot appliances

    2. Use well-designed, safe car seats or restraints

    3. Turn all handles of pots and pans in toward the stove, away from the child's reach

    4. Cover electrical outlets with protective plastic caps

    5. Do not allow the child to play with the bathtub faucets; do not leave the child unattended in the bathtub or shower

    6. Keep all medications and poisonous substances out of the child's reach (preferably in a locked cabinet)

    7. Know the number and location of the nearest poison control center and hospital

    8. Put up gates at the top and bottom of stairwells

    9. Choose well-made toys appropriate for the child's age, without sharp edges or small removable pieces

    10. Store all guns, dangerous tools, and equipment in a locked cabinet

    11. Teach the toddler about common dangers such as "hot" items, looking "both ways" before crossing the street, and water safety

Preschool Age (Ages 3 to 5)
NORMAL GROWTH AND DEVELOPMENT
Physical Development

A. Growth is slow during the preschool years; children gain 3 to 5 lb (1 to 2 kg) and 2 to 3 inches (5 to 7.5 cm) in height each year

B. Deciduous teeth are being replaced by permanent teeth; there is a definite need for proper dental hygiene and dental checkups at this age level and throughout childhood

C. Visual development continues; visual acuity is not fully developed until 6 to 8 years of age

D. Language development of preschoolers is rapid; 3-year-olds talk to themselves and their toys; 4-year-olds begin to talk and communicate more with other people

Psychosocial Development

A. Preschoolers are in Erikson's stage of "initiative vs. guilt"; at this age level they learn how to interact with other children and adults; they also learn the difference between proper and improper behavior, and the rewards and disciplines associated with each; without proper adult guidance, preschoolers can learn improper behavior and develop a sense of guilt and inferiority rather than a sense of initiative and accomplishment

B. Preschoolers begin to develop their imaginations; they use "magical thinking" and have difficulty distinguishing fantasy from reality

C. Preschoolers become acutely aware of their sexuality, including their roles as boys or girls and their sex organs; parents must work with their children in a positive way to help them develop healthy attitudes toward themselves and their bodies

D. Preschoolers continue to learn through play; they still use parallel play but also begin to use associative play (play with other children) and imitative play (play by imitating the actions of adults or other children)

HEALTH PROMOTION

A. Immunizations started in infancy and toddlerhood should continue according to schedule (see Table 9-2)

B. Nutrition should be appropriate to age, keeping in mind that growth is slow during this period; preschoolers should be eating foods from all four basic food groups

HEALTH PROBLEMS
Communicable Diseases

See Appendix E

Respiratory Disorders: Tonsillitis and Adenoiditis

A. Definition: inflammation of the tonsils and adenoids caused by chronic upper respiratory infections

B. Symptoms: sore throat, difficulty in swallowing and breathing ("mouth breathers"), hoarseness, harsh cough

C. Diagnosis: based on the symptoms and the presence of swelling and redness of the tonsils and adenoids on examination

D. Treatment/nursing interventions

    1. Acute infections are treated with antibiotics as ordered, increased oral fluids, and warm saltwater gargles

    2. If chronic infections continue after antibiotic treatment, surgery is often indicated (tonsillectomy and adenoidectomy); however, surgery is less common today than in the past

    3. Postoperative nursing care measures include keeping the child in a prone position with head to the side until fully awake; monitoring vital signs frequently; checking the throat and nares for active bleeding; keeping the suction equipment at the bedside for emergency use; observing the child for frequent swallowing (this may indicate oozing of blood in the nasopharynx or pharynx); and encouraging cool, clear oral fluids after the nausea subsides

Genitourinary Disorders
Nephrotic Syndrome

A. Definition: idiopathic damage to the glomeruli of the kidneys, causing edema and loss of large amounts of protein in the urine

B. Symptoms: edema of the face, extremities, and abdomen; proteinuria, hypoalbuminemia, respiratory distress; malnutrition; irritability; increased susceptibility to infection

C. Diagnosis: based on decreased serum protein levels and increased proteinuria, edema, and hypercholesterolemia

D. Treatment/nursing interventions

    1. Nephrotic syndrome is a chronic disorder, with remissions and exacerbations, usually lasting 12 to 18 months; treatment measures continue for an extended period

    2. Corticosteroids as ordered to reduce the edema

3. Frequent urine testing for protein and albumin
4. Recording of intake and output
5. Diuretics as ordered
6. Low-salt diet during exacerbations
7. Antibiotics as ordered during exacerbations
8. Parent teaching for home care regarding medications, diet, and follow-up

Acute Glomerulonephritis

A. Definition: inflammation of the glomeruli and nephrons of the kidney that occurs as a reaction to infections (usually streptococcal infections, such as in the throat)
B. Symptoms: hematuria, fever (103° to 105° F; 39.4° to 40.5° C), vomiting, slight edema, oliguria, elevated blood urea nitrogen (BUN), creatinine levels, and uric acid levels; these symptoms usually occur 1 to 3 weeks after the initial infection
C. Diagnosis: based on the symptoms and a positive recent history of streptococcal infections
D. Treatment/nursing interventions
   1. Bed rest for 2 to 4 weeks until the symptoms subside
   2. Antibiotics as ordered; see Chapter 4, Pharmacology
   3. Liquid diet, progressing to a regular, low-salt diet
   4. Measurement of intake and output and observation of color of urine
   5. Frequent checking and recording of blood pressure
   6. Urine testing for protein and specific gravity

Circulatory Disorders
Hemophilia

A. Definition: an X-linked recessive disorder of metabolism that results in a delayed coagulation of blood; hemophilia is typed according to which clotting factor is affected
B. Symptoms: prolonged bleeding and clotting times; easy bruising and bleeding into tissues and joints; joint pain
C. Diagnosis: based on the symptoms, as well as family health history, and a prolonged clotting time
D. Treatment/nursing interventions
   1. Observations for any signs of internal bleeding and shock
   2. Transfusions as ordered with fresh frozen plasma, cryoprecipitate, and/or the missing clotting factor
   3. Frequent laboratory tests, such as partial thromboplastin time (PTT), clotting time, complete blood count (CBC); screening for HIV (from receiving contaminated transfusions or clotting factors)
   4. Corticosteroids and nonsteroidal antiinflammatory drugs as ordered
   5. Exercise and physical therapy to strengthen muscles around joints
   6. Protection of the child from injuries as much as possible
   7. Emotional support and counseling for the child and parents
   8. Parent teaching regarding follow-up physical examinations, protection of the child from physical harm, the need for immediate care if any injury occurs, and administration of the clotting factor to the child
   9. Referrals to community resources, such as the National Hemophilia Foundation
   10. Genetic counseling for parents

Leukemia

A. Definition: blood disorder in which normal white blood cells (WBCs) decrease while immature, abnormal white cells (called blasts) are formed in large numbers in the spleen, liver, and bone marrow; also known as cancer of the blood-forming tissues
B. Symptoms: lethargy, pallor, anorexia, fever, pain in the bones and joints; anemia, petechiae, easy bruising, and sores in the mouth
C. Diagnosis: made on the basis of history, symptoms, an elevated WBC count, and presence of immature leukocytes and blast cells in a bone marrow biopsy or aspiration
D. Treatment/nursing interventions
   1. Leukemia is a chronic, sometimes fatal disease with remissions and exacerbations; the child and family need a great deal of emotional support from the physician and nursing staff
   2. Chemotherapy drugs and corticosteroids as ordered (see Chapter 4, Pharmacology)
   3. IV fluids and blood transfusions as ordered
   4. Administration of pain medications as ordered; joint pain during exacerbations may be severe, especially in the more advanced stages; higher than normal doses are often required
   5. Proper skin and mouth care
   6. Providing proper nutrition as the child's condition allows
   7. Prevention of infections whenever possible; chemotherapy drugs lower the WBC count, which in turn decreases the child's resistance to infection
   8. Observation for possible side effects of chemotherapy drugs
   9. Bone marrow transplants may be ordered in certain types of leukemia to replace unhealthy bone marrow; an exact "match" is often difficult to find

School Age (Ages 6 to 12)
NORMAL GROWTH AND DEVELOPMENT
Physical Development

A. Growth is slow in children between the ages of 6 and 10 years; the child gains 6 to 7 lb (2.5 to 3 kg) and 2 to 3 inches (5 to 7.5 cm) per year
B. Bone growth is slow; the cartilage is replaced by bone at the bone epiphyses

Psychosocial Development

A. School-age children are in Erikson's stage of "industry vs. inferiority"; an eagerness to develop new skills and interests, and the processes of cooperating and competing with other children are characteristics of this age that engender a sense of accomplishment rather than a sense of inferiority and poor self-worth
B. Children ages 7 to 10 start to become more influenced by their peer group than by their parents; they develop "best friends" and start to separate into boy and girl groups

HEALTH PROMOTION

A. Communicable disease prevention is accomplished by timely immunizations, proper rest and diet, and frequent medical and dental check-ups

B. Accident prevention remains a major factor at this age level; safety measures should now include rules for bicycle and skateboard safety (helmets) and for safety in competitive sports such as baseball, football, and soccer

C. Sex education should begin at this age level and should be presented by the parents in simple, honest terms; audiovisual aids such as books and pictures are available to assist parents in presenting the information on the child's level

D. Promotion of a balanced diet continues to be important at this age level; high-calorie, low-nutrition snacks are popular with school-age children but often lead to excess weight gain

HEALTH PROBLEMS
Respiratory Disorders: Allergic Conditions
Asthma

A. Definition: an obstructive airway disease caused by spasms of bronchial tubes; results from hypersensitivity of the airways, accompanied by inflammation and edema of the bronchial mucosa and increased production of bronchial mucus; it is often caused by an allergic response to allergens such as pollen, animal fur, or food; attacks can also be triggered by emotional upsets

B. Symptoms: wheezing, dyspnea, harsh, dry cough, retractions, and cyanosis

C. Diagnosis: based on the symptoms, physical examination, the child's history, family history, chest x-ray films that rule out other respiratory diseases, and pulmonary function studies

D. Treatment/nursing interventions
1. Bronchiodilator medications as ordered (administered by inhalation, by mouth, or by injection); (epinephrine is the drug of choice for an acute asthma attack); see Chapter 4, Pharmacology
2. Steroid medications as ordered to reduce lung inflammation
3. Chest physiotherapy and inhalation therapy
4. IV fluids as ordered
5. Liquid diet, progressing to a regular diet
6. Identification and removal of the allergens if possible
7. Parent and child teaching regarding home care including medications, removal of any potential allergens, and follow-up examinations

Allergic Rhinitis (Hay Fever)

A. Cause: an allergy to some pollen, dust, or animal fur

B. Symptoms: sneezing, runny nose, postnasal drip, and watery, itchy eyes

C. Diagnosis: based on the symptoms and results of allergy testing done to discover specific allergen

D. Treatment/nursing interventions
1. Find and remove the allergen if possible
2. Antihistamines or decongestants as ordered

Gastrointestinal Disorders
Appendicitis

A. Definition: inflammation of the appendix, often following an infection elsewhere in the body

B. Symptoms: pain in the right lower quadrant of the abdomen, nausea and vomiting, fever, and constipation

C. Diagnosis: based on the symptoms and usually an elevated WBC count

D. Treatment/nursing interventions
1. Removal of the inflamed appendix (appendectomy), preferably before it ruptures and spreads the infection throughout the abdomen, causing peritonitis
2. Routine postoperative care, including monitoring of vital signs, frequent observation of the incision or dressing for bleeding, careful recording of intake and output, and administration of IV fluids as ordered
3. Antibiotics may be ordered if there is a possibility of infection (especially with a ruptured appendix)
4. Pain medication as ordered

Pinworms

A. Definition: worms that affect the intestine; the worms or eggs are swallowed and are spread easily from person to person by the hands, linen, or food

B. Symptoms; itching around the anus, anorexia, and diarrhea

C. Diagnosis: made by the cellophane tape test; the eggs are captured from the anal area during the night or early morning hours by placing a tongue blade covered with cellophane tape at the anal opening; the worms come out of the intestine at night to lay their eggs, and the eggs are picked up on the tape

D. Treatment/nursing interventions
1. Good handwashing technique to prevent spread of the worms and reinfection
2. Frequent changes of underwear and linen
3. Administration of vermifuge medications as ordered; see Chapter 4, Pharmacology
4. Examination and treatment of family members (if affected)

Nervous System Disorder: Epilepsy

A. Definition: a convulsive disorder of unknown cause; the seizures can be general or localized (focal)

B. Symptoms: classification of seizures (see the box to the right)

C. Diagnosis: based on the evidence of seizures; differentiation of the type of seizure by physical examination, neurologic assessment, patient history, and changes in the electroencephalogram (EEG) (changes in the brain wave patterns)

D. Treatment/nursing interventions
1. Anticonvulsant medications as ordered; see Chapter 4, Pharmacology
2. Parent and child education regarding medications and the necessity of taking them as prescribed; safety factors; actions to take if the child has a seizure at home; and the importance of follow-up physical examinations and laboratory work (to measure blood levels of anticonvulsants)
3. Community referrals to support groups such as the National Epilepsy Foundation

Musculoskeletal Disorders
Scoliosis

A. Definition: a lateral S-shaped curvature of the spine that occurs from rapid growth; most often seen in young girls

---

International Classification of Epileptic Seizures

I. Partial seizures (seizures beginning locally)
  A. Simple partial seizures (with elementary symptoms; consciousness unimpaired)
   • With motor symptoms
   • With somatosensory or special sensory symptoms
   • With autonomic symptoms
   • Compound forms (with psychic symptoms)
  B. Complex partial symptoms (temporal lobe or psychomotor; generally with impaired consciousness)
   • With impairment of consciousness only
   • With cognitive symptoms
   • With affective symptoms
   • With psychosensory symptoms
   • With psychomotor symptoms
   • Compound forms
  C. Partial seizures, secondarily generalized
II. Generalized seizures (bilaterally symmetric; without local onset; with impairment of consciousness)
   • Tonic-clonic (grand mal) seizures
   • Tonic seizures
   • Clonic seizures
   • Absence (petit mal) seizures
   • Atonic seizures
   • Myoclonic seizures
   • Infantile spasms
   • Akinetic seizures
III. Unilateral seizures (those involving one hemisphere)
IV. Unclassified epileptic seizures (incomplete data)

Modified from Commission on Classification and Terminology of the International League Against Epilepsy: Proposal for revised clinical and electroencephalographic classification of epileptic seizures, *Epilepsia* 22:489-501, 1981.

B. Symptoms: poor posture; uneven length of legs; uneven shoulders and hips
C. Diagnosis: based on symptoms and x-ray films
D. Treatment/nursing interventions
  1. A brace (Milwaukee brace) or splint is often used to prevent the curvature from increasing (rarely corrects curve); may be used as the only treatment or before surgery
  2. Spinal fusion may be necessary to correct severe scoliosis; postoperative care as indicated

Muscular Dystrophy

A. Definition: a hereditary disease (recessive trait) characterized by gradual degeneration of muscle fibers, which is evidenced by muscle wasting and weakness and increasing disability and deformity
B. Symptoms: gradual muscle weakness including difficulty walking, standing up, a "waddle" gait, and mild mental retardation; most symptoms appear in children between 3 and 5 years of age
C. Diagnosis: based on the history of the symptoms, family history, muscle biopsy to determine muscle degeneration, electromyography (EMG), and serum enzyme measurement
D. Treatment/nursing interventions

  1. There is no cure for muscular dystrophy, so treatment is supportive
  2. Encouragement of the child to be as active and to lead as normal a life as possible
  3. Range-of-motion exercises and physical therapy as ordered to prevent contractures
  4. Use of walkers, crutches, braces, and wheelchairs as needed
  5. Emotional support for the parents and child; this is a progressive disease, and the family requires ongoing support by the health care team
  6. Frequent medical checkups to observe for progressive symptoms such as respiratory distress
  7. Genetic counseling for the parents

Integumentary Disorders
Ringworm

A. Definition: a fungal infection transferred from person to person or from animal to person; it can occur on the scalp (tinea capitis), the body (tinea corporis), and the feet (tinea pedis) (Fig. 9-11)
B. Symptoms: small papules, dry, scaly skin, and itching on the affected part
C. Diagnosis: based on the symptoms
D. Treatment/nursing interventions
  1. Washing of the affected areas with soap and water and removal of crusts
  2. Antifungal ointment to affected areas as ordered
  3. Antifungal oral medication as ordered; see Chapter 4, Pharmacology

Pediculosis

A. Definition: infestation by lice of the scalp and hairy areas of the body
B. Symptoms: severe itching in the affected area and appearance of lice on the hair or clothing
C. Diagnosis: based on the symptoms
D. Treatment/nursing interventions
  1. Special shampoo to the hair and scalp as ordered
  2. Washing of all linens and clothing in hot water to destroy the nits (small lice) and eggs of the lice
  3. Emphasis on importance of follow-up treatment to prevent reinfestation
  4. Examination and treatment of other family members (if affected)
  5. Report to school, daycare facility

Hives (Urticaria)

A. Definition: an allergic reaction on the skin, usually caused by an allergy to food or drugs
B. Symptoms: bright red, raised patches on the skin and itching of the affected areas
C. Diagnosis: based on the symptoms; allergy testing may be done to determine the specific allergen
D. Treatment/nursing interventions
  1. Determination and removal of the allergen
  2. Antihistamines as ordered to decrease the swelling and inflammation
  3. Cool-water soaks to the affected areas to decrease the itching
  4. Keeping the child's nails short to avoid scratching and possible infection

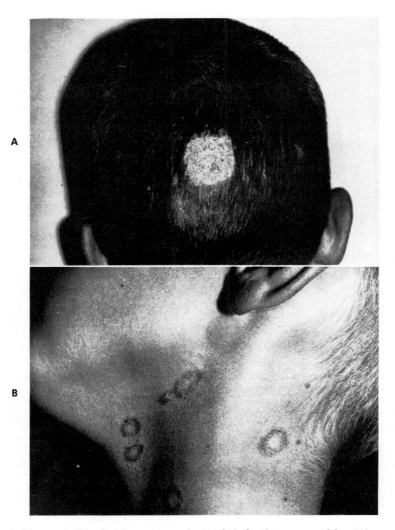

FIG. 9-11. A, Tinea capitis. **B,** Tinea corporis. Both infections caused by *Microsporum canis,* the "kitten" or "puppy" fungus. (From Stewart WD, Danto JL, Maddin S: *Dermatology: diagnosis and treatment of cutaneous disorders,* ed 4, St Louis, 1978, Mosby.)

Rheumatic Fever

A. Definition: a chronic disease affecting the connective tissue of the heart, lungs, brain, and joints; it follows a streptococcal infection that occurred elsewhere in the body
B. Symptoms: begin 1 to 5 weeks after the initial streptococcal infection; lethargy, anorexia, muscle and joint pain, fever, polyarthritis, chorea (muscle tremors and emotional upset), and carditis
C. Diagnosis: based on the symptoms; specific diagnosis based on the Jones criteria (see the box on p. 287)
D. Treatment/nursing interventions
  1. Bed rest to decrease the workload on the heart and help prevent or ease the carditis
  2. Feeding meals to the child during strict bed rest
  3. Medications as ordered including salicylates for pain, steroids to decrease inflammation of the muscle and connective tissue, and antibiotics to fight infection (penicillin is the drug of choice); see Chapter 4, Pharmacology
  4. Emotional support and nonstressful diversion for the child during bed rest
  5. Monitoring of frequent laboratory tests, including the WBC count and the erythrocyte sedimentation rate (ESR) (elevated in inflammatory diseases)
  6. Parent and child teaching for home care, including the need for rest, proper administration of medications, and the need for prophylactic antibiotic therapy before dental work and invasive procedures

Insulin-Dependent Diabetes Mellitus (IDDM)

A. Definition: in insulin-dependent (formerly juvenile-onset) diabetes the beta cells of the pancreas stop producing insulin, which is necessary for the metabolism of fats, carbohydrates, and proteins
B. Symptoms: rapid onset of symptoms, including easy fatigability, polydipsia (excessive thirst), polyphagia (increased appetite), polyuria (increased urine output), glycosuria (glucose in the urine), and weight loss
C. Diagnosis: based on the symptoms, blood glucose levels,

Guidelines for the Diagnosis of Initial Attack of Rheumatic Fever (Jones Criteria, 1992 Update)*

Major manifestations

Carditis
Polyarthritis
Chorea
Erythema marginatum
Subcutaneous nodules

Minor manifestations

Clinical findings
   Arthralgia
   Fever
Laboratory findings
   Elevated acute phase reactants
      Erythrocyte sedimentation rate
      C-reactive protein
   Prolonged PR interval

Supporting evidence of antecedent group A streptococcal infection

Positive throat culture or rapid streptococcal antigen test
Elevated or rising streptococcal antibody titer

From Guidelines for the diagnosis of rheumatic fever, *JAMA* 268:2070, 1992. Copyright 1992, American Medical Association.
*If supported by evidence of preceding group A streptococcal infection, the presence of two major manifestations or of one major and two minor manifestations indicates a high probability of acute rheumatic fever.

and the presence of glucose and ketones in the urine

D. Treatment/nursing interventions
1. Insulin injections as ordered to control blood sugar levels
2. American Diabetes Association diet as ordered
3. Routine urine testing for glucose and ketones
4. Routine blood sugar monitoring; Chemstrips, Accu-check, or one-touch glucometers are commonly used for this
5. Child and parent teaching regarding insulin injection technique, diet, exercise, urine testing, blood glucose monitoring, signs of hypoglycemia and hyperglycemia, and need for regular follow-up visits to the pediatrician
6. Support group for parents and child

Adolescence (Ages 13 to 19 Years)
NORMAL GROWTH AND DEVELOPMENT
Physical Development

A. During the adolescent period there is a "growth spurt." This accelerated growth includes an increase in both height and weight. In girls, this occurs between 9 and 11 years of age; in boys it occurs between 11 and 13 years of age
B. Secondary sex characteristics also develop during early adolescence
1. In girls the pelvis widens, the breasts develop and enlarge, and body hair starts to appear
2. In boys the penis and scrotum enlarge and pubic and facial hair start to appear, puberty in boys officially begins with the first nocturnal emission

Psychologic and Emotional Development

A. Adolescence is the time of transition from childhood to adulthood. Adolescents are in Erikson's stage of "identity vs. role confusion." They are in the process of developing a self-image or a sense of identity about who they are and what they want in life. If they do not develop a positive self-image and identity, they may develop a sense of inferiority, or a negative self-image
B. Development of a positive self-image and healthy personality depends a great deal on the adolescents' relationships with their peer group as well as with their family
C. Body image is the major part of adolescents' self-concept; sexuality and sexual feelings are a new part of their body images; physical appearance is important to how they perceive themselves as being accepted by their peer group
1. Boys' responses to puberty include pleasure at becoming a "man" as evidenced by enlargement of the sex organs, being able to shave, and the sexual feelings they begin to have during this stage; because of their strong sex drive, they often masturbate to relieve themselves of strong sexual tension
2. Girls' responses to puberty include a developing awareness of their bodily changes, both internal and external (such as hormonal changes and menstruation); the sex drive in girls is not as strong as it is in boys

HEALTH PROMOTION

A. Immunizations and physical examinations should continue according to schedule
B. Counseling and sex education, especially concerning AIDS, venereal disease, and birth control, should be made available to all adolescents
C. Counseling regarding drug and alcohol abuse should be presented and readily available to all adolescents who are in need of it
D. Emotional stress is high during adolescence; psychiatric counseling is necessary for some adolescents to work through their stresses and fears
E. Proper nutrition needs may not be met because of increased snacking, especially on high-calorie, high-fat foods; nutritional counseling may be helpful

HEALTH PROBLEMS
Substance Abuse (Drugs, Alcohol)

A. Definition: abuse of alcohol or mood-altering drugs, usually because of peer pressure or increased tension and stress
B. Signs of abuse: increased school absences, poor academic performance, changes in behavior patterns, wearing dark glasses inside, wearing long-sleeved shirts/blouses every day, and a sloppy, unclean appearance
C. Diagnosis: based on the symptoms (signs of abuse)
D. Substances abused
1. Alcohol
2. Narcotics
3. Psychedelic drugs (LSD, marijuana, PCP)
4. Hypnotics (barbiturates, methaqualone [Quaalude])
5. Amphetamines
6. Cocaine

7. Analgesics (codeine)
8. Heroin
9. Valium
10. Organic solvents (e.g., glue, cleaning fluids)
11. Stimulants
12. Amphetamines ("speed")
E. Treatment/nursing interventions
   1. Prevention of the problem is of course the best treatment
   2. Emergency measures when necessary (such as cardiopulmonary resuscitation [CPR] and gastric lavage)
   3. Psychiatric counseling as needed for the adolescent and family
   4. Follow-up health care; group support and counseling as needed for adolescent and family

Suicide

A. Definition: the act of taking one's own life voluntarily
B. Etiology: suicide usually does not occur without warning; the adolescent usually has a history of emotional problems, difficult relationships, and emotional upsets including such things as divorce in the family, death of a family member or friend, or a self-identity crisis
C. Treatment/nursing interventions
   1. Prevention is the best treatment; listen for verbal clues, such as "after tomorrow, it won't matter anymore"; and watch for warning signs
   2. Psychiatric counseling to determine the reasons for the adolescent's actions; this should also include the family members
   3. Follow-up medical care as needed
   4. Emotional support and counseling for the family members, especially during the crisis stages

Anorexia Nervosa and Bulimia

A. Definition (these disorders can occur together or separately)
   1. Anorexia nervosa is a disorder characterized by severe weight loss without physical cause; it is most often seen in adolescent females
   2. Bulimia is a disorder characterized by overeating or "binge" eating, followed by induced vomiting immediately after eating
B. Symptoms
   1. With anorexia nervosa there are three basic psychologic disturbances: the inability to correctly perceive body size, the absence of hunger or inability to perceive hunger, and feelings of inadequacy or lack of self-esteem; other symptoms include amenorrhea, constipation, dry skin, low blood pressure, anemia, and lanugo (fine, soft hair) on the back and arms
   2. With bulimia many of these same symptoms may occur
C. Diagnosis: based on the symptoms, family history, and psychologic evaluation
D. Treatment/nursing interventions
   1. The adolescent is usually hospitalized to correct the malnutrition and to identify and treat the psychologic cause
   2. Behavior modification techniques are often used to assist in changing the adolescent's behavior; for ex-

ample, privileges or visitors are withdrawn until the adolescent begins to gain weight
   3. Psychologic counseling for the adolescent and family members to determine the cause

Crohn's Disease

A. Definition: a chronic, recurrent inflammatory disorder of the intestines; it occurs most often in upper-middle-class men and women, aged 15 to 35 years
B. Symptoms: regional ileitis causing acute low abdominal pain, fever, chronic diarrhea, weight loss, abdominal tenderness and distention, and anemia
C. Diagnosis based on the symptoms, x-ray films of the intestine (barium enema), endoscopy and mucosal biopsy of the intestines
D. Treatment/nursing interventions
   1. The goal of treatment is to relieve the symptoms and discomfort
   2. Adequate rest and relaxation to alleviate stress
   3. Soft, low-fiber diet
   4. Steroid drugs as ordered to decrease inflammation of the intestines
   5. Antidiarrheal drugs as ordered
   6. Antispasmodic drugs as ordered to relieve intestinal spasms
   7. Emotional support and psychologic counseling as needed to decrease the stress level

Mononucleosis

A. Definition: an acute viral infectious disease causing an increase in mononuclear WBCs and signs of general infection; it is usually thought to be only mildly contagious and is spread by oral contact (known as the "kissing disease")
B. Symptoms: general malaise, sore throat, fever, enlarged lymph glands, lack of energy, headache, red, flat rash on the body, and tonsillitis
C. Diagnosis: based on the symptoms, an elevated WBC count, and a positive Monospot blood test (which indicates increased agglutinins in the blood count)
D. Treatment/nursing interventions
   1. Antibiotics as ordered
   2. Antipyretics to relieve fever and discomfort
   3. Increased oral fluids; IV fluids may be ordered for severe dehydration
   4. Gargles or lozenges as ordered for sore throat
   5. Adequate rest and sleep
   6. Diet as tolerated; if the patient can only tolerate fluids, high-calorie fluids should be provided
   7. Patient teaching regarding follow-up care, including the need for adequate rest and sleep

Acne Vulgaris

A. Definition: a disorder of the sebaceous glands; the glands become irritated with the secretion of sebum and the interaction of the sebum with the hormones; the glands become impacted with sebum and form comedones (noninflamed) and papules and pustules (inflamed)
B. Symptoms: the appearance of the comedones, papules, and pustules on the face; they can also appear on other places on the body such as the chest and back
C. Diagnosis: based on the symptoms

D. Treatment/nursing interventions
1. Cleaning the affected areas with soap or soap substitute and water daily
2. A diet low in greasy foods, chocolate, and nuts may help decrease the amount of oil in the skin
3. Nonprescription topical creams and lotions have limited effectiveness; retinoic acid and antibacterial agents when used together are the most effective
4. Encouraging the adolescent to keep stress levels to a minimum when possible may help in keeping acne to a minimum
5. Patient teaching: papules and pustules should not be squeezed; they can become infected and spread
6. Counseling for the adolescent to maintain a positive body image

The Battered Child Syndrome

A. Definition: abuse of children by parents or other caregivers; the abuse can be physical, sexual, nutritional, or emotional
B. Characteristics of battered children
1. They are often from an unplanned pregnancy
2. Many of them were premature, had a low birth weight, or had major birth defects
3. They sometimes resemble a person that the parents disliked

C. Characteristics of abusive parents
1. One parent often has a previous emotional problem
2. The abuse is usually done by one parent; the other parent knows about the abuse but usually does not report it
3. Abusive parents often have very high expectations of their children; if they do not "perform" up to these expectations, they are "punished"
4. Abusive parents are often substance abusers
5. The most common characteristic of abusive parents is that often they were abused themselves as children; however, this is not always true
6. They come from all socioeconomic levels
D. Identifying the battered child
1. The child has many unexplained scars, bruises, and injuries; many of these markings are characteristic of abuse (Fig. 9-12)
2. Bone fractures may be seen on x-ray examination at various stages of healing
3. The child exhibits signs of physical neglect: malnourishment or improper or dirty clothing
4. The parents' explanations of the child's injury are inconsistent; one parent's explanation differs from the other's, or it changes from one time to the next
5. The child withdraws when approached by the parents, nurse, or physician

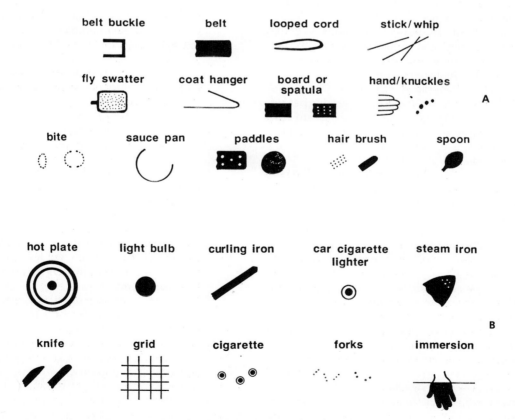

FIG. 9-12. Characteristic markings often seen in child abuse. **A,** Marks from objects. **B,** Marks from burns. (From Reece RM, Smith MK, editors: Inflicted injury versus accidental injury, *Pediatr Clin North Am,* Aug 1990.)

6. The parents' emotional reaction is inconsistent with the extent of the child's injury
E. Nursing interventions for the battered child and parents
   1. Interview the parents calmly regarding the history of the incident
   2. Nursing personnel must control their own feelings and attitudes toward the parents to work effectively with the family
   3. Provide physical care for the child as needed
   4. Emotional care for the child should include providing a safe environment, explaining all procedures, providing toys and familiar belongings while the child is hospitalized, and physical cuddling and holding when appropriate
   5. Referrals should be made to the hospital social worker, the local department of children and family services, the police, and the psychologist as needed

Acquired Immunodeficiency Syndrome (AIDS)

A. Definition: an immune disorder caused by a retrovirus, the human immunodeficiency virus (HIV)
   1. The AIDS virus is known to be transmitted by blood, and body fluids containing blood (see Chapter 6, Medical-Surgical Nursing)
   2. Three primary modes of transmission of the AIDS virus in children are prenatal exposure to infected mothers, blood transfusion, and engaging in high-risk activities (sexual or IV drug use, specifically with adolescents)
   3. The majority of pediatric cases have occurred in children under 2 years of age
B. Symptoms: recurrent or chronic infections including meningitis, pneumonia, and urinary tract infections; fever; weight loss; failure to thrive; anemia; hepatosplenomegaly; persistent lymphadenopathy
C. Diagnosis: abnormal laboratory values, including abnormal T-cell ratio, decreased T-lymphocytes and hypergammaglobulinemia; history of possible exposure to AIDS virus; positive HIV test; and history of recurrent infections
D. Treatment/nursing interventions
   1. There is no cure for AIDS, so treatment and nursing care measures are supportive and designed to prevent and alleviate opportunistic infections
   2. The drug azidothymidine (AZT) (zidovudine) to assist in controlling the progression of the disease (see Chapter 4, Pharmacology)
   3. Antibiotics/antifungal drugs as ordered (see Chapter 4, Pharmacology)
   4. Drugs such as acyclovir and IV gamma-globulin to help reduce overwhelming viral infections
   5. Adequate nutrition and fluid intake
   6. Use of "Universal Precautions" when caring for the child in the hospital or clinic
   7. Maintenance of an environment as free from infection as possible
   8. Promotion of normal development of the child
   9. Education and emotional support for the child and family
E. Prognosis: poor, especially in children with AIDS who are under 1 year of age

HOSPITALIZATION AND THE CHILD

A. Preparation for hospitalization
   1. The rationale for preparing children for hospitalization is based on the theory that fear of the unknown is more severe than fear of the known
   2. Preadmission preparation can be done by both parents and professionals (nurses and physicians) honestly at a level the child can understand
   3. Hospital admission procedures include the admission history, blood tests, chest x-ray studies when necessary, physical examination, and placement in the child's room and bed; these should be explained to the child during preadmission preparation
   4. In preparing the child for any hospital procedure the nurse or parent should include all necessary information regarding the procedure and any necessary preparation; time should be allowed for questions by the child and parents
B. Hospitalization as a crisis
   1. Children are more vulnerable to the crisis of illness and hospitalization because stress is a change from their usual state of health and routine, and children have a limited number of coping mechanisms to deal with stressful events
   2. Their reactions to stress differ in each developmental age group
      a. Infants and preschoolers: their major stress is separation anxiety (fear of being separated from their parents and family)
      b. Preschoolers: their major stresses are separation anxiety and fear of loss of body control and of bodily injury and pain
      c. School-age children: their major stresses are fear of separation (sometimes more from peers than from family), of loss of body control, and of bodily injury, mutilation, pain, and death
      d. Adolescents: their major stresses are fear of separation from their peer group; of loss of body control, independence and identity; and of bodily injury and pain, especially concerning sexual changes
   3. Nursing measures that can be used to minimize the hospitalized child's fears and stresses
      a. Open visiting for parents and siblings; visiting by peers in the school-age and adolescent groups should be encouraged
      b. Explain procedures or preparation for procedures at the child's age level
      c. Allow the child to have favorite toys and games from home
      d. Nursing personnel should not lie to the child about the parents' visits; the visits should not be used as rewards or as something to be withheld if the child does not cooperate or "behave"
      e. Allow the child as much physical freedom as his or her condition will allow
      f. Allow the child to participate in decision making as much as possible, especially regarding treatments and procedures; for example, don't ask, "Do you want your shot?"; instead ask, "Do you want your shot now, or in 10 minutes?"; this allows the child some control in the situation

g. Encourage the parents to visit as much as possible; explain all procedures to them and encourage them to assist in their child's care if they are comfortable in doing so

h. Instruct the parents not to lie to the child; lying only sets up a sense of mistrust among the child, the parents, and the hospital staff

i. Administer pain medications as ordered whenever necessary; a child's pain response is affected by developmental level

j. Expect some regressive behavior during the child's hospital stay; tell the parents that this is normal during stressful periods

C. Use of play during hospitalization

1. Play in the hospital helps relieve tension and anxiety, lessens the stress of separation and feelings of homesickness, and helps the child to relax and feel more secure

2. The play activities should be based on the child's age, interests, and limitations

3. Play can be used for diversion, recreation, and to play out the child's fears and anxieties over his illness and treatment

4. Toys can come from home or from the hospital play area; they can even be adapted from hospital "stock" supplies

5. Play therapy can be used to teach the child about procedures and surgery, as well as to help the child work through fears and anxieties about hospitalization

D. Preparation and teaching for discharge

1. Preparation for discharge should begin during the admission by setting long-term goals concerning discharge

2. Discharge planning should include several areas

   a. Parent-child teaching regarding home care procedures and medication regimen

   b. Follow-up care including physician appointments and the importance of keeping them

   c. Referrals to community agencies, public health nurses, and other resources as needed

Nursing Care of the Hospitalized Child

A. Safety factors

1. Side rails should be kept up at all times when the child is in bed; if the bed is adjustable, it should be kept in the low position

2. When restraints are used, they should be applied securely to the child; extremities should be checked frequently for impaired circulation caused by tight restraints; appropriate charting should be done

3. Small toys, game pieces, and other small objects should be kept away from infants and toddlers who may swallow them

4. Toddlers and young children should not be left unattended in their rooms or hallways; if they are out of bed, they should be observed continuously to avoid accidents and injuries

5. Medications, needles, and syringes should be kept out of the reach of all children

B. Medication administration

1. General guidelines in giving medications to children

   a. Approach the child with a cheerful, positive attitude and explain what you are going to do

   b. Be honest when talking to the child; tell the child it is medicine, not "juice" or "candy"

   c. When necessary, use foods or liquids to disguise the taste of bad-tasting medications

   d. Oral syringes or syringes without needles may be used to deliver oral medications to infants and young children

   e. Allow the child some control in the situation; don't ask, "Do you want your shot?" but ask, "Do you want your shot in your leg or your hip?"; make sure the question you ask the child is appropriate to the child's age level and the situation

   f. Intramuscular (IM) injections are safer and easier to give to a young child if a second person helps restrain the child

   g. Tell the child that it is all right to cry if the shot "hurts"

   h. Teach the child to "say no" to street drugs but that the drugs received in the hospital are okay to take

2. Safe IM injection technique includes the same steps used for IM injections in adults

   a. In infants the lateral thigh (vastus lateralis muscle) should be used

   b. In toddlers and preschoolers, the ventrogluteal area is the preferred site (lateral thigh can also be used)

   c. In older children and adolescents, other regularly used injection sites may be used (ventrogluteal muscle is the safest; deltoid and dorsogluteal muscles may also be used) (Fig. 9-13)

C. Assisting with treatments and procedures

1. All tests and procedures should be explained to the child in an honest, simple manner; older children and adolescents should be allowed to ask questions and receive answers

2. All children should be allowed to say "ouch," or to cry if the procedure is a painful one; rewards are often given after a painful procedure (a reward "sticker," toy, or special food treat)

3. The child may need to be held or restrained in certain positions for procedures; all equipment should be assembled before the procedure is started so that the nurse can stay with the child as much as possible

D. Preoperative teaching

1. Patient teaching in pediatrics should include the child (preschool age and older) and the parents; both should be involved in the teaching and preparation for surgery

2. Use words that the child can understand; audiovisual aids (pictures, dolls, puppets, and bandages) are extremely useful in helping the child understand the procedure or surgery

3. Be honest with the child, especially regarding procedures or treatments that may be uncomfortable or painful

4. Tell the child that he or she will not feel any pain during the surgery because of the "special sleep" of anesthesia and that he or she will "wake up" after surgery is over in the recovery room

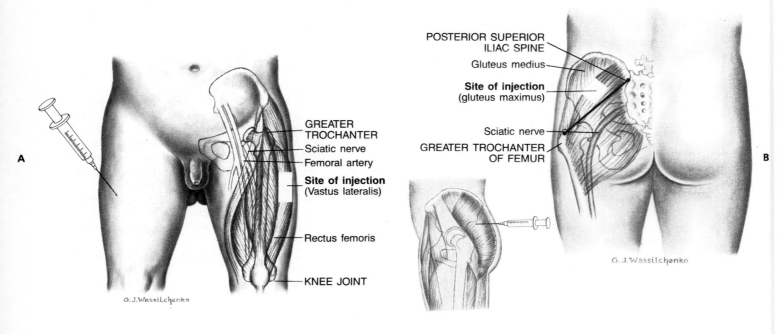

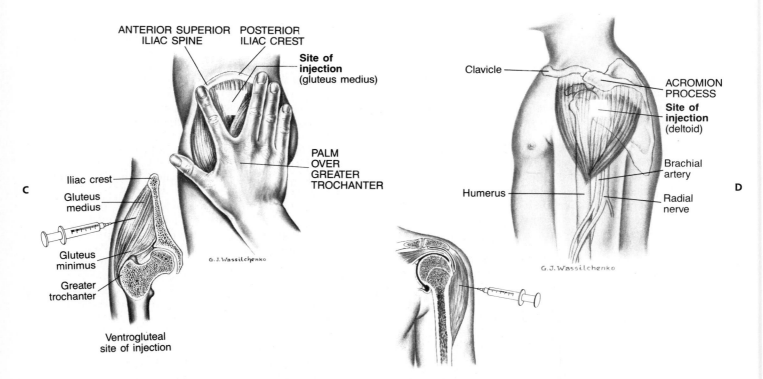

FIG. 9-13. Acceptable intramuscular sites in children. **A,** Vastus lateralis. **B,** Dorsogluteal. **C,** Ventrogluteal. **D,** Deltoid. (From Whaley LF, Wong DL: *Nursing care of infants and children,* ed 4, St Louis, 1991, Mosby.)

5. Include details specific to the child's surgery such as dressings, tubes, IV fluids, medications, the specific site of the pain or discomfort, and the diet restrictions before and after surgery

E. General postoperative care

1. Basic postoperative care is similar to nursing care of adult postoperative patients
   a. Frequent vital signs
   b. Observation of the incision or dressings
   c. Level of consciousness

d. Intake and output, IV fluids, Foley catheter, nasogastric (NG) tube
e. Administer pain medications as needed (IV, IM, PO)
2. Allow the child's parents to assist in the child's care if they desire to do so
3. Explain all postoperative procedures before doing them
F. Care of the child in a cast
1. The cast should be handled lightly with open palms while it is still damp to avoid indentations
2. Observe and record the condition of the skin at the edges of the cast for color, warmth, irritation, sensation, and edema
3. Check the color of the nail beds below the cast; check the pulse in the area below the cast if it is in an accessible area (radial or pedal pulse)
4. Teach the child not to put anything inside the cast or to "scratch" the skin beneath the cast
5. Check the cast for drainage or discoloration; any drainage should be marked, timed, and dated
6. Protect the cast from water, urine, and stool
7. "Petal" the edges of the cast before the patient goes home (if cast is damp, teach parents the proper way to do it)
G. Care of the child in traction
1. Types of traction
a. Skeletal: uses pins, wires, and tongs

b. Skin: uses tape, plastic, and bandages attached to the skin
c. Bryant's: a type of skin traction; it is most commonly used in infants and toddlers for treatment of a fractured femur and congenital hip dislocation (Fig. 9-14)
2. Nursing care measures for the child in traction
a. Explain the traction apparatus to the child; allow the child to participate in his or her care as much as possible
b. Maintain traction alignment; be sure that all ropes are in the center tracks of the pulleys and that the weights are hanging freely
c. Provide proper skin care; observe for reddened, irritated areas at the edges of the tape and elastic bandages, as well as at other pressure sites
d. Observe skeletal pin sites for bleeding, inflammation, and signs of infection; provide pin-site care as ordered
e. Observe affected extremity for skin color, nail bed color, and changes in sensation and mobility
f. Administer pain medications as ordered and keep the child as comfortable as possible
g. Provide range-of-motion exercises to the unaffected body parts to help prevent contractures and muscle atrophy
h. Provide toys and activities appropriate to the child's age level and limited mobility

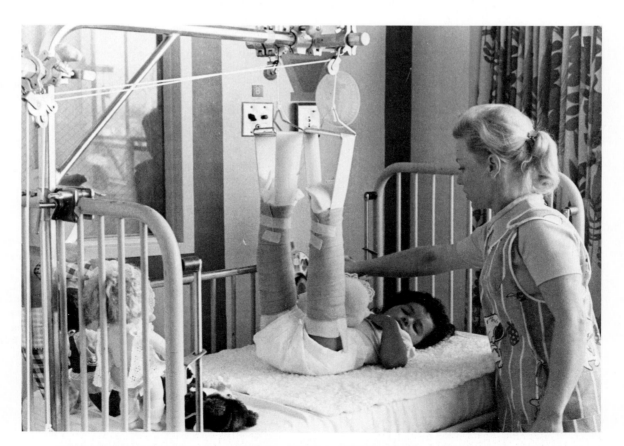

FIG. 9-14. Bryant's traction. (From Whaley LF, Wong DL: *Nursing care of infants and children,* ed 3, St Louis, 1987, Mosby.)

Suggested Reading List

Caspe WB: Guidelines for the care of children and adolescents with HIV infection, *J Pediatr* 119(suppl):S1-S68, 1991.

Feeg VD, Harbin RE: *Pediatric nursing care curriculum and resource manual,* Pitman, NJ, 1991, Anthony J Janetti.

Hamilton PM: *Basic pediatric nursing,* ed 6, St Louis, 1991, Mosby.

Ingalls AJ, Salerno MC: *Maternal and child health nursing,* ed 7, St Louis, 1991, Mosby.

Kline MW, Shearer WT: A national survey on the care of infants and children with HIV infection, *J Pediatr* 118:817-821, May 1991.

Lowrey GH: *Growth and development of children,* ed 8, Chicago, 1986, Mosby.

Physicians' desk reference, Montvale, NJ, Medical Economics (published annually).

Pizzo PA, Wilfert CM: *Pediatric AIDS: the challenge of HIV infection in infants, children and adolescents,* Baltimore, 1991, Williams & Wilkins.

Reece RM, Smith MK: Child abuse, *Pediatr Clin North Am* 37:905-922, Aug 1990.

Whaley LF, Wong DL: *Nursing care of infants and children,* ed 4, St Louis, 1991, Mosby.

Wong DL: *Whaley and Wong's essentials of pediatric nursing,* ed 4, St Louis, 1992, Mosby.

Pediatric Nursing Review Questions

Answers and rationales begin on p. 444.

1. A Wilms' tumor is an adenosarcoma found in the:
   ① Brain
   ② Small intestine
   ③ Colon
   ④ Kidney
2. Infancy is that period from:
   ① Birth to 6 weeks of age
   ② Birth to 1 year of age
   ③ 4 weeks to 1 year of age
   ④ 4 weeks to 2 years of age
3. The physician orders Demerol 20 mg with Atropine 0.08 mg IM as a preoperative medication. The Demerol is supplied at 50 mg/ml, the Atropine at 0.2 mg/ml. The nurse should draw up a total volume of:
   ① 0.4 ml
   ② 0.8 ml
   ③ 1.0 ml
   ④ 1.2 ml
4. Your neighbor Sarah, age 7 years, has developed a red, raised rash on her face, neck, and trunk. She also has a temperature of 101.4° F (38.5° C) and whitish spots on the back of her throat. From these symptoms, you know Sarah has:
   ① Chickenpox
   ② Measles (rubeola)
   ③ Mumps
   ④ German measles (rubella)

Situation: Karen, age 4, was admitted with a diagnosis of possible epiglottitis.

5. If the nurse suspects Karen has epiglottitis, she should:
   ① Check her throat carefully with a flashlight
   ② Increase her oral intake
   ③ Direct warm steam toward the patient
   ④ Have emergency tracheostomy equipment immediately available
6. The most important nurse caring for Karen is:
   ① Taking Karen's vital signs
   ② Maintaining a patent airway
   ③ Keeping Karen in her croup tent
   ④ Providing fluids for her to drink
7. Karen has to have blood drawn for a CBC. When she asks you if it will hurt to have the blood drawn, the best response would be:
   ① "No, of course it won't hurt!"
   ② "It might hurt for a minute, but I will be here with you, and you can hold my hand if you want to."
   ③ "If you are a big girl, the blood test won't hurt you."
   ④ "It might hurt, but you have to have it done, so try not to cry."
8. The symptoms of epiglottitis are caused by:
   ① A bacterial infection; usually *H. influenzae*
   ② Inflammation of the trachea and esophagus
   ③ Spasms of the epiglottis
   ④ Viral upper respiratory infection (URI)

9. Christina, age 3, has an order for Gantrisin 750 mg po q AM. On hand, you have Gantrisin 0.5 g/5 ml. You give Christina:
   ① 2 ml
   ② 4 ml
   ③ 1½ tsp
   ④ 2 tsp

10. Adolescence begins when:
   ① The growth rate increases rapidly
   ② The child develops a positive self-image
   ③ Secondary sex characteristics appear
   ④ The child starts to be attracted to the opposite sex

11. Hospitalized teenagers have the most difficulty with:
   ① Dependency vs. independency
   ② Trust vs. autonomy
   ③ Reality vs. fantasy
   ④ Initiative vs. guilt

12. According to Erikson's theory of psychosocial development, preschoolers are in the stage of:
   ① Trust vs. mistrust
   ② Industry vs. inferiority
   ③ Autonomy vs. shame and doubt
   ④ Initiative vs. guilt

13. The best way for the pediatric nurse to establish a good working relationship with parents is to:
   ① Avoid contact whenever possible
   ② Answer their questions honestly
   ③ Refer all questions to the physician
   ④ Keep them out of their child's room as much as possible

14. Rheumatic fever is caused by:
   ① A fungus
   ② *Staphylococcus* bacteria
   ③ A virus
   ④ *Streptococcus* bacteria

15. The most serious complication of rheumatic fever is:
   ① Endocarditis
   ② Pneumonia
   ③ Arthritis
   ④ Meningitis

16. A drug used to reduce overwhelming viral infections in the child with AIDS is:
   ① Cimetidine
   ② Penicillin
   ③ Neostigmine
   ④ Acyclovir

Situation: Kelly is an 11-year-old child with cystic fibrosis. She was admitted to the hospital for treatment of a respiratory infection.

17. Which of the following pathophysiologic mechanisms is responsible for respiratory alterations seen in children with cystic fibrosis?
   ① Decreased ciliary action causing stasis of mucus in lungs
   ② Edema of the epiglottis causing upper airway occlusion
   ③ Excessive production of thick mucus leading to airway obstruction
   ④ Laryngeal stricture leading to bronchospasm

18. Kelly also takes pancreatic enzymes with each meal. The purpose of this therapy is to facilitate:
   ① Absorption of vitamins A, C, and K
   ② Increased carbohydrate metabolism for growth
   ③ Digestion and absorption of fats and proteins
   ④ Sodium excretion and electrolyte balance

19. Aerosol treatment, chest physiotherapy, and postural drainage are ordered for Kelly to:
   ① Decrease respiratory effort and mucous production
   ② Dilate the bronchioles and clear secretions
   ③ Increase efficiency of the diaphragm and gas exchange
   ④ Stimulate coughing and arterial oxygen consumption

20. One of the major physical characteristics of the child with Down's syndrome is:
   ① Hypertonic musculature
   ② A single transverse crease on palms
   ③ Inflexibility of the joints
   ④ Janeway spots on the palms and soles

21. In caring for a child with Down's syndrome, the nurse should be aware that a frequent accompanying defect is:
   ① Congenital heart disease
   ② Congenital hip dysplasia
   ③ Central auditory imperception
   ④ Pyloric stenosis

22. Which one of the following statements is *not* appropriate when giving medications to 5-year-old Cindy?
   ① "Hi, Cindy. It's time for your medicine. I know you don't like the flavor of the medicine, so I brought some juice for you to drink with the medicine to help cover up the bad taste."
   ② "Cindy, are you finished with breakfast? I have some candy pills for you to take. They taste just like peppermint."
   ③ "Cindy, I have a shot to give you. I know shots hurt, but you need to have the medicine in the shot to make you better. Would you like me to give it to you now or in 5 minutes?"
   ④ "Hi Cindy. It's time for your medicine. Let me check your arm band so I can check your name."

23. The safest place to give an infant an intramuscular (IM) injection is the:
   ① Deltoid muscle
   ② Vastus lateralis muscle
   ③ Ventrogluteal muscle
   ④ Dorsogluteal muscle

24. Celiac disease is characterized by disturbance in the absorption of:
   ① Proteins
   ② Carbohydrates
   ③ Vitamins
   ④ Fats

25. Symptoms of celiac disease include which of the following?
   ① Constipation, anorexia, and malnutrition
   ② Malnutrition, distended abdomen, constant appetite for sweets
   ③ Distended abdomen, constipation, anorexia
   ④ Bulky, greasy stools, distended abdomen, and malnutrition

26. The infant with diagnosed celiac disease should be given which cereal?
    1. Rice
    2. Wheat
    3. Oat
    4. Barley

27. The best, most reliable method of assessing for pinworms in a child is by:
    1. The history, symptoms, and a stool culture
    2. A blood culture
    3. Capturing the eggs from the anal edge on cellophane tape
    4. Sending a stool culture to the laboratory

28. Two-year-old Stephanie is diagnosed as having leukemia. The most common signs and symptoms of leukemia related to bone marrow involvement are:
    1. Headache, papilledema, and irritability
    2. Muscle wasting, weight loss, and fatigue
    3. Decreased intracranial pressure, psychosis, and confusion
    4. Petechiae, joint pain, and lethargy

29. The most common method of treatment for an infant weighing more than 30 lb with a simple fractured femur is:
    1. Surgery and placement of a pin to set the fracture
    2. Putting the child in skeletal traction
    3. Immediate setting and casting of the fractured leg
    4. Putting the child in Bryant's traction

30. The lateral S-shaped curvature of the spine that often occurs in school-age girls is:
    1. Scoliosis
    2. Nephrosis
    3. Lordosis
    4. Kyphosis

Situation: Joshua, age 17 months, is admitted to the hospital with a diagnosis of meningitis.

31. Which of the following findings would be noted relative to Joshua's cerebrospinal fluid (CSF)?
    1. Reduced protein level
    2. Elevated glucose level
    3. Reduced pressure
    4. Cloudy color

32. The most notable symptoms the nurse would observe in Joshua would be:
    1. Weak or absent cry, coma
    2. Bulging fontanel, irritability
    3. Absent reflexes, rigid digits
    4. Dilated and fixed pupils

33. While you are caring for Joshua, he has a complex febrile seizure in his crib. What is the most important nursing activity at this time?
    1. Place a seizure stick between Joshua's jaws
    2. Prepare the suction equipment
    3. Observe the seizure and protect Joshua from harm
    4. Restrain Joshua to prevent injury

34. John, age 2, is admitted to the hospital for a bilateral myringotomy because of frequent occurrences of otitis media. Otitis media occurs more frequently in young children than in older children because of the different position and shape of the young child's:
    1. Esophagus
    2. Tympanic membranes
    3. External ear canals
    4. Eustachian tubes

35. When performing a procedure on an uncooperative small child, which of the following actions would be the best for the nurse to try first?
    1. Sedate the child
    2. Use wrist and ankle restraints
    3. Allow a parent to assist
    4. Bring in another nurse to assist

Situation: Michael, age 3, has asthma. He was brought to the emergency clinic while having an acute asthma attack.

36. During this attack, Michael's breathing is most likely to be characterized by:
    1. Loud inspiratory stridor
    2. Loud audible wheezing
    3. Coarse rales in lower lobes
    4. Frequent crowing cough

37. Which of the following is responsible for airway-narrowing characteristic of an asthma episode?
    1. Laryngeal edema, dehydration, and anxiety
    2. Bronchospasm, respiratory mucosal edema, and increased production and accumulation of mucus
    3. Increased negative pleural pressure, laryngospasm, and mucus plugging
    4. Carbon dioxide retention, pharyngeal hyperemia, and alveolar collapse

38. The drug of choice for Michael during this acute attack is:
    1. Epinephrine
    2. Corticosteroids
    3. Ephedrine
    4. Cough syrup with codeine

39. You are caring for a child who weighs 25 lb. The usual dose for Ampicillin for children is 100 mg/kg/day. Which of the following would be an appropriate order for this child?
    1. Ampicillin 25 mg q4h
    2. Ampicillin 250 mg qid
    3. Ampicillin 100 mg q6h
    4. Ampicillin 100 mg qid

40. The physician orders Ampicillin 300 mg IVPB. Ampicillin is supplied as 500 mg/2 ml. What volume of Ampicillin would you draw up from the vial?
    1. 0.6 ml
    2. 0.8 ml
    3. 1.2 ml
    4. 1.4 ml

41. Bulimia is an eating disorder characterized by:
    1. Severe weight loss
    2. "Binge" eating followed by induced vomiting
    3. Sudden weight gain
    4. Chronic diarrhea

42. The childhood disease that exhibits symptoms of lethargy, muscle pain, polyarthritis, and chorea, and is diagnosed by using the Jones criteria is:
    1. Infectious mononucleosis
    2. Muscular dystrophy
    3. Cystic fibrosis
    4. Rheumatic fever

Situation: Brian is a 3-month-old infant admitted to the pediatric unit for treatment of bronchiolitis. Brian's vital signs are: temperature, 101.6° F; apical pulse, 160 beats per minute; and respirations, 70 per minute. He is irritable, fussy, and coughs frequently.

43. Oxygen therapy is ordered for Brian primarily to:
    1. Reduce fever
    2. Allay anxiety and restlessness
    3. Liquify secretions
    4. Relieve dyspnea and hypoxemia

44. Intravenous fluids are given to Brian through a peripheral venipuncture. Fluids by mouth were initially contraindicated for Brian because of feeding difficulty caused by:
    1. Tachypnea
    2. Bradycardia
    3. Irritability
    4. Fever

45. The stage of development where "parallel play" takes place is:
    1. Infancy
    2. Toddler
    3. Preschool age
    4. School age

46. The disorder characterized by a malfunction of the motor centers of the brain (because of lack of oxygen to the brain) is:
    1. Down's syndrome
    2. Scoliosis
    3. Osteomyelitis
    4. Cerebral palsy

47. Which of the following statements about pain in children is true?
    1. A child's behavioral response to pain is affected by his or her age and developmental stage
    2. Recovery from a painful experience occurs at a faster rate in children than in adults
    3. Narcotic use in children is dangerous because of the increased risk of addiction and respiratory depression
    4. Immaturity of the nervous system in young children provides them with increased thresholds for pain

48. The average 2- to 3-month-old infant:
    1. Babbles
    2. Has a crude pincer grasp
    3. Has a closed posterior fontanel
    4. Has one lower incisor

49. About 90% of all sudden infant death syndrome (SIDS) cases occur:
    1. In the first 10 weeks of life
    2. In the first 3 months of life
    3. In the first 6 months of life
    4. Between 6 and 12 months of age

50. The first immunizations an infant receives at 2 months of age are:
    1. DTP only
    2. PPD, OPV
    3. DTP, OPV, HbCV vaccine
    4. DTP, OPV

51. The leading cause of death in children between 1 and 14 years of age is
    1. Meningitis
    2. Leukemia
    3. Accidents
    4. Polio

52. A disorder caused by an obstruction of cerebrospinal fluid drainage is:
    1. Opisthotonos
    2. Wilms' tumor
    3. Hydrocephalus
    4. Meningitis

53. Characteristics of an infant diagnosed as failure to thrive (FTT) include all *except*:
    1. Listlessness, floppy body posture
    2. Little eye-to-eye contact
    3. Stiff or rigid body posture
    4. Prolonged periods of sleep

54. A baby with gastroesophageal reflux and FTT is classified as:
    1. Organic FTT
    2. Nonorganic FTT
    3. Idiopathic FTT
    4. Unstable FTT

55. In caring for a child in a full leg cast, which of the following findings should the nurse report to the physician *immediately?*
    1. The cast is still damp after 4 hours
    2. The child's pedal pulse is 80
    3. The child complains of pain in his leg
    4. The child is unable to move his toes

56. Of the following, the most important criterion on which to base the decision to report suspected child abuse is:
    1. Inappropriate parental concern for the degree of injury
    2. Absence of the parents for questioning about the child's injuries
    3. A complaint other than the one associated with the signs of abuse
    4. Incompatibility between the history given and the injury observed

57. When starting an infant on new foods, it is best to instruct the mother to:
    1. Mix the new food with one that the infant already likes
    2. Mix the new food with breast milk or formula
    3. Feed the infant one new food at a time, to observe likes and dislikes
    4. Try a new food at each feeding

58. By the end of the school-age years, a child should have developed a sense of:
    1. Initiative, purpose
    2. Industry, competence
    3. Identity, role
    4. Intimacy, fidelity

59. Laura is 2 years old. Her favorite word is "No!" She is in Erikson's developmental stage of:
    1. Trust vs. mistrust
    2. Initiative vs. guilt
    3. Autonomy vs. shame and doubt
    4. Industry vs. inferiority

60. A 5-week-old infant is brought to the pediatrician's office with symptoms of irritability, weight loss, and projectile vomiting. On physical examination the infant appears dehydrated. From these symptoms you know that the infant probably has:
    1. Hirschsprung's disease
    2. Pyloric stenosis
    3. Esophogeal atresia
    4. Intussusception

61. Laura is a 12 month old with sickle cell anemia. She has been admitted in sickle cell crisis. Her symptoms might include:
    1. Fever, seizures, coma
    2. Abdominal pain; swollen, painful joints
    3. Polycythemia
    4. Severe itching

62. Nursing intervention for the child in sickle cell crisis is directed primarily toward:
    1. Maintaining active range of motion
    2. Oxygen therapy
    3. Administration of blood
    4. Maintaining adequate hydration

63. A Denis Browne splint is a common method of treatment for:
    1. Scoliosis
    2. Congenital clubfoot
    3. Developmental dysplasia of the hip (DDH)
    4. Fractured femur

64. Preparation of a child for surgery should include all of the following *except*:
    1. Explaining all procedures and treatments before they occur
    2. Telling the child not to cry but to "be brave" if something hurts
    3. Explaining anesthesia as a "special sleep"
    4. Explaining where the incision or dressings will be after surgery

65. The physician has ordered an IV of D5.2NS to be infused at 100 ml/hr. If the IV tubing delivers 10 gtt/ml, at what rate would you infuse the IV fluid?
    1. 10 gtt/min
    2. 12 gtt/min
    3. 16 gtt/min
    4. 18 gtt/min

CHAPTER 10

Gerontologic Nursing

The percentage of the population over age 65 has topped 13% and continues to constitute our fastest growing age group. As the life expectancy of Americans continues to lengthen, we should be increasingly aware that by the year 2020 one of every five individuals in our society will be an older adult.

It is nursing's challenge to meet the care needs of our elders, who are so vulnerable to the biases of our fast-paced, youth-oriented society. As nurses we have an opportunity to play a significant role in determining whether these will be years of continued growth and development, years of happiness and accomplishment, or years of forced shame, illness, and neglect.

Refer to Chapter 12, Current Trends in Nursing and Health Care in the United States and Canada, for discussion of ethical and legal issues. This chapter focuses on aging as a normal process and strives to increase the practitioner's knowledge of and understanding for a stage of life we will all pass through.

"For age is opportunity no less than youth itself, though in another dress."

Longfellow

GOVERNMENT RESOURCES FOR THE ELDERLY
Income

A. Social Security (Federal Old-Age, Survivors, and Disability Insurance, FOASDI)
1. Funded by employee and employer payroll taxes
2. Entitlement determined by United States Social Security Administration; benefits are granted in accordance with
   a. Age
   b. Lifetime earnings record
   c. Free earnings credits for active military service
   d. Whether required number of work credits have been earned (work credits are measured in quarters)
3. Specific maximum benefit amount with cost-of-living protection against inflation
4. Retirement benefits may start at age 62
5. Railroad workers have a separate retirement system; workers who have less than 10 years of railroad service may transfer earnings to Social Security and count toward Social Security benefits
6. Federal employees are covered under the Civil Service Retirement System, Federal Employees Retirement System, and the Thrift Savings Plan
7. Social Security benefits are reduced according to monies earned over a stated maximum annual allowable income
8. No reduction in Social Security benefits for fulltime employees over the age of 70

9. Payments are indexed according to inflation rate
B. Supplemental Security Income (SSI)
1. Funded from general tax revenues
2. Cash assistance program
3. Administered by Social Security Administration
4. Designed to provide for disabled, blind, or aged with limited incomes and resources
5. Medicaid eligibility in many states is based on SSI eligibility

Health

A. Medicare (Title XVIII of Social Security Act)
1. Administered by Health Care Financing Administration
2. Designed to help those over 65 years of age and certain disabled people under 65 who are eligible under Social Security to meet medical care costs regardless of income
3. Major insurance companies in each state handle claims (e.g., Travelers Insurance Company in New York)
4. Do not have to be retired to receive benefits
5. Financed by employee and employer payroll taxes
6. Everyone over 65 who is entitled to Social Security benefits receives hospital insurance without paying premium charges
7. Automatic hospital insurance is provided to disabled persons who have been entitled to Social Security disability benefits for 24 consecutive months

8. Deductible is applied to each benefit period
9. Two parts
   a. Part A designed as hospital insurance that has certain exclusions
   b. Part B covers physician services and outpatient services, which has exclusions and excess charges
   c. If subscribing to part A, automatically enrolled in part B
B. Medicaid (Title XIX of Social Security Act)
   1. Purposes
      a. To cover specific expenses not provided for by Medicare
      b. To reduce expenses of those who have exhausted their Medicare benefits
      c. To defray medical expenses of those who cannot afford Medicare premiums
   2. Federally funded
   3. State-operated program
   4. Eligibility usually determined by eligibility for SSI but varies from state to state

Housing

A. Department of Housing and Urban Development
   1. Rent Supplement Program: rent-subsidized apartments for elderly, disabled, or low-income families
      a. Utility and rent costs in existing buildings
      b. Renovations of existing units
      c. Building of new units
   2. Provides home improvement loans
   3. Provides mortgage insurance
   4. Age, asset, income eligibility requirements
B. Elderly and handicapped housing (Housing Act of 1959)
   1. Funding to private, nonprofit organizations for renovation or building of units for the elderly and handicapped
   2. Low-interest federal loans for same
C. National Housing Act (Housing and Urban Development Act, 1968): funding to private corporations for construction of low- and middle-income housing
D. National Housing Act of 1952: funding to private, profit or nonprofit groups for nursing home construction or renovation

Title XX of the Social Security Act

A. Federal monies for social programs
B. State administered
C. Individual must be eligible for SSI
D. Many of the programs are suitable and available for the elderly

Food Stamp Program

A. Administered by U.S. Department of Agriculture
B. Eligibility requirement
C. State welfare department determines eligibility
D. Components
   1. Home-delivered meals
   2. Grocery store food purchases

Administration on Aging

A. State, regional, area, and local units: area units responsible for providing program coordination and development expertise
B. Major services
   1. Nutritional programs
      a. On-site meals
      b. Home-delivered meals
   2. Senior centers
      a. Services
      b. Programs
   3. Home care
      a. Homemaker
      b. Home health aide
      c. Home visits
      d. Telephone calls
      e. Chore maintenance
   4. Information and referral
   5. Transportation
      a. Urban Mass Transit Act
      b. Area agencies on aging

THEORIES OF AGING
Sociologic Theories

A. Disengagement
   1. Controversial
   2. Mutual withdrawal from social interaction by aged individual or society
   3. Engagement meaning active occupation and devotion
   4. Supports leisure as a form of activity
   5. Respects individual initiated withdrawal
B. Activity
   1. Individual remains active and interacts with society's events
   2. Pursues new interests, friends, and roles to substitute for lost roles
   3. Supports social activity as beneficial
C. Continuity or development
   1. Lifelong personality characteristics and coping strategies continue
   2. Sense of "inferiority" develops
   3. Supportive network of relationships established
D. Passages: life cycle changes can be identified, predicted, planned for, and managed

Biologic Theories

A. Wear-and-tear
   1. Stress and use deplete the body cells of repair ability
   2. Coping mechanisms decline because of decrease in available energy
B. Collagen
   1. Most abundant body protein
   2. Collagen molecules held together by bonds
   3. Chemical reactions cause a switching of bonds between collagen molecules, resulting in structural changes characteristic of the aging process
C. Lipofuscin accumulation
   1. Lipofuscins or age pigments are insoluble end products of cell metabolism
   2. Accumulate in the cell, altering the cell's ability to function normally
D. Immunologic responses
   1. Aging is an autoimmune disease process
   2. Cells change, and the body does not recognize its own cells

3. Autoimmune responses damage the cells, causing cell death
E. Cell death of genetic programming
   1. Cell reproduction is programmed
   2. The programming determines the rate and time a given species ages and dies
F. Stress adaptation
   1. Damage from stress accumulates
   2. System's resistance to stress steadily declines, leading to death
G. Free radical
   1. Molecules that have an extra electron are free radicals
   2. Free radicals attach to other molecules altering function or structure
   3. There are internal and external sources of free radicals
   4. Believed that the free radicals do damage membrane function and structure
H. Mutation and error
   1. Cell division errors occur progressively over time
   2. Mutated cells are altered in their function and effectiveness
   3. Error theory expands mutation theory to include errors in interpretation of cell messages

Psychologic Theories

A. Freud: did not recommend psychoanalysis for the aged population (see Chapter 7, Mental Health Nursing)
B. Sullivan: see Chapter 7, Mental Health Nursing
C. Maslow: see Chapter 2, Basic Nursing Concepts and the Nursing Process
D. Erikson: see Chapter 7, Mental Health Nursing

1. Eighth stage (65 to 100 years of age) identified as "integrity vs. despair" (Fig. 10-1)
2. Older adult who views own life as having no meaning ends life's stages in despair; older adult who can review his or her accomplishments and errors derives a sense of integrity
E. Peck
   1. Expanded Erikson's developmental theory
   2. Expanded Erikson's eighth stage into three stages to focus on new roles, alternatives to preoccupation with body changes and illness, thereby achieving life satisfaction (Fig. 10-2)

ROLE CHANGES

A. Types
   1. Crisis
      a. Sudden
      b. Not able to plan for appropriate replacement
      c. Substitute not readily available
      d. Stress producing
   2. Gradual
      a. Develops slowly
      b. Time available for preparation, which eases transition
      c. Control over whether to develop a substitute
B. Sufficient preparation and adequate support determine adjustment success or failure
C. Role changes that occur to the older adult are predominantly crisis oriented
   1. Forced retirement
   2. Alteration in income
   3. Loss of spouse
   4. Illness

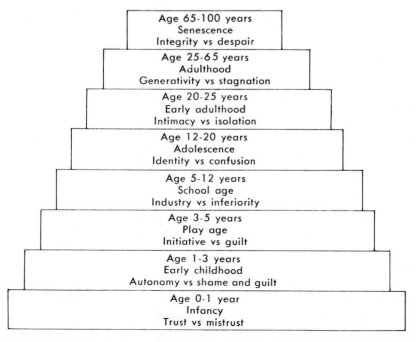

FIG. 10-1. Erikson: Eight stages of man. (From Forbes ES, Fitzsimmons VM: *The older adult: a process for wellness,* St Louis, 1981, Mosby.)

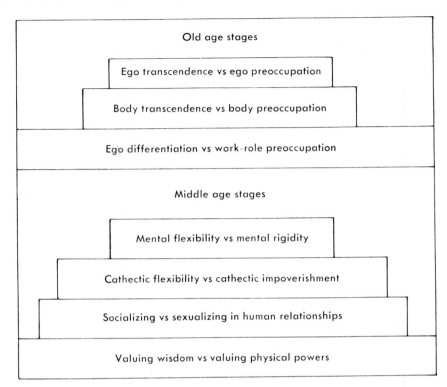

FIG. 10-2. Peck: Stages of middle age and old age. (From Forbes ES, Fitzsimmons VM: *The older adult: a process for wellness,* St. Louis, 1981, Mosby.)

5. Friends move away or die
6. Family members relocate, assume new roles, have increasingly less time for relationships
7. Society's assigned role of decreased psychologic and physiologic functioning
D. Role losses
  1. Work
    a. No longer the breadwinner
    b. Job-related companionship
    c. Usefulness, competence, identity
    d. Income
    e. Sense of purpose
    f. Self-esteem
  2. Family
    a. Usually no longer the decision maker
    b. Not held in the same esteem
    c. Loss of independence
E. Role gains
  1. Grandparenthood or great-grandparenthood
  2. Family support roles assumed
    a. Economic
    b. Child care
    c. Caring role in illness
    d. House care
  3. Community activities
  4. Religious activities
  5. Recreational activities
  6. Clubs, organizations, and associations
  7. Advisory roles
  8. New friends

9. Adult education
10. Volunteerism

ALTERATIONS IN LIFE-STYLE
Employment
A. Society emphasizes the employed as valuable and the unemployed as useless
B. Increase in the number of older women working
C. Decrease in the number of older men working
D. Part-time employment more common
E. Trend toward early retirement
F. Serial careers emerging in keeping with interest changes
G. More women are joining the work force at a time when men are winding down their working lives
H. Older worker possesses involuntary limitations
  1. Health problems
  2. Sensory or perceptual alterations, for example, in vision and auditory acuity
  3. Decline in physical strength, endurance, and speed
I. Older workers possess innumerable strengths
  1. Reliability
  2. Dependability
  3. Knowledge
  4. Expertise
  5. Experience

Retirement
A. Mandatory retirement in federal employment eliminated
B. Mandatory retirement age raised to 70 in private employment

C. More people taking advantage of early retirement
D. Health problems are primary reason for voluntary retirement
E. Increase in leisure time
F. Stress-producing event at a time when one's ability to handle stress is diminished
G. Creates tremendous anxiety
H. Some derive an initial feeling of relief, but for most it's a loss that comes at a time of meaningful productivity
I. Adjustment depends on previously established patterns of adjustment, degree of financial security, state of health, and future outlook
J. For most it creates an additional series of losses and problems at a time in life when coping and problem-solving abilities are fragile
K. Job loss
  1. Loss of daily routine
    a. Alters household routine
    b. Alters life-style
    c. Creates discouragement, depression, and loneliness
    d. Alters family relationships
  2. Loss of income
    a. Relocation
    b. Daily decision making determined by economics
    c. Decreases self-esteem
    d. Increases fear and anxiety
    e. Increases insecurity
L. Welcome changes
  1. New friends
  2. New activities
  3. New interests
  4. Renewal of marriage
  5. Seek new and different employment
  6. Find purpose and opportunity
  7. Rest and relaxation

Economic Changes

A. Most elderly live on fixed incomes
B. Of elderly persons, 1 out of 10 lives below the nation's poverty level
C. Independence declines as costs increase and buying power decreases
D. For many Social Security is the sole source of income
E. Many elderly are not receiving the assistance to which they are entitled
  1. Lack of resource knowledge
  2. Inability to find out about resources
    a. Lack of mobility
    b. Health problems
F. Supplemental Social Security: may qualify for in addition to or instead of Social Security benefits
G. Economic penalties: limit on the amount a Social Security beneficiary can earn annually without losing some monthly payments
H. Income tax reforms: once-in-a-lifetime capital gains tax exemption on sale of personal residence for person over 55 years of age
I. Income sources
  1. Public
    a. Social Security (Federal Old-Age, Survivors, and Disability Insurance)
    b. Supplemental Social Security income

  2. Private (e.g., pensions and investments)
  3. Other (e.g., Railroad Retirement System, Federal Employee's Retirement System, and Civil Service Retirement System)

Health

A. Most elderly have more than one chronic disease
B. Health care needs increase with age
C. Cost of health care is increasing as financial income is either decreasing or fixed
D. Elderly account for one third of the nation's health care costs

Housing

A. Most elderly prefer to remain independent as long as family and friends live nearby
B. Most live with spouse, alone, or with family
C. Large percentage continue to own their own home and prefer this life-style
  1. Security
  2. Privacy
  3. Independence
  4. Sense of purpose
  5. Familiarity
  6. Household activities
  7. Pride
  8. Socialization
D. Other housing alternatives
  1. Mobile homes
    a. Convenient
    b. Economical
  2. Retirement communities
    a. Minimum age requirement
    b. Different cost levels, for example, houses, apartments, and condominiums
  3. Foster home
  4. Life care facilities: living, recreational, medical facilities on the premises
  5. Nursing homes
  6. Homes for the aged
  7. Convalescent homes
  8. Rest homes
  9. House sharing
  10. Public housing
  11. Rooming houses
  12. Hotels: SROs (single room occupancy)
E. Special assistance needs of the elderly that enable them to remain in their own homes longer
  1. Transportation
    a. Reliable
    b. Nearby
    c. Inexpensive
    d. Safe
  2. Meals available in the event of illness or disability
  3. Health hotlines: most elderly are institutionalized because of health needs and lack of convenient community health services
  4. Housecleaners
  5. Homemaker services
  6. Social services
  7. Home care services
  8. Neighborhood safety

Recreation

A. Elderly have more time for recreation, but deterring factors exist
   1. Cost
      a. Transportation
      b. Special equipment
      c. Special clothing
      d. Fees for membership and use of facilities
   2. Health problems
   3. Diminished energy level
   4. Lack of incentive
   5. Sensory losses
   6. Lack of environmental aids
   7. Lack of conveniently located facilities, for example, rest rooms
B. Most elderly depend on a family as the major source of activity and interaction
C. Alternatives
   1. Religious activities
   2. Community activities, for example, volunteerism
   3. Day care
   4. Senior citizen centers
   5. Clubs, organizations, and associations
   6. Recreation centers
   7. Adult education
   8. Shopping
   9. Cultural events

Social Isolation

A. Four classifications (Ebersole and Hess, 1985)
B. Attitudinal: that which is self-imposed and that imposed by society
   1. Self-imposed aloneness, loneliness
   2. Society imposes myths about the aged, perceptions of aging
C. Presentational: set apart or sets one apart
D. Behavioral: exhibits behaviors that are not acceptable to a youth-oriented society, for example, confusion, eccentricity
E. Geographic
   1. Lack of resources to relocate
   2. Psychological safety and security at present location
   3. Fear of being victims of crime
   4. Distance from family and friends who have moved away

Drug Use

A. Largest users of prescription medications are those over the age of 65
B. Tendency to self-medicate
C. Higher frequency of hospital admissions that are drug-related than that for other age groups
D. Self-administration errors are common
E. Slower ingestion of drug into the system as a result of a decline in gastric acid secretion and decreased gastric motility
F. Circulatory alterations affect drug distribution
G. Drug metabolism altered by such factors as a diminished rate of body metabolism
H. Drug excretion time reduced by illness, disease, and the aging process
I. Management
   1. Patient education

2. Medication administration times more compatible with life-style
   3. Color coding
   4. Larger print on labels
   5. Easily removable bottle and vial caps
   6. Monitoring of drug effectiveness and compatibility

Alcohol Abuse

A. Tolerance to alcohol decreases with age
B. System does not excrete and detoxify as rapidly as that of a younger adult
C. Substitution for unmet psychological needs and untreated physiological problems
D. Cause of accidents, nutritional deficiencies, drug incompatibilities, self-neglect, alterations in self-esteem, psychosocial and physiological health care problems
E. Statistics inaccurate as clients are protected by family
F. Significant number of alcohol abusers are over age 60
G. High-risk group for alcoholism
H. Adult men have a higher incidence of abuse than adult women

Elder Abuse (Table 10-1)

A. Physical
   1. Battering
   2. Neglect

Table 10-1. Profile of the violent family relevent to elder abuse

Elder abuse		
Identifying data	Abuser	Victim
Age	40 to 60 yr	60 yr and older
Sex	Female	Not a factor; more elder are female
Relationship	Son/daughter, relative, or caretaker	Parent of abuser most often
Marital status	Married	Widowed
History of childhood physical sexual abuse	Data not widely available; positive history in some cases	Positive history in some cases; repeated victimization
Socioeconomic status (SES)	Not a factor: evident at all SES levels; founded cases mostly lower to middle class and found through health care systems	
Occupation	Professional or semi-skilled	Not employed
Employment status	Least violence in homes of retired men; victim often physically or mentally impaired	
Race	Highest, American Indians, orientals, minorities; blacks = 12%, whites = 88%; also reported as no difference	
Religion	Protestant	
Education	High school diploma or some college	
Residence	Limited data, evenly distributed with more reports in large cities Not Southern phenomenon	

Adapted from Stuart GW, Sundeen S: Profile of the violent family. In *Principles and practices of psychiatric nursing,* ed 3, St Louis, 1987.

3. Sexual abuse
4. Confinement or restraint

B. Psychologic: threatened or forced
1. Relinquishment of assets
2. Institutionalization
3. Loss of control over independent functioning
4. Social isolation
5. Sensory deprivation

C. Prevention
1. Acquire knowledge of family abuse and patterns of violence
2. Identify predisposing factors
3. Incorporate assessment tools into interviewing and counseling strategies
4. Increase public awareness and education
5. Identify actual and potential sources of emergency protection
6. Acquire knowledge of community resources

PHYSIOLOGIC ALTERATIONS (NORMAL AGING PROCESS) AND SELECTED DISORDERS (ABNORMAL)

Normal aging changes are gradual and begin in early middle age.

Integumentary System Alterations

1. Moisture loss; dryness
2. Epithelial layer thinning; fragility
3. Shrinkage and rigidity of elastic collagen fibers: sagging and wrinkling
4. Sweat glands decrease in number, activity, and size: less efficient body cooling system
5. Subcutaneous fat loss: deepening of hollows and more prominent contours
6. Loss of capillaries and melanocytes: skin sallowness
7. Peripheral circulation loss: thick, brittle, split nails
8. Skin pigmentation increases: keratoses (scaly, raised areas), senile lentigines (liver spots: brown or yellow spots)
9. Hair changes in color (gray, white), changes in texture (becomes fine or coarse), and thins (balding)
10. Appearance of facial hair for women; decrease in facial hair for men

Musculoskeletal System

A. Alterations
1. Loss of lean muscle mass and muscle cells: decreased muscle strength, size, and tone
2. Loss of elastic fibers in muscle tissue: increased stiffness and decreased flexibility
3. Thinning of long bones: brittle, porous bones
4. Thinning of intervertebral disks: height loss and changes in posture

B. Selected disorders
1. Contributing factors
   a. Poor nutritional patterns
   b. Endocrine system changes: decreased estrogen and testosterone
   c. Gastrointestinal system changes: decreased absorption of vitamins and minerals
   d. Cardiovascular system changes: poor circulation
   e. Neurologic deficits causing safety hazards
   f. Decreased level of activity and periods of prolonged bed rest
   g. Side effects of medications, for example, steroids

2. Resulting problems
   a. Increased susceptibility to fractures
   b. Altered body image
   c. Pain and discomfort
   d. Decreased mobility
   e. Impaired ability to perform activities of daily living (ADL)
   f. Increasing feelings of dependency
   g. Calcium deposits in blood vessels and renal structures
   h. Weakened muscles affecting other systems
      (1) Diaphragm
      (2) Bladder
      (3) Myocardium
      (4) Abdominal wall

3. Nursing management
   a. Handle patient gently
   b. Reduce environmental safety hazards
   c. Encourage mobility and exercise
   d. Allow extra time for performing activities
   e. Assist with ADL and exercises as needed
   f. Provide encouragement and support for accomplishments
   g. Prevent deformities
      (1) Proper positioning
      (2) Exercises such as range of motion (ROM)
   h. Alleviate pain
      (1) Rest periods
      (2) Positioning
   i. Encourage liberal fluid intake

Pulmonary System

A. Alterations
1. Structural alterations (scoliosis, kyphosis, osteoporosis): decrease in lung expansion
2. Alveoli enlarge and thin out: decreased oxygen and carbon dioxide diffusion
3. Loss of bronchiole elasticity: decreased breathing capacity, increased residual air
4. Diaphragm becomes fibrotic and weakened; diminished efficiency
5. Respiratory muscle structure and function decreases: diminished strength for breathing and coughing
6. Changes in larynx: weaker, higher-pitched voice
7. Decrease in ciliary function: increased susceptibility to upper respiratory tract infection

B. Selected disorders
1. Contributing factors
   a. Decreased resistance to infection
   b. Musculoskeletal system changes: weakened muscles and postural changes
   c. Longer history of smoking and exposure to pollutants
   d. Periods of prolonged bed rest
   e. Cardiovascular system changes
   f. Side effects of medications, for example, sedatives and hypnotics

2. Resulting problems
   a. Dyspnea

b. Chronic cough
c. Fatigue and debilitation
d. Cerebral hypoxia
  (1) Confusion
  (2) Restlessness
  (3) Behavioral changes
e. Decreased activity tolerance
f. Cardiovascular problems, for example, congestive heart failure
g. Anorexia
3. Nursing management
  a. Assist with ADL as necessary
  b. Encourage breathing exercises
  c. Administer oxygen therapy and intermittent positive pressure breathing (IPPB)
  d. Change position frequently
  e. Encourage liberal fluid intake
  f. Discourage smoking
  g. Position for maximum comfort and efficiency of respiration, for example, extra pillows, Fowler's position
  h. Allow rest periods
  i. Assess pulmonary status when assessing behavioral changes

Cardiovascular System

A. Alterations
  1. Decrease in enzymatic stimulation: longer and less forceful contractions
  2. Increase in fat and collagen amounts: decline in cardiac output
  3. Increase in oxygen demands of coronary arteries and brain: decreased peripheral circulation
  4. Loss of elasticity of vessel walls; decrease in contraction and recoiling responses
  5. Reduced or unaltered heart rate at rest
  6. Mild tachycardia on activity
B. Selected disorders
  1. Contributing factors
    a. Poor nutritional patterns
    b. Anxiety and stress
    c. Decreased activity level
    d. Arteriosclerosis and hypertension
    e. Pulmonary system changes
    f. Side effects of medications
  2. Resulting problems
    a. Fatigue and decreased activity tolerance
    b. Increased anxiety
    c. Edema
    d. Hypertension: increased risk of cerebrovascular accident (CVA)
    e. Behavioral changes
    f. Poor circulation to other systems and extremities: delayed healing
  3. Nursing management
    a. Assist with ADL prn
    b. Encourage moderate activity and exercise
    c. Patient teaching considerations
      (1) Confusion
      (2) Forgetfulness
      (3) Resistance to change
    d. Avoid excess pressure on the skin
      (1) Change position frequently

(2) Sheepskin; water mattress
(3) Bed cradle
e. Assess cardiovascular status when assessing behavioral changes
f. Avoid tight, constrictive clothing and shoes
g. Special foot care
  (1) Prevent trauma
  (2) Prevent infection

Gastrointestinal System

A. Alterations
  1. Muscle atrophy in the tongue, cheeks, mouth
  2. Esophageal wall thinning
  3. Decrease in ptyalin and amylase secretion by salivary gland: alkaline saliva
  4. Decrease in saliva secretion: thicker mucus and dryness
  5. Oral sensitivity loss
  6. Ill-fitting dentures, periodontal disease, lack of teeth: nutritional deficiencies
  7. Shrinkage of bony structure of mouth
  8. Gastric mucosa shrinks: decline in digestive enzyme secretion leads to delayed digestion
  9. Decrease in lipase secretion: fat intolerance
  10. Decrease in gastric acid: diminished ability to use calcium
  11. Decrease in intrinsic factor: pernicious anemia
  12. Decrease in iron absorption: iron deficiency anemia
  13. Internal sphincter muscle tone loss: alterations in bowel evacuation
B. Selected disorders
  1. Contributing factors
    a. Decreased level of activity
    b. Dental problems
    c. Poor nutritional patterns
    d. Weakened muscles
    e. Nervous system changes
    f. Overuse of laxative and enemas
    g. Anorexia
    h. Side effects of medications; for example, opiates and steroids
  2. Resulting problems
    a. Discomfort
    b. Constipation and impaction
    c. Fecal incontinence
    d. Anorexia
    e. Increased risk of aspiration
  3. Nursing management
    a. Promote nutritional intake
      (1) Consistency of food
      (2) Ability to manage utensils
      (3) Allow extra time for feeding (oral and tube)
    b. Provide good oral hygiene
    c. Encourage mobility and exercise
    d. Provide adequate fluid intake
    e. Educate patient regarding constipation and laxative abuse
    f. Check bowel habits regularly
    g. Give prompt assistance to bathroom or with bedpan
    h. Prevent skin and mucosal breakdown

(1) Prompt, thorough cleansing of anal area
(2) Extra gentleness when inserting rectal and feeding tubes

Renal System

A. Alterations
   1. Decrease in kidney size
   2. Decline in renal blood flow
   3. Reduced ability of nephron to filter urine: decreased clearance
   4. Reduced ability of tubule cells to selectively secrete and reabsorb: fluid and electrolyte alterations
   5. Bladder capacity decreases: frequency and urgency
   6. Loss of muscle tone of bladder and uterus
   7. Loss of pelvic muscle tone
   8. Decreased urine concentration ability
   9. Prostate gland enlargement
B. Selected disorders
   1. Contributing factors
      a. Periods of prolonged bed rest
         (1) Increased urinary stasis
         (2) Renal calculi formation
      b. Cardiovascular system changes, for example, decreased renal perfusion
      c. Nervous system changes
      d. Decreased fluid intake
      e. Muscle weakness
      f. Social withdrawal and apathy, for example, sensory deprivation
      g. Side effects of medication, for example, diuretics, antiparkinsonian drugs
   2. Resulting problems
      a. Hyperglycemia
      b. Behavioral changes, for example, confusion, elevated BUN, electrolyte imbalance
      c. Interference with sleep and recreational patterns
         (1) Urinary frequency
         (2) Urinary urgency
         (3) Nocturia
      d. Increased chance of skin breakdown; for example, incontinence
      e. Feelings of embarrassment, rejection, and withdrawal
   3. Nursing management
      a. Prevent urinary stasis
         (1) Encourage liberal fluid intake
         (2) Encourage frequent change of position
         (3) Encourage ambulation
      b. Prevent skin breakdown: prompt and thorough cleansing
      c. Bladder retraining
      d. Promptly respond to call for bathroom or bedpan
      e. Leave night-light on if patient experiencing nocturia
      f. Assess renal status when assessing behavior changes
      g. Early recognition of urinary tract infection

Neurologic System

A. Alterations
   1. Decrease in weight and size of brain
   2. Decline in number of neurons
   3. Diminished nerve conduction speed
      a. Voluntary movement slower
      b. Increased reaction time
      c. Delayed decisions
   4. Alterations in sleep-wake cycle
      a. Less rapid eye movement (REM) sleep
      b. Less deep sleep: tendency to catnap
      c. Easily awakened
      d. Difficulty falling asleep
      e. Average 5 to 7 hours
   5. Brain tissue atrophy and meningeal thickening: short-term memory loss
B. Selected disorders
   1. Contributing factors
      a. Poor nutrition patterns
      b. Cardiovascular system changes, for example, decreased circulation
      c. Pulmonary system changes, for example, cerebral hypoxia
      d. Sensory deprivation
      e. Side effects of medications, for example, sedatives
   2. Resulting problems
      a. Safety hazards
         (1) Impaired senses, for example, vision, hearing, pain, and temperature
         (2) Forgetfulness and confusion
      b. Anorexia, for example, decreased taste buds
      c. Social isolation and rejection
      d. Impaired ability to perform ADL
         (1) Decreased coordination
         (2) Safety hazards
      e. Increased sense of dependency
      f. Incontinence
      g. Altered self-image and declining confidence
      h. Behavioral changes, for example, forgetfulness, and confusion
   3. Nursing management
      a. Provide for safety
      b. Establish means of communication if patient has hearing impairment
      c. Assess all systems when assessing behavioral changes
      d. Maintain sense of independence when possible
      e. Assist with ADL only when necessary; allow extra time
      f. Encourage socialization
      g. Provide sensory stimulation
      h. Consider forgetfulness and confusion when teaching
         (1) Be consistent
         (2) Provide repetition when necessary
         (3) Be patient
         (4) Provide positive reinforcement and encouragement
      i. Assess other symptoms carefully when assessing for infection and trauma: decreased temperature control and pain perception mask these symptoms
      j. Carefully check temperature of bath water and forms of heat therapy to avoid burns: discrepancy in sensation of heat and cold
      k. Maximize use of environmental aids

Endocrine System

A. Alterations
  1. Decline in growth hormone secretion
  2. Estrogen secretion diminishes
  3. Uterus becomes smaller
  4. Fallopian tubes decrease in size and motility
  5. Vagina loses elasticity
  6. Vulva and external genitalia shrink with loss of subcutaneous fat
  7. Vaginal secretions diminish
  8. Response to sexual stimulation takes longer
  9. Elasticity of breast tissue is reduced
  10. Testosterone secretion decreases
  11. Testes become smaller and less firm
  12. Sperm production is slowed
  13. Erection takes longer to achieve and subsides more rapidly
  14. Ejaculation is shorter and less forceful
  15. Time between erection and orgasm lengthens
  16. Basal metabolism rate is decreased
  17. Woman loses ability to procreate
  18. Glucose metabolism diminishes
  19. Pancreatic secretions decrease
B. Selected disorders
  1. Contributing factors: glandular changes as result of aging process
  2. Resulting problems
    a. Adult-onset diabetes mellitus
    b. Musculoskeletal system changes
    c. Hypothyroidism
  3. Nursing management of diabetes mellitus: special considerations
    a. Poor vision
    b. Lack of coordination
    c. Poor nutritional patterns
    d. Forgetfulness and confusion
    e. Resistance to change
    f. Masking of symptoms by physiologic changes of aging and disease
    g. Decreased activity level
    h. Stress and anxiety
    i. Increased susceptibility to complications

Autoimmune System

A. Alterations
  1. Diminshed immunoglobulin production
  2. Weakened antibody response
  3. Atypical signs and symptoms frequently a response to infection, for example, subnormal temperature, behavior changes, and decreased pain sensation
B. Selected disorders
  1. Contributing factors
    a. Weakened antibody response
    b. Reduced immunoglobulin production
      (1) Thymus gland wasting
      (2) Reticuloendothelial system alterations
  2. Resulting problems
    a. Self-destructive autoaggressive phenomenon
    b. Increased susceptibility to infection
    c. Increased susceptibility to disease
    d. Misdiagnosis
  3. Nursing management
    a. Be careful in observation and assessment
    b. Be aware that atypical symptoms of infection are common among the elderly; for example, with otitis media, difficulty in hearing is too often dismissed as a typical aging problem
    c. Use early nursing intervention

Sense Organs

A. Vision
  1. Alterations
    a. Pupil size diminshes: loss of responsiveness to light
    b. Decline in peripheral vision
    c. Accommodation ability decreases, causing presbyopia (farsightedness)
    d. Decrease in tear production
    e. Decrease in lens transparency and elasticity
    f. Decline in ability to focus quickly
    g. Decline in color discrimination
    h. Difficulty in adjusting to dark-light changes
  2. Selected disorders
    a. Cataracts
    b. Glaucoma
    c. Senile macular degeneration
B. Auditory alterations
  1. Progressive loss of hearing, starting with high-frequency tones
    a. Presbycusis (loss of sound perception)
    b. Otosclerosis (bone cell overgrowth)
    c. Cerumen accumulation
  2. Eardrum thickens and becomes more opaque
C. Taste bud alterations
  1. Number of taste buds decline
  2. Taste sensation is dulled
  3. Taste detection declines with bitter, sour, salty, flavors
  4. Sweet flavor awareness remains intact
D. Olfactory alterations
  1. Olfactory nerve fibers decrease
  2. Sense of smell diminishes
E. Tactile alterations
  1. Sense of touch dulled
  2. Pain threshold higher
  3. Sense of vibration diminished
F. Vestibular/kinesthetic alterations
  1. Diminished proprioception
  2. Decrease in coordination
  3. Decline in equilibrium

SPECIAL CONSIDERATIONS
Nutrition

A. Diet
  1. Nutrition needs same as those of other adults
  2. Decreased need for calories
  3. Adequate protein to prevent muscle wasting and weakness
  4. Adequate fats for padding, insulation, and energy
  5. Adequate carbohydrates from unprocessed foods for energy: elderly have a tendency to buy high-carbohydrate, empty-calorie foods because they are
    a. Less costly
    b. Filling
    c. Easy to chew
    d. Require minimal preparation

6. Ethnic, cultural, and life-style preferences should be encouraged for identity reinforcement and appetite stimulation
7. Fluid intake should be 2500 to 3000 ml per day: tendency is to reduce intake because of urinary frequency, urgency, and incontinence
8. Vitamin supplements to prevent deficiencies
9. Lactose deficiency common: calcium can be obtained from other sources, for example, spinach, asparagus, broccoli, and sardines
10. Fiber, roughage, bulk to aid elimination
11. Consistency and preparation in accordance with chewing, swallowing, and digestive abilities
12. Small, frequent meals are easier to digest and conserve energy

B. Unhurried atmosphere to increase appetite and incentive to eat
C. Caution against food fads and megavitamin therapy
D. Assess facilities for appropriateness
   1. Storage
   2. Cooking
   3. Refrigeration
E. Financial assistance and planning
F. Transporation to and from grocery store
G. Assistance with packages because of weakness and physical disabilities
H. Mealtime socialization
I. Assistance for the confused, forgetful, and ill
J. Encourage regular meals—elderly have a tendency to skip meals
K. Education classes on purchasing healthful foods on limited income

Hygiene

A. Skin
   1. Water temperature 100° to 105° F (37.7° to 40.5° C)
   2. Daily baths not necessary
   3. Oil-base or emollient lotion
   4. Alcohol and dusting powder not appropriate because they dry out the skin
   5. Avoid friction
   6. Avoid pressure
   7. Neutral-reaction or oil-based soap
   8. Susceptible to bruising and skin tears
B. Nose: blunt-end scissors to trim nasal hairs that extend beyond nares
C. Oral hygiene
   1. Dentures
      a. Take out at night and reinsert the next morning to prevent tissue swelling
      b. Frequent cleaning
      c. Proper storage
      d. If patient is institutionalized, make sure dentures are labeled
   2. Soft nylon toothbrush, electric toothbrush, or adaptive toothbrush
   3. Half-strength hydrogen peroxide rinses
   4. Lanolin to lips
   5. Encourage semiannual dental visits
   6. Frequent mouth inspection for food accumulation, injury, disease, and infection

D. Ears
   1. Clean with warm, soapy water and dry with towel
   2. Do not use cotton swabs because they force cerumen back against the tympanum
   3. Trim ear hair growth in men
   4. Hearing aids
      a. Wash mold and receiver with mild soap and warm water
      b. Check cannula for patency, and clean and dry with pipe cleaner
      c. Remove batteries when aid is not in use
      d. Store batteries in refrigerator to retain freshness
      e. Turn aid to off position when inserting in patient's ear
      f. Turn aid on to adjust volume
      g. Store aid in its original box away from cold, heat, and sunlight
E. Eyes
   1. More frequent cleaning of eyeglasses required
   2. Use cool water to clean eyeglasses
   3. Store only in eyeglass case
   4. If patient is institutionalized, make sure glasses are labeled
F. Nails
   1. Daily care
   2. Use moisturizer on nails and cuticles
   3. Encourage circulation with buffing of nails
   4. File with emery board (cutting makes them more brittle and risks injury)
G. Hair
   1. Use mild shampoo that is not irritating to the eyes
   2. Remove facial hair from women with tweezers or waxing
   3. Use of a shaving brush is recommended for men
   4. Moisturizers are beneficial for men's facial skin
H. Feet
   1. Give daily care
   2. Inspect between and under toes for abrasions, cracking, lacerations, and scaling
   3. Clip toenails straight across
   4. Pumice stone should be used to remove dry, hard skin
   5. Discourage use of irritants
   6. Avoid elastic-top socks or knee-high stockings
   7. Emphasize the danger of roll garters
   8. Recommend properly fitting shoes with low, broad, rubber heels for safety, comfort, and fatigue reduction

Safety

A. Susceptibility to accidents increased by
   1. Decline in sensory acuity
   2. Decreased ability to interpret environment
   3. Increased reflex time
   4. Postural change sensitivity
   5. Gait disturbances
   6. Muscular weakness
   7. Urinary urgency and frequency
   8. Confusion
   9. Judgment alterations
   10. Forgetfulness
   11. Proprioceptive inadequacies
   12. Improper footwear

13. Depression
14. Environmental hazards
15. Medications that cause drowsiness
B. Accident prevention
  1. Attire
    a. Short or three-quarter-length sleeves as opposed to long, loose-fitting sleeves
    b. Avoid long garments
  2. Furniture
    a. Proper height
    b. Chairs with arms
  3. Floors
    a. No-slip wax
    b. No scatter rugs or deep pile carpeting
    c. Avoid clutter
    d. Rubber tips on ambulation aids
  4. Kitchen
    a. Tong reachers instead of foot stools, chairs, and step ladders
    b. Temperature-controlled faucets
    c. Electric rather than gas stoves
    d. Stoves with controls on the front
    e. Shelves within comfortable reach
    f. Wall cabinets at comfortable height instead of floor-based cabinets to avoid bending and stooping
    g. Avoid trash accumulation
  5. Bathroom
    a. Nonskid strips or rubber mats in tub and shower
    b. Temperature-controlled faucets
    c. Good soap containers
    d. Tub and toilet handrails
    e. Bathtub seats
    f. Shower chairs
    g. High toilet seats
    h. Colored toilet seats
    i. Night-light
  6. Bedroom
    a. Bedside commode
    b. Side rails
    c. Night-light
    d. Telephone next to bed
  7. General
    a. Proper lighting
    b. Railings on stairways
    c. Safe electric appliances
    d. No overloading of electric outlets
    e. No frayed wiring
    f. Securely taped cords
    g. Emergency telephone numbers readily available at telephone
    h. Smoke detectors
    i. Crime prevention assessment and implementation
    j. Medications
      (1) Separate from those of other household members
      (2) Internal and external medications in different locations
      (3) Large print labels
      (4) Color coded labels
      (5) Daily supply containers
      (6) Calendar or alarm clock reminders
      (7) Discard outdated medications and prescriptions

Vision

A. Bright, diffused light is best
B. Place items on better-vision side
C. Avoid glare
D. Strips on stairs improve depth perception
E. Glasses should be kept clean (the elderly frequently forget or ignore this)
F. Use colors that increase visal acuity, for example, red, orange, and yellow
G. Avoid night driving
H. Use resources and aids for visually handicapped
I. Preserve independence
J. Visual losses increase susceptibility to illusions, disorientation, confusion, and isolation
K. Place objects directly in front of individual with decreased peripheral vision
L. Stimulate other senses

Hearing

A. Elderly usually do poorly on hearing tests because of their cautious responsiveness
B. Reduce distractions
C. Do not fatigue with unnecessary noise and talk
D. Speak in a normal tone of voice; shouting is misinterpreted by those who have normal hearing
E. Observe for signs of developing hearing loss
  1. Leaning forward
  2. Inappropriate responses
  3. Cupping ear when listening
  4. Loud speaking voice
  5. Requests to repeat what has been said
F. Reduce background noise before speaking, for example, television and radio
G. Hearing deficits increase social isolation, suspiciousness, and fears
H. Speak toward the better ear
I. Be sure to have the person's attention before speaking
J. Use resources and aids for the hearing impaired, for example, television and telephone amplifiers, sound lamps, and alarm clocks that shake the bed

Activities of Daily Living

A. Elderly may ignore appearance because of fatigue, unawareness, or lack of incentive
B. Clean clothing is essential for maintaining pride and dignity
C. Choosing what to wear provides a source of control over one's life, fosters independence, and increases self-confidence and self-esteem
D. Lifelong sleeping attire or lack of attire should be encouraged
  1. Reinforces individuality
  2. Reduces sleep interference
E. Standard clothing sizes no longer fit; loose-fitting, comfortable clothing should be encouraged
F. Front closures are more easily managed
G. Cotton socks absorb perspiration
H. Zippers, velcro, and large buttons make dressing easier
I. Layering provides warmth in cold weather
J. Daily exercise should be encouraged and paced

K. Increase self-awareness with mirrors
L. Use daily living resources and aids
    1. Zipper aids
    2. Extralong shoehorns
    3. Shoelace tiers
    4. Adaptive utensils

Sexuality

A. Cultural stereotypes deny freedom of sexual expression for the elderly
B. Lifelong sexual adjustment will determine how the elderly person deals with sexual needs
C. Partner availability is made difficult
    1. More elderly women than men
    2. Social and business roles change
D. Physiologic alterations affect self-image and foster non-participation
E. Families of elderly persons tend to discourage sexual relationships because of stereotypes and inheritance threats
F. Sexual focus shifts to companionship
G. Older persons continue to enjoy sexual activity; decrease is primarily a result of declining health or lack of available partner

Speech

A. Elderly tend to rely on speech more than action
B. Speak slowly and clearly
C. Allow sufficient time for comprehension and response
D. Speak to and treat the individual as an adult
E. Explanations will reduce fear
F. Recovery of speech is influenced by multiimpairments and dependency

NEUROLOGIC SYSTEM (SELECTED DISORDERS)
Organic Mental Syndromes (see box)

A. Onset may be rapid or progressive
B. Cognitive function alterations
    1. Judgment
    2. Memory
    3. Intellect
    4. Orientation
    5. Affect
C. Associated factors (Table 10-2)
D. Cognitive dysfunction: dementia

Dementia

A. Alzheimer's disease: progressive, deteriorating, chronic dementia
    1. Types
        a. Senile dementia Alzheimer's type (SDAT): onset over age 65
        b. Presenile dementia: onset between ages 40 to 60
    2. Cerebral pathophysiology
        a. Senile plaques
        b. Neurofibrillary tangles
        c. Neurotransmitter abnormalities
        d. Atrophy
    3. Diagnosis confirmed by above findings on autopsy
    4. Assessment
        a. Personality changes
        b. Memory changes
        c. Behavioral changes

Organic Mental Syndromes

Delirium

A reduced ability to maintain attention to external stimuli and to appropriately shift attention to new external stimuli; disorganized thinking, as manifested by rambling, irrelevant, or incoherent speech; reduced level of consciousness; sensory misperceptions; disturbances of the sleep-wake cycle and level of psychomotor activity; disorientation to time, place, or person; memory impairment

Dementia

Impairment of short- and long-term memory; changes in abstract thinking; impaired judgment

Amnestic syndrome

Impairment in a short- and long-term memory that is attributed to a specific organic factor; immediate memory is not impaired

Organic delusional syndrome

Delusions resulting from specific organic factor such as amphetamine use or cerebral lesions of the right hemisphere

Organic hallucinosis

Hallucinations that are persistent or recurrent and caused by a specific organic factor such as use of hallucinogens that produce visual hallucinations, or alcohol, which induces auditory hallucinations

Organic mood syndrome

Persistent depressed, elevated, or expansive mood caused by a specific organic factor such as a toxic effect of substances, including reserpine or methyldopa, an endocrine disorder such as hyperthyroidism, or structural brain disease that results from hemispheric strokes

Organic anxiety syndrome

Recurrent panic attacks or generalized anxiety caused by a specific organic factor such as endocrine disorder, use of psychoactive substances, brain tumors in the vicinity of the third ventricle, vitamin B_{12} deficiency, aspirin intolerance, heavy metal intoxication

Organic personality syndrome

Persistent personality disturbance caused by a specific organic factor such as structural damage to the brain caused by neoplasms, head trauma, cerebrovascular disease

Intoxication

Maladaptive behavior and a substance-specific syndrome caused by the recent ingestion of a psychoactive substance such as alcohol, cannabis, amphetamine, cocaine

Withdrawal

Development of a substance-specific syndrome that follows the cessation of, or reduction in, intake of a psychoactive substance that the person previously used regularly

Adapted from Haber J et al: *Comprehensive psychiatric nursing*, ed 4, St Louis, 1992, Mosby, p 610.

Table 10-2. Factors associated with organic mental syndromes and disorders

Influential factors	Examples
Volatile agents	Gasoline, aerosols, glues, paint removers, solvents, lacquers, varnishes, dry-cleaning agents; home cleaning products alone or when mixed
Heavy metals	Lead paints, ceramic glazes, moonshine whiskey, mercury, arsenic, manganese
Insecticides	DDT, parathion, malathion, diazine
Brain trauma	Concussion, contusion, hemorrhage, thrombosis, penetrating wounds, blast effects, electrical trauma; exposure to repeated courses of electroconvulsive therapy; oxygen deprivation
Drugs	Alcohol, barbiturates, opioids, cocaine, amphetamines, cannabis, hallucinogens such as lysergic acid diethylamide (LSD) and phencyclidine (PCP)
Infections	Tuberculous and fungal meningitis, viral encephalitis, neurosyphilis (tabes dorsalis), Jakob-Creutzfeld disease, human immunodeficiency virus (HIV) related disorders (AIDS, ARC)
Neoplasms, tumors	Astrocytoma, medulloblastoma, meningioma
Metabolic and endocrine disorders	Hepatic disease, uremic encephalopathy, porphyria; thyroid, parathyroid and adrenal dysfunction; Wernicke-Korsakoff syndrome
Nutritional deficiencies	Lack of protein; deficiencies in vitamin C and the B vitamins (folic acid, niacin, pyridoxine, riboflavin, thiamine, B_{12}); fluid and electrolyte imbalance
Seizures	Petit mal, grand mal, focal seizures, psychic seizures
Hypoxia-ischemia	Anoxia related to delayed or prolonged cardiopulmonary resuscitation
Neurologic disease (possible genetic influence)	Huntington chorea, multiple sclerosis, Pick's disease, cerebral degeneration, Parkinson's disease
Cerebral changes associated with Alzheimer's disease	Loss of neurons, plaques, neurofibrillary degeneration, tangles, amyloid deposits, loss of dentritic tree, choline acetyl transferase, CAT defects, degeneration of basal forebrain, elevated platelet fluidity, inherited genetic factor

From Haber et al: *Comprehensive psychiatric nursing,* ed 4, St Louis, 1992, Mosby, p 608.

  d. Impaired cognition
  e. Late-stage physical alterations affecting mobility and swallowing
  5. Nursing intervention/management
    a. Support independence with ADL
    b. Provide structured, consistent environment
    c. Facilitate sleep-activity balance
    d. Promote bowel and bladder continence
    e. Provide reality orientation, remotivation, reminiscence
    f. Provide for patient safety
      (1) At risk for wandering
      (2) Becomes lost easily
      (3) Fails to recognize environmental hazards
    g. Encourage socialization, because withdrawal and social isolation are common
    h. Reduce anxiety-provoking situations
    i. Provide for nutritional needs
    j. Recognize self-concept needs
    k. Encourage verbal communications
    l. Monitor effectiveness of medications, for example, antidepressants
B. Multi-infarct dementia: cognitive impairment caused by cerebrovascular disease
C. Psychoactive substance-induced mental disorders: chemically induced organic disease

Parkinson's Disease
  Progressive neurologic movement disorder
A. Characteristics
  1. Tremors
  2. Bradykinesia
  3. Muscular rigidity
B. Assessment
  1. Slowness of movement
  2. Waxlike rigidity of extremities

  3. Facial masking
  4. Tremors while at rest—characteristic pill-rolling motion
  5. Muscular weakness
  6. Shuffling gait
  7. Stature alterations
  8. Drooling
  9. Cognitive impairment
  10. Mood swings
C. Nursing intervention/management
  1. Foster independence with ADL
  2. Maintain physical mobility
  3. Provide adequate nutrition
    a. Keep swallowing difficulties in mind
    b. May require suction; prone to aspiration
    c. Monitor weight weekly
    d. Provide adaptive eating devices
    e. Provide thick liquids
  4. Prevent constipation
  5. Encourage communication
    a. Be attentive: speech is soft and low pitched
    b. Allow time: speech is slow and monotonous
  6. Enhance self-concept
    a. Focus on patient's strengths
    b. Encourage activities that foster success
    c. Give positive feedback
    d. Establish realistic goals
    e. Encourage verbalization of feelings
  7. Monitor effectiveness of medications in controlling tremors and rigidity and alleviating characteristic depression
    a. Tricyclic antidepressants; monoamine oxidase inhibitors (MAOI)
    b. Antihistamines
    c. Anticholinergics
    d. Levodopa

PSYCHOLOGIC ALTERATIONS (NORMAL AGING PROCESS)
Self-image
A. Physiologic alterations
B. Youth-oriented society
C. Retirement
D. Income alterations
E. Role changes
F. Sexual expression alterations

Intelligence
A. Verbal ability and retained information remain unchanged
B. Abstract thinking and performance response decline
C. Performance of activities involving neuromuscular learning decline
D. Attention span shortens
E. Literal approach to problem-solving affects ability
F. Fluid intelligence declines after adolescence
G. Crystallized intelligence continues to increase throughout life
H. Learning capacity continues

Memory
A. Short term: concentration and retention decline
B. Long term: minimal impairment
C. Remote
    1. Remote memory is better than short-term memory
    2. Involved in reminiscence

Motivation
A. Not risk takers
B. Do not actively seek change
C. Possess fear of failure
D. Self-fulfilling prophecies
E. Competitiveness declines
F. Energy levels decline

Attitudes, Beliefs, Interests
A. General attitude realignment
B. Interests either narrow or expand
C. Tend to keep lifelong beliefs amid rapidly changing society

Personality
A. Basically unchanged
B. Some exaggeration of behavioral responses is evident
C. Adaptive capacities are diminished
D. Reduced ability to handle stress

PSYCHOLOGIC DISORDERS (ABNORMAL)
Depression
A. Reaction to loss of
    1. Independence
    2. Status
    3. Spouse, relatives, and friends
    4. Possessions
B. Medications can cause depression (e.g., digitalis)
C. Physical illness and changes
    1. Lowered self-esteem
    2. Self-concept alterations
    3. Feelings of hopelessness and worthlessness

D. Types
    1. Exogenous
      a. Referred to as neurotic; external, caused by outside events
      b. Common in the elderly
      c. Usually a reaction to losses
    2. Endogenous
      a. Referred to as psychotic; caused by internal events
      b. Characterized by
        (1) Guilt
        (2) Reduced self-regard
        (3) Early morning awakening
        (4) Slowing of thought, verbalization, and level of activity
      c. Classifications
        (1) Unipolar: life history of depression
        (2) Bipolar (manic-depressive psychosis)
          (a) Mood swings from depression to euphoria
          (b) More likely to have hallucinations and delusions
E. Symptoms: Table 10-3
F. Nursing intervention
    1. Encourage self-expression; increase self-esteem
    2. Improve appearance
    3. Provide structure, routine
    4. Assist with maintaining or regaining control
    5. Have kind, understanding attitude
    6. Provide physical care as needed; encourage independence
    7. Provide safety, security
    8. Reduce environmental stimuli and stress

Table 10-3. Symptoms of depression as observed in cognitive, affective, and somatic changes

Cognitive	Affective	Somatic
Indecisiveness	Fear*	Tearful
Confusion*	Anxiety	Crying spells
Impaired thinking*	Sadness	Agitation*
Poverty of thought	Irritability	Anorexia
Hopelessness/emptiness	Anger*	Weight loss
Suicidal ideation*	Feels distant from others*	Constipation
Guilt	Depersonalized*	Palpitations
Inability to concentrate		Fatigue/weakness
Worry		Insomnia
Believes self a failure*		Restlessness*
Believes self causing harm to others*		
Believes self going crazy*		
Believes self deserving of punishment*		

From Ebersole P, Hess P: *Toward healthy aging: human needs and nursing response,* ed 2, St Louis, 1985, Mosby. Data from Morris J, Wolf R, Kerman L: *J Gerontol* 30:209, 1975; Zung W: *Arch Gen Psychiatry* 29:328, 1973.
*Presence of clinically significant depression.

9. Continuously test reality perception
10. Ascertain emotional support network
11. Prevent isolation and avoidance
12. Realize potential for suicide exists
    a. Suicide is an act that stems from depression
    b. Approximately 25% of suicides occur in persons over age 65
    c. White males over age 75 have the highest rate
    d. Refer to Chapter 7, Mental Health Nursing, for suicidal risk assessment, crisis intervention, and nursing interventions

Aggressive Behavior

A. Abnormal anger, rage, or hostility, which if turned inward would lead to depression and if turned outward would lead to aggressiveness
B. Response to
    1. Anxiety
    2. Stress
    3. Guilt
    4. Insecurity
    5. Loss of self-esteem
    6. Loss of control of destiny
    7. Forced dependency
C. Clinical manifestations
    1. Lack of cooperation
    2. Irritability
    3. Demanding
    4. Hostility
    5. Demonstration of coping mechanisms characteristically used to decrease stress, for example, rationalization and repression
    6. Altered interpersonal relationships
    7. Altered reality testing
D. Nursing intervention
    1. Reduce stress source and sensory overload
    2. Encourage ventilation
    3. Set realistic, reachable goals
    4. Respond to questions directly and briefly
    5. Allow ample time for task completion
    6. Meet physical needs as necessary
    7. Encourage environmental participation and activity involvement
    8. Positively recognize attainments
    9. Set limits on activities
    10. Anticipate hostile, demanding behavior
    11. Allow only the degree of independence that can be successfully handled
    12. Avoid responses and action that could lead to guilt, feelings of rejection, bother, or dislike
    13. Increase feeling of self-worth
    14. Medication
    15. Therapy if indicated

Regression

The display of regressive behavior, an ego defense mechanism, is not an uncommon response in the elderly to external stressors. This return to an earlier behavioral stage (e.g., temper tantrums, rocking, or incontinence) requires prevention, early detection, and prompt intervention (remove source of stress and reverse the behavior).

Paranoid Behavior

A. Inappropriate attempt of coping with stress
B. Response to
    1. Physical impairments
    2. Sensory deprivation
    3. Loss
    4 Loneliness
    5. Medications
    6. Environmental changes
    7. Isolation
    8. Vision alterations
    9. Auditory alterations
C. Clinical manifestations
    1. Secretiveness
    2. Mistrust
    3. Mood disturbances
    4. Oversensitivity
    5. Insecurity
    6. Superiority attitude
    7. Alterations in behavior
    8. Delusions
    9. Withdrawal
    10. Fearfulness
    11. Aloofness
    12. Refusal to take medications, eat, or carry out normal self-care activities
D. Nursing intervention
    1. Attempt to allay anxiety
    2. Allow patient to refuse treatments
    3. Don't argue with patient
    4. Try not to take patient's anger personally
    5. Administer medication
    6. Don't make promises to patient
    7. Look for alterations in ADL as cues to whether the patient's verbalizations are of real concern or are for attention
    8. Be aware of events precipitated by environment
    9. Stress management techniques
    10. Patient-predicted events that do not occur should be brought to patient's attention
    11. Encourage independence

REHABILITATION
Reality Orientation (Table 10-4)

A. First used with disoriented, confused elderly at Veterans Administration Hospital in Tuscaloosa, Alabama, in 1965
B. Emphasizes orientation to time, place, and person
C. Reality orientation boards are used to provide contact with reality; for example, time, date, locations, weather, last meal, and next meal
D. Program success depends on total staff commitment and 24-hour implementation
E. Many facilities that care for the elderly have implemented modified programs
F. Program implementation not limited to an institutional setting
G. Components
    1. Small groups
    2. Formal classroom sessions
        a. 20 to 30 minutes
        b. Morning sessions recommended (elderly are more alert in the morning)

Table 10-4. Differences between remotivation and reality orientation

Reality orientation	Remotivation
1. Correct position or relation with the existing situation in a community. Maximum use of assets	1. Orientation to reality for community living; present oriented
2. Called reality orientation and classroom reality orientation program	2. Called remotivation
3. Structured	3. Definite structure
4. Refreshments or food may be served for identification	4. Refreshments not served
5. Appreciation of the work of the world. Constantly reminded of who they are, where they are, why they are here, and what is expected of them	5. Appreciation of the work of the group stimulates the desire to return to function in society
6. Class range from 3 to 5 patients, depending on degree/level of confusion or disorientation from any cause	6. Group size: 5 to 12 patients
7. Meeting ½ hour daily at same time in same place	7. Meeting once to twice weekly for an hour
8. Planned procedures: reality-centered objects	8. Preselected and reality-centered objects
9. Consistence of approach response of resident responsibility of teacher	9. No exploration of feelings
10. Periodic reality orientation test pertaining to residents' level of confusion or disorientation	10. Progress ratings
11. Emphasis on time, place, person orientation	11. Topic: no discussion of religion, politics, or death
12. Use of portion of mind function still intact	12. Untouched area of the mind
13. Residents greeted by name, thanked for coming, and extended hand shake and/or physical contact according to attitude approach in group	13. No physical contact permitted. Acceptance and acknowledgment of everyone's contribution
14. Conducted by trained aides and activity assistants	14. Conducted by trained psychiatric aides

From Barns E, Sack A, Shore H. Reprinted by permission of *The Gerontologist* 13:513, 1973.

    c. Reality orientation board, calendars, clocks, and other materials used according to instructor plan
    d. Positive verbal feedback emphasized
    e. Confusion never reinforced
H. All personnel who come in contact with patients participating in the program are expected to use reality orientation
    1. Address patient by name and title
    2. Orient patient to time, place, and person
    3. Give positive verbal feedback
    4. Do not reinforce confusion

Remotivation (see Table 10-4)

A. Similar to reality orientation
B. Normal behavior reinforced through structured group program
C. Stimulating participation and interest in the environment are key components
D. Sessions average 20 minutes
E. Visual aids used, for example, items that stimulate sensory responses
F. Client behavior recorded
G. Staff support and involvement essential

Reminiscence (Table 10-5)

A. Small group sessions
B. Based on life review process
C. Elderly with cognitive dysfunction retain long-term memory and through reminiscence can adapt to the aging process
D. Purposes
    1. Conflict resolution
    2. Sharing of memories
    3. Sense of identity and self-importance achieved

    4. Focus is on a life that has meaning as opposed to a life viewed as a waste of time
    5. Natural for elderly persons to reminisce
        a. Feel comfortable
        b. They're good at it
        c. Reinforces sense of belonging (everyone talks about life's trials and tribulations)
    6. Therapeutic relationship with leader more likely to develop as patients realize their memories are important and valued
    7. Depressed patients find a caring listener and an opportunity to externalize their anger
    8. Psychologically disturbed patients receive acceptance, group validation, and a forum for expression: encourage active exploration of past strengths
    9. Strive to change outlook on the past rather than establishing new future directions
    10. Psychologic assessment tool (e.g., insight into past coping mechanisms)
    11. Reduces isolation, insecurity, and negative self-esteem
    12. Confused patients can be assisted to explore a memory that will stimulate latent thoughts, become more oriented, and improve ability to focus
    13. Current circumstances are often reflected through memories
E. If patients have difficulty focusing their thoughts, assist by selecting a specific memory
F. Stimulation of dormant thoughts to the surface decreases disorientation
G. Patients who are reluctant to talk can usually be stimulated with topics of food, movies, or music
H. Program implementation is not limited to institutional settings

Table 10-5. Suggestions for reminiscent group strategies

	Cognitively impaired	Psychologically disturbed	Depressed
Patient selection	No more than 5 members Age cohorts Both sexes	10 members Varied ages Both sexes	8 to 10 members Those with similar problems, for example, grieving, retired Both sexes
Structure	Consistent place and time Frequent, 30 minute meetings Coleaders	Consistent place and time Biweekly, 1-hour meetings One leader consistently	Varied meeting places Weekly, 1-hour meeting Variable leadership
Process	Connect specific events, things, and places common to group	Connect members through shared feelings and survival strategies	Focus members on successful coping during life span; encourage mutuality
Goals	Stimulate memory Enhance identity Raise self-esteem Increase socialization skills	Recognition of feelings and meaning of suppressed conflicts Enlarge coping strategies Integrate self-view Promote universality	Reduce feelings of hopelessness Restore personal control Increase affectual responsiveness Develop a sense of integrity and acceptance of life as lived Promote caring between members
Nurse's function	1. Provide a comfortable, mildly stimulating environment 2. Select props that will stimulate memories 3. Assist members by giving specific information, reminders, and clues 4. Give praise and recognition for any participation	1. Establish a private meeting and a closed group 2. Plan to focus on specific developmental stages or critical life events 3. Accept and validate all expressions of feeling 4. Clarify multiple meanings of events 5. Reduce anxiety	1. Provide a comfortable, stimulating environment 2. Appeal to sensory memories 3. Focus member's attention on evidence of caring and sharing 4. Demonstrate a caring attitude 5. Allow time to verbalize feelings, complain, etc.

Adapted from Ebersole P, Hess P: *Toward healthy aging: human needs and nursing response,* ed 2, St Louis, 1985, Mosby.

Cognitive Training

A. Consists of memory exercises, problem-solving situations, and memory training
B. Leader must be familiar with patient's past leisure time utilization, hobbies, and occupations
C. Individual, small, or large groups
D. Purpose is to maintain mental activity

Relaxation Therapy

A. Promotes sense of physical well-being, reduces stress, releases tension
B. Small groups
C. Involves rhythmic breathing, tension-relaxation exercises, and altered state of consciousness

Bladder Retraining: Urinary Incontinence

A. Causes
  1. Physiologic changes
    a. Decline in muscle support of pelvis
    b. Reduction in bladder's capacity to hold urine
    c. Sphincter weakness
  2. Behavioral alterations
    a. Regression
    b. Insecurity
    c. Rebellion
    d. Attention seeking
    e. Dependency
    f. Sensory deprivation
  3. Drugs
  4. Consciousness alterations
  5. Disease
  6. Obstruction
  7. Trauma
  8. Immobility
  9. Bedpans and urinals
  10. Lack of privacy
  11. Lack of time
B. Types
  1. Stress or passive
    a. Bladder outlet weakness
    b. Involuntary
    c. Frequency when sneezing, coughing, laughing, and lifting
  2. Paradoxical or overflow
    a. Uncontrollable contraction waves
    b. Bladder does not empty
    c. Frequency accompanied by retention
  3. Total
    a. Constant dribbling
    b. Storage problem
C. Elderly susceptible to
  1. Urinary tract infections
  2. Urgency
  3. Frequency
D. Patient reactions to incontinence
  1. Insecurity
    a. Social withdrawal
    b. Isolation
    c. Sensory deprivation
    d. Avoidance of previously developed relationships

2. Depression
   a. Embarrassment
   b. Guilt
   c. Shame
E. Intervention
   1. Pelvic exercises
      a. Bearing down
      b. Push-ups from a chair
   2. Indwelling catheter as a last resort if skin integrity threatened
   3. Condom drainage
   4. Absorbent, waterproof underpants
   5. Keep patient clean and dry
   6. Skin care
   7. Retraining
      a. Assess and record voiding pattern for minimum of 72 hours
         (1) Time
         (2) Place
         (3) Quantity
         (4) Activity
         (5) Patient awareness
         (6) Significant medications
         (7) Character of urine
         (8) Presence or absence of constipation or discharge
         (9) Problems: for example, clothing and ambulation hindrances
      b. Reestablish voiding pattern
         (1) First scheduled voiding of the day should be attempted immediately after awakening in the morning even if bed is wet
         (2) Voiding should be attempted at intervals determined from the assessment period (usually at 1-, 2-, or 3-hour periods; goal is every 4 hours)
         (3) Patient takes one or two 8-oz (240 ml) glasses of fluid 1 hour before attempting to urinate
         (4) No fluids should be taken between 6 PM and 6 AM if no urinating is desired
         (5) Fluid intake should be at least 2000 ml per day
         (6) Alcoholic drinks contraindicated
         (7) Soft drinks, tea, and coffee should be avoided
         (8) All fluid intake should be measured and recorded
         (9) All urine output should be measured and recorded

Bowel Retraining: Fecal Incontinence

A. Causes
   1. Physiologic changes
      a. External anal sphincter relaxation
      b. Perineal relaxation
      c. Muscle atony
   2. Behavioral alterations
      a. Regression
      b. Rebellion
      c. Dependency
      d. Sensory deprivation
   3. Central nervous system injury
   4. Obstruction
   5. Impaction
   6. Consciousness alterations
   7. Immobility
   8. Trauma
B. Intervention
   1. Keep patient clean and dry
   2. Absorbent, waterproof underpants
   3. Skin care
   4. Retraining
      a. Bowel retraining is easier than bladder retraining; if patient is incontinent of urine and stool, start bowel retraining program first
      b. Use no laxatives
      c. Ensure adequate fluid intake (2 L per day)
      d. Fluids and solids that promote patient's bowel movements (e.g., bran and orange juice) and roughage should be included in the diet
      e. Encourage physical activity
      f. Obtain bowel history
      g. Procedure
         (1) Establish regular day(s) and time to assist patient to the toilet for evacuation; preferably after a meal
         (2) After 20 minutes if patient has not had a bowel movement, insert a lubricated glycerine suppository
            (a) Do not use directly from refrigerator
            (b) Do not insert into a bolus of stool (ineffective)
            (c) After ascertaining that patient requires the suppository for training, it can be inserted 1 to 2 hours before the scheduled training time and after a meal
         (3) Digital stimulation is recommended after 48 hours if the above procedure is not successful
         (4) Take patient to the bathroom at the scheduled time daily, even if he or she has had a bowel movement between scheduled times

Suggested Reading List

Burggraf V, Stanley M, editors: *Nursing the elderly,* Philadelphia, 1989, JB Lippincott.

Ebersole P, Hess P: *Toward healthy aging: human needs and nursing response,* ed 3, St Louis, 1990, Mosby.

Eliopoulos C: *Gerontological nursing,* Philadelphia, 1987, JB Lippincott.

Haber J et al: *Comprehensive psychiatric nursing,* ed 4, St Louis, 1992, Mosby.

Smeltzer SC, Bare BG: *Brunner and Suddarth's textbook of medical surgical nursing,* ed 7, Philadelphia, 1992, JB Lippincott.

Stuart GW, Sundeen SJ: *Principles and practice of psychiatric nursing,* ed 4, St Louis, 1991, Mosby.

Gerontologic Nursing Review Questions

Answers and rationales begin on p. 447.

Situation: 71-year-old Mr. Yarnes has osteoarthritis and is admitted to the hospital for a total knee replacement.

1. Of the following baseline data, which is most important for the nurse to obtain?
   ① Extent of knee flexion and extension
   ② Food likes and dislikes
   ③ Mental health status and history
   ④ Usual sleeping habits

2. Preoperative teaching for Mr. Yarnes should include which of the following?
   ① Cast brace application
   ② Continuous passive motion (CPM) device
   ③ Principles of Buck's extension
   ④ Russell traction

3. Routine nursing care for Mr. Yarnes after the total knee replacement should include which of the following?
   ① Elevating affected knee when out of bed
   ② Keeping the head of the bed elevated up to 45 degrees
   ③ Keeping the affected leg in abduction
   ④ Using wedge pillows between his legs

4. Which of the following statements is accurate regarding ice application to the affected knee following a total knee replacement?
   ① Increases circulation and movement
   ② Reduces the chance of infection
   ③ Reduces edema and bleeding
   ④ Reduces fluid accumulation in the joint

5. Which of the following signs/symptoms would be the earliest indication of a postoperative infection following a total knee replacement?
   ① Fever
   ② Joint pain
   ③ Purulent drainage
   ④ Swelling

6. The discharge teaching plan for Mr. Yarnes should reinforce which of the following measures?
   ① Full weight bearing in the affected leg
   ② Non–weight bearing in the affected leg
   ③ Weight bearing only as prescribed by his physician
   ④ Weight bearing only as tolerated by Mr. Yarnes

---

7. Mrs. Russell is 89 years old, alert, and active. On annual physical examination, she complains of hemorrhoids and annoying constipation. Her physician instructs her to increase her fluid and dietary fiber intake. Which of the following snacks, if selected by Mrs. Russell, would indicate that she can identify food sources high in fiber?
   ① Apple juice
   ② Small banana
   ③ Raspberries
   ④ Cucumber

8. 62-year-old Mr. Ruff has a diagnosis of Type I or sliding hiatal hernia. Which of the following nursing measures should be included in his case?
   ① Eat three good meals a day
   ② Eat high-protein, high-fat foods
   ③ Lie down for 1 to 2 hours after meals
   ④ Sleep with the head of the bed elevated

Situation: Mr. Peck is 67 years old. His family reports that his personality has changed. He has become tactless, short tempered, and withdrawn. After a thorough history, physical examination, and laboratory testing, his family physician suspects senile dementia Alzheimer's type (SDAT).

9. A positive diagnosis of Alzheimer's disease can be obtained through which of the following procedures?
   ① Computer tomography scanning (CT)
   ② Positron emission tomography (PET)
   ③ Neural tissue evaluation on autopsy
   ④ Serial evaluations of neuropsychologic testing

10. Mr. Peck is admitted to a nursing home. He's not there very long when the nurse notices him heading for the exit door. She catches up with him and asks if he needs help. Mr. Peck responds, "You can leave me alone. I'm going home." Which of the following nursing actions would be most appropriate?
    ① Call the security department
    ② Go with Mr. Peck
    ③ Engage him in an activity
    ④ Physically prevent him from leaving

11. Mr. Peck becomes restless and agitated. Which of the following activities should the nurse engage him in?
    ① Listening to music
    ② Taking a nap
    ③ Taking a walk
    ④ Watching television

12. Mr. Peck demonstrates increasing difficulty with planning and decision making. Which of the following activities would be most appropriate for him?
    ① Hoeing in the garden
    ② Planning the dinner menu
    ③ Sorting the laundry
    ④ Writing out the grocery list

13. Mr. Peck continues to demonstrate progressive personality changes. When he becomes hostile and combative the nurse should include which of the following measures in her plan of care?
    ① Decrease environmental stimuli
    ② Simplify daily activity
    ③ Secure doors leading from the house
    ④ Use memory aids

14. When caring for the elderly, the nurse must know that the most common and easily reversed cause of dementia is:
    ① AIDS
    ② Alzheimer's disease
    ③ Drug toxicity
    ④ Parkinson's disease

---

15. 82-year-old Mr. Jones has periods of confusion and disorientation. He also has difficulty remembering where the bathroom is. Which of the following nursing actions would be most helpful to Mr. Jones?
    ① Take him to the bathroom every hour
    ② Place a sign saying *Here it is* on the door
    ③ Place a picture of a toilet on the bathroom door
    ④ Tell him if he can't find the bathroom he'll have to wear diapers

16. Mr. Jones' nutritional intake is poor. He eats a few mouthfuls and then gets up and leaves the table. Which of the following approaches by the nurse would be most appropriate?
    ① Apply a vest restraint during meals
    ② Have a staff member feed him his meals
    ③ Offer five to six small feedings daily
    ④ Provide him with a variety of finger foods

17. 79-year-old Mr. Walters is confused. When planning his care, which of the following nursing measures would be most therapeutic?
    ① Explain the planned daily activities to him each morning
    ② Leave him alone and let him do what he wants
    ③ Place a weekly activity calendar in his room
    ④ Speak clearly, calmly, and in short sentences

18. Mr. Walters' physician has ordered a vest restraint to be applied and released according to agency policy when Mr. Walters becomes agitated. Which of the following statements by the nurse indicates the *best understanding* of Mr. Walter's needs?
    ① All agitated patients should be restrained for their own safety
    ② The use of restraints causes decubiti
    ③ The use of restraints can increase a patient's agitation level
    ④ The use of restraints fosters incontinence

19. You are assigned to care for Mr. Walters. His nursing care plan indicates that his first name is Jake. When you enter Mr. Walters' room you recognize him as the school crossing guard everyone calls "Pops." Which of the following greetings would be most appropriate?
    ① "Hi, aren't you Pops, the school crossing guard."
    ② "Hi Jake. I'm your nurse, Karen."
    ③ "Hi there, Mr. Walters, remember me?"
    ④ "Mr. Walters. Hello. I'm your nurse, Miss Oats."

20. Mr. Walters put on his call bell for the nurse. When the nurse responded she found Mr. Walters standing at the bedside in a puddle of urine and his pajamas soaked. Which of the following is the best response for the nurse to make?
    ① "Let me help you to the bathroom where you can wash up and put on clean pajamas."
    ② "Next time wait for help before getting out of bed. That's what we're here for."
    ③ "Not again. It's diapers for you for sure now."
    ④ "Now look what you've done. I just changed you ten minutes ago."

Situation: Mr. Simms has Parkinson's disease and his physician orders Sinemet 10/100 po tid.

21. His daughter asks what the drug will do. Which of the following explanations by the nurse would be most accurate?
    ① It can decrease his tremors and improve his gait
    ② It's really very complicated and not necessary for you to know
    ③ It's the carbidopa-levodopa content ratio of the drug
    ④ You'll have to discuss that with the physician

22. Which of the following assessments would indicate possible drug toxicity in Mr. Simms?
    ① Akinesia and drooling
    ② Muscle stiffness and rigidity
    ③ Muscle and eyelid twitching
    ④ Slow movements and handwriting changes

23. After 2 weeks. Mr. Simms' daughter tells the nurse that she sees no improvement in her father since the Sinemet was started and perhaps another drug should be tried. Which of the following responses by the nurse would be most helpful to Mr. Simms' daughter?
    ① "I'll let the physician know you want a medication change."
    ② "It frequently takes several months to achieve maximum effect."
    ③ "What makes you say he's not improving?"
    ④ "Why don't you call the physician? He's in his office now."

24. Mr. Simms doesn't seem to want his meals and occasionally vomits when he does eat. To reduce the gastrointestinal side effects of Sinemet and enhance the absorption, which of the following nursing measures should be included in his care?
    ① Administer the medication before meals
    ② Administer the medication after meals
    ③ Crush the medication and mix with his food
    ④ Recommend a lower dosage to the physician

25. Which of the following explanations by Mr. Simms' daughter would indicate a basic understanding of her father's disease?
    ① Autosomal dominant genetic disorder
    ② Chronic progressive hereditary disease of the nervous system
    ③ Progressive damage to neurons that regulate and control movement
    ④ Progressive, fatal disease caused by a virus

Situation: Mrs. Jacobs is a 66-year-old resident in a SNF (Skilled Nursing Facility). She has rheumatoid arthritis resulting in severe deformities of both hands and a history of paranoid behavior. Her medications consist of prednisone 5 mg po qd and Ridaura 2 mg po tid.

26. Mrs. Jacobs refuses her qd po dose of prednisone. Which of the following actions should the nurse take?
    ① Call the physician and get an order for an injectable adrenocorticosteroid
    ② Chart the refusal in the nurses' notes and inform the head nurse
    ③ Return to Mrs. Jacobs in an hour and offer her the medication again
    ④ Chart *refused* on the medication sheet and report it to the physician

27. When planning care for Mrs. Jacobs, which of the following behaviors would *not* be especially important for the staff to be alert to?
    ① Verbalized hallucination
    ② Demonstrated superiority
    ③ Refusal of meals and treatments
    ④ Verbalized oversensitivity

28. The nurse is busy caring for another resident, and Mrs. Jacobs demands that she be taken to the bathroom immediately. It is correct for the nurse to:
    1. Stop what she's doing and attend to Mrs. Jacobs
    2. Inform Mrs. Jacobs that she will be with her shortly
    3. Tell Mrs. Jacobs to ask someone else who's free
    4. Tell Mrs. Jacobs that she is busy and will come back in 10 minutes

29. The nurse brings Mrs. Jacobs her breakfast tray and she says, "Take it away, I don't want it." The nurse's best response would be:
    1. "I'll tell the dietitian you don't like the food here."
    2. "I'll call the kitchen and order something else for you."
    3. "I'll leave the tray here just in case you change your mind."
    4. "I'll throw it out and record that you refused your breakfast."

30. Mrs. Jacobs reports that nobody does anything for her and that the staff ignores her needs but takes care of all the other residents. The nurse knows this to be inaccurate and understands that Mrs. Jacobs is:
    1. Looking to cause trouble
    2. Experiencing active hallucinations
    3. Demonstrating manifestations of paranoia
    4. Attempting to manipulate the staff

31. The staff decides that Mrs. Jacobs needs an activity. Which recommendation should the nurse pursue as therapeutic for Mrs. Jacobs?
    1. Operating the Resident Gift Shop
    2. Making her own bed daily
    3. Independently preparing her meal tray
    4. Participating daily in arts and crafts

Situation: Mr. Fiore is 80 years old. He takes the subway to and from his job as a proofreader Monday through Friday. He lives in a two-bedroom, fourth-floor walk up and faithfully attends to his four cats. His wife passed away a month ago; he sees his married daughter once a week and his divorced son once every 2 weeks. Mr. Fiore is bothered by spinal and bilateral hand arthritis and has a history of an old healed gastric ulcer and a healed left wrist fracture.

32. Mr. Fiore's children want him to move to a ground-floor, smaller apartment. He refuses and says he'll stay where he is until he dies. It is important that Mr. Fiore's children recognize that their father is:
    1. Becoming paranoid
    2. Displaying eccentricity
    3. Afraid to move
    4. Feeling secure where he is

33. Mr. Fiore falls in the street and is taken to the hospital by EMS (Emergency Medical Service). Physical examination and diagnostic testing reveal a mild concussion and a fractured left radius. Mr. Fiore is rather sullen and snippy and is only interested in going home, because he's worried about his cats. Which of the following actions should the nurse take?
    1. Speak with Mr. Fiore's children about arranging care for his cats
    2. Remind Mr. Fiore that cats are independent and can care for themselves
    3. Tell Mr. Fiore that he has too many cats and to give them to the ASPCA
    4. Offer to go to Mr. Fiore's apartment once a day to care for the cats

Situation: Mr. Dorman, a 78-year-old widower, is brought to the local emergency room by the police, who found him wandering aimlessly about the street. He is confused, disoriented, and hospitalized for pneumonia.

34. The nurse should recognize that the cause of Mr. Dorman's confusion and disorientation is:
    1. Arteriosclerosis
    2. Organic brain syndrome
    3. Infection
    4. Unknown

35. Mr. Dorman's nutritional intake is poor. The nurse should know that his appetite will probably improve if:
    1. He is served small meals frequently
    2. His food is blenderized
    3. All liquids are served warm
    4. A roll is served with each meal

36. Each time a member of the hospital staff enters Mr. Dorman's room he asks the time. The nurse should know that this is characteristic of
    1. Confusion
    2. Disorientation
    3. Memory deficit
    4. Impaired judgment

37. Mr. Dorman has wet the bed. The most appropriate response by the nurse would be to:
    1. Admonish Mr. Dorman for soiling himself and the bed
    2. Tell Mr. Dorman that now he'll have to wear diapers
    3. Offer Mr. Dorman the urinal
    4. Proceed with making Mr. Dorman clean and dry

38. The nurse notes that Mr. Dorman has not had a bowel movement in 3 days and identifies the problem as constipation. Constipation in the elderly is frequently the result of:
    1. Too much fiber in the diet
    2. Too much bulk in the diet
    3. Lack of daily laxatives
    4. Poor eating habits

39. Mr. Dorman's bedside stand is found to be full of packets of sugar, salt, jelly, napkins, and straws. These items he has removed from his meal trays and stored. The nurse should understand this indicates:
    1. Decreased self-esteem
    2. Increased insecurity
    3. Increased confusion
    4. Increased disorientation

40. The night staff expresses their concern that Mr. Dorman is awake most of the night. The most appropriate response by the nurse would be:
    1. "Mr. Dorman requires less sleep at night as he rests often throughout the day."
    2. "I'll get a physician's order for a sedative."
    3. "As people get older they require less sleep."
    4. "We'll increase his day activities."

CHAPTER 11

Emergency Nursing

This chapter emphasizes the nursing assessments and interventions essential to preserving the lives of victims of acute illness or injury. Rapid clinical assessment emphasizing airway, breathing, and circulation, establishment of care priorities, and implementation of lifesaving measures should be instituted until emergency medical care is available. The most serious and life-threatening injuries should be treated first, and all first aid measures carried out before transporting the victim(s).

Concurrent with emergency management is the practitioner's recognition and understanding of the victim's emotional state. The feelings of the victim's significant others should be acknowledged and responded to realistically, gently, and as expeditiously as possible.

Nurses should be familiar with the extent of protection and legal limitations of practice under the Good Samaritan Act, which varies from state to state.

The incidence of AIDS and hepatitis B indicates that nurses should consider all patients potentially infected; have access to equipment that minimizes the need for mouth-to-mouth, mouth-to-nose, and mouth-to-stoma resuscitation; and implement universal infection control precautions.

Current cardiopulmonary resuscitation literature raises the issues of cardiac pump theory versus thoracic pump theory; the effectiveness of abdominal compressions; and whether synchronized or interposed abdominal and chest compressions are more effective than chest compressions. To date, no new cardiopulmonary resuscitation guidelines specific to these issues have been released by the American Heart Association.

BASIC LIFE SUPPORT
Artificial Respiration

A. Simultaneously shake victim and shout to establish unconsciousness
B. Activate the EMS system (call 9-1-1) immediately when the victim is an adult; if an infant or child, call for help (even if you do not see anyone in the immediate vicinity), give 1 minute of CPR (20 cycles), check for pulse, and then activate EMS.
C. Quickly place victim in supine position
D. Establish airway using the head tilt–chin lift maneuver or head tilt–jaw thrust maneuver (Fig. 11-1) if additional forward displacement of the jaw is required; for patients with possible neck or spine injuries, use only jaw thrust maneuver (Fig. 11-2)
   1. Infant: maintain neck in neutral position
   2. Child: maintain neck slightly further back
E. Put your ear near victim's mouth and look, listen, and feel for breathing
F. Commence mouth-to-mouth, mouth-to-nose, or mouth-to-stoma resuscitation by delivering two breaths (1½ to 2 sec/breath) at the lowest possible pressure
G. Allow for victim's exhalation between breaths by removing your mouth; check the carotid pulse (brachial for infant) for 5 seconds

H. In the presence of a pulse continue to deliver one breath every 5 seconds (12 breaths/min) for the adult and every 3 seconds (20 breaths/min) for the infant and for a child until breathing is restored.

Cardiopulmonary Resuscitation (CPR)

A. Follow steps A to G above; be sure victim is on a firm surface
B. In the absence of a pulse, place the heel of one hand on top of the other two finger-breadths above the victim's xiphoid process (Fig. 11-3)
   1. Child (1 to 8 years old): place heel of one hand one finger-breadth above the notch where the ribs and breast bone meet and deliver 100 compressions per minute
   2. Infant (less than 1 year old): place two fingers one finger-breadth below an imaginary line drawn between the nipples and deliver 100 compressions per minute
C. Compress the adult sternum 1½ to 2 inches (child 1 to 1½ inches, infant ½ to 1 inch) for 15 compressions; then deliver two breaths
D. Continue the 15 compressions and two breaths sequence; 5 compressions and one breath for infants and children

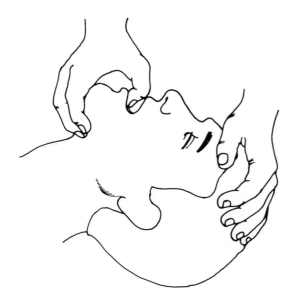

FIG. 11-1. Head tilt—jaw thrust maneuver. Pull mandible forward using thumb and forefingers. (From Budassi SA, Barber J: *Mosby's manual of emergency care: practices and procedures,* ed 2, St Louis, 1984, Mosby.)

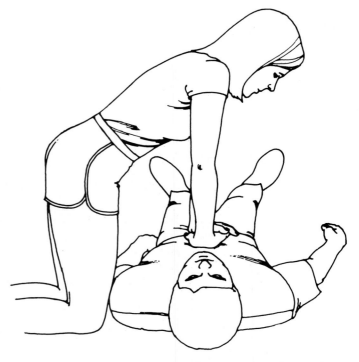

FIG. 11-3. External cardiac compression. With knees close to patient and shoulders parallel to patient's sternum, apply pressure to sternum with elbows straight and in locked position. (From Budassi SA, Barber J: *Mosby's manual of emergency care: practices and procedures,* ed 2, St Louis, 1984, Mosby.)

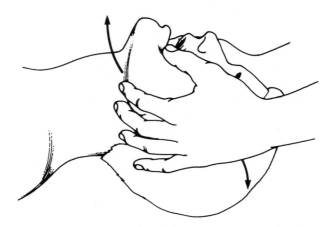

FIG. 11-2. Jaw thrust maneuver.(From Budassi SA, Barber J: *Mosby's manual of emergency care: practices and procedures,* ed 2, St Louis, 1984. Mosby.)

E. With two rescuers deliver 5 compressions and one breath
F. Check the carotid pulse after four cycles (1 minute), child after 20 cycles; brachial pulse in infant after 20 cycles
G. If no pulse, resume CPR. If there is a pulse but no breathing resume artificial respiration (rescue breathing)

Heimlich Maneuver

The Heimlich maneuver is used for management of foreign body airway obstruction (FBAO). Do not interfere if victim can cough, speak, or breathe
A. Conscious adult victim
   1. Stand behind the victim, encircle his or her waist

with your arms, place your fist above the umbilicus and below the xiphoid process with your thumb against victim's abdomen; grasp your fist with your other hand and apply pressure with an inward and quick upward motion (Fig. 11-4)
   2. Repeat the thrusts until the obstruction is relieved, or switch to procedure for conscious victim who loses consciousness
B. Conscious adult victim who loses consciousness
   1. Place victim in supine position, call for help, and activate Emergency Medical Service (EMS)
   2. Perform tongue-jaw lift and carefully sweep your curved finger in one direction along the back of the victim's throat to retrieve object
   3. Establish airway using the head tilt—chin lift maneuver
   4. Deliver two breaths
   5. Kneel at level of victim's hips or straddle victim to deliver five abdominal thrusts by placing the heel of one hand above the umbilicus and below the xiphoid process; place your second hand on top of the first hand and apply pressure with an inward and upward motion
   6. Perform the tongue-jaw lift and carefully sweep curved finger in one direction along the back of the victim's throat to retrieve object
   7. Establish airway using the head tilt—chin lift maneuver

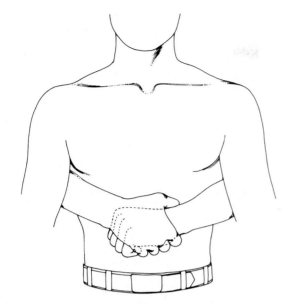

FIG. 11-4. Heimlich (abdominal thrust) maneuver. Place both arms around victim's waist; place fleshy part of fist below xiphoid and above navel. Place other hand on top. Apply quick firm upward and inward motion. (From Budassi SA, Barber J: *Mosby's manual of emergency care: practices and procedures,* ed 2, St Louis, 1984, Mosby.)

    8. Attempt to ventilate
    9. Continue repeating abdominal thrusts, finger sweeps, and breathing attempts in rapid sequence
C. Unconscious adult victim
    1. Simultaneously shake victim and shout to establish unconsciousness
    2. Activate EMS
    3. Quickly place victim in supine position
    4. Establish airway using the head tilt–chin lift maneuver
    5. Put your ear near victim's mouth and look, listen, and feel for breathing
    6. Deliver two breaths
    7. If no response, reposition head and again attempt to deliver two breaths
    8. Repeat steps 5 to 8 of *conscious adult victim who loses consciousness* until effective
D. Child
    1. Same as adult, except
    2. Provide 1 minute of rescue support, then activate EMS
    3. Do not perform finger sweeps; use tongue-jaw lift and remove object only if visualized
E. Obese victim and later stages of pregnancy
    1. Conscious victim: deliver chest thrusts (place thumb side of fist on middle of breast bone) until foreign body is expelled or victim becomes unconscious
    2. Unconscious victim
       a. Deliver chest thrusts with victim in supine position by placing heel of hand on lower half of sternum with other hand on top (CPR position)
       b. Follow Heimlich maneuver–finger sweep–ventilate sequence

F. Conscious infant
    1. Supporting head and neck, position infant face down with head lower than trunk along rescuer's forearm
    2. Administer five back blows between the shoulder blades with heel of hand
    3. Continue to support head and turn infant over, keeping head lower than trunk
    4. Compression location is directly below the point where the sternum is bisected by an imaginary line between the nipples
    5. Administer five chest thrusts with the ring and middle fingers
    6. Continue to administer back blows and chest thrusts until airway is cleared or infant becomes unconscious
G. Conscious infant who loses consciousness
    1. Place in supine position, call for help, and activate EMS
    2. Perform tongue-jaw lift and remove object only if you see it (do not perform finger sweeps)
    3. Establish airway using the head tilt–chin lift maneuver
    4. Attempt to deliver two breaths, reposition head, and repeat
    5. Administer five back blows
    6. Administer five chest thrusts
    7. Perform tongue-jaw lift and remove object only if you see it
    8. Establish airway using head tilt–chin lift maneuver and deliver two breaths
    9. Continue repeating back blows, chest thrusts, tongue-jaw lift, and breathing until effective
H. Unconscious infant
    1. Simultaneously shake and tap victim to establish unconsciousness
    2. Call for help even if you do not see anyone in the immediate vicinity
    3. Quickly place infant in supine position while supporting the head and neck
    4. Establish airway using head tilt–chin lift maneuver but do not tilt too far
    5. Put your ear near victim's mouth and look, listen, and feel for breathing
    6. Administer two breaths
    7. If no response, reposition head and again deliver two breaths
    8. Activate EMS
    9. Administer five back blows
    10. Administer five chest thrusts
    11. Perform tongue-jaw lift and remove object only if you see it
    12. Attempt to ventilate
    13. Repeat steps 9 through 12 until effective

HEMORRHAGE

A. Types
    1. Venous: dark color; steady flow
    2. Arterial: bright color; spurts
    3. Capillary: red; oozes
B. Assessment
    1. Restlessness
    2. Anxiety

3. Rapid, weak pulse
4. Cool, moist, pale skin
5. Rapid respirations
6. Thirst
7. Nausea/vomiting
8. Alteration in level of consciousness
9. Hypotension
C. Intervention: external
1. Apply direct pressure with a clean cloth for at least 6 minutes (use gloves if available)
2. Elevate injured part above heart level
3. If arterial bleeding does not respond to direct pressure, attempt to control by applying direct pressure on supply artery (Fig. 11-5)
4. Tourniquets are not recommended unless an extremity is amputated or severely mutilated
   a. Leave tourniquet exposed
   b. Tag or label victim with location of tourniquet
   c. Apply proximal to wound
   d. Tourniquet should not be removed except by a physician
5. Treat for shock
D. Usual medical care: replacement of fluids intravenously

SHOCK

A. Description: depressed state of vital body functions that, if untreated, could result in death
B. Types
1. Hypovolemic: decrease in circulating blood volume, for example, hemorrhage
2. Vasogenic: disturbance in tissue perfusion caused by circulating blood volume alterations
3. Cardiogenic: faulty pumping resulting in reduced cardiac output, for example, insect venom
4. Neurogenic: disruption of vasomotor tone resulting in decrease of circulating blood volume, for example, spinal cord injury
5. Septic: massive bacterial infection, for example, gram-negative organisms
C. Assessment
1. Shallow, rapid respirations
2. Cool, pale, clammy skin
3. Thirst
4. Tachycardia
5. Decreased blood pressure
6. Weak, thready pulse
7. Restlessness
8. Decreased urine output
9. May become confused or disoriented
D. Intervention
1. Ensure adequate airway and ventilation
2. Control bleeding if present
3. Place in supine position with legs elevated unless contraindicated (e.g., head injuries)
4. Insert urinary catheter
5. Monitor vital signs
6. Cover victim to conserve body heat
E. Usual medical care
1. IV fluids
2. Administer oxygen
3. Medications depending on the type of shock

ANAPHYLACTIC REACTION

A. Description: rapidly developing allergic reaction; more likely to occur in outdoor environments
B. Assessment
1. Pallor
2. Diaphoresis
3. Tachycardia or bradycardia
4. Hypotension
5. Wheezing, dyspnea
6. Anxiety, restlessness
7. Urticaria
8. Edema
9. Pruritis
10. Rash
11. Possible respiratory distress
12. Diffuse erythema
C. Intervention
1. Ensure adequate airway and ventilation

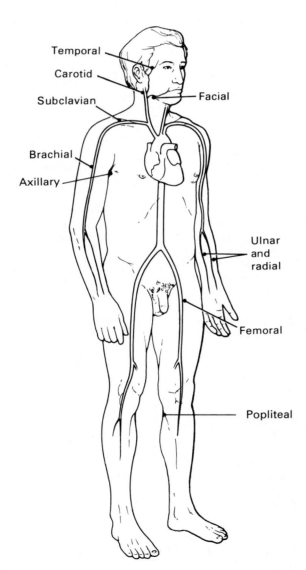

Temporal
Carotid
Subclavian
Facial
Brachial
Axillary
Ulnar and radial
Femoral
Popliteal

FIG. 11-5. Pressure points for control of hemorrhage. (From Lewis SM, Collier IC: *Medical-surgical nursing: assessment and management of clinical problems,* ed 3, St Louis, 1992, Mosby.)

2. Elevate feet slightly, unless contraindicated (e.g., head injuries)
D. Usual medical care
   1. Administer oxygen
   2. Epinephrine
   3. Antihistamines
   4. Steroids
   5. IV fluids
   6. Drug therapy for cardiovascular support
E. Preventive measures
   1. Allergy history
   2. Medical identification tag for high-risk persons
   3. Sting emergency medical kits
   4. Skin testing when possible
   5. Question previous allergic reactions before administering medications

HEAD INJURIES

Trauma to the head can result in scalp, skull, and brain injuries

Scalp Injury

Type	Intervention
Abrasion	Wash with soap and water
Hematoma	Apply ice
Contusion	Apply ice
Laceration	Stop bleeding by compression (only if no depression present)
	Treat for shock
	Shave around laceration
	Clean wound
	Suture

Skull Fracture

A. Simple: skull surface crack
   1. Observation for alteration of respiration, vision, consciousness, pupils, motor strength, and speech
   2. X-ray examination
B. Depressed: bone fragments driven into the skull, resulting in pressed-in appearance
   1. Intervention
      a. Ensure adequate airway and ventilation
      b. Administer oxygen
      c. Control bleeding
      d. Treat for shock
      e. Observe for alteration of respiration, vision, consciousness, pupils, motor strength, and speech
      f. Maintain body temperature
   2. Usual medical care
      a. Surgical intervention
      b. Antibiotic therapy
C. Basilar: fracture located along skull base
   1. Assessment
      a. Periorbital ecchymosis (black eyes)
      b. Cerebrospinal fluid (CSF) leak
      c. Discoloration behind ears (Battle's sign)
      d. Blood behind eardrum (hemotympanum)
   2. Intervention: observe for alterations of respiration, vision, consciousness, pupils, motor strength, and speech
   3. Usual medical care
      a. X-ray examination (although usually not visible)
      b. Antibiotic therapy if CSF leak is present

Brain Injury

A. Concussion: temporary alteration of neurologic functioning caused by a blow to the head, which results in jarring of the brain
   1. Assessment
      a. Nausea and vomiting
      b. Headache
      c. Possible brief period of unconsciousness and memory loss
      d. Possible skull fracture
      e. Confusion
   2. Intervention
      a. Observe for alteration of respiration, vision, consciousness, pupils, motor strength, and vision
      b. Administer nonnarcotic analgesics as ordered
      c. Maintain hydration
B. Contusion: brain surface bruise
   1. Assessment
      a. Nausea and vomiting
      b. Visual alterations
      c. Neurologic alterations
   2. Intervention
      a. Maintenance of adequate airway and ventilation
      b. Observation
   3. Usual medical care
      a. Hospitalization
      b. Antiemetics

EYE INJURIES
Foreign Body in Eye

A. Evert eyelid
B. Touch particle gently with sterile swab moistened in sterile saline solution or water (do not remove if particle is on the cornea or if there is eyeball penetration)
C. Apply an eye patch after ensuring that the eye is closed

Foreign Body in Conjuctiva

A. Invert eyelid
B. Remove particle as described above
C. Irrigate with saline solution or water
D. Eye patch may be applied

Contusion

A. Cold compresses or ice pack intermittently for the first 24 hours
B. Warm compresses after 48 hours
C. Bilateral eye patches if intraocular hemorrhage is present

Corneal Abrasion

A. Assessment
   1. Pain
   2. Photosensitivity
   3. Spasms of the eyelid
   4. Tearing
B. Intervention: patch injured eye
C. Usual medical care: local antibiotics

Burns

A. Chemical
   1. If action of chemical is not enhanced by water, immediately flush area with copious amounts of water for 15 minutes (damage increases with length of chemical contact)

2. The following solutions will neutralize the following types of burns
   a. Acid: sodium bicarbonate 2% solution
   b. Lime: ammonium tartrate 5% solution
   c. Alkali: boric or citric acid solution
B. Thermal
   1. Irrigate with saline solution or water
   2. Apply bilateral eye patches
C. Radiation
   1. Assessment
      a. Excessive blinking
      b. Tearing
      c. Feeling that something is in the eye
      d. Pain
   2. Intervention
      a. Cold compresses
      b. Bilateral eye patches
   3. Usual medical care
      a. Topical antibiotics
      b. Cycloplegics
      c. Analgesics

Penetrating Injuries

A. Place a protective shield, such as a paper cup, over the eye to prevent further damage by pressure (Fig. 11-6)
B. Apply eye patch to the uninjured eye
C. See an ophthalmologist immediately

SPINAL CORD INJURIES

Vertebrae	Number	Injury produces
Cervical	7	Paralysis of trunk and all four extremities
		C-4 level injury: respiratory difficulty
Thoracic	12	Paraplegia
Lumbar	5	Lower extremity paralysis
Sacral	5 (fused)	Paraparesis

A. Assessment
   1. Pain, tenderness
   2. Numbness, tingling
   3. Weakness
   4. Alterations of sensation and motor function below level of injury
   5. Possible signs and symptoms of shock
B. Intervention
   1. Ensure adequate airway and ventilation; if helmet is on victim, leave it in place if airway is accessible
   2. Treat for shock
   3. Immobilization (movement may cause further damage)
   4. Maintain body temperature
   5. When help arrives, place victim on board without flexing neck or back

CHEST INJURIES
Fractured Rib

A. Assessment
   1. Chest pain (increases on inspiration), tenderness
   2. Shortness of breath, shallow breathing
   3. Tachycardia
   4. Hypotension
   5. Ecchymosis

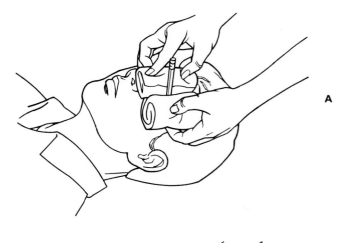

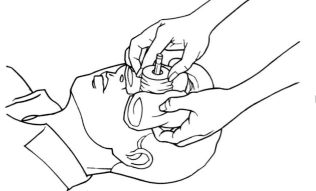

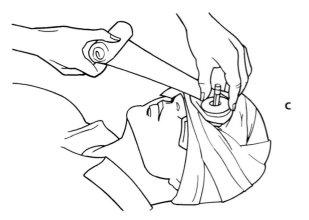

FIG. 11-6. A, Do not remove an object impaled in the eye. Place sterile dressings around the object. **B,** Support the object with a paper cup and carefully bandage the cup in place. **C,** Cover the other eye to keep blood, fluid, and dirt out. (Courtesy American Red Cross: *First aid: responding to emergencies,* St Louis, 1991, Mosby.)

B. Intervention
   1. Immobilization
   2. Apply ice for 24 hours, then apply heat locally
   3. Observe for signs and symptoms of pneumothorax
   4. Encourage deep breathing
   5. Administer analgesics sparingly

Flail Chest

A. Fracture of several ribs resulting in loss of chest wall stability
B. Assessment
   1. Pain
   2. Difficulty breathing
   3. Shallow, rapid, noisy respirations
   4. Chest moves in opposite from normal direction: moves in on inspiration, out on expiration
   5. Cyanosis
   6. Possible bruises
C. Intervention
   1. Ensure adequate airway and ventilation
   2. Stabilize chest wall with hands
   3. Apply pressure dressing
   4. Position victim on affected side in semi-Fowler's position
D. Usual medical care
   1. Pain control
   2. Possible intubation and ventilation with severe flail

Simple Pneumothorax

A. Description: air enters the pleural cavity; negative pressure is lost resulting in partial or total lung collapse
B. Assessment
   1. Chest pain
   2. Shortness of breath
   3. Decreased breath sounds
C. Intervention
   1. Ensure adequate airway and ventilation
   2. Place victim in sitting position
   3. Administer oxygen
D. Usual medical care: possible chest tube placement

Tension Pneumothorax

A. Description: air enters the pleural cavity on inspiration and is trapped during exhalation, creating pressure
B. Assessment
   1. Extreme shortness of breath
   2. Trachea deviation
   3. Mediastinal shift
   4. Neck vein distention
   5. Hypotension
   6. Tachycardia
   7. Restlessness
   8. Cyanosis
   9. Distant breath sounds
C. Intervention
   1. Ensure adequate airway, breathing, and circulation
   2. Administer oxygen
D. Usual medical care
   1. Needle thoracotomy
   2. Chest tube placement
   3. Intravenous fluids

Open Pneumothorax (Sucking Chest Wound)

A. Description
   1. One-way flap: air enters pleural space but cannot escape (tension pneumothorax)
   2. Two-way flap: air enters and leaves pleural space
B. Assessment
   1. Audible sucking noise
   2. Shortness of breath
   3. Cyanosis
   4. Shock
   5. Possible signs and symptoms of tension pneumothorax
C. Intervention
   1. Ensure adequate airway, breathing, and circulation
   2. Cover wound with air-tight dressing
   3. Administer oxygen
D. Usual medical care
   1. Chest tube placement
   2. Antibiotic therapy
   3. Treat for shock

Spontaneous Pneumothorax

A. Description: no evidence of trauma; frequently occurs during strenuous physical activity; air from injured lung enters pleural cavity
B. Assessment
   1. Sudden, sharp chest pain
   2. Shortness of breath
   3. Diaphoresis
   4. Anxiety
   5. Hypotension
   6. Tachycardia
   7. Cessation of normal chest movement on affected side
C. Intervention
   1. Ensure adequate airway and ventilation
   2. Keep victim quiet
   3. Place in semi- or high-Fowler's position
D. Usual medical care
   1. Needle aspiration
   2. Chest tube
   3. IV fluids
   4. Oxygen

Hemothorax

A. Description: blood in the pleural space
B. Assessment
   1. Chest pain
   2. Shortness of breath
   3. Distant breath sounds
   4. Anxiety
   5. Shock
   6. Cyanosis
C. Intervention
   1. Ensure adequate airway and ventilation
   2. Treat for shock
D. Usual medical care: chest tube placement; thoracentesis

Pulmonary Embolism

A. Description: thrombus or other foreign matter lodged in a pulmonary arterial vessel
B. Assessment
   1. Sudden, sharp chest pain
   2. Shortness of breath
   3. Pallor, possible cyanosis
   4. Anxiety
   5. Tachycardia
   6. Rapid, shallow respirations
   7. Possible hypotension, elevated temperature
   8. Possible cough, wheeze, hemoptysis
   9. Possible sudden death if large blood vessel is blocked

C. Intervention
   1. Ensure adequate airway, breathing, and circulation
   2. Treat for shock
   3. Administer oxygen
   4. Keep victim quiet
   5. Place patient in semi- to high-Fowler's position if vital signs permit
D. Usual medical care
   1. Anticoagulant therapy
   2. IV fluids

Intraabdominal Injuries
Penetrating Wound
A. Assessment
   1. Hypotension
   2. Shock
   3. Diminished bowel sounds
   4. Pain
   5. Tenderness
   6. Progressive abdominal distention
   7. Nausea or vomiting
B. Intervention
   1. Do not move victim
   2. Ensure adequate airway, breathing, circulation
   3. Control bleeding
      a. Look for entrance and exit wounds
      b. Apply compression for external bleeding
      c. Look for chest injuries
   4. Cover wounds with wet, sterile, or nonadhesive dressing(s) (e.g., saline or plastic wrap)
   5. Monitor vital signs
   6. Treat for shock
   7. Keep victim NPO
C. Usual medical care
   1. IVs
   2. Oxygen
   3. Tetanus prophylaxis
   4. Antibiotics
   5. Analgesics
   6. Indwelling catheter
   7. Nasogastric tube
   8. X-ray examination
   9. Possible surgery

Blunt Wound
A. Assessment
   1. Diminished bowel sounds
   2. Abdominal distention
   3. Pain
   4. Tenderness
   5. Guarding
B. Intervention
   1. Do not move victim
   2. Ensure adequate airway, breathing, circulation
   3. Observe for hemorrhage
   4. Observe for chest injuries
   5. Monitor vital signs
   6. Treat for shock
C. Usual medical care
   1. Oxygen
   2. Nasogastric tube
   3. X-ray examination

   4. Peritoneal lavage
   5. Possible surgery

BURNS
A. Depth classification

Depth	Degree	Assessment
Superficial	First degree	Pain; red; minimal or no edema
Partial thickness	Second degree	Pain; mottled color; blistering; edema; wet appearance
Full thickness	Third degree	Gray, white, brown, leathery, or charred appearance; edema; minor or no pain

B. Surface area classification
   1. The greater the body surface area (BSA) affected, the more serious the damage
   2. Use rule of nines (Fig. 11-7) to estimate percent of BSA affected

Major Burns
A. Burns are considered major or critical if they fulfill the following criteria
   1. In adults: greater than 25% of BSA has received second-degree burns
   2. In children: greater that 20% of BSA has received second-degree burns
B. Intervention
   1. Lay victim flat (standing forces him or her to breathe flames and smoke; running fans flames)

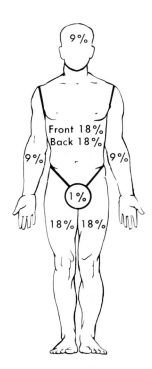

FIG. 11-7. Rule of nines is used to estimate amount of skin surface burned. (From Phipps WS, Long BC, Woods NF, editors: *Medical-surgical nursing: concepts and procedures,* ed 3, St Louis, 1988, Mosby.)

2. Roll victim in carpet or blankets or use water to extinguish fire
3. Remove any smoldering clothing that is nonadherent
4. Ensure adequate airway and ventilation
5. Administer oxygen
6. Assess for inhalation burns
7. Remove nonadherent, tight-fitting clothing
8. Remove tight jewelry
9. Apply cold soaks
10. Cover burns with moist, sterile dressings or clean cloth
11. Elevate affected parts if possible
12. Cover victim
13. Insert indwelling catheter
14. Treat burned areas as ordered by physician

C. Usual medical care
1. Tetanus prophylaxis
2. Central venous pressure line
3. Pain management
4. Nasogastric tube
5. Reverse isolation
6. Intravenous therapy
7. Antibiotic therapy

D. Warnings
1. *Do not use salves, ointments, or oils*
2. *Do not soak large burns unless you can maintain body warmth*
3. *Do not use ice or ice water on partial- or full-thickness burns*

Chemical Burns

A. Powdered chemicals: sweep off skin
B. Nonpowered chemicals: irrigate with copious amounts of water
C. Cover loosely with a clean cloth

Electrical Burns

A. Assessment
1. Discoloration
2. Edema
3. Cardiac irregularities
4. Entrance and exit sites of current visible
5. Confusion
6. Unconsciousness
7. Respiratory distress

B. Intervention
1. Do not touch the victim
2. Remove electrical source with a nonconductor or shut off current source
3. If victim has no pulse and is not breathing, institute cardiopulmonary resuscitation
4. Check victim for other injuries
5. Monitor cardiac and renal function

Radiation Burns

A. Intervention: apply cool, moist compresses
B. Usual medical care: possibly antipyretics

Smoke Inhalation

A. Assessment
1. Singed hair in nares
2. Mouth burns
3. Brassy cough
4. Respiratory distress

B. Intervention
1. Ensure adequate airway and ventilation
2. Administer oxygen
3. Be prepared to initiate cardiopulmonary resuscitation

WOUNDS

A. Open (break in skin)
1. Laceration: jagged cut through the skin and underlying tissue
2. Abrasion: skin scrape
3. Avulsion: flap of skin and subcutaneous tissue torn loose
4. Puncture: tissue penetration by a sharp object
5. Abscess: localized pus formation

B. Closed (no break in skin; e.g., contusion): injury to underlying tissue by blunt object

C. General management
1. Stop bleeding
   a. Apply pressure dressing
   b. Elevate affected part
   c. Use digital pressure on supply artery
   d. Apply tourniquet only as a lifesaving measure and leave tourniquet visible
2. Treat shock
3. Control infection
   a. Wounds requiring medical care: it is generally recommended not to clean them until they are seen by a physician
   b. Cover open wounds with a clean, nonadhesive dressing
   c. Apply ice during the first 24 to 48 hours for closed wounds
   d. Minor wounds being treated at home: clean well with soap and water; thoroughly rinse; approximate wound edges with adhesive; cover with a clean dressing; seek medical care for signs of infection
4. Puncture wounds
   a. Impaled object should be stabilized and left in place
   b. Medical attention should be sought

D. Special wounds
1. Human bites
   a. May be self-inflicted or inflicted by another; evidenced by teeth marks and often by knuckle lacerations
   b. Intervention
      (1) Clean with soap and water
      (2) Rinse thoroughly
      (3) Apply clean dressing
      (4) Keep injured part elevated
   c. Usual medical care
      (1) Tetanus prophylaxis
      (2) Antibiotic therapy
2. Animal bites
   a. Dog bites are most common and usually produce puncture marks
   b. Intervention
      (1) Clean minor wounds with soap and water

(2) Rinse thoroughly

(3) Flush with povidone-iodine (Betadine)

(4) Apply clean dressing

NOTE: major wounds (severe bleeding) require control of bleeding and medical attention

  c. Usual medical care

    (1) Antibiotic therapy for large, contaminated bites

    (2) Tetanus prophylaxis

    (3) Rabies prophylaxis if necessary

3. Snakebites

  a. Assessment

    (1) Teeth marks; possibly fang marks

    (2) Edema

    (3) Pain

    (4) Ecchymosis

    (5) Bleeding

    (6) Numbness of affected part

  b. Intervention

    (1) Have victim lie quietly in shaded area

    (2) Clean wound

    (3) Suction

      (a) Do not use mouth suction if you have open sores in your mouth

      (b) Suction wound using snakebite kit

      (c) Only use mouth suction if no other means is available

    (4) Apply clean dressing

    (5) Immobilize affected limb

    (6) Affected limb should be in dependent position

  c. Usual medical care

    (1) Analgesics

    (2) IV fluids

    (3) Tetanus prophylaxis

    (4) Antivenom therapy

4. Insect bites (bees, wasps, hornets)

  a. Assessment

    (1) Pruritus

    (2) Burning

    (3) Swelling

  b. Intervention

    (1) Remove the stinger by scraping; do not pull out because this releases more toxin; do not squeeze

    (2) Clean with soap and water

    (3) Apply ice

    (4) Apply ammonia diluted with warm water or a paste of baking soda and water

  c. Usual medical care

    (1) Epinephrine

    (2) Antihistamines

    (3) Steroids

5. Tick

  a. Attaches to host with its teeth

  b. Releases a toxin that may cause tick paralysis or Lyme disease

  c. Squeezing tick releases more toxin

  d. If paralysis progresses to bulbar, respiratory failure and subsequent death may occur

  e. Paralysis will disappear after tick is removed

  f. Intervention

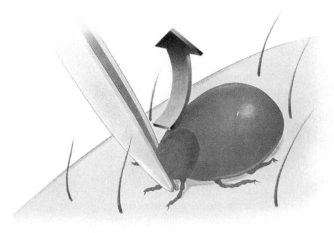

FIG. 11-8. Remove a tick by pulling steadily and firmly with fine-tipped tweezers. (Courtesy American Red Cross: *First aid: responding to emergencies,* St Louis, 1991, Mosby.)

    (1) Grasp tick with tweezers and pull slowly and steadily (Fig. 11-8)

    (2) Wash with soap and water

    (3) Seek medical treatment

FRACTURE

A. Description: a complete or incomplete break in bone continuity

1. Fracture without displacement presents normal alignment despite the fracture

2. Fracture with displacement presents a separation of bone fragments at fracture site

3. Compound or open: bone protrusion through skin

4. Simple or closed: no bone protrusion through the skin

5. Incomplete: part of bone is broken

6. Complete: breakage producing two fragments

B. Types by line of fracture

1. Transverse: break is straight across a bone

2. Oblique: fracture line is at an oblique angle to the bone shaft

3. Comminuted: fragmented into three or more pieces

4. Green-stick: splintering; occurs mainly in children

5. Telescoped: end of one bone jams together with the end of another bone

6. Spiral: partial encirclement of bone by fracture lines

C. Assessment

1. Localized pain, tenderness

2. Ecchymosis

3. Swelling

4. Deformity, possible limb shortening and external rotation

5. Alterations in sensation and function

6. Spasms

7. Characteristic grating sound (crepitus)

8. Possible bone snap heard by victim

9. Possible paralysis

10. External bleeding

D. Intervention

1. Control bleeding

2. Treat for shock
3. Immobilize affected part
4. Splint above and below the fracture
5. Apply ice
6. Elevate affected part, if possible
7. Observe for changes in sensation, temperature, and color (indicate nerve injury or circulation interference)

E. Usual medical care
  1. X-ray examination
  2. Possible cast application
  3. Possible surgery
  4. Analgesics
  5. Traction

DISLOCATION

A. Description: joint injury and bone displacement
B. Assessment
  1. Pain, tenderness
  2. Swelling
  3. Deformity
  4. Alterations in function
  5. Discoloration
C. Intervention
  1. Control hemorrhage
  2. Immobilize the affected part
  3. Apply sterile dressing to open wounds
  4. Splint in the position found above and below the site
  5. Apply ice
  6. Elevate affected part, if possible
  7. Check for fractures
  8. Monitor neurologic status (check pulses distal to the injury)

SPRAIN

A. Description: stretched or ruptured ligaments; *sprain should be considered a fracture until proven otherwise by x-ray examination*
B. Assessment
  1. Pain, tenderness
  2. Discoloration
  3. Swelling
  4. Alterations in function
C. Intervention
  1. Elevate affected part
  2. Apply ice intermittently for 72 hours
  3. Apply elastic (Ace) bandages
  4. Immobilize affected part

STRAIN

A. Description: muscle or tendon damage caused by overstress or overstrain
B. Assessment
  1. Pain
  2. Discoloration
C. Intervention
  1. Bed rest
  2. Heat application

HYPERTHERMIA
Heat Stroke

A. Description: body's mechanism for heat regulation breaks down, and excessive body heat is retained

B. Assessment
  1. Hyperpyrexia to 106° or 107° F (41.1° to 41.6° C)
  2. Flushed, hot, dry skin
  3. Dizziness
  4. Headache
  5. Confusion
  6. Nausea
  7. Tachycardia
  8. Hypotension
  9. Cessation of sweating
  10. Seizures
  11. Possible consciousness alterations
  12. Shallow, rapid breathing
  13. Delirium
C. Especially at risk are
  1. The elderly
  2. The obese
  3. Individuals with cardiovascular problems
  4. Strenuous exercisers
  5. Individuals taking medications that decrease perspiration, decrease thirst, or alter heat production
D. Intervention
  1. Ensure adequate airway, breathing, and circulation
  2. Move victim out of sun
  3. Loosen or remove clothing
  4. Provide rapid cooling, for example, immerse in cold water; apply towels soaked in cold water; air conditioning, fanning, and cool-water sponge
  5. If conscious, provide cool water
  6. Control shivering (this causes body temperature to increase)
  7. Advise victim to avoid reexposure and warn of possible lowered tolerance to heat for a long time or indefinitely
E. Usual medical care
  1. Oxygen
  2. IV therapy

Heat Exhaustion

A. Description: excessive fluid loss and exposure to heat without sufficient fluid and electrolyte replenishment
B. Assessment
  1. Headache
  2. Dizziness, faintness
  3. Nausea and vomiting
  4. Marked diaphoresis
  5. Cool, pale, damp skin
  6. Muscle cramps
  7. Possible temperature elevation
  8. Orthostatic hypotension
  9. Tachycardia
  10. Dehydration
C. Especially at risk are
  1. The elderly
  2. The very young
D. Intervention
  1. Move victim to cool area
  2. Administer salted water if vomiting absent
  3. Provide rest
  4. Relieve muscle cramps (firm pressure against muscle with palm of hand)
  5. Advise victim of preventive measures

COLD INJURIES
Frostbite

A. Classification
   1. Superficial: superficial tissue below the skin freezes
   2. Deep: deep subcutaneous tissue freezes, and temperature of affected part is lowered
B. Most frequently affected areas: ears, nose, cheeks, fingers, and toes
C. Assessment
   1. Superficial
      a. Numbness, tingling, burning
      b. Gray-white appearance of affected parts
   2. Deep
      a. Hyperemic skin
      b. Edema
      c. Blister formation
      d. Discoloration
      e. Numbness
D. Intervention
   1. Superficial
      a. Remove wet, constricting clothing
      b. Give warm-water soaks
      c. Advise victim of preventive measures
   2. Deep
      a. Remove wet, constricting clothing
      b. Give warm-water soaks only if continuously available; otherwise keep area dry, place sterile gauze between affected fingers and toes, cover, and elevate frozen part
      c. If conscious, give warm liquids
      d. Do not allow use of frostbitten part
   3. Usual medical care
      a. Tetanus prophylaxis
      b. Analgesics
      c. Antibiotic therapy
E. Warnings
   1. *Do not rub area with snow or ice*
   2. *Do not massage*

Immersion Foot

A. Cause: wet foot in continuous contact with cold temperatures
B. Assessment: shriveled appearance to foot
C. Intervention
   1. Dry footwear
   2. Warm-water soaks

Chilblain

A. Description: localized inflammation caused by exposure to cold
B. Commonly affected areas: fingers, toes, and earlobes
C. Prevention: avoidance of cold, damp climates

Accidental Hypothermia

A. Description: exposure to cold resulting in heat loss and reduction in body temperature below the average normal range
B. Assessment (Table 11-1)
C. Intervention
   1. Ensure adequate airway and ventilation
   2. Administer oxygen
   3. Remove wet clothing and cover victim

Table 11-1. Signs and symptoms of hypothermia

Temperature	Signs and symptoms
96°-99° F (35.6°-37.2° C)	Shivering, loss of manual coordination
91°-95° F (32.8°-35° C)	Violent shivering, slurred speech, amnesia
86°-90° F (30°-32.2° C)	Shivering decreases but is replaced by strong muscular rigidity and cyanosis
Below 86° F (30° C)	Possibility of developing rewarming shock
81°-85° F (27.2°-29.4° C)	Irrational, stuporous; pulse and respirations decrease
78°-80° F (25.6°-26.7° C)	Coma, erratic heartbeat
Below 81° F (27.2° C)	Possibility of ventricular fibrillation
Below 78° F (25.6° C)	Cardiopulmonary arrest

From Budassi SA, Barber J: *Mosby's manual of emergency care: practices and procedures,* ed 2, St Louis, 1984, Mosby, p 279.

   4. Warm the body gradually; use heating pad or hot-water bottles wrapped in a towel
   5. Give warm beverages high in sugar content
D. Usual medical care
   1. IV fluids
   2. Possible steroid therapy
E. Warnings: *do not rub or massage the skin*

POISONING
Food

A. Cause: pathogenic organisms tranferred to victim from contaminated food; illness is caused by toxins produced by the organism
B. Botulism *(Clostridium botulinum)*
   1. Causes
      a. Improperly canned food
      b. Improperly cured food
   2. Assessment
      a. Headache
      b. Fatigue
      c. Nausea and vomiting
      d. Double vision
      e. Muscle incoordination
      f. Difficulty swallowing, talking, and breathing
   3. Intervention
      a. Ensure adequate airway and ventilation
      b. Be prepared to administer cardiopulmonary resuscitation
      c. Induce vomiting if consumption was recent, victim has clinical and neurologic symptoms, no seizure activity, and no alterations in level of consciousness
      d. Usual medical care: antitoxin
C. *Staphylococcus aureus*
   1. Causes
      a. Respiratory tract and skin of food handlers
      b. Unrefrigerated cream-filled foods
      c. Fish
      d. Meat

2. Assessment
    a. Nausea and vomiting
    b. Diarrhea
    c. Abdominal cramps
    d. Weakness
3. Intervention
    a. Fluids
    b. Bed rest
4. Usual medical care
    a. Possible IV therapy
    b. Antiemetics
    c. Antidiarrheals
D. *Salmonella*
    1. Causes: inadequately cooked meat, poultry, and eggs
    2. Assessment
        a. Nausea and vomiting
        b. Diarrhea
        c. Weakness
        d. Abdominal pain
        e. Elevated temperature
        f. Chills
    3. Intervention
        a. Bed rest
        b. Fluids
    4. Usual medical care
        a. Possible IV therapy
        b. Antiemetics
        c. Antidiarrheals

Chemical Ingestion

A. Corrosive
    1. Assessment
        a. Burning
        b. Vomiting
        c. Pain
    2. Intervention
        a. Ensure adequate airway and ventilation
        b. Treat for shock
        c. Take seizure precautions
        d. Call local poison control center: give name of poison, amount ingested, and time ingested
        e. Do not induce vomiting if victim has swallowed strong acid or alkali corrosive or hydrocarbon solvent
        f. Give antidote if known, if victim is conscious and free of airway swelling
            (1) For acids: give milk, milk of magnesia, or water
            (2) For alkalies: give diluted vinegar, fruit juice, milk, or water
B. Noncorrosive
    1. Give milk or water
    2. Induce vomiting
        a. Keep head down and to the side to reduce risk of aspiration
        b. Give syrup of ipecac
        c. Insert index finger at back of throat
    3. Call local poison control center

Inhaled Poison

A. Assessment
    1. Coughing
    2. Choking

B. Intervention
    1. Carry victim to fresh-air source
    2. Ensure adequate airway and ventilation
    3. Loosen constrictive clothing
    4. Keep victim warm and quiet

Carbon Monoxide

A. Assessment
    1. Headache
    2. Drowsiness
    3. Bright red skin (late indicator)
    4. Dizziness
    5. Weakness
    6. Consciousness alterations
    7. Possible seizures
B. Intervention
    1. Remove victim from source
    2. Establish airway
    3. Administer 100% oxygen
    4. If victim is not breathing but has a pulse, commence artificial respiration
    5. Keep victim warm
C. Usual medical care
    1. Possibly hyperbaric oxygenation
    2. IV fluids

DIABETES MELLITUS AND HYPOGLYCEMIA
Ketoacidosis (Acute Insulin Deficiency)

A. Assessment
    1. Polydipsia
    2. Weak, rapid pulse
    3. Hypotension
    4. Dry, warm, flushed skin
    5. Pallor
    6. Diaphoresis
    7. Acetone odor on breath
    8. Kussmaul's respiration
    9. Nausea and vomiting
    10. Alterations in consciousness
    11. Dehydration
    12. Weakness
    13. Headache
B. Intervention
    1. Ensure adequate airway and ventilation
    2. Monitor vital signs, fluid intake and output, and level of consciousness
    3. Provide fluids if conscious, for example, broth, orange juice
C. Usual medical care
    1. Regular insulin
    2. IV therapy: normal saline solution or 0.45% saline solution
    3. Monitor blood sugar

Hypoglycemia (Low Blood Sugar; Insulin Reaction)

A. Assessment
    1. Weakness
    2. Pallor
    3. Hunger
    4. Nervousness; irritability
    5. Cool, moist skin

6. Tachycardia
7. Tremors
8. Dizziness, syncope
9. Headache
10. Visual disturbances
11. Drowsiness
12. Confusion
B. Intervention
1. Assure adequate airway and ventilation
2. Administer quick-acting carbohydrate, for example, orange juice with sugar, honey, lump sugar, cola beverage, candy
C. Usual medical care: if unconscious
1. IV therapy: 50% glucose
2. Monitor blood sugar

DROWNING

A. Description: asphyxiation that results when one cannot stay afloat in water
B. Causes
1. Accidental, for example, exhaustion, inability to swim, panic, injury, medical incident such as a seizure
2. Intentional: suicide attempt
C. Intervention
1. Remove victim from water
2. If victim is not breathing, commence artificial respiration (may need to be instituted while victim is being removed from the water)
3. If there is no carotid pulse, commence cardiopulmonary resuscitation
4. Observe for pulmonary edema

DRUG ABUSE

A. Description: physical and psychologic dependence on the effects of mind-altering drugs
B. Assessment
1. Needle marks on the body along the veins (many addicts wear long-sleeved shirts to conceal mainlining)
2. Anorexia
3. Abdominal cramping
4. Constipation
5. Nutritional deficiencies
6. Watery, reddened eyes
7. Runny nose
8. Dilated or constricted pupils
9. Central nervous system alterations
10. Poor personal hygiene
11. History of difficulty in school, on job, with interpersonal relationships
12. Accident-prone
13. History of personality change
14. Possibly hepatitis
C. Effects of frequently abused drugs (Table 11-2)
D. Intervention
1. Ensure airway, breathing, and circulation
2. Administer oxygen
3. Insert indwelling catheter
4. Monitor vital functions and neurologic status
5. Take seizure precautions

E. Usual medical care
1. Arterial blood gases
2. Specific drug antagonist (e.g., naloxone hydrochloride [Narcan])
3. IV therapy
4. Central venous pressure line
5. Possible dialysis
6. High-protein, high-calorie diet
7. Vitamin supplements
8. Psychotherapy
9. Withdrawal treatment: methadone (Dolophine) hydrochloride
   a. Legal synthetic drug addiction
   b. Supervised administration
10. Rehabilitation

ACUTE ALCOHOLISM

A. Description: large alcohol intake in a short time
B. Assessment
1. Alcohol on breath
2. Slurring of speech
3. Drowsiness
4. Ataxia
5. Agitation
6. Belligerence
C. Intervention
1. Protect airway
2. Observe for respiratory embarrassment
3. Monitor cardiac status
4. Assess for head injury
D. Usual medical care
1. Hydration
2. Vitamin supplements
3. High-protein diet
4. Analeptics to control or prevent seizures

MILD ALCOHOL WITHDRAWAL

A. Assessment
1. Nausea and vomiting
2. Shaking
3. Headache
4. Ataxia
B. Intervention
1. Rest
2. Quiet environment
C. Usual medical care
1. Analgesics
2. Hydration

DELIRIUM TREMENS

A. Assessment
1. Tachycardia
2. Hypotension
3. Tremors
4. Anxiety
5. Fear
6. Agitation
7. Hallucinations
8. Seizures
B. Intervention
1. Ensure adequate airway and ventilation

Table 11-2. Effects of frequently abused drugs

Drug	Psychologic effects	Physiologic effects	Effects of overdose	Withdrawal syndrome
Stimulants Cocaine, amphetamines, methylphenidate, phenmetrazine, other stimulants	Elation, psychomotor agitation, grandiosity, talkativeness, ↑ alertness, mood swings	Dilated pupils, ↑ blood pressure, ↑ TPR, diaphoresis, nausea, vomiting, insomnia, loss of appetite	Agitation, increased body temperature, hallucinations, convulsions, possible death	Severely depressed mood, prolonged sleep, apathy, irritability, disorientation
Depressants Chloral hydrate, barbiturates, methaqualone, benzodiazepines, alcohol	Disorientation, euphoria, emotional lability, ↑ sexual and aggressive drives with intoxication (↓ with increased doses), talkativeness	Slurred speech, staggering, constricted pupils, ↓ respirations, sedation, nausea	Shallow respiration, cold and clammy skin, weak and rapid pulse, coma, possible death	Anxiety, insomnia, tremors, delirium, convulsions, possible death
Narcotics Opium, morphine, codeine, heroin, methadone, other narcotics	Euphoria, ↓ sexual and aggressive drives	↓ Respiratory rate, nausea, "nodding out," insensitivity to pain, constricted pupils	Slow and shallow breathing, clammy skin, constricted pupils, coma, possible death	Watery eyes, runny nose, yawning, loss of appetite, tremors, panic, chills and sweating, cramps, nausea
Hallucinogens LSD, psilocybin, mescaline, peyote, amphetamine variants, phencyclidine	Hallucinations, illusions, altered body and time perception, mood swings, suspiciousness, confusion, anxiety, panic, intense emotions, depersonalization	Lack of coordination, dilated pupils, ↑ blood pressure, tremors, blurred vision, nausea, dizziness, ↓ weakness response to pain	More prolonged episodes, possibly resembling psychotic states	N/A
Cannabis Marijuana, tetrahydrocannabinol, hashish	Euphoria, impaired memory and attention, relaxation, poor judgment, apathy, abrupt mood changes, slowed time sensation	↑ Appetite, tachycardia, reddened eyes	Fatigue, paranoia; hallucinogen-like psychotic state (at very high doses)	Insomnia, hyperactivity (rare syndrome)
Inhalants Glues, aerosols, cleaning solutions, nail polish removers, lighter fluids, paints and paint thinners, other petroleum products, halothane, nitrous oxide, amyl nitrite, butyl nitrite	Giddiness, light-headedness, decreased inhibitions, floating sensation, illusions, clouding of thoughts, drowsiness, amnesia	Eye irritation, sensitivity to light, double vision, ringing in ears, irritation in lining of nose and mouth, cough, nausea, vomiting, diarrhea, faint heart beat, cardiac irregularities or dysrhythmias	Anxiety, mental impairment, depressed respiration, cardiac dysrhythmias, sudden death	No clinically relevant syndrome, development of tolerance likely at high doses

From Lewis SM, Collier IC: *Medical-surgical nursing: assessment and management of clinical problems*, ed 3, St Louis, 1992, Mosby, p 1786.
↑, Increased; *TPR*, temperature, pulse, respirations; ↓, decreased; *LSD*, lysergic acid diethylamide; *N/A*, no data available.

2. Treat for shock
3. Hydration
4. Monitor vital signs
5. Crisis counseling
C. Usual medical care
   1. Treatment for seizures
   2. Anticonvulsant drugs
   3. IV therapy
   4. Sedation
   5. Vitamin therapy
   6. High-protein diet

DISULFIRAM (ANTABUSE) REACTIONS

A. Assessment
   1. Nausea and vomiting
   2. Diaphoresis
   3. Hypotension
   4. Consciousness alterations
   5. Tachycardia
   6. Headache
   7. Facial flushing
   8. Reddened conjunctiva
B. Intervention
   1. Ensure adequate airway, breathing, and circulation
   2. Administer oxygen
C. Usual medical care
   1. IV therapy
   2. Diphenhydramine hydrochloride (Benadryl)
   3. Chlorpheniramine maleate (Chlor-Trimeton)
   4. Ascorbic acid

SEXUAL ASSAULT

A. Victim should be examined and treated as quickly as possible
B. Victim should not be left alone
C. Victims should be asked who they wish to have stay with them; offer to call family member, friend, or rape crisis center advocate
D. Provide immediate privacy
E. Kindness and support are crucial
F. Obtain history
G. Assess acuteness of physical and psychologic needs
H. Assess victim's readiness for physical examination
I. Explain all procedures and encourage questions
J. Obtain necessary written permissions
K. Assist victim to undress
L. Observe for and ask about other possible injuries
M. Assist with physician's examination
   1. A water-moistened speculum is used
   2. History will indicate the body orifices from which specimens for semen analysis will be required
   3. Pubic hair is combed for foreign hairs
   4. Clothing is usually saved for analysis, and replacement clothing will be necessary
   5. Venereal disease prophylaxis
   6. Pregnancy prophylaxis if contraception not in effect at time of attack: DES (diethylstilbestrol) treatment and side effects should be thoroughly explained

7. If possible and desired, offer accommodations for bathing and douching
8. Care for tissue trauma: immediate and follow-up
9. Care for psychologic trauma: immediate and follow-up
10. If present, family and friends often require assistance and counseling
11. Notify police

DISASTER

A. Definition: catastrophic event
   1. Natural, for example, flood, earthquake, hurricane
   2. Man-made, for example, riot, fire, train accident
B. May involve as few as 10 or more than 100 victims
C. Prevention
   1. Community planning
   2. Public education
D. Assessment
   1. Civilian triage: care priority to those whose life is threatened
   2. Military triage: care priority to those most likely to survive
E. Planning: the most capable person is designated to sort casualties
F. Intervention
   1. First aid should be rendered before victims are transported
   2. Care priorities
      a. Ensure airway, breathing, and circulation
      b. Control bleeding
      c. Treat for shock
         (1) Whole blood
         (2) IV fluids
         (3) Parenteral medications
         (4) Pain relief
         (5) Emergency wound care
      d. Preserve motor and sensory functioning
      e. Provide psychologic support
      f. Treat and transport

Suggested Reading List

American Heart Association: *Heartsaver manual*, Dallas, 1993, The Association.

American Red Cross: *First aid, responding to emergencies*, St Louis, 1991, Mosby.

Coleman: Cardiac issues in CPR: What the future might hold, *Nursing 92*, 22(4):54, 1992.

Hafen BQ, and Karren KJ: *Emergency care first aid handbook*, ed 4, Englewood, CO, 1990, Morton.

Ignatavicius DD, Bayne MV: *Medical-surgical nursing: a nursing process approach*, Philadelphia, 1991, WB Saunders.

Smeltzer SC, Bare BG: *Brunner and Suddarth's textbook of medical surgical nursing*, ed 7, Philadelphia, 1992, JB Lippincott.

Stuart GW, Sundeen SJ: *Principles and practice of psychiatric nursing*, ed 4, St Louis, 1991, Mosby.

Thygerson AL: *First aid and emergency care workbook*, Portola Valley, Calif, 1987, Jones & Bartlett.

Emergency Nursing Review Questions

Answers and rationales begin on p. 449.

1. Susan Sawyer, a motor vehicle accident (MVA) victim, is admitted to the hospital with an unstable fracture of the pelvis. In the initial assessment of Ms. Sawyer, the nurse would identify which of the following?
   ① Bowel sounds
   ② External rotation
   ③ Pain on defecation
   ④ Symphysis pubis tenderness

2. While caring for Ms. Sawyer, the nurse notices blood in her stool. Which of the following nursing actions would demonstrate the best judgment?
   ① Notify the physician of the observation
   ② Perform a stool guaiac reaction test
   ③ Request a physician's order for a stool softener
   ④ Send the next stool specimen to the lab

3. Tom Korn was in a motorcycle accident and knocked to the pavement. As you approach him you notice that his helmet is cracked. In caring for Mr. Korn, which of the following should receive priority?
   ① Maintain an open airway
   ② Maintain normal body temperature
   ③ Minimize movement of the head
   ④ Monitor breathing

4. The presence of Human Immunodeficiency Virus infection is increasing. Which of the following measures is essential for the nurse to incorporate into her care?
   ① Ask the patient his or her HIV status
   ② Have an HIV-positive health care worker attend to the patient
   ③ Strictly adhere to universal infection control precautions
   ④ Take infection control precautions only if exposure to blood or body fluids is obvious

5. You are caring for a rape trauma survivor. Your initial assessment indicates that the patient appears calm and very much in control. Which characteristic psychologic reaction best describes the patient's behavior?
   ① Denial
   ② Humiliation
   ③ Hyperalertness
   ④ Reorganization

6. For the rape survivor treated in the emergency room, an appropriate short-term expected outcome (goal) would be to:
   ① Initiate social interation
   ② Regain control over her life before she leaves the ER
   ③ Return to her pretrauma level of functioning
   ④ Verbalize two methods of stress management

7. In caring for an unconscious victim of an airway obstruction, the nurse should take which of the following actions *first*?
   ① Immediately start cardiopulmonary resuscitation
   ② Open the airway using the head tilt–chin lift maneuver
   ③ Place victim in supine position on a firm, flat surface
   ④ Remove any foreign object obstructing the airway

8. While making midmorning rounds the nurse finds Mr. Meshel, a 60-year-old diabetic patient, unconscious on the floor next to his bed. The nurse's *immediate* action should be to:
   ① Call the physician and prepare IV glucose
   ② Establish an airway
   ③ Administer regular insulin
   ④ Commence mouth-to-mouth resuscitation

9. In the presence of a pulse and a patent airway but the absence of respirations, which of the following actions would be *most appropriate* on an adult?
   ① Compress the sternum 1½ to 2 inches (3.75 to 5 cm)
   ② Turn the patient on his or her side
   ③ Sweep the back of the patient's throat
   ④ Continue to deliver breaths

10. After administering mouth-to-mouth resuscitation for a full minute, the nurse should:
    ① Reassess for presence of pulse and respirations
    ② Give two quick, full breaths
    ③ Initiate a sharp chest blow
    ④ Give four abdominal thrusts

11. When one rescuer is performing cardiopulmonary resuscitation on an adult, the rate of cardiac compressions is:
    ① 80 times per minute
    ② 5 times per minute
    ③ 60 times per minute
    ④ 15 times per minute

12. When one rescuer is performing cardiac compressions, the hands should be placed:
    ① Directly over the xiphoid process
    ② 2 inches below the xiphoid process
    ③ Two finger breadths above the xiphoid process
    ④ Two finger breadths to the left of the xiphoid process

13. When two rescuers are performing cardiopulmonary resuscitation, the ratio of compressions to respirations is:
    ① 15:2
    ② 5:2
    ③ 15:1
    ④ 5:1

14. When performing adult mouth-to-mouth resuscitation, the rescuer should deliver breaths that are:
    ① Full and quick
    ② Deep and forceful
    ③ Every 4 seconds
    ④ Every 5 seconds

15. While you are in a restaurant, you observe the man at the next table coughing and then clutching his throat. Which of the following actions should you take?
    ① Ask him if he is choking
    ② Encourage him to cough harder
    ③ Perform the Heimlich maneuver
    ④ Smack him on the back several times

16. Which of the following patients would be most at risk for mortality following burn injury?
    ① 5-year-old male
    ② 38-year-old female
    ③ 12-year-old female
    ④ 78-year-old male

17. 10-year-old Timothy is stabbed in the abdomen in the school playground. You respond to the other children's cries for help. By the time you reach Timothy he has a rapid pulse, his lips are cyanotic, and he is pale and diaphoretic. Your priority nursing action would be to:
    ① Elevate his feet to promote venous return
    ② Ensure a patent airway and maintain breathing
    ③ Administer fluids rapidly to restore blood volume
    ④ Cover him with a jacket to maintain body temperature

18. Your neighbor shouts to come quickly, that her child has been stung by a bee. Which of the following skin manifestations would indicate that a general systemic reaction is developing?
    ① Body itching
    ② Facial pallor
    ③ Localized redness
    ④ Localized swelling

19. Emergency Medical Service (EMS) arrives, and the child is given a subcutaneous injection of epinephrine. Why is epinephrine administered for anaphylactic reactions?
    ① To provide a sedative effect
    ② To provide relief of hypersensitivity reaction
    ③ To prevent recurrences of the reaction
    ④ To reduce the child's anxiety

20. Jake Barnes sustains a crush injury to his left lower arm in a tractor accident. Unable to palpate a radial pulse, you should take which of the following actions?
    ① Check for a pulse in another major artery
    ② Commence cardiopulmonary resuscitation
    ③ Prepare to commence rescue breathing
    ④ Run to the phone and call 9-1-1

21. Mr. Barnes begins to bleed profusely from the injured site. Emergency management of hemorrhage requires the nurse to implement which of the following actions *first*?
    ① Apply pressure to the bleeding area
    ② Apply a pressure dressing to the bleeding area
    ③ Elevate the injured area
    ④ Immobilize the injured area

Situation: You're out of state on vacation, driving alone on a scenic country road, and you come across a child lying in the middle of the road. On further observation you see an overturned bicycle on the side of the road. You estimate the child's age to be between 12 and 15 years.

22. Which of the following nursing actions should you take *immediately*?
    ① Keep driving to the nearest gas station and telephone for an ambulance
    ② Turn around and go back to the nearest main highway and hail a police car
    ③ Proceed with a rapid clinical assessment with emphasis on airway, breathing, and circulation
    ④ Check with local authorities for specifics on the state's Good Samaritan law

23. The child has a bleeding occipital laceration; pain, discoloration and swelling of the right ulna; and right-sided chest pain that increases on inspiration. Which of the following nursing actions will have the *highest priority*?
    ① Immobilization of the right arm
    ② Elevation of the right arm and head
    ③ Applying ice to the right side of the chest
    ④ Stopping the bleeding and treating for shock

24. Reassessment of the child's condition reveals tachycardia; cool, pale, clammy skin; and shallow, rapid respirations. You should recognize these symptoms as those of shock and immediately:
    ① Cover the child to prevent loss of body heat
    ② Maintain airway patency and elevate the lower extremities
    ③ Elevate the upper extremities and cover the child to prevent loss of body heat
    ④ Administer clear fluids to prevent shock

25. To stop the bleeding from the occipital laceration the *best* nursing action would be to:
    ① Apply pressure to the site
    ② Apply ice to the site
    ③ Elevate the child's head
    ④ Elevate the child's extremities

26. Reassessment of the right ulna should include which of the following actions?
    ① Ascertaining range-of-motion (ROM) limitations
    ② Observing for changes in sensation, temperature, and color
    ③ Determining the presence of crepitus
    ④ Preventing limb shortening

27. An acquaintance known to be taking lithium and under psychiatric care has taken cocaine. She telephones you with abdominal cramps and extreme anxiety and asks you what to do. Your *best* response would be to:
    ① Refer her to the local emergency room
    ② Refer her to her psychiatrist
    ③ Refer her to the cocaine hotline number
    ④ Tell her you cannot get involved right now

28. Which individual is especially at risk for heat exhaustion?
    ① 78 year old
    ② 20 year old
    ③ 31 year old
    ④ 52 year old

29. Running to catch a bus, you trip, fall, and sprain your wrist. Which of the following nursing interventions would be *most appropriate*?
    ① Application of dry heat
    ② Splinting above and below the wrist
    ③ Application of ice for 24 hours
    ④ Observation for sensation changes

30. You come across a multiple trauma scene. Priority care should be given to:
    ① The victim with cyanosis of earlobes and nailbeds
    ② The victim who is hemorrhaging
    ③ The victim who appears to be in a daze
    ④ The victim with a suspected fracture of the femur

31. Which of the following would be your priority nursing concern for a victim with severe burns?
    ① Administering cardiopulmonary resuscitation
    ② Relieving pain
    ③ Stopping the burning process
    ④ Tetanus prophylaxis

32. The mother of 3-year-old Dawn tells you that her daughter has swallowed bleach, which was stored under the kitchen sink. A rapid assessment reveals no evidence of acute airway swelling. Which of the following interventions should the nurse take?
    ① Absorb the poison with activated charcoal
    ② Give nothing by mouth
    ③ Give water or milk
    ④ Induce vomiting with syrup of ipecac

33. A laboratory employee has sustained chemical burns to his left forearm, thigh, and foot. Which of the following nursing actions should be taken initially?
    ① Apply ice to the burns immediately
    ② Cover the burns with dry, sterile dressings
    ③ Flush burns with cool, running water
    ④ Treat the victim for shock and tend to the burns later

34. The nurse knows that oils or ointments are not applied to severe burns. What is the chief purpose of this principle?
    ① Burn areas should be left open to the air
    ② These products impede ice application to burn areas
    ③ These products prevent blisters from being broken
    ④ These products seal in heat

35. Two teenagers are playing frisbee in the park. Suddenly one of them sustains a blow to the nose from the frisbee, resulting in rapid epistaxis. To prevent aspiration of blood, the victim should be placed in which of the following positions?
    ① Side lying
    ② Supine
    ③ Upright with head tilted backward
    ④ Upright with head tilted forward

CHAPTER 12

Current Trends in Nursing and Health Care in the United States and Canada

This text emphasizes the role responsibilities of the licensed practical/vocational nurse (LP/VN) as a member of the health care team. This chapter reviews the history of practical/vocational nursing and functions of the professional organizations; explores ethical and legal aspects, focusing on professional obligations and patients' rights; and discusses the delivery of health care and the changes within the system as they relate to the LP/VN.

PRACTICAL/VOCATIONAL NURSING
History

A. Practical/vocational nursing evolved to provide better use of nursing personnel and to ease the shortage of nurses
B. The first school to train practical/vocational nurses was the Ballard School in New York City, founded in 1893. This 3-month program taught care of chronic invalids, elderly persons, and children
C. In 1907 the Thompson School was founded in Brattleboro, Vermont. The Household Nursing Association School of Attendant Nursing was founded in Boston in 1918. The Thompson School is still in existence
D. These first training programs prepared the practical/vocational nurse for home care. Courses included cooking, care of the house, dietetics, and simple nursing procedures
E. In the 1940s there were about 50 approved programs
F. During the 1950s the number of schools of practical/vocational nursing grew. Most programs were extended to 12 months, and placed emphasis on integrating class instruction with clinical experience
G. In 1956 Public Law 911 appropriated millions of dollars for the improvement and expansion of practical/vocational nurse training. The United States Office of Education established a practical nurse education service
H. Today practical/vocational nursing schools are located in hospitals, colleges, and vocational-technical schools
I. In 1990 there were 1069 practical/vocational nursing programs, with a student enrollment of 52,749
J. Today approximately 887,800 licensed practical/vocational nurses are working in the United States—the second largest group of health care providers in the nation's system

Education

A. Practical/vocational nursing programs must meet requirements and be approved by the state board of nursing
B. Practical/vocational nursing schools of high standards

may voluntarily apply for national accreditation by the National League for Nursing
C. Admission requirements to practical/vocational nursing programs vary, but generally applicants must
1. Be at least 17 years of age
2. Have a high school diploma or equivalent
3. Have good physical and mental health
4. Be of good moral character
D. The curriculum incorporates content and concepts from the biologic and physical sciences, behavioral sciences, and principles and practices of nursing
E. The curriculum includes nursing theory and clinical practice, which provide the students with learning opportunities to meet physical and psychosocial needs of mothers and infants, children, medical-surgical patients, the elderly, and patients with long-term illnesses
F. Graduates receive a diploma or certificate and are eligible to take the practical/vocational nurse licensing examination
G. Practical/vocational nursing is the entry level into the practice of nursing

Role Responsibilities

A. The licensed practical/vocational nurse (LP/VN) has a vital and effective role as a member of the health care team
B. The LP/VN provides direct nursing care to patients whose conditions are stable under the supervision and direction of a registered nurse or physician
C. The LP/VN assists the registered nurse with the care of patients whose conditions are unstable and complex
D. The LP/VN, adhering to the nursing process, observes, assesses, records, reports, and performs basic therapeutic, preventive, and rehabilitative procedures
E. LP/VNs work in acute and long-term care hospitals, nursing homes, physician's offices, ambulatory care facilities, home health agencies, community agencies, and industries
F. To identify the abilities of the beginning practitioner in

practical/vocational nursing, see the statement by the National Association for Practical Nurse Education and Service in the box to the right

Continuing Education

A. Each LP/VN has the responsibility to maintain competency and increase level of knowledge
B. The rapid growth of nursing and medical knowledge and advances in technology require nurses to keep up-to-date
C. The LP/VN must take advantage of learning opportunities through in-service programs where employed; attending seminars and workshops available through institutions, school, official, or voluntary organizations; and reading professional journals
D. Membership in nursing organizations provides continuing education opportunities, usually at a lower cost to their members

THE PATIENT'S CARE
Nurse-Patient Relationship

A. The nurse-patient relationship must always be professional
B. Phases of a nurse-patient relationship
    1. Initiation phase: during this stage boundaries are established and goals are defined
        a. Begins as soon as the nurse and patient meet
        b. Important to build trust and instill confidence
        c. Preparation for termination begins during this stage
    2. Working phase
        a. Begins when trust has been established
        b. LP/VN uses interpersonal skills to foster communication
    3. Termination phase: period preceding the permanent separation
        a. Time to say good-bye; important to prepare in advance
        b. Can be difficult for both nurse and patient
C. Developing a relationship first requires knowing and understanding self as a person, including attitudes, values, and beliefs
D. Important part of nursing is developing a therapeutic relationship by
    1. Meeting the patient's needs promptly
    2. Accepting patient as a worthy human being
    3. Conveying a nonjudgmental manner
    4. Treating patient as a whole person
    5. Providing empathy not sympathy
    6. Listening to patient: involves hearing and interpreting what is heard
    7. Having concern for patient's preferences

Health Care Team

A. Members of the health care team vary depending on the patient's needs and goals
B. Constant team members are
    1. Physicians: diagnose and prescribe
    2. Nurses: plan and carry out nursing care
    3. Patient and family: participate in planning care
C. Other team members include physical therapists, social workers, occupational therapists, respiratory therapists, dietitians, clergy, and others

---

National Association for Practical Nurse Education and Service, Statement of Practical/Vocational Nursing Entry Level Competencies

Assessment

Uses basic communication skills in a structured care setting
Obtains specific information from patients through goal-directed interviews
Participates in the identification of physical, emotional, spiritual, cultural, and overt learning needs of patients by collecting appropriate data
Analyzes data collected in relation to patients' pathophysiology

Planning

Determines priorities and plans nursing care accordingly
Formulates and/or collaborates in developing written nursing care plans
Participates in developing preventive or long-term health plans for patients and/or families

Implementation

Protects the rights and dignity of patients and families
Uses basic communication skills in a structured care setting
Safely performs therapeutic and preventive nursing procedures, incorporating fundamental biologic and psychologic principles in giving individualized care
Observes patients and communicates significant findings to the health care team
Conducts incidental teaching and supports and reinforces the teaching plan for a specific patient and/or family

Evaluation

Evaluates, with guidance if necessary, the care given and makes necessary adjustments
Records evaluations of the results of nursing actions
Identifies own strengths and weaknesses and seeks assistance for improvement of performance

Professional responsibilities

Recognizes the LP/VN's role in the health care delivery system and articulates that role with those of other health care team members
Maintains accountability for own nursing practice within ethical and legal framework
Serves as a patient advocate
Accepts role in maintaining and developing standards of practice in providing patient care
Participates in nursing organizations
Seeks further growth through educational opportunities

D. Successful nursing care depends on the interaction and cooperation of all members of the team
E. The LP/VN collaborates with team members

Delivery of Nursing Care

A. Functional method: each nursing team member is assigned specific tasks (e.g., obtaining and recording all vital signs, administering all medications)
B. Team nursing: a group of patients are cared for by a team consisting of professional nurses, practical/vocational nurses, nurses' aides, and student nurses

C. Primary nursing
 1. One nurse assigned to patient from admission to discharge, usually registered nurse
 2. Total responsibility for care on all shifts
 3. Coordinates care with other health workers, for example, LP/VN, aide

LEGISLATION RELATED TO PRACTICE OF LP/VN
Nurse Practice Act

A. Nursing is subject to laws passed by the state's legislature
B. Laws pertaining to nursing are in the state's nurse practice act
C. The nurse practice act varies from state to state. Some states define the practice of nursing, whereas others describe what a nurse may or may not do in the practice of nursing
D. The nurse practice act also provides for some type of nursing board to regulate nursing practice and procedures for
 1. Approval of nursing schools and curriculum requirements
 2. Licensure and renewal
 3. Grounds for suspension and revocation of licensure
E. The LP/VN must practice nursing within the legally defined scope of her state's nurse practice act

State Boards of Nursing

A. Administer the state nurse practice act
B. Membership on the board varies from state to state, usually consists of RNs, LP/VNs, and consumers appointed by the governor
C. In most states, both professional and practical/vocational nursing practice are under the same board; some states have two boards, one for each
D. Functions
 1. Enforces established educational requirements of schools of nursing
 a. Surveys program to determine if preestablished standards are being met
 b. Approves new programs that meet standards
 c. Withholds or withdraws approval from programs that do not meet standards
 2. Controls licensure
 a. Administers the official licensure examination
 b. Grants license to authorized applicants
 c. Renews license
 d. Denies, suspends, or revokes license for cause
 3. Conducts investigations and hearings relating to charges of unsafe nursing practice
 4. Interpret the nurse practice act based on past practice, standard of care, and information from other states

Licensure

A. Protects the public from unqualified practitioners
B. A license is mandatory to practice nursing
C. Permits use of title LPN or LVN
D. Qualifications vary from state to state but most require
 1. Graduation from an approved program in practical/vocational nursing
 2. Proof of moral character

 3. Attaining a minimum score on the nationally administered examination
E. License must be renewed for a small fee at regular intervals
F. Many states require LP/VN to submit proof of continuing education before license will be renewed
G. License may be revoked or suspended for acts of misconduct or incompetence such as drug addiction or conviction of a felony
H. Licensure by endorsement occurs when a state board of nursing reviews the credentials of a nurse licensed in another state and determines that the nurse meets the qualifications of their state

Examination

A. All states as of October 1986 administer the National Council of State Boards of Nursing (NCSBN) examination, called the NCLEX-PN (National Council Licensure Examination for Practical Nurses)
B. Used to determine if LP/VN candidate is prepared to practice nursing safely by testing knowledge of nursing care and the ability to apply that knowledge in a clinical situation
C. Given twice a year: April and October
D. All states administer examination on same day
E. Passing score determined by the National Council of State Boards of Nursing

ETHICAL PRINCIPLES: CODE OF ETHICS

A. Principles established by professional group as a means of self-regulation
B. Each LP/VN is responsible for upholding the professional standards of conduct and ethics

LEGAL IMPLICATIONS FOR THE LP/VN
Responsibilities

A. Function within the scope of state nurse practice act
B. Maintain standards of care (see the standards of practice for the LP/VN in the box to the right)
C. Function according to employer or agency policy
D. Apply the skills and knowledge that a prudent LP/VN with comparable training would apply in a similar situation
E. Maintain complete and accurate patient records
F. Maintain confidentiality

Illegal Actions

A. Torts—civil law
 1. An act or wrong committed by one person against another that results in injury or damage
 2. Can be either the commission or omission of an act
 3. Acts of negligence include
 a. Professional misconduct
 b. Performing care incorrectly
 c. Illegal or immoral conduct
 d. Examples include
 (1) Administration of wrong medication
 (2) Administration of medication or treatment to wrong patient
 (3) Failure to ensure safety through use of side rails or restraints as ordered by the physician

Standards of Practice for the LP/VN

The LP/VN provides individual and family-centered nursing care

Follow principles of nursing process in meeting specific needs of patients of all ages in the areas of safety, hygiene, nutrition, medication, elimination, psychosocial, cultural, and respiratory needs

Apply appropriate knowledge, skills, and abilities in providing safe, competent care

Apply principles of crisis intervention in maintaining safety and making appropriate referrals when necessary

Use effective communication skills

- Communicate effectively with patients, family, significant others, and members of the healthcare team
- Maintain appropriate written documentation

Provide appropriate health teaching to patients and significant others in the areas of

- Maintenance of wellness
- Rehabilitation
- Use of community resources

Serve as a patient advocate

- Protect patient's rights
- Consult with appropriate others when necessary

The LP/VN fulfills the professional responsibilities of the practical/vocational nurse

Know and apply the ethical principles underlying the profession

Know and follow the appropriate professional and legal requirements

Follow the policies and procedures of the employing institution

Cooperate and collaborate with all members of the health care team to meet the needs of family-centered nursing care

Demonstrate accountability for own nursing actions

Maintain current knowledge and skills in the area of employment

Adapted from Standards of Practice for LP/VN.
Adopted in 1985 by the National Association for Practical Nurse Education and Service.

(4) Failure to prevent injury while applying heat
  e. Gross negligence: patient's life is endangered or lost—often results in criminal action
B. Intentional torts
  1. Legal liability exists even if no damage occurs to the other person
  2. May not be covered by malpractice insurance
  3. Assault and battery
    a. Assault
      (1) Definition: threat or attempt to make bodily contact with another person without that person's consent with intent to injure
      (2) Example: threatening to restrain or physically punish patient if he or she does not cooperate
    b. Battery
      (1) Definition: act of making unauthorized contact
      (2) Example: nurse actually restrains patient

4. False imprisonment
  a. Definition: unwarranted restriction of another person by force or threat of force
  b. Example detaining patient in hospital against his or her will; unwarranted use of restraints
  c. Patient who wishes to leave hospital against advice of physician may be asked to sign a release; cannot detain patient if he or she refuses to sign
5. Invasion of privacy
  a. Definition: unauthorized disclosures about a patient even if information is true
  b. Examples
    (1) Release of patient's medical information
    (2) Exposure of patient during procedures or transportation
6. Defamation
  a. Definition: attack on the name, business, or professional reputation of another through false and malicious statements to a third person
  b. Types
    (1) Slander: oral statements
    (2) Libel: written statement

Other Legal Aspects

A. Good Samaritan laws
  1. Laws that give certain persons legal protection when giving aid at the scene of an accident; not all states cover nurses
  2. Purpose: to encourage people to give assistance at the scene of an emergency
  3. These laws do not make it legally necessary for a nurse to assist
  4. When nurses do assist, they are expected to use good judgment in deciding whether an emergency exists
  5. The LP/VN is expected to give a standard of care that a reasonable LP/VN with comparable training would give in similar circumstances
B. Child abuse
  1. All states have laws that require reporting known or suspected cases of child abuse
  2. The laws grant immunity from civil suits to those who are required to report child abuse
C. Narcotics
  1. The Federal Controlled Substances Act of 1970 is a federal law that regulates the manufacture, sale, prescription, and dispensing of narcotics and other harmful drugs
  2. Violation of the law by a nurse is a felony and will result in revocation of the LP/VN license
D. Wills
  1. A legal declaration of how a person (testator) wishes to dispose of his or her property after death
  2. For a will to be valid, the testator must be of sound mind and acting without force
  3. No legal reason for the nurse not to witness a will; the witness is only witnessing the person's signature, not the contents of the will
  4. A beneficiary of the will must not witness it
E. Malpractice insurance
  1. Professional liability policies cover liability arising out of the rendering of or failure to render professional service

2. Policy is safeguard against suits for damages; can be expensive to prove innocence
3. Can be purchased from nursing organizations, bargaining organizations, and private insurance companies
4. Provides monetary award of damages within specified limits of the policy, also legal fees, court costs, and payment of bond
5. Employer's insurance only protects employee while on duty

PATIENTS' RIGHTS
Bill of Rights

A. Patients have the right to courteous, individual care given without discrimination as to race, color, religion, sex, marital status, national origin, or ability to pay
B. A patient's bill of rights is a statement of what the patient can expect from the institution
C. The following is paraphrased from the Patient's Bill of Rights adopted by the American Hospital Association. The patient should
   1. Be given considerate and respectful care
   2. Obtain from the physician complete current information concerning diagnosis, treatment, and prognosis in terms he or she can be reasonably expected to understand
   3. Receive from the physician information necessary to give informed consent prior to the start of any procedure or treatment
   4. Be allowed to refuse treatment to the extent permitted by law and be informed of the medical consequences of that action
   5. Be given every consideration of privacy concerning his or her own medical care program
   6. Expect that all communications and records pertaining to his or her care be treated as confidential
   7. Expect that within its capacity a hospital must make reasonable response to the request of a patient for services
   8. Obtain information as to any relationships of the patient's hospital to other health care and educational institutions insofar as his or her care is concerned
   9. Be advised if the hospital proposes to engage in or perform human experimentation affecting the patient's care or treatment
   10. Expect reasonable continuity of care
   11. Examine and receive an explanation of the bill regardless of the source of payment
   12. Know what hospital rules and regulations apply to the patient's conduct

Standard of Care

A. Patients are entitled to a safe, competent standard of nursing care no matter who administers it (RN, LP/VN, student)
B. The LP/VN is accountable for her own actions and must ensure that the patient receives qualified care
C. If the LP/VN thinks that the patient assignment is beyond her ability, the LP/VN must discuss the matter with the registered nurse before carrying it out

D. Standard of care is established by
   1. State nurse practice act
   2. Institution's job description
   3. Hospital policies and procedures
   4. Patient's nursing care plan

Patient Advocate

A. An advocate acts on behalf of another person and stands up or speaks up on behalf of that person
B. Patient has the right to information needed to make informed decisions freely and without pressure
C. The responsibility of the LP/VN is to
   1. Maintain standard of care
   2. Support patients in the decisions they make
   3. Inform physician when the patient apparently does not understand what is going to happen to him or her
   4. Observe and speak out regarding instances of incompetent, unethical, or illegal practice by any member of the health care team
   5. Know hospital policy regarding procedure to follow when patients' rights are being violated
D. Many hospitals employ a patient representative who serves as a liaison between patient and institution and who has the power to act to resolve patients' problems

Consent Forms

A. Before any procedure can be performed, the patient must give written consent, except in extreme emergency when failure to treat may be considered negligence
B. Patient must be fully informed of the extent of the proposed procedure, risks and benefits, alternatives, and their consequences
C. Consent must be obtained by the physician, whose duty it is to advise the patient
D. Consent may be withdrawn by the patient prior to the procedure

Patient's Medical Records

A. The chart is a legal document
B. Provides a written account of the patient's hospitalization
C. May be used as evidence in courts of law; records only information related to patient's health problem
D. Information contained in records must be held in confidence
E. Only authorized persons should have access to patient's records
F. Most states consider medical records the property of the hospital, and the contents the property of the patient

NURSING ORGANIZATIONS

A. Membership
   1. LP/VN has the responsibility to join a professional organization and support practical/vocational nursing by becoming an active member
   2. Membership provides
      a. Fellowship and interaction with other LP/VNs
      b. Opportunity to enhance and strengthen role of LP/VN
      c. Means to keep current on issues relating to practical/vocational nursing

d. A voice in planning policies of the association

e. Continuing education opportunities

B. National Association for Practical Nurse Education and Service (NAPNES)*

1. NAPNES was organized in 1941 to promote the development of sound practical/vocational nursing education and to promote advancement and recognition of the LP/VN as a member of the health team

2. Membership includes

a. Regular members: LP/VNs, practical nursing educators, other registered nurses, general educators, physicians, hospital and nursing home administrators, practical nursing students, and interested laypersons

b. Student members: students in state-approved schools of practical/vocational nursing

c. Agency members: hospitals, nursing homes, schools of practical nursing, alumni groups, civic organizations, and other institutions or groups in harmony with NAPNES' objectives

3. Functions and activities listed by NAPNES

a. Serves as clearing house for information about practical/vocational nursing, including information about functions and roles of LP/VNs

b. Publishes *Journal of Practical Nursing*, a monthly magazine

c. Prepares publications useful to faculties in schools of practical/vocational nursing

d. Sponsors workshops and seminars for LP/VNs and practical nursing educators in conjunction with state LP/VN associations, universities, and national organizations

e. Engages in activities aimed at protecting and strengthening position of LP/VNs and cooperates with state LP/VN associations in activities of this kind

f. Provides consultation to state LP/VN constituencies on matters relating to their organization and programs

C. National Federation of Licensed Practical Nurses (NFLPN)†

1. NFLPN was organized in 1949 to foster high standards in practical nursing and to promote practical nursing

2. Membership limited to LP/VNs and student practical/vocational nurses

3. Affiliate membership is available to individuals who are not LP/VNs or students but are interested in the work of NFLPN

4. There are state associations in many states

5. Functions of the NFLPN

a. Provides leadership for LP/VNs employed in the US

b. Fosters high standards of practical/vocational nursing education and practice

c. Encourages every LP/VN to make continuing education a priority

d. Achieves recognition for LP/VNs and advocates

the effectiveness of LP/VNs in every type of health care facility

e. Interprets the role and function of the LP/VN for the public

f. Represents practical/vocational nursing through relationships with other national nursing, medical, and allied health organizations, legislators, government officials, health agencies, educators, and other professional groups

g. Serves as the central source of information on the new and changing aspects of practical/vocational nursing education and practice

D. National League for Nursing (NLN)*

1. The NLN was organized in 1952 by combining the National League for Nursing Education and six other national nursing organizations

2. Membership includes

a. Individual membership: anyone interested in nursing; registered nurses, LP/VNs, student nurses, consumers

b. Agency membership: hospitals, nursing homes, public health agencies, schools of nursing

3. Functions are

a. Defining and furthering good standards for all nursing service

b. Defining and promoting good standards for institutions giving nursing education on all levels

c. Helping to extend facilities to meet these services when necessary

d. Helping in proper distribution of nursing education and nursing service

e. Working to improve organized nursing services in hospitals, public health agencies, nursing homes, and other agencies; accrediting community public health nursing services; developing criteria and other self-evaluation tools

f. Working to improve nursing education programs; acting as an accrediting agency for all levels of nursing education

g. Constructing, processing, and providing preadmission, achievement, and qualifying tests

h. Gathering and publishing information about trends in nursing, personnel needs, community nursing services, and schools of nursing

4. Official journal is *Nursing and Health Care*

5. In 1984 the NLN Council of Practical Nursing Programs adopted a resolution that recognized the NFLPN as the official organization for LP/VNs

E. National Council of State Boards of Nursing (NCSBN)†

1. Established in 1978 to strengthen and coordinate the credentialing of nurses nationally

2. Membership open to any state board of nursing; presently composed of 53 state boards

3. Maintains a liaison with national organizations that represent nursing

4. Controls the NCLEX, which prepares the LP/VN and RN licensure examinations

*1400 Spring Street, Suite 310, Silver Spring, MD 20910.
†PO. Box 18088, 3948 Browning Place, Raleigh, NC 27619.

*350 Hudson Street, New York, NY, 10014.
†676 N St Clair, Suite 550, Chicago, Ill 60611.

National League for Nursing Statement Supporting Practical/Vocational Nursing and Practical/Vocational Nursing Education*

The Executive Committee of the Council of Practical Nursing Programs of the National League for Nursing believes that practical/vocational nursing is a vital component of the occupation of nursing and supports those who elect practical/vocational nursing as a permanent career choice. The minimal educational credential for entry into practical/vocational nursing is a diploma or certificate.

Nursing is an occupation that exists on a continuum, and education for nursing can be developed at different levels of knowledge and skills required to fulfill identified yet different nursing roles. The nursing profession has an obligation to society to develop sound and efficient patterns for nursing education that meet the varied nursing needs of society and permit educational options for those who wish them.

Practical/vocational nurses are involved in the nursing process. Practical/vocational nurses, with the supervision and direction of a registered nurse or physician, utilize the nursing process to give direct care to patients whose conditions are considered to be stable. This care encompasses observation, assessment, recording, reporting to appropriate persons, and performing basic therapeutic, preventive, and rehabilitative procedures. When patients' conditions are unstable and complex, the practical/vocational nurse assists and collaborates with the registered nurse in the provision of care.

The practical/vocational nurse is prepared for employment in health care settings in which the policies and protocols for providing patient care are well defined and in which supervision and direction by a registered nurse or physician are present. These settings may be acute or long-term care hospitals, nursing homes, home health agencies, and ambulatory care facilities.

Practical/vocational nurses function within the definition and framework of the regulations set forth by the nurse practice act of the state in which they are employed. The practice of practical/vocational nursing requires licensure, which is the responsibility of the board of nursing in each state, in order to protect the public and safeguard nursing practice.

Education of the practical/vocational nurse is characterized by its consistent emphasis on the clinical practice experience necessary to meet common nursing problems. The curriculum—based on concepts from the physical and biologic sciences that underlie nursing measures and the behavioral science concepts necessary to individualize care—is a planned sequence of correlated theory and clinical experience.

On completion of the program of study in practical/vocational nursing, the graduate demonstrates the specific competencies related to assessment, planning, implementation, and evaluation of nursing care as identified by the Council of Practical Nursing Programs.

The licensed practical/vocational nurse is responsible for maintaining and updating her or his competencies. Adequate orientation and continuing inservice education are responsibilities of the employing agency. However, the practical/vocational nurse must take advantage of other opportunities for continuing self-improvement and, if desired, career advancement.

Opportunities for career mobility without undue penalty must exist in the system of nursing education to provide for changing career goals.

*Issued in 1982, reaffirmed in 1987.

F. American Nurses Association (ANA)*
   1. National organization for registered nurses formed in 1896 as the Nurses Association Alumnae; renamed ANA in 1911
   2. Concerned with standard of nursing practice and promoting general welfare of the professional nurse
   3. Membership limited to registered nurses
   4. Publishes *American Journal of Nursing (AJN),* a monthly magazine
G. Alumni associations
   1. Organization of graduates from the LP/VN's respective school
   2. Membership provides a means of
      a. Keeping informed of school's progress
      b. Offering suggestions to improve programs
      c. Providing continuing education
      d. Facilitating social activities with classmates and other graduates
      e. Offering scholarships to future students

CONCEPT OF HEALTH AND ILLNESS

A. The World Health Organization (WHO) defines health as "a state of complete physical, mental and social well-being and not just the absence of disease and infirmity"
B. Health and illness continuum
   1. The continuum is an abstract horizontal line, with optimum health functioning at one end, and death at the other
   2. The continuum allows for levels of wellness
   3. Level of wellness depends on internal and external factors, the person's ability to adapt, and the level of adaptation that is achieved
   4. Level of wellness is continually changing
   5. High-level wellness is functioning at one's best
C. Many factors influence levels
   1. Physical disabilities
   2. Heredity
   3. Age
   4. Environment
   5. Socioeconomic status
   6. Level of education
   7. Religious affiliation
   8. Culture/background
   9. General life-style
D. Stress: many diseases are related to stress
   1. A certain amount of stress is beneficial to life
   2. Stress factors may be internal or external
   3. Stresses may be physical, psychologic, cultural, or social
   4. Stress affects health when coping mechanism is insufficient
E. Leading causes of death in United States
   1. Heart disease
   2. Cancer
   3. Cerebrovascular disease
   4. Accidents

TRENDS IN DELIVERY OF HEALTH CARE

A. Traditionally the health care focus was on diagnosis and treatment of disease

*600 Maryland Avenue, SW, Suite 100 West, Washington, DC. 20024.

B. Trends
   1. Emphasis on prevention of illness and maintenance of health
   2. Decrease in length of hospital stay
   3. Rise in home health care
C. Reason for changes in delivery of health care
   1. Technologic advances: scientific knowledge has provided early diagnosis and effective treatment of diseases
   2. Consumer movement: the public has exerted pressure for the right to health at an affordable price through legislative action
   3. Population change: life expectancy has significantly increased with an increase in the number of elderly and a declining birth rate
   4. Nature of disease pattern is changing: decrease in acute diseases with an increase in chronic and degenerative diseases
   5. Continuing scrutiny of health care costs
D. Related health problems
   1. Growing technology and use of complex scientific equipment has caused
      a. Increase in cost of health care; even a short hospitalization can be financially crippling
      b. Fragmentation of care caused by increased number of health workers required by technology
   2. Increased population has caused health problems related to air, noise, and water pollution with overcrowding and unsanitary living conditions
   3. Aging population: more likely for elderly persons to become ill and to develop chronic and degenerative diseases
   4. Uneven distribution of health care facilities and resources available for
      a. Elderly, poor, and minorities
      b. Rural areas and inner cities

PREVENTION AND MAINTENANCE OF HEALTH
Barriers to Preventive Health Care

A. High cost
   1. Preventive measures not always covered under insurance plan
   2. Lower economic group unable to finance cost
B. Inconvenience
   1. Clinics usually open during day
   2. Difficult to get appointment with physician
C. Unpleasantness of diagnostic or treatment measures accompanied by fear of pain
D. Fear of findings causes many to seek care only after symptoms are acute

Levels of Health Care

A. Primary
   1. Promotion of health and prevention of disease including
      a. Immunization against infectious diseases
      b. Health education such as nutrition counseling
      c. Physical fitness program
      d. Research to find cause of disease
   2. Primary care takes place in prenatal centers, well-baby centers, schools, and health maintenance organizations

B. Secondary
   1. Early diagnosis and treatment to stop progress of disease
   2. Prevention of complications
   3. The largest and most expensive segment of the health care delivery system
   4. Secondary care usually takes place in hospitals, but also occurs in clinics and physicians' offices
C. Tertiary
   1. Rehabilitation after illness to return the patient to a level of maximum functioning
   2. Involves assessing patient's strengths and weaknesses, assisting the patient to increase strengths and cope with limitations, assisting with rehabilitation measures, and encouraging self-care
   3. Agencies providing tertiary care are rehabilitation hospitals, skilled nursing homes, and hospices
   4. Other groups involved with rehabilitation are special interest groups such as Alcoholics Anonymous and Reach to Recovery

Role of LP/VN

A. To act as a role model by promoting personal health
   1. Assess own health status through regular physical and dental examinations
   2. Observe basic principles of personal hygiene and avoid products known to be harmful to health such as tobacco and drugs
   3. Provide for adequate rest, sleep, and nutrition
   4. Participate in primary care programs
   5. Obtain treatment of any infection or injury
B. LP/VN functions within the health care system
   1. Promote health: patient teaching
   2. Prevention of disease: provide safe environment for patients; encourage and participate in screening programs
   3. Discovery and treatment of disease by assisting physician with patient's physical examination, making observations, collecting specimens and data, and performing procedures as ordered
   4. Rehabilitation: assist patients with rehabilitation procedures

HEALTH CARE AGENCIES

A. The LP/VN should know what resources are available, what services they provide, and how to make use of the services
B. International agency
   1. WHO is an agency of the United Nations established in 1948
   2. WHO assists nations to strengthen and improve their health services by providing advisory service in disease control
C. Official agencies in the United States—federal, state, and local—are supported by tax dollars and are accountable to the public
   1. Department of Health and Human Services (DHHS)
      a. Administration of federal programs relating to health is under the jurisdiction of the DHHS
      b. The DHHS has five divisions
         (1) Social Security Administration (SSA): administers the national system of health, old age, survivor, and disability insurance

(2) Health Care Financing Administration: created in 1977 to oversee the Medicare and Medicaid programs

(3) Office of Human Development Services: administers programs on aging, children, youth and families, and native Americans

(4) Public Health Service (PHS): involved with improving and protecting the health and environment of the United States; the major components of the PHS include

    (a) Centers for Disease Control

    (b) Food and Drug Administration

    (c) Health Resources and Services Administration

    (d) National Institutes of Health

    (e) Alcohol, Drug Abuse, and Mental Health Administration

(5) Family Support Administration

2. State health departments

  a. Supported by tax funds from the state

  b. Functions vary among the states; usually responsible for licensing of hospitals, nursing homes, and undertakers; health education materials; vital statistics; and communicable disease control

3. Local health department functions also vary; the general functions include

  a. Keeping vital statistics

  b. Reporting communicable diseases

  c. Maternal and child health service

  d. Environmental sanitation; inspecting food establishments

D. Voluntary agencies

1. Depend on voluntary contributions for funds

2. Concerned with prevention and solution of specific health problem

3. Provide funds for research and educational projects

4. National organizations function through state or local chapters; examples of voluntary agencies are

  a. The American Cancer Society

  b. The American Diabetes Association

  c. The American Heart Association

  d. The American Red Cross

  e. The National Society for the Prevention of Blindness

E. Health service providers: presently a realignment of services is shifting care from acute hospital setting to ambulatory and home care

1. Hospitals

  a. Short-term facilities provide acute care for patients undergoing treatment for health problems

  b. Long-term facilities provide service over an extended period for patients with chronic or long-term health problems; rehabilitation as well as recreational and occupational therapy are stressed

2. Nursing homes, also called long-term or extended care facilities; the federal government has established two categories of nursing homes

  a. Skilled nursing facility (SNF), which provides 24-hour nursing service for the recuperating resident who no longer needs intensive nursing but still requires skilled nursing

  b. Intermediate care facility (ICF), which provides regular nursing care, but not around the clock, for residents not capable of living by themselves

3. Hospices

  a. Care provided to assist the terminally ill patient to achieve the highest possible quality of life

  b. The goal is to maintain the patient in his or her own environment

  c. Care is provided in the home by home care nurses

4. Home care

  a. Provides continuity and comprehensive health service for individuals who do not need to be hospitalized but who require more than ambulatory care

  b. Services provided vary from homemaker services to skilled nursing care

  c. Estimated skilled nursing care may be provided at one third of the cost of hospitalization

5. Ambulatory care: care provided on outpatient basis

6. Geriatric day-care centers: patients are cared for during the day at the center and returned home during the evening

F. Financing health care

1. Health maintenance organizations (HMOs)

  a. Provide comprehensive health services to participants on a prepaid basis

  b. Emphasize primary care to prevent costly illness and hospitalization

  c. Does not cover illness outside service area

2. Medicare and Medicaid are government-supported health insurance programs created in 1965 by an amendment to the Social Security Act

  a. Medicare, title XVIII, provides medical care to the elderly receiving Social Security benefits regardless of their need, to people with permanent disabilities, and to those with end stages of renal disease

  b. Medicaid, title XIX, was designed to defray expenses that Medicare did not provide for the elderly in need; it also provides services for the poor; program is jointly sponsored with matching funds from federal and state governments; today the states contribute a larger share than the federal govenment

3. Diagnosis-related groups (DRGs)

  a. In 1983 a public law (PL98:21) was passed that reformed the Medicare reimbursement system, establishing a prospective payment system (PPS) based on DRG categories

  b. All in-hospital admissions are divided into DRGs, and payment is made prospectively based on the cost averages of each individual DRG

  c. Hospital will know in advance what they will be paid; if treatment costs less, hospital keeps the difference; if treatment cost exceeds payment, hospital will have to absorb cost

  d. Built into the DRG system is the Professional Standards Review Board (PSRB), which reviews admissions, discharge practice, and quality of care to protect against abuses in the system

  e. The PPS provides an incentive for hospitals to be efficient and economical in patient care

f. The PPS affects patient census because hospitals discharge patients sooner to be cost efficient; the demand for long-term care and home care will continue to increase

g. Many states have implemented prospective payment for all acute hospital cost reimbursement

PRACTICAL/VOCATIONAL NURSING IN CANADA
History

A. There has always been a person working as an assistant to the professional nurse

B. During and following World War II there was a shortage of nurses; to meet this need, hospitals began a variety of short courses on the job

C. In response to these many and varied short courses, the Canadian Nurses Association developed a syllabus for a course to be used as a guide by provincial nursing associations, with the aim of standardizing courses

D. The title for graduates suggested by the CNA was "nursing assistant"

E. In 1940 Ontario was the first province to pass legislation protecting the title "certified nursing assistant"

F. In 1941 the Registered Nurses Association of Ontario opened a demonstration school in London, Ontario, to determine the feasibility of training an auxiliary group; the course lasted 6 months and had a grade 8 admission requirement

G. Following the war, arrangements were made through the Department of Veterans Affairs, the national and provincial nursing associations, and the departments of health and education in each province to organize courses to meet the needs of people released from the armed services

H. Standardized courses developed across the country were offered to the public in such places as hospitals, secondary schools, and technical/vocational schools, as well as independent schools

I. Each province assumed responsibility for supervising the course of instruction, evaluating the programs, and registering/licensing the graduates, plus designating their title: this accounts for the variation in title, program lengths, and responsibilities of the nursing assistant across the country

J. In 1971 the Ontario Association for Nursing Assistants began discussions with the other provinces to form a national organization

K. In 1975 the Canadian Association of Practical Nursing Assistants was incorporated; all provinces are affiliated except Quebec

L. There are currently approximately 84,000 practical/vocational nurses in Canada

Education

A. Practical/vocational nursing programs must meet requirements of the registering/licensing body in each province/territory

B. There is no national accreditation body for nursing in Canada

C. Admission requirements vary from province to province and the territories; a high school diploma or its equivalent is usually required

D. The curriculum incorporates content and concepts from the biologic and psychosocial sciences, as well as principles and practice of nursing

E. The curriculum includes nursing theory and clinical practice, which provide the students with learning opportunities to meet physical, psychosocial, and spiritual needs of patients across the lifespan

F. Graduates receive a diploma or certificate and are eligible to take the certification/licensing examination in their jurisdiction

Responsibilities of the Canadian Practical/ Vocational Nurse

A. The practical/vocational nurse has a vital and effective role as a member of the health care team

B. The practical/vocational nurse provides direct nursing care to patients whose conditions are stable under the supervision and direction of a registered nurse or physician

C. The practical/vocational nurse aids the registered nurse with the care of patients whose conditions are unstable and complex

D. The practical/vocational nurse, using the nursing process, observes, assesses, records, reports, and performs basic therapeutic, preventive, and rehabilitative procedures

E. The practical/vocational nurse works in acute and long-term care hospitals, nursing homes, physicians' offices, ambulatory care facilities, home health agencies, public health agencies, community agencies, and industry

F. The practical/vocational nurse uses the nursing process, that is, assessment, planning, implementation, and evaluation, in delivering nursing care in all settings

G. The practical/vocational nurse practices within the legal and ethical boundaries for the province/territory

Continuing Education

A. Each practical/vocational nurse has the responsibility to maintain competency and increase level of knowledge

B. The rapid growth of medical knowledge and advances in technology make it necessary that practical/vocational nurses keep up-to-date

C. The practical/vocational nurse must take advantage of learning opportunities through in-service programs where employed; attending seminars and workshops available through institutions and school, official, or voluntary organizations; and reading professional journals

D. Membership in nursing organizations provides continuing education opportunities, usually at a lower cost to their members

Legislation Related to Practice of Practical/ Vocational Nursing in Canada

A. Legislation
   1. Nursing is subject to legislation passed by each province/territory
   2. Laws pertaining to nursing are specific to each province/territory
   3. The regulating body is designated through legislation in each province/territory
   4. Each province/territory designates a body to approve and review nursing schools

B. Regulatory body: each province/territory has either an

independent body such as a council or a college or a professional association responsible for the practice of its members

C. Certification/registration/licensure
   1. Each province/territory determines the title held by the practical/vocational nurse in that jurisdiction
   2. Certification, registration, and licensure ensure the public of a minimum standard of safe nursing care
   3. Registration protects the title of the registrant only; licensure also protects the practice of nursing
   4. Certificates/licenses are usually renewed annually
   5. Certificates/licenses may be revoked or suspended for acts of misconduct, negligence, or incompetence as outlined in legislation
D. Examination
   1. All provinces and territories except Quebec purchase the Canadian Nurses Association examinations
   2. The CNA examination for practical/vocational nurses is held three times a year, in March, June, and October
   3. All provinces and territories administer the examination on the same day
   4. Passing scores are determined by each province or territory; 350 is generally required
   5. Quebec administers its own examinations

Canadian Nursing Organizations

A. Canadian Association of Practical Nursing Assistants (CAPNA)*: all provincial associations are affiliated with CAPNA except Quebec
B. Membership
   1. The practical/vocational nurse has the responsibility to join a professional organization and support practical/vocational nurses by becoming an active member
   2. Membership provides
      a. Fellowship and interaction with other practical/vocational nurses
      b. Opportunity to enhance and strengthen role of practical/vocational nurse
      c. Means to keep current on issues relating to the practical/vocational nurse
      d. A voice in planning and policies of the association
      e. Continuing education opportunities

Suggested Reading List

Arbeiter J: A buyer's guide to malpractice insurance, *RN* 49:22, 1986.

Becker BG, Fendler DT: *Vocational and personal adjustments in practical nursing,* ed 6, St Louis, 1990, Mosby.

Bernzweig EP: *The nurse's liability for malpractice: a programmed course,* ed 5, St Louis, 1990, Mosby.

Morris JJ: *Canadian nurses and the law,* Markham, & Vancouver, 1991, Butterworth's Canada.

Raatikainen R: Values and ethical principles in nursing, *J Adv Nurs* 14:92, 1989.

Wills-Long SL: Off-duty emergency care . . . do you know your legal risks? *Nurs Life,* 8(1)31-33, 1988.

---

*13209 95th Street, Edmonton, Alberta T5E 3Y2.

Current Trends in Nursing and Health Care Review Questions

Answers and rationales begin on p. 451.

1. Practical/vocational nursing programs must be approved by:
   ① National Association for Practical Nurse Education and Service (NAPNES)
   ② National League for Nursing (NLN)
   ③ The Health Resources and Services Administration
   ④ That state's board of nursing

2. Practical/vocational nursing programs must be accredited by:
   ① National Association for Practical Nurse Education and Service
   ② National League for Nursing
   ③ The Health Resources and Services Administration
   ④ The state board of nursing

3. Continuing education for LP/VNs is:
   ① An obligation of the individual LP/VN
   ② Difficult to obtain
   ③ Required by all states
   ④ Required by the NLN

4. Which of the following is *not* usually considered the role of the LP/VN?
   ① Assisting in the care of unstable patients
   ② Providing direct care to stable patients
   ③ Working as the night charge nurse on a psychiatric unit
   ④ Working as a nurse in a physician's office

5. The functions of the LP/VN are determined by the:
   ① American Nurses Association (ANA)
   ② National Council of State Boards of Nursing (NCSBN)
   ③ National League for Nursing
   ④ State nurse practice act

6. The patient's chart, which provides a written account of a patient from admission to discharge, is:
   ① Shown on request to the family
   ② Discarded after discharge
   ③ Given to the patient on discharge
   ④ A legal document

7. On your nursing unit, the RN carries out the treatments, and you administer the medications. This method of delivering patient care is known as:
   ① District
   ② Functional
   ③ Primary
   ④ Team

8. Establishing trust in the nurse-patient relationship occurs during which phase?
   ① Initiation
   ② Interim
   ③ Working
   ④ Termination

9. To establish a nurse-patient relationship the LP/VN must first:
   ① Greet the patient warmly
   ② Know own self
   ③ Know the patient's strengths and weaknesses
   ④ Read the patient's chart

10. The aspect of health care with which the LP/VN is most concerned is:
    ① Critical care nursing
    ② Bedside nursing
    ③ Cardiac arrest team
    ④ Charge nurse in an acute care facility

11. The responsibility for upholding professional standards of conduct and ethics rests with the:
    ① ANA
    ② Individual LP/VN
    ③ NLN
    ④ State Nurses Association

12. Causing injury to a patient by omitting a medication dose would legally be considered:
    ① Assault
    ② A tort
    ③ Battery
    ④ Imprudence

13. The current definition of health is:
    ① A state of complete absence of physical illness
    ② No evidence of acute or chronic disease
    ③ No evidence of handicap or physical disability
    ④ A state of complete mental, physical, and social well-being, not merely the absence of illness

14. Today the focus of health care as practiced in the United States is:
    ① The treatment of contagious diseases
    ② Promoting hospitalization of chronically ill patients
    ③ Preventive medicine and home care
    ④ Longer hospital confinement for routine surgery

15. Mrs. Clayton sees her physician because she has been urinating frequently. Diabetes mellitus is diagnosed and treatment is begun. This level of health care is known as:
    ① Primary
    ② Secondary
    ③ Restorative
    ④ Tertiary

16. Primary health care is defined as:
    ① Treatment in skilled nursing homes
    ② Rehabilitation
    ③ Preventive medicine
    ④ Treatment of acute disease

17. John is seen in an ambulatory clinic for physical therapy after a fractured ankle has healed. This level of health care is known as:
    ① Primary
    ② Secondary
    ③ Restorative
    ④ Tertiary

18. High-level wellness indicates:
    ① An absence of disease
    ② An absence of physical symptoms
    ③ The individual is physically well
    ④ The individual is enjoying a state of well-being

19. The misuse of restraints or the detention of a patient may be termed:
    ① False imprisonment
    ② Justifiable detention
    ③ Unordered restraints
    ④ True imprisonment

20. The purpose of the team-nursing method of delivering patient care is to:
    ① Maximize abilities of all nursing personnel
    ② Challenge all nurses to provide good nursing care
    ③ Teach student nurse to give orders, make assignments, and administer treatments
    ④ Lessen the work load of all employees

21. The nurse observes multiple bruises on the back and extremities of a 3-year-old patient who is having a cast applied to a fractured forearm. The nurse directs the physician's attention to the bruises because:
    ① The child appears shy and doesn't communicate in response to questions about the bruises
    ② The child's mother commented that her daughter is accident-prone and is always falling
    ③ All states have reporting laws for known or suspected cases of child abuse
    ④ The nurse is making sure the physician observed the bruises

22. The Patient's Bill of Rights has been established to protect and inform patient of:
    ① What is expected of hospital and staff
    ② What activities are planned for entertainment
    ③ What dietary specialties are available from which to choose
    ④ Which physicians are staff members and members of the American Medical Association

23. To legally witness a will, the LP/VN must:
    ① Have a lawyer
    ② Not be a beneficiary
    ③ Know the contents of the will
    ④ Seek permission of the nursing supervisor

24. In 1941 an organization was formed for the purpose of extending and improving the education of practical/vocational nurses. This organization is still active today and is called:
    ① National League for Nurses
    ② National Association for Practical Nurse and Education Service
    ③ National Federation of Licensed Practical Nurses
    ④ American Nurses Association

25. Relating to a patient's visitor that the patient has gone to the operating room for biopsy of a breast lump would be legally considered:
    ① Defamation
    ② Invasion of privacy
    ③ Libel
    ④ Slander

26. A hospital representative serving as a liaison between patient and institution acts to:
    ① Support family
    ② Resolve patient's problems
    ③ Explain hospital charges
    ④ Arrange home care

27. One key aspect to being covered by a Good Samaritan law is:
    ① Asking the victim's permission to give assistance
    ② Determining that a true emergency exists
    ③ Doing anything necessary to save a life
    ④ Giving no statement to the press

28. An LP/VN is sued by a neighbor who claims the LP/VN gave incorrect advice. The LP/VN's employee malpractice insurance does not cover this situation because:
    1. Employee insurance only covers the LP/VN while on duty
    2. Malpractice insurance doesn't cover incorrect advice
    3. This is gross negligence and is not covered by malpractice insurance
    4. This situation would fall under a Good Samaritan law

29. One reason for joining an LP/VN nursing organization is that membership:
    1. Can provide opportunities for continuing education
    2. May be required by the state board
    3. May be required for renewal of license
    4. Reduces the premium on malpractice insurance

30. The nursing organization to which only LP/VNs may belong is:
    1. NAPNES
    2. NCSBN
    3. NFLPN
    4. NLN

31. If involved in a lawsuit, the nurse should first notify the:
    1. Director of Nursing
    2. State board of nursing
    3. Insurance company
    4. American Nurses Association

32. The *American Journal of Nursing (AJN)* is published by the:
    1. AHA
    2. ANA
    3. NAPNES
    4. NFLPN

33. DRG pertains to:
    1. Drug-related group
    2. Diagnosis-related group
    3. Disease-related group
    4. Discharge rating group

34. The American Cancer Society is a/an:
    1. Local health agency
    2. Official United States agency
    3. Part of the Public Health Service
    4. Voluntary agency

35. If a registered nurse or physician asked the LP/VN to do a duty not within the limits of LP/VN's nurse practice act and the patient sustains an injury the:
    1. Hospital is liable
    2. LP/VN is liable
    3. Registered nurse is liable
    4. Physician is liable

Review Questions on Canadian Content

36. Canadian certification/registration/licensure is regulated by:
    1. Federal legislation
    2. Provincial legislation
    3. Local regulatory bodies
    4. Local professional associations

37. Each Canadian province has responsibility to monitor:
    1. Admission requirements
    2. Nursing curricula
    3. Standards of practice
    4. All of the above

38. Which of the following descriptions best reflects the role of the Canadian practical/vocational nurse?
    1. Able to work independently in all settings
    2. Works as an integral part of the health care team
    3. Works under the direct supervision of an RN
    4. Cares for only those patients whose conditions are stabilized

39. The purpose of registration is to protect the:
    1. Public
    2. Individual registrant
    3. Title of the registrant
    4. Level of nursing practice

40. Which of the following is a responsibility of the provincial regulating bodies in Canada?
    1. Setting and administering examinations
    2. Passing laws pertaining to the practice of nursing
    3. Establishing minimum levels of safe nursing care
    4. Reporting acts of criminal negligence to the appropriate authorities

Appendices

APPENDIX A

NANDA-Approved Nursing Diagnoses (Through the 10th Conference, 1992)*

Activity intolerance
Activity intolerance, high risk for
Adjustment, impaired
Airway clearance, ineffective
Anxiety
Aspiration, high risk for
Body image disturbance
Body temperature, altered, high risk for
Bowel incontinence
Breast-feeding, effective
Breast-feeding, ineffective
Breast-feeding, interrupted
Breathing pattern, ineffective
Cardiac output, decreased
Caregiver role strain
Caregiver role strain, high risk for
Communication, impaired verbal
Constipation
Constipation, colonic
Constipation, perceived
Coping, defensive
Coping, family: potential for growth
Coping, ineffective family: compromised
Coping, ineffective family: disabling
Coping, ineffective individual
Decisional conflict (specify)
Denial, ineffective
Diarrhea
Disuse syndrome, high risk for
Diversional activity deficit
Dysfunctional ventilatory weaning
    response (DVWR)
Dysreflexia
Family processes, altered
Fatigue
Fear
Fluid volume deficit (1)
Fluid volume deficit (2)
Fluid volume deficit, high risk for
Fluid volume excess
Gas exchange, impaired
Grieving, anticipatory

Grieving, dysfunctional
Growth and development, altered
Health maintenance, altered
Health-seeking behaviors (specify)
Home maintenance management,
    impaired
Hopelessness
Hyperthermia
Hypothermia
Incontinence, functional
Incontinence, reflex
Incontinence, stress
Incontinence, total
Incontinence, urge
Infant feeding pattern, ineffective
Infection, high risk for
Injury, high risk for
Knowledge deficit (specify)
Mobility, impaired physical
Noncompliance (specify)
Nutrition, altered: less than body
    requirements
Nutrition, altered: more than body
    requirements
Nutrition, altered: high risk for more
    than body requirements
Oral mucous membrane, altered
Pain
Pain, chronic
Parental role conflict
Parenting, altered
Parenting, altered, high risk for
Peripheral neurovascular dysfunction,
    high risk for
Personal identity disturbance
Poisoning, high risk for
Posttrauma response
Powerlessness
Protection, altered
Rape-trauma syndrome
Rape-trauma syndrome, compound
    reaction

Rape-trauma syndrome, silent reaction
Role performance, altered
Self-care deficit, bathing/hygiene
Self-care deficit, dressing/grooming
Self-care deficit, feeding
Self-care deficit, toileting
Self-esteem disturbance
Self-esteem, chronic low
Self-esteem, situational low
Self-mutilation, high risk for
Sensory/perceptual alterations (specify)
    (visual, auditory, kinesthetic, gustatory,
    tactile, olfactory)
Sexual dysfunction
Sexuality patterns, altered
Skin integrity, impaired
Skin integrity, impaired, high risk for
Sleep pattern disturbance
Social interaction, impaired
Social isolation
Spiritual distress (distress of the human
    spirit)
Stress syndrome, relocation
Suffocation, high risk for
Swallowing, impaired
Therapeutic regimen (individual), ineffec-
    tive management of
Thermoregulation, ineffective
Thought processes, altered
Tissue integrity, impaired
Tissue perfusion, altered (specify type)
    (renal, cerebral, cardiopulmonary,
    gastrointestinal, peripheral)
Trauma, high risk for
Unilateral neglect
Urinary elimination, altered patterns
Urinary retention
Ventilation, inability to sustain sponta-
    neous
Violence, high risk for: self-directed or
    directed at others

*Adapted from the proceedings of the 10th National Conference of the North American Nursing Diagnosis Association (1992).

APPENDIX   B

Guide to common drug interactions

Drug	Interacting drug	Effect
Over-the-counter drugs and substances		
Antacids		
Alumina and magnesia Dihydroxaluminum sodium carbonate Magnesia	Dicumarol	Effects of dicumarol may be faster and/or increased
	Digoxin	Effects of digoxin may be reduced

	Tetracyclines
	  Doxycycline
	  Tetracycline
		Effects of tetracyclines may be reduced
		Should be taken 1 to 3 hours apart

Painkillers		
Acetaminophen Buffered acetaminophen	Alcoholic beverages	May cause liver damage

	Blood-thinning drugs
	  Dicumarol
	  Warfarin sodium
		High doses of acetaminophen may increase blood-thinning effects of these drugs

	Tetracycline	Buffered form may cancel the effects of tetracycline Should be taken 1 hour apart
Ibuprofen	Alcoholic beverages	May cause internal bleeding or ulcers

	Blood-thinning drugs
	  Dicumarol
	  Heparin
	  Warfarin sodium
		May cause internal bleeding or ulcers

	Salicylates
	  Aspirin
	  Aspirin and caffeine
	  Buffered aspirin
		May cause stomach upset without relieving symptoms

Salicylates
  Aspirin
  Aspirin and caffeine
  Buffered aspirin
	Alcoholic beverages	May cause stomach ulcers or internal bleeding

	Antidiabetics
	  Chlorpropamide
	  Tolazamide
		May cause blood sugar level to drop too low

	Blood-thinning drugs
	  Dicumarol
	  Heparin
	  Warfarin sodium
		Increases risk of internal bleeding

	Ibuprofen	May cause stomach upset without relieving symptoms
	Tetracycline	Effects of tetracycline are reduced
Other substances		
Alcoholic beverages	Acetaminophen Buffered acetaminophen	May cause liver damage

	Antidiabetics
	  Chlorpropamide
	  Tolazamide
		Stomach upset, vomiting, cramps, headaches, low blood sugar

	Antiseizure drugs
	  Carbamazepine
	  Chlordiazepoxide
	  Diazepam
	  Phenytoin
		May cause extreme drowsiness

Adapted from *Mosby's medical, nursing, & allied health dictionary*, ed 3, St Louis, 1990, Mosby.
This table includes only common over-the-counter and prescription drugs. Some of these drugs may also interact with less common drugs and substances not described.
When using any drug, always consult your physician or pharmacist about possible interactions with other drugs, substances, or foods.

Continued.

Guide to common drug interactions—cont'd

Drug	Interacting drug	Effect
Other Substances Alcoholic beverages—cont'd	Barbiturates Pentobarbital Phenobarbital Secobarbital Secobarbital and amobarbital	May cause drowsiness, increase effects of either drug, cause breathing to fail, or cause blood pressure to drop too low
	Ibuprofen	May cause internal bleeding or ulcers
	Narcotic analgesics Acetaminophen and codeine Meperidine Propoxyphene	May depress nervous system and breathing or cause blood pressure to drop too low
	Reserpine	May increase effects of alcohol and reserpine
	Salicylates Aspirin Aspirin and caffeine Buffered aspirin	May cause stomach ulcers or internal bleeding
	Tricyclic antidepressants Amitriptyline Amoxapine Doxepin	May cause extreme drowsiness
Sodium chloride (salt)	Lithium	Low-salt diet causes lithium to build up in body and is not advised
Tobacco (smoking)	Birth control pills Norethindrone with ethinyl estradiol Norethynodrel with mestranol	May increase chances of blood clot or heart attack
Tyramine-containing foods Avocados, bananas, beer, caffeine, cheese, chicken liver, chocolate, fava beans, fermented sausages (salami, pepperoni, bologna, etc.), canned figs, pickled herring, pineapple, raisins, red wine, sauerkraut, soy sauce, yeast extract, yogurt	MAO inhibitors Isocarboxazid Phenelzine Tranylcypromine	May cause severe and sometimes fatal high blood pressure Headache, vomiting, fever, and high blood pressure are warning signals
Prescription drugs **Antibiotics** Erythromycins Erythromycin Erythromycin lactobionate Penicillins Amoxicillin Ampicillin	Penicillins Amoxicillin Ampicillin	Could interfere with the effects of penicillins
	Birth control pills Norethindrone with ethinyl estradiol Norethynodrel with mestranol	May interfere with and result in unplanned pregnancy or menstrual problems
	Blood-thinning drugs Dicumarol Warfarin sodium	May increase blood thinning effects of these drugs
	Erythromycins Erythromycin Erythromycin lactobionate	May interfere with effects of penicillins
	Tetracyclines Doxycycline Tetracycline	May interfere with effects of penicillins

Drug	Interacting drug	Effect

Tetracyclines
  Doxycycline
  Tetracycline
	Acetaminophen
	Buffered acetaminophen	

	Antacids
	  Alumina and magnesia
	  Dihydroxaluminum sodium carbonate
	  Magnesia
		May decrease effects of tetracyclines and should be taken 1 to 3 hours apart

	Barbiturates
	  Pentobarbital
	  Phenobarbital
	  Secobarbital
	  Secobarbital and amobarbital
		May decrease effects of doxycycline
		Other tetracyclines can be used

	Penicillins
	  Amoxicillin
	  Ampicillin
		May interfere with effects of penicillins

	Salicylates
	  Aspirin
	  Aspirin and caffeine
	  Buffered aspirin
		Effects of tetracyclines are reduced

Antidepressants Lithium	Sodium chloride (salt)	Low-salt diet causes lithium to build up in body and is not advised

	Thiazide diuretics
	  Cyclothiazide
	  Furosemide
	  Methyclothiazide
		May cause lithium to have toxic effect

Tricyclic antidepressants
  Amitriptyline
  Amoxapine
  Doxepin
	Alcoholic beverages	May cause extreme drowsiness

	Antiseizure drugs
	  Carbamazepine
	  Chlordiazepoxide
	  Diazepam
	  Phenytoin
		Effects of antiseizure drug may be decreased
		Dosage should be adjusted

	Blood-thinning drugs
	  Dicumarol
	  Warfarin sodium
		May cause internal bleeding

	MAO inhibitors
	  Isocarboxazid
	  Phenelzine
	  Tranylcypromine
		Severe seizure and death could result
		
		Should be taken 14 days apart

	Narcotic analgesics
	  Acetaminophen and codeine
	  Meperidine
	  Propoxyphene
		May depress nervous system and breathing and cause blood pressure to drop too low

Antidiabetics Chlorpropamide Tolazamide	Alcoholic beverages	May cause stomach upset, vomiting, cramps, headaches, low blood sugar

	Beta-adrenergic blockers
	  Metoprolol
	  Propranolol
		May increase risk of either high or low blood sugar levels
		May mask symptoms

	Blood-thinning drugs
	  Dicumarol
	  Warfarin sodium
		Blood-thinning effect will be increased at first, later it will be decreased
		May also cause low blood sugar and become toxic

Continued.

Guide to common drug interactions—cont'd

Drug	Interacting drug	Effect
Antidiabetics Chlorpropamide Tolazamide—cont'd	MAO inhibitors Isocarboxazid Phenelzine Tranylcypromine	Can cause extreme low blood sugar level
	Salicylates Aspirin Aspirin and caffeine Buffered aspirin	May cause blood sugar level to drop too low
Isophane insulin suspension	Beta-adrenergic blockers Metoprolol Propranolol	These may mask symptoms of low blood sugar
	Birth control pills Norethindrone with ethinyl estradiol Norethynodrel with mestranol	May increase risk of high blood sugar levels Dosages should be adjusted
	MAO inhibitors Isocarboxazid Phenelzine Tranylcypromine	May cause extreme low blood sugar level
Antiseizure drugs Carbamazepine Chlordiazepoxide Diazepam Phenytoin	Alcoholic beverages	May cause extreme drowsiness
	Beta-adrenergic blockers Metoprolol Propranolol	Could decrease the effect of beta-blockers
	Birth control pills Norethindrone with ethinyl estradiol Norethynodrel with mestranol	Phenytoin and carbamazepine may interfere and increase risk of unplanned pregnancy May increase effect of diazepam
	Tricyclic antidepressants Amitriptyline Amoxapine Doxepin	Effects of antiseizure drug may be decreased Dosage should be adjusted
Barbiturates Pentobarbital Phenobarbital Secobarbital Secobarbital and amobarbital	Alcoholic beverages	May cause drowsiness, increase effects of either drug, cause breathing to fail, or cause blood pressure to drop too low
	Birth control pills Norethindrone with ethinyl estradiol Norethynodrel with mestranol	Barbiturates may interfere with and result in unplanned pregnancy
	Blood-thinning drugs Dicumarol Warfarin sodium	May decrease blood-thinning effects of these drugs
	Doxycycline	May decrease effects of doxycycline Other tetracyclines can be used

Drug	Interacting drug	Effect

Birth control pills
Norethindrone with ethinyl estradiol
Norethynodrel with mestranol
	Antiseizure drugs
	  Carbamazepine
	  Chlordiazepoxide
	  Diazepam
	  Phenytoin
		Will increase the sedative effects of these drugs
		May decrease the effects of other antiseizure drugs

	Barbiturates
	  Pentobarbital
	  Phenobarbital
	  Secobarbital
	  Secobarbital and amobarbital
		Barbiturates may interfere with birth control pills and result in unplanned pregnancy

	Isophane insulin suspension	May increase risk of high blood sugar levels; dosages should be adjusted

	Penicillins
	  Amoxicillin
	  Ampicillin
		May interfere with birth control pills and result in unplanned pregnancy

	Tobacco (smoking)	May increase chances of blood clot or heart attack

Blood pressure drugs
Thiazide diuretics
  Cyclothiazide
  Furosemide
  Methyclothiazide
	Beta-adrenergic blockers
	  Metoprolol
	  Propranolol
		Can cause extremely low blood pressure

	Digitalis glycosides
	  Digitalis
	  Digoxin
		Can cause irregular heartbeat, which can be fatal
		Can cause extremely low blood pressure

	Lithium	May cause lithium to have toxic effect
	Reserpine	Can cause extremely low blood pressure
Rauwolfia alkaloids Reserpine	Alcoholic beverages	May increase effects of alcohol May increase effects of rauwolfia alkaloids

	Beta-adrenergic blockers
	  Metoprolol
	  Propranolol
		May cause extremely slow heartbeat and low blood pressure

	Digitalis glycosides
	  Digitalis
	  Digoxin
		May cause irregular heartbeat

	MAO inhibitors
	  Isocarboxazid
	  Phenelzine
	  Tranylcypromine
		May cause slight to sudden and severe high blood pressure
		May cause extreme high fever
		Either effect could be life-threatening

	Thiazide diuretics
	  Cyclothiazide
	  Furosemide
	  Methyclothiazide
		Can cause extreme low blood pressure

Blood-thinning drugs Dicumarol Warfarin sodium	Acetaminophen Buffered acetaminophen	High doses of acetaminophen may increase blood-thinning effects of these drugs

	Antacids
	  Alumina and magnesia
	  Dihydroxyaluminum sodium carbonate
	  Magnesia
		Effects of dicumarol may be faster and may also be increased

	Antidiabetics
	  Chlorpropamide
	  Tolazamide
		Blood-thinning effect will be increased at first, later it will be decreased
		May also cause low blood sugar and become toxic

Continued.

Guide to common drug interactions—cont'd

Drug	Interacting drug	Effect
	Barbiturates Pentobarbital Phenobarbital Secobarbital Secobarbital and amobarbital	Decreases blood-thinning effect
	Heparin	May cause increased risk of internal bleeding
	Ibuprofen	May cause internal bleeding or ulcers
	Penicillins Amoxicillin Ampicillin	May increase blood-thinning effects of these drugs
	Salicylates Aspirin Aspirin and caffeine Buffered aspirin	Blood-thinning effects will be increased May cause ulcers or internal bleeding
	Tricyclic antidepressants Amitriptyline Amoxapine Doxepin	May cause internal bleeding
Heparin	Blood-thinning drugs Dicumarol Warfarin sodium	May cause increased risk of internal bleeding
	Salicylates Aspirin Aspirin and caffeine Buffered aspirin	Blood-thinning effects will be increased May cause ulcers or internal bleeding
Heart drugs Beta-adrenergic blockers Metoprolol Propranolol	Antidiabetics Chlorpropamide Tolazamide	May increase risk of either high or low blood sugar levels May mask symptoms
	Antiseizure drugs Carbamazepine Chlordiazepoxide Diazepam Phenytoin	Could decrease the effect of beta blockers
	Digitalis glycosides Digitalis Digoxin	May cause extremely slow heartbeat with a chance of heart block
	Isophane insulin suspension	Beta blockers may mask symptoms of low blood sugar May also cause low blood sugar
	Reserpine	May cause extremely slow heartbeat and low blood pressure
	Thiazide diuretics Cyclothiazide Furosemide Methyclothiazide	Can cause extremely low blood pressure

Drug	Interacting drug	Effect
Digitalis glycosides Digitalis Digoxin	Antacids Alumina and magnesia Dihydroxyaluminum sodium carbonate Magnesia	Effects of digoxin may be reduced
	Beta-adrenergic blockers Metoprolol Propranolol	May cause extremely slow heartbeat with a chance of heart block
	Reserpine	May cause irregular heartbeat
	Thiazide diuretics Cyclothiazide Furosemide Methyclothiazide	May cause extreme low blood pressure; may cause digitalis to become toxic
Monoamine oxidase inhibitors (MAO inhibitors) Isocarboxazid Phenelzine Tranylcypromine	Antidiabetics Chlorpropamide Isophane insulin suspension Tolazamide	Can cause extreme low blood sugar level
	Narcotic analgesics Acetaminophen and codeine Meperidine Propoxyphene	May cause severe and sometimes fatal reactions
	Reserpine	May cause slight to sudden and severe high blood pressure May cause extreme high fever Either effect could be life threatening
	Tricyclic antidepressants Amitriptyline Amoxapine Doxepin	Severe seizure and death could result Should be taken 14 days apart
	Tyramine-containing foods Avocados, bananas, beer, caffeine, cheese, chicken liver, chocolate, fava beans, fermented sausages (salami, pepperoni, bologna, etc.) canned figs, pickled herring, pineapple, raisins, red wine, sauerkraut, soy sauce, yeast extract, yogurt	May cause severe and sometimes fatal high blood pressure. Headache, vomiting, fever, and high blood pressure are warning signals
Painkillers Narcotic analgesics Acetaminophen and codeine Meperidine Propoxyphene	Alcoholic beverages	May depress nervous system and breathing May cause blood pressure to drop too low
	MAO inhibitors Isocarboxazid Phenelzine Tranylcypromine	May cause many severe and sometimes fatal reactions
	Tricyclic antidepressants Amitriptyline Amoxapine Doxepin	May depress nervous system and breathing May cause blood pressure to drop too low

Comparison of selected effects of commonly abused drugs

Drug category	Physical dependence	Characteristics of intoxication
Opiates	Marked	Analgesia with or without depressed sensorium; pinpoint pupils (tolerance does not develop to this action); patient may be alert and appear normal; respiratory depression with overdose
Barbiturates	Marked	Patient may appear normal with usual dose, but narrow margin between doses needed to prevent withdrawal symptoms and toxic dose is often exceeded and patient appears "drunk," with drowsiness, ataxia, slurred speech, and nystagmus on lateral gaze; pupil size and reaction normal; respiratory depression with overdose
Nonbarbiturate sedatives: glutethimide (Doriden)	Marked	Pupils dilated and reactive to light; coma and respiratory depression prolonged; sudden apnea and laryngeal spasm common
Antianxiety agents ("minor tranquilizers")	Marked	Progressive depression of sensorium as with barbiturates; pupil size and reaction normal; respiratory depression with overdose
Ethanol	Marked	Depressed sensorium, acute or chronic brain syndrome, odor on breath, pupil size and reaction normal
Amphetamines	Mild to absent	Agitation, with paranoid thought disturbance in high doses; acute organic brain syndrome after prolonged use; pupils dilated and reactive; tachycardia, elevated blood pressure, with possibility of hypertensive crisis and CVA; possibility of convulsive seizures
Cocaine	Absent	Paranoid thought disturbance in high doses, with dangerous delusions of persecution and omnipotence; tachycardia; respiratory depression with overdose
Marijuana	Absent	Milder preparations; drowsy, euphoric state with frequent inappropriate laughter and disturbance in perception of time or space (occasional acute psychotic reaction reported); stronger preparations such as hashish: frequent hallucinations or psychotic reaction; pupils normal, conjunctivas injected (marijuana preparations frequently adulterated with LSD, tryptamines, or heroin)
Psychotomimetics: LSD, STP, tryptamines, mescaline, morning glory seeds	Absent	Unpredictable disturbance in ego function, manifest by extreme lability of affect and chaotic disruption of thought, with danger of uncontrolled behavioral disturbance; pupils dilated and reactive to light
Phencyclidine	Unknown	Disinhibition, agitation, confusion, chaotic thought disturbance, unpredictable behavior, hypertension, meiosis, respiratory collapse, cardiovascular collapse, death
Anticholinergic agents	Absent	Nonpsychotropic effects such as tachycardia, decreased salivary secretion, urinary retention, and dilated, nonreactive pupils plus depressed sensorium, confusion, disorientation, hallucinations, and delusional thinking
Inhalants*	Unknown	Depressed sensorium, hallucinations, acute brain syndrome; odor on breath; often glassy-eyed appearance

Adapted from *Mosby's medical, nursing, & allied health dictionary*, ed 3, St Louis, 1990, Mosby.

*The term *inhalant* is used to designate a variety of gases and highly volatile organic liquids, including the aromatic glues, paint thinners, gasoline, some anesthetic agents and amylnitrite. The term excludes liquids sprayed into the nasopharynx (droplet transport required) and substances that must be ignited before administration (such as marijuana).

Characteristics of withdrawal	"Flashback" symptoms	Masking of symptoms of illness or injury during intoxication
Rhinorrhea, lacrimation, and dilated, reactive pupils, followed by gastrointestinal disturbances, low back pain, and waves of gooseflesh; convulsions not a feature unless heroin samples were adulterated with barbiturates	Not reported	An important feature of opiate intoxication, resulting from analgesic action, with or without depressed sensorium
Agitation, tremulousness, insomnia, gastrointestinal disturbances, hyperpyrexia, blepharoclonus (clonic blink reflex), acute brain syndrome, major convulsive seizures	Not reported	Only in presence of depressed sensorium or after onset of acute brain syndrome
Similar to barbiturate withdrawal syndrome, with agitation, gastrointestinal disturbances, hyperpyrexia, and major convulsive seizures	Not reported	Same as in barbiturate intoxication
Similar to barbiturate withdrawal syndrome, with danger of major convulsive seizures	Not reported	Same as in barbiturate intoxication
Similar to barbiturate withdrawal syndrome, but with less likelihood of convulsive seizures	Not reported	Same as in barbiturate intoxication
Lethargy, somnolence, dysphoria, and possibility of suicidal depression; brain syndrome may persist for many weeks	Infrequently reported	Drug-induced euphoria or acute brain syndrome may interfere with awareness of symptoms of illness or may remove incentive to report symptoms of illness
Similar to amphetamine withdrawal	Not reported	Same as in amphetamine intoxication
No specific withdrawal symptoms	Infrequently reported	Uncommon with milder preparations; stronger preparations may interfere in same manner as psychotomimetic agents
No specific withdrawal symptoms; symptoms may persist for indefinite period after discontinuation of drug	Commonly reported as late as 1 year after last dose	Affective response or psychotic thought disturbance may remove awareness of, or incentive to report, symptoms of illness
No specific withdrawal symptoms	Occasionally reported	Same as in LSD intoxication
No specific withdrawal symptoms; mydriasis may persist for several days	Not reported	Pain may not be reported as a result of depression of sensorium, acute brain syndrome, or acute psychotic reaction
No specific withdrawal symptoms	Infrequently reported	Same as in anticholinergic intoxication

Commonly used medications: generic to trade name listing

Generic name	Trade name	Generic name	Trade name
acetaminophen	Tylenol, Datril, Anacin-3	cefapirin	Cefatrex
acetazolamide	Diamox, Diamox Sequels	cefazolin	Ancef, Kefzol
acetohexamide	Dymelor	cefoperazone	Cefobid
acetylcysteine	Mucomyst	cefoxitin	Mefoxin
acetylsalicylic acid (ASA)	aspirin	ceftizoxime	Cefizox
acyclovir	Zovirax	cephalexin	Keflex
albuterol	Proventil, Ventolin	cephalothin	Keflin
allopurinol	Zyloprim	cephapirin	Cefadyl
alprazolam	Xanax	cephazolin	Ancef, Kefzol
aluminum hydroxide gel	Amphogel	cephradine	Anspor, Velosef
aluminum-magnesium suspension	Maalox, Mylanta, Gelusil	chloral hydrate	Noctec
amikacin	Amikin	chlorambucil	Leukeran
amiloride	Midamor	chloramphenicol	Chloromycetin, Chloroptic
aminoglutethimide	Cytadren	chlorazepate, dipotassium	Tranxene
amitriptyline	Elavil, Endep	chlorazepate, monopotassium	Azene
amobarbital	Amytal	chlordiazepoxide	Librium, Libritab
amoxicillin	Amoxil, Larotid, Polymox	chlordiazepoxide and amitriptyline	Limbitrol
amphotericin B	Fungizone	chlordiazepoxide and clidinium	Limbrax
ampicillin	Amcil, Omnipen, Polycillin	chloroquine	Aralen
ascorbic acid	vitamin C	chlorothiazide	Diuril
aspirin, buffered	Bufferin	chlorotrianisene	Tace
aspirin, enteric coated	Ecotrin	chlorpheniramine	Chlortrimeton
atenolol	Tenormin	chlorpromazine	Thorazine
baclofen	Lioresal	chlorpropamide	Diabinese
beclomethasone	Vanceril, Beclovent	chlorprothixene	Taractan
belladonna alkaloids and phenobarbital	Donnatal	chlorthalidone	Hygroton
		cholestyramine	Questran
benzocaine	Americaine, Hurricaine	cimetidine	Tagamet
benzquinamide	Emeta-Con	cinoxacin	Cinobac
benztropine	Cogentin	cisplatin	Platinol
betamethasone	Celestone, Valisone	clemastine	Tavist
bethanechol chloride	Urecholine	clidinium	Quarzan
biperiden	Akineton	clindamycin	Cleocin-T
bisacodyl	Dulcolax	clofibrate	Atromid-S
bleomycin	Blenoxane	clonazepam	Clonopin
bretylium tosylate	Bretylol	clonidine	Catapres
bromocriptine	Parlodel	colestipol	Colestid
brompheniramine	Dimetane	conjugated estrogens	Premarin
bumetanide	Bumex	corticotropin	ACTH, Acthar
busulfan	Myleran	cortisone acetate	Cortone
butabarbital	Butisol	cromolyn	Intal
butorphanol	Stadol	cyclizine	Marezine
calcitonin	Calcimar	cyclophosphamide	Cytoxan
calcium carbonate	Tums, Titralac, Alka-2	cyproheptadine	Periactin
camphorated tincture of opium	Paregoric	dactinomycin	Cosmegen
captopril	Capoten	dantrolene sodium	Dantrium
caramiphen and phenylpropanolamine	Tuss-Ornade	demeclocycline	Declomycin
		desipramine	Norpramin, Pertofrane
carbamazepine	Tegretol	deslanoside	Cedilanid-D
carbenicillin	Geocillin, Geopen, Pyopen	dexamethasone	Decadron, Hexadrol
carbidopa	Lodosyn	diazepam	Valium
carbidopa and levodopa	Sinemet	diazoxide	Hyperstat, Proglycem
carmustine	BiCNU	dibucaine	Nupercaine, Nupercainal
cefaclor	Ceclor	dicyclomine	Bentyl
cefamandol	Mandol	diethylstilbestrol	Stilbestrol, DES

Adapted from *Mosby's medical, nursing, & allied health dictionary*, ed 3, St Louis, 1990, Mosby.

Generic name	Trade name	Generic name	Trade name
diflunisal	Dolobid	hydralazine	Apresoline
digitoxin	Crystodigin	hydrochlorothiazide	HydroDiuril, Esidrex
digoxin	Lanoxin	hydrochlorothiazide and	Aldactazide
dimenhydrinate	Dramamine	spironolactone	
dioctyl calcium sulfosuccinate (DOCS)	Surfak	hydrochlorothiazide and timolol	Timolide
dioctyl sodium sulfosuccinate (DSS)	Colace	hydrochlorothiazide and triamterene	Dyazide
dioctyl sodium sulfosuccinate with casanthranol	Pericolace	hydrocodone	Dicodid
diphenhydramine	Benadryl	hydrocodone and homatropine	Hycodan
diphenoxylate HCl with atropine	Lomotil	hydrocortisone	Solu-Cortef
dipyridamole	Persantine	hydromorphone	Dilaudid
disopyramide	Norpace	hydromorphone and guaifenesin	Dilaudin cough syrup
disulfiram	Antabuse	hydroxyzine HCl	Atarax
dobutamine	Dobutrex	hydroxyzine pamoate	Vistaril
docusate calcium	Surfak	ibuprofen	Advil, Motrin, Rufen
docusate sodium (DSS)	Colace	idoxuridine	Stoxil, Herplex
dopamine	Intropin	imipramine	Tofranil
doxapram	Dopram	indomethacin	Indocin
doxepin HCl	Adapin, Sinequan	INH (isoniazid)	Nydrazid
doxorubicin HCl	Adriamycin	iron dextran	Imferon
doxycycline	Vibramycin	isoetharine HCl	Bronkosol
dyphylline	Lufyllin	isoproterenol	Isuprel
edrophonium	Tensilon	isosorbide dinitrate	Isordil, Sorbitrate
ephedrine	Vaponefrin	isotretinoin	Accutane
epinephrine	Adrenalin, Sus-Phrine	isoxsuprine HCl	Vasodilan
ergoloid mesylates	Hydergine	kanamycin	Kantrex
ergonovine	Ergotrate	kaolin-pectin	Kaopectate
ergotamine	Ergomar, Ergostat	ketoconazole	Nizoral
erythromycin	Erythrocin, Ilotycin	labetalol	Normodyne, Trandate
erythromycin estolate	Ilosone	lactulose syrup	Chronulac
estrogens, conjugated	Premarin	lanatoside C	Cedilanid
ethacrynic acid	Edecrin	levarterenol	Levophed
ethchlorvynol	Placidyl	levodopa	Dopar, Larodopa
fentanyl	Sublimaze	levorphanol	Levo-Dromoran
ferrous fumarate	Femiron	levothyroxine	Synthroid
ferrous gluconate	Fergon	lidocaine	Xylocaine
ferrous sulfate	Moliron, Feosol	lindane	Kwell
flucytosine	Ancobon	liothyronine	Cytomel
fludrocortisone	Florinef	liotrix	Euthroid, Thyrolar
fluocinolone acetonide	Synalar	lithium carbonate	Lithane, Lithobid
fluocinonide	Lidex	lomustine	Cee Nu
fluphenazine HCl	Prolixin	loperamide HCl	Imodium
flurazepam	Dalmane	lorazepam	Ativan
folic acid	Folvite	loxapine succinate	Loxitane
folinic acid	Leucovorin calcium	magaldrate	Riopan
furosemide	Lasix	magnesium sulfate	Epsom salt
gemfibrozil	Lopid	maprotiline	Ludiomil
gentamicin	Garamycin	mazindol	Sanorex
glycopyrrolate	Robinul	mebendazole	Vermox
griseofulvin	Fulvicin P/G	mecamylamine	Inversine
guaifenesin (glyceryl guaiacolate)	Robitussin	mechlorethamine	Mustargen, nitrogen mustard
guanabenz	Wytensin	meclizine HCl	Antivert, Bonine
guanethidine	Ismelin	melphalan	Alkeran
haloperidol	Haldol	menadiol	Synkayvite, vitamin K
haloprogin	Halotex	meperidine	Demerol
halothane	Fluothane	mephenytoin	Mesantoin
heparin	Lipo-Hepin, Liquaemin	mephobarbital	Mebaral
hetacillin	Versapen	meprobamate	Miltown, Equanil
hyaluronidase	Wydase	mesoridazine	Serentil
		metaproterenol	Alupent

Continued.

Commonly used medications: generic to trade name listing—cont'd

Generic name	Trade name	Generic name	Trade name
metaraminol	Aramine	paraldehyde	Paral
methadone	Dolophine	pargyline	Eutonyl
methandrostenolone	Dianabol	pemoline	Cylert
methenamine hippurate	Hiprex, Urex	penicillamine	Cuprimine
methenamine mandelate	Mandelamine	penicillin and benzathine	Bicillin
methicillin	Staphcillin	penicillin G potassium	Pfizepen, Pentid
methimazole	Tapazole	penicillin procaine	Duracillin, crysticillin, Wycillin
methocarbamol	Robaxin	penicillin V potassium	PEN-VEE K, V-cillin K
methoxyflurane	Penthrane	pentaerythritol tetranitrate	Peritrate
methyldopa	Aldomet	pentazocine	Talwin
methylphenidate	Ritalin	pentobarbital	Nembutal
metoclopramide	Reglan	perphenazine	Trilafon
metolazone	Zaroxolyn	phenazopyridine HCl	Pyridium
metoprolol	Lopressor	phenazopyridine and sulfisoxazole	Azo-Gantrisin
metronidazole	Flagyl	phenelzine sulfate	Nardil
miconazole	Monistat	pentoxifylline	Trental
milk of magnesia (MOM)	magnesium hydroxide	phenmetrazine	Preludin
mineral oil emulsion	Kondremul	phenobarbital	Luminal
minocycline	Minocin	phenolphthalein	Ex-Lax, Feen-A-Mint
minoxidil	Loniten	phenoxymethyl penicillin	V-Cillin, PENICILLIN VK
mithramycin	Mithracin	phenylbutazone	Butazolidin, Azolid-A
mitotane	Lysodren	phenylephrine	Neosynephrine
molindone HCl	Moban	phenytoin	Dilantin
moxalactam	Moxam	phosphate enema	Fleet enema
nadolol	Corgard	phosphated carbohydrate solution	Emetrol
nalbuphine	Nubain	physostigmine	Antilirium
nalidixic acid	Neg Gram	phytonadione (vitamin K₁)	Mephyton, Aquamephyton
naloxone	Narcan	pilocarpine	Isoptocarpine
naproxen	Naproxyn	piroxicam	Feldene
naproxen sodium	Anaprox	potassium chloride	Klor, Kaon, Cl, Slow K,
neostigmine	Prostigmin		Micro K, Klorvess
niacin (nicotinic acid)	Nicobid, Nicolar	potassium gluconate	Kaon
nifedipine	Procardia	povidone-iodine	Betadine
nitrofurantoin	Furadantin	prazosin	Minipress
nitrogen mustard	Mustargen	prednisolone	Meticortelone, Delta Cortef
nitroglycerin	Nitrobid, Nitrospan, Nitrostat	primidone	Mysoline
nitroprusside	Nipride	probenecid	Benemid
norepinephrine	Levophed	procainamide	Pronestyl
norethindrone	Norlutin	procaine	Novocain
norethindrone acetate	Norlutate	procarbazine	Matulane
nortriptyline	Aventyl, Pamelor	prochlorperazine	Compazine
nylidrin	Arlidin	procyclidine	Kemadrin
nystatin	Mycostatin, Nilstat	promazine	Sparine
orphendrine	Norflex	promethazine	Phenergan
oxacillin	Prostaphlin	propantheline	Probanthine
oxazepam	Serax	propoxyphene	Darvon
oxtriphylline	Choledyl	propoxyphene, napsylate,	Davocet-N
oxycodone, ASA	Percodan	acetaminophen	
oxycodone, acetaminophen	Percocet	propranolol	Inderal
oxymetazoline, nasal	Afrin, Dristan Long Lasting	psyllium hydrocolloid	Effersyllium
oxyphenbutazone	Tandearil	pyridostigmine	Mestinon
oxytetracycline	Terramycin	pyrvinium pamoate	Povan
oxytocin	Pitocin	quinacrine	Atabrine
pancrelipase	Cotazym, Viokase	quinidine gluconate	Quinaglute
pancuronium	Pavulon	quinidine sulfate	Quinora
papaverine	Pavabid, Cerespan	quinine sulfate	Auinamm

Generic name	Trade name	Generic name	Trade name
racepinephrine	Vaponefrin, Asthmanefrin	ticarcillin disodium	Ticar
ranitidine	Zantac	timolol maleate	Biocadren, Timoptic
rauwolfia serpentina	Raudixin	tobramycin	Nebcin, Tobrex
reserpine	Serpasil	tocainide	Tonocard
rifampin	Rimactane, Rifadin	tolazamide	Tolinase
ritodrine	Yutopar	tolbutamide	Orinase
salsalate	Disalcid	tranylcypromine sulfate	Parnate
scopolamine	Transderm-Scop	trazodone	Desyrel
secobarbital	Seconal	triamcinolone	Kenacort, Aristocort
selenium sulfide	Selsun Blue, Selsun	triamterene	Dyrenium
senna	Senokot	triamterene and	Dyazide, Maxzide
silver sulfadiazine	Silvadene	hydrochlorothiazide	
simethicone	Mylicon	triazolam	Halcion
sodium polystyrene sulfonate	Kayexalate	trifluoperazine	Stelazine
spironolactone	Aldactone	trihexyphenidyl HCl	Artane, Tremin
streptokinase	Streptase	trimethadione	Tridione
succinylcholine	Anectine	trimethaphan	Arfonad
sucralfate	Carafate	trimethobenzamide	Tigan
sulfamethoxazole	Gantanol	trimethoprim	Proloprim, Trimpex
sulfamethoxazole and	Bactrim, Septra	undecylenic acid	Desenex
trimethoprim		urokinase	Breokinase
sulfasalazine	Azulfidine	valproic acid	Depakene
sulfisoxazole	Gantrisin	vancomycin	Vancocin
sulfisoxazole and phenazopyridine	Azo-Gantrisin	vasopressin	Pitressin
sulindac	Clinoril	verapamil	Calan, Isoptin
tamoxifen	Nolvadex	vidarabine	Vira-A
temazepam	Restoril	vinblastine	Velban
terbutaline	Brethine, Bricanyl	vincristine	Oncovin
tetanus immune globulin	Hyper-tet	vitamin B_6	Pyridoxine, Hexabetalin
tetracaine	Pontocaine	vitamin B_{12}	cyanocobalamin, Redisol
tetracycline	Achromycin, Sumycin	vitamin C	ascorbic acid
theophylline	Elixophyllin, Theo-Dur	vitamin D	Deltalin
thioridazine	Mellaril	vitamin K_1	phytonadione
thiothixene	Navane	warfarin	Coumadin
thyroglobulin	Proloid		

APPENDIX   **E**

To prevent the spread of infection, any person with symptoms suggestive of a communicable disease should be kept away from others. Measures for control of communicable diseases are established either by law or regulation in various states and communities. As these may vary, practical nurses should keep in touch with local health authorities and cooperate with them in preventing the spread of disease.

Common communicable diseases

Disease	How spread	Prevention	How long from exposure to onset
Chickenpox	Directly from person to person; indirectly through articles freshly soiled by discharges from skin and mucous membrane of infected persons	No immunization available; avoid exposure; one attack usually gives immunity	2 to 3 weeks
Common cold	Contact with discharges from nose and throat; directly from person to person; indirectly through articles freshly soiled by discharges	No specific prevention; maintain body resistance and avoid chilling and exposure to illness	12 to 72 hours
Diphtheria	Contact with discharges from nose and throat or other infected membranes; by carriers as well as by sick persons; milk may carry germs of disease	Immunization in infancy, with reinforcing doses periodically; adults exposed to infection should be given Schick test to determine susceptibility before immunization; second attacks possible	2 to 5 days, sometimes longer
Dysentery	Contact with discharges from bowels of infected persons; contaminated food and water; flies	No immunization; avoidance of known sources; personal cleanliness; proper sanitation; periodic examination of food handlers	1 to 7 days or 3 to 4 weeks
Encephalitis (sleeping sickness)	Mosquitoes; ticks	Personal cleanliness; strict isolation of patient; spray mosquitoes' breeding places; window screens; insect repellents	4 to 15 days
German measles (rubella)	Contact with discharges from throat and mouth; easily communicable	Immunization available; second attacks rare; especially important to guard women in early pregnancy against exposure	5 to 21 days
Gonorrhea	Contact with fresh discharges from genital tract of infected persons or from other infected areas such as eyes; most frequently through sexual intercourse	No immunization; avoidance of contact; medicine put in eyes of newborn babies; one attack does not confer immunity; case-finding; early diagnosis and treatment	1 to 14 days; usually 3 to 5 days
Infectious hepatitis	Contact with infected feces, serum, and contaminated food and water	Passive immunity with gamma globulin; avoid contact with infected feces, food, water, and blood serum	2 to 6 weeks
Serum hepatitis	Contact with contaminated needle or solution containing blood serum	Cleanliness and sterilization of syringes and needles; careful history of blood donors	1½ to 6 months

*Not communicable. Infection that precedes this disease is communicable but has usually subsided by time symptoms of rheumatic fever appear.
†Bacteria causing scarlet fever (hemolytic streptococci) may also cause other diseases such as streptococcal sore throat, erysipelas, and "childbed fever" (puerperal fever).

Common symptoms	How long communicable	Some possible complications
Small reddish pimples or blisters, usually more abundant on covered than exposed parts of body, which become itchy; slight fever; headache	Probably not more than 1 day before or more than 6 days after pimples first appear; highly communicable during early stages	Rarely, skin eruptions may become infected
Tickling, dry sensation in throat; slight fever; chilliness; sick feeling; cough and runny nose	Usually limited to early stage of disease	Bronchitis; laryngitis; pneumonia; middle ear infection in children
Inflammation of tonsils, throat, and nose, with grayish white patches; fever	Until germs have disappeared as shown by tests, usually 2 weeks or less	Damage to heart and throat muscles; otitis media; bronchial pneumonia; peripheral neuritis
Diarrhea; fever; stools may contain mucus or blood; abdominal cramps	As long as stools contain infecting agent as checked by laboratory tests, sometimes weeks	Often recurs
Slow or sudden onset of fever, headache, vertigo, joint pains, confusion, drowsiness, and paralysis; nausea, vomiting; convulsions; hiccoughs; cranial nerve involvement	Unknown	Disturbed mental and physical functions for some time after infection
Slight cold followed by red rash on face and body; slight fever (frequently confused with scarlet fever)	From onset and for at least 4 days, possibly 7 days	None usually; serious for women during early pregnancy as may result in defect of baby if mother contracts measles during first trimester
Pus discharge from mucous membrane of genital tract or of eyes; pain and burning on urination	As long as germs appear in discharges, as checked by laboratory tests	Arthritis; sterility, infection of eyes of newborn infants; salpingitis or epididymitis
Anorexia; upper abdominal distress; sudden onset of chills, headache, fever, and jaundice; constipation or diarrhea; pain in or about the eyes; pruritus	As long as the virus is in the feces and blood	Liver damage; changes in mental state; bleeding from a body orifice; mild case can suddenly become serious, leading to death
Slow onset; afebrile; weakness; easily fatigued; anorexia; nausea; jaundice	As long as the virus is in the blood serum	Liver damage

Continued.

Common communicable diseases — cont'd

Disease	How spread	Prevention	How long from exposure to onset
Impetigo	Contact with moist discharges from sores on skin; possible nose and throat discharges	No immunization; reinfection possible; personal cleanliness; prevention of excessive scratching in such conditions as chickenpox and scabies	Perhaps 2 to 5 days
Infantile paralysis (poliomyelitis)	Contact with nose and throat and bowel discharges or infected persons or carriers	Salk and Sabin (oral) vaccines; adults have more immunity than children; one attack usually confers immunity; good sanitation and personal hygiene	Usually 7 to 14 days (may be from 3 to 35 days)
Influenza	Contact with discharges from nose and mouth and articles freshly soiled with discharges	Immunization available; repeated attacks are possible	24 to 72 hours
Measles (rubeola)	Contact with discharges of nose and throat; easily spread	Immunization available; attack may be lightened or prevented in children exposed to measles if immune serum globulin given; babies of immune mothers usually immune for first few months of life; one attack usually confers immunity	Usually about 10 days from exposure to onset of fever; 13 to 15 days to the appearance of rash; as long as 21 days if immune serum globulin has been given
Epidemic meningitis	Contact with discharges of nose and throat; carriers	No immunization; avoid contact, droplet infection, and overcrowding; stress personal cleanliness	2 to 10 days; usually 7 days
Mumps	Contact with saliva of infected persons	Immunization; second attacks have been known but are rare	12 to 26 days; usually 18 days
Rheumatic fever*	Unknown	No immunization; disease recurs; immediate and proper care of "strep" infections	Unknown; it may be several days to 8 weeks after infection before symptoms appear; average is 3 weeks
Ringworm	Contact with sores, discharges from sores, or clothing in contact with sores; contact with infected cats or dogs	No immunization; repeated attacks common; cleanliness; proper sanitation	Not known
Salmonellosis (food poisoning)	Improper refrigeration of foods; foods contaminated by excreta of infected rodents; pet turtles may be carriers	Clean, well-preserved, and well-cooked foods; examination of leftover food for foul odor and color or decomposition; examination of food handlers	6 to 48 hours

Common symptoms	How long communicable	Some possible complications
Running sores on face and hands or body, later showing crusts	As long as sores are unhealed	Occasional infection of sores; may result in death in infants
Many cases not recognized; fever, headache, drowsiness, stiff neck and back, and irritability	Not exactly known, probably latter part of incubation period and first week of acute illness; virus may be found in feces for months	Paralysis of affected parts of body
Sudden onset; fever, aching limbs and back, runny nose, sore throat, bronchitis, and prostration; fatigue; sweating	Uncertain	Pneumonia
Fever, runny eyes and nose, eruption in mouth, followed by rash; branny peeling of skin during convalescence	During period of running eyes and nose, usually about 9 days (from 4 days before to 5 days after rash appears)	Inflammation of middle ear; pneumonia; encephalitis
Usually sudden onset; fever, headache, nausea, and vomiting; rash occasionally; dizziness, stiff neck, and delirium	Until germs disappear from discharges, as checked by laboratory tests	Spread of infection to tissue of brain; eye and ear infections; hydrocephalus
Fever and swelling of salivary glands in cheeks and under tongue	From 1 to 2 days before the symptoms appear until swelling of glands has disappeared	Inflammation of ovaries or testicles in persons past puberty
Slow onset; fever, joint, and muscle pains; nosebleed and petechiae; rapid pulse out of proportion to temperature; loss of appetite, irritability; profuse irritating perspiration; listlessness	See footnote*	Serious damage to heart; chorea
Round, scaly patches on scalp or body; likely to appear on feet, and between toes as well; itching	As long as fungus or spores remain around sores	Occasional secondary infection of sores
Abrupt onset of nausea and vomiting; diarrhea with offensive odor; abdominal cramps and tenderness; may or may not have fever, dizziness, apprehension, delirium, and coma	Not communicable	Prostration; death

Continued.

Common communicable diseases — cont'd

Disease	How spread	Prevention	How long from exposure to onset
Scabies	Contact with an infected person or articles in contact with an infected person	Avoid contact; repeated infestation common; cleanliness; proper sanitation	24 to 48 hours
Scarlet fever†	Contact with discharges of nose, throat, or ears of infected person; carriers; contaminated milk or other foods	No immunization; pasteurization of milk; avoidance of contact with ill persons	1 to 5 days
Smallpox (variola)	Contact with nose and throat discharges and sores on bodies of patients	Vaccination gives protection if rules are followed; one attack usually prevents another	7 to 16 days, occasionally longer; commonly 12 days
Staphylococcal infections	Contact with infected blood, exudates, sputum, stool, etc.; airborne carriers	Asepsis and isolation; reevaluation and enforcement of basic hospital procedures and techniques	2 to 3 days
Syphilis	Contact with discharge from known sores or those hidden on mucous membrane and skin; usually contracted through sexual intercourse; blood of infected persons	No immunization; one attack does not prevent another; case-finding; recognition and treatment of early cases; health education	10 days to 3 weeks or longer
Tetanus	Infected soil, street dust, and animal feces introduced through break in skin, especially through puncture wounds such as those made by nails	Tetanus toxoid — requires enforcing at certain intervals; one attack does not protect; antitoxin given in presence of suspected wound	4 days to 3 weeks
Tuberculosis, pulmonary	Contact with discharges of nose and throat from "active" tuberculous case; occasionally by milk from tuberculous cattle	BCG vaccine given to tuberculin nonreactors; one attack does not prevent another; pasteurization of milk; killing of tuberculous cattle	Variable; probably not less than 1 month and possible longer
Typhoid fever	Contact with infected feces and urine; contaminated water or food, especially milk	Typhoid vaccine gives immunity for about 2 years; one attack usually prevents another	3 to 38 days; usually 7 to 14 days
Undulant fever (brucellosis)	Contact with infected animals; milk of infected animals	No immunization; boiling or pasteurization of milk	6 to 30 days or more
Whooping cough	Contact with infected discharges of nose and throat	Immunization giving considerable protection available; one attack usually prevents another; reinforcing doses of vaccine may be advisable within year and at 2 or 3 years of age	7 to 21 days

Common symptoms	How long communicable	Some possible complications
"Burrows" or lines of sores (row of black dots); severe itching, particularly between fingers	Until itch mite and eggs destroyed	Occasional infection of sores
Sore, inflamed throat; strawberry tongue; fever, nausea, and vomiting; later rash, usually beginning on neck and chest	Not known; 2 weeks at least	Inflammation of middle ear; damage to heart and kidneys; rheumatic fever
Abrupt onset of high fever, vomiting, headache, severe backache, delirium, convulsions, or chills, followed by eruption 1 to 5 days later; crusts fall off in 10 to 40 days; the disease may vary from mild to very severe, with high death rate	From first symptom to disappearance of crusts of eruption; most communicable in early stages of illness	Pitting of skin; occasional blindness; bronchitis; ear infection; abscesses on skin
Depends on location of infection	As long as *staphylococcus* can be cultured	Depends on location of infection
Sore at point of contact, which will heal but may recur during next 5 years after infection; rash, sore throat, headache; in congenital syphilis, only late manifestations, such as those listed under complications, occur	From onset and, if untreated, up to 5 years	Damage to heart and central nervous system including brain, unless treated early
Restlessness and irritability; unreasonable disposition; severe headache; difficulty in urination; profuse sweating; painful muscular movements; pain in cheek or neck muscles on chewing or swallowing; infection of umbilical cord in newborn infant	Not passed on to another person	Rare under proper treatment and prevention — highly fatal if not treated promptly; serum sickness; urticaria
Usually no noticeable symptoms until disease moderately advanced; then fatigue, loss of weight, chronic cough, loss of appetite, and afternoon rise in temperature; night sweats	For duration of active state of disease as shown by tests and x-ray study	Meningitis; miliary (general) tuberculosis; laryngitis; bronchiectasis; hemoptysis; spontaneous pneumothorax
Fever, headache, diarrhea, and stomachache; later rose spots on trunk; mouth and tongue coated with thick "fur"; pulse rapid, out of proportion to temperature	As long as typhoid germs appear in discharges from bowels as checked by laboratory tests	Hemorrhage; bronchitis; pneumonia; perforation and hemorrhage of intestine
Slow onset; irregular fever, sweating, chills, and pain in joints and muscles	Not communicable from human to human	Disease may be prolonged through months and years
Typical "whooping" cough develops from ordinary cough in 1 to 2 weeks; suspect any cough when disease known to be present in neighborhood	From onset to 3 weeks	Bronchitis; bronchial pneumonia; frequently fatal to young babies; convulsions

Tables of weights and measures

Metric system

Length

meter (m) basic unit

1 micrometer (μm)	= 0.000001 meter
1 millimeter (mm)	= 0.001 meter
1 centimeter (cm)	= 0.01 meter
1 decimeter (dm)	= 0.1 meter
1 dekameter (Dm)	= 10 meters
1 hectometer (Hm)	= 100 meters
1 kilometer (km)	= 1000 meters

Weight

gram (g or gm) basic unit

1 microgram (mgc or μg)	= 0.000001 gram
1 milligram (mg)	= 0.001 gram
1 centigram (cg)	= 0.01 gram
1 decigram (dg)	= 0.1 gram
1 dekagram (Dg)	= 10 grams
1 hektogram (Hg)	= 100 grams
1 kilogram (kg)	= 1000 grams

Volume

liter (L) basic unit

1 milliliter* (ml)	= 0.001 liter
1 centiliter (cl)	= 0.01 liter
1 deciliter (dl)	= 0.1 liter
1 dekaliter (Dl)	= 10 liters
1 hektoliter (Hl)	= 100 liters
1 kiloliter (kl)	= 1000 liters

Apothecaries' system

Weight

20 grains (gr)	= 1 scruple (Э)
3 scruples (Э)	= 1 dram (ʒ)
8 drams (ʒ)	= 1 ounce (ʒ)
12 ounces (ʒ)	= 1 pound (lb)

Volume

60 minims (♏)	= 1 fluidram (fʒ or ʒ)
8 fluidrams (fʒ)	= 1 fluidounce (fʒ or ʒ)
16 fluidounces (fʒ)	= 1 pint (O or pt)
2 pints (O)	= 1 quart (qt)
4 quarts (qt)	= 1 gallon (C, Cong, or gal)

Household equivalents

1 teaspoonful (tsp)	= 5 milliliters (ml)
1 dessertspoonful	= 10 milliliters (ml)
1 tablespoonful (tbsp)	= 15 milliliters (ml) or ½ ounce (ʒ)
1 teacupful	= 120 milliliters (ml) or 4 ounces (ʒ)
1 cupful	= 240 milliliters (ml) or 8 ounces (ʒ)

Other commonly used equivalents (approximate)

Weight

1 grain (gr)	= 60 to 65 milligrams (mg)
15 grains (gr)	= 1 gram (g)
1 kilogram (kg)	= 2.2 pounds (lb)

Volume

1 minim (♏)	= 0.06 milliliter (ml)
16 minims (♏)	= 1 milliliter (ml)
1 fluidram (fʒ)	= 1 teaspoonful (tsp)†
1 fluidounce (fʒ)	= 30 milliliters (ml)
1 pint (pt)	= 500 milliliters
1 quart (qt)	= 1000 milliliters (ml)

* 1 ml is considered equivalent to 1 cubic centimeter (cc).

† In medication orders, ʒi is commonly used to designate 1 tsp (5 ml).

Food and Nutrition Board, National Academy of Sciences—National Research Council Recommended Daily Dietary Allowances, Revised 1980 Designed for the Maintenance of Good Nutrition of Practically All Healthy People in the USA Mean Heights and Weights and Recommended Energy Intake

Category	Age (years)	Weight		Height		Energy needs (with range)	
		kg	lb	cm	in	kcal	MJ
Infants	0.0-0.5	6	13	60	24	kg × 115 (95 − 145)	kg × .48
	0.5-1.0	9	20	71	28	kg × 105 (80 − 135)	kg × .44
Children	1-3	13	29	90	35	1300 (900-1800)	5.5
	4-6	20	44	112	44	1700 (1300-2300)	7.1
	7-10	28	62	132	52	2400 (1650-3300)	10.1
Men	11-14	45	99	157	62	2700 (2000-3700)	11.3
	15-18	66	145	176	69	2800 (2100-3900)	11.8
	19-22	70	154	177	70	2900 (2500-3300)	12.2
	23-50	70	154	178	70	2700 (2300-3100)	11.3
	51-75	70	154	178	70	2400 (2000-2800)	10.1
	76+	70	154	178	70	2050 (1650-2450)	8.6
Women	11-14	46	101	157	62	2200 (1500-3000)	9.2
	15-18	55	120	163	64	2100 (1200-3000)	8.8
	19-22	55	120	163	64	2100 (1700-2500)	8.8
	23-50	55	120	163	64	2000 (1600-2400)	8.4
	51-75	55	120	163	64	1800 (1400-2200)	7.6
	76+	55	120	163	64	1600 (1200-2000)	6.7
Pregnancy						+300	
Lactation						+500	

From Recommended Dietary Allowances, Revised 1980. Food and Nutrition Board, National Academy of Sciences—National Research Council, Washington, DC.

The data in this table have been assembled from the observed median heights and weights of children . . . together with desirable weights for adults . . . for the mean heights of men (178 cm) and women (163 cm) between the ages of 18 and 34 years as surveyed in the US population (HEW/NCHS data).

The energy allowances for the young adults are for men and women doing light work. The allowances for the two older age groups represent mean energy needs over these age spans, allowing for a 2% decrease in basal (resting) metabolic rate per decade and a reduction in activity of 200 kcal/day for men and women between 51 and 75 years, 500 kcal for men over 75 years and 400 kcal for women over 75. The customary range of daily energy output is shown for adults in parentheses, and is based on a variation in energy needs of ±400 kcal at any one age, emphasizing the range of energy intakes appropriate for any group of people.

Energy allowances for children through age 18 are based on median energy intakes of children these ages followed in longitudinal growth studies. The values in parentheses are 10th and 90th percentiles of energy intake, to indicate the range of energy consumption among children of these ages (see original text).

Recommended daily dietary allowances,[a] revised 1980

Category	Age (years)	Weight		Height		Protein (g)	Fat-soluble vitamins		
		kg	lb	cm	in		Vitamin A (μg RE)[b]	Vitamin D (μg)[c]	Vitamin E (mg α TE)[d]
Infants	0.0-0.5	6	13	60	24	kg × 2.2	420	10	3
	0.5-1.0	9	20	71	28	kg × 2.0	400	10	4
Children	1-3	13	29	90	35	23	400	10	5
	4-6	20	44	112	44	30	500	10	6
	7-10	28	62	132	52	34	700	10	7
Men	11-14	45	99	157	62	45	1000	10	8
	15-18	66	145	176	69	56	1000	10	10
	19-22	70	154	177	70	56	1000	7.5	10
	23-50	70	154	178	70	56	1000	5	10
	51 +	70	154	178	70	56	1000	5	10
Women	11-14	46	101	157	62	46	800	10	8
	15-18	55	120	163	64	46	800	10	8
	19-22	55	120	163	64	44	800	7.5	8
	23-50	55	120	163	64	44	800	5	8
	51 +	55	120	163	64	44	800	5	8
Pregnant						+30	+200	+5	+2
Lactating						+20	+400	+5	+3

[a]The allowances are intended to provide for individual variations among most normal persons living in the United States under usual environmental stresses. Diets should be based on a variety of common foods to provide other nutrients for which human requirements have been less well defined.

[b]1 RE (retinol equivalent) = 1 μg retinol or 6 μg β parotene.

[c]As cholecalciferol. 10 μg cholecalciferol = 400 IU vitamin D.

[d]1αTE (tocopherol equivalent) = 1 mg d-α-tocopherol.

Water-soluble vitamins							Minerals					
Vitamin C (mg)	Thiamin (mg)	Ribo-flavin (mg)	Niacin (mg NE)[e]	Vitamin B_6 (mg)	Folacin[f] (μg)	Vitamin B_{12} (μg)	Calcium (mg)	Phos-phorus (mg)	Mag-nesium (mg)	Iron (mg)	Zinc (mg)	Iodine (μg)
35	0.3	0.4	6	0.3	30	0.5[g]	360	240	50	10	3	40
35	0.5	0.6	8	0.6	45	1.5	540	360	70	15	5	50
45	0.7	0.8	9	0.9	100	2.0	800	800	150	15	10	70
45	0.9	1.0	11	1.3	200	2.5	800	800	200	10	10	90
45	1.2	1.4	16	1.6	300	3.0	800	800	250	10	10	120
50	1.4	1.6	18	1.8	400	3.0	1200	1200	350	18	15	150
60	1.4	1.7	18	2.0	400	3.0	1200	1200	400	18	15	150
60	1.5	1.7	19	2.2	400	3.0	800	800	350	10	15	150
60	1.4	1.6	18	2.2	400	3.0	800	800	350	10	15	150
60	1.2	1.4	16	2.2	400	3.0	800	800	350	10	15	150
50	1.1	1.3	15	1.8	400	3.0	1200	1200	300	18	15	150
60	1.1	1.3	14	2.0	400	3.0	1200	1200	300	18	15	150
60	1.1	1.3	14	2.0	400	3.0	800	800	300	18	15	150
60	1.0	1.2	13	2.0	400	3.0	800	800	300	18	15	150
60	1.0	1.2	13	2.0	400	3.0	800	800	300	10	15	150
+20	+0.4	+0.3	+2	+0.6	+400	+1.0	+400	+400	+150	[h]	+ 5	+25
+40	+0.5	+0.5	+5	+0.5	+100	+1.0	+400	+400	+150	[h]	+10	+50

[e]1 NE (niacin equivalent) is equal to 1 mg of niacin or 0 mg of dietary tryptophan.

[f]The folacin allowances refer to dietary sources as determined by *Lactobacillus casei* assay after treatment with enzymes ("conjugases") to make polyglutamyl forms of the vitamin available to the test organism.

[g]The RDA for vitamin B_{12} in infants is based on average concentration of the vitamin in human milk. The allowances after weaning are based on energy intake (as recommended by the American Academy of Pediatrics) and consideration of other factors such as intestinal absorption.

[h]The increased requirement during pregnancy cannot be met by the iron content of habitual American diets nor by the existing iron stores of many women; therefore the use of 30 to 60 mg of supplemental iron is recommended. Iron needs during lactation are not substantially different from those of nonpregnant women, but continued supplementation of the mother for 2 to 3 months after parturition is advisable to replenish stores depleted by pregnancy.

Vitamins

Vitamin	Function	Deficiency	Source
Fat-soluble			
A	Essential for growth Helps eyes to adjust from light to dark Ensures healthy skin and mucous membranes	Retarded growth Night blindness Dry skin and mucous membranes	Fish-liver oils Yellow vegetables and fruits Cream and fortified margarine
D	Needed for normal growth Regulates absorption and use of calcium by body	Soft bones Poor tooth and bone formation Rickets	Fish-liver oils Sunlight Fortified and irradiated foods
E	Normal growth Normal reproduction	Unknown	Seed-germ oils, such as wheat Vegetable greens
K	Normal clotting of blood Normal liver function	Hemorrhages	Green vegetables Medication if grave deficiency
Water-soluble			
C	Normal growth Normal cell activity Blood vessels' strength Healthy gums	Scurvy Sore and bleeding gums; bleed easily	Citrus fruits, tomatoes, potatoes, raw vegetables, and melons
B_1 (thiamine)	Normal growth Carbohydrate metabolism Heart, nerve, and muscle function	Retarded growth Loss of appetite Impaired digestion Neuritis (nerve disorders)	Pork, liver, milk, green vegetables, eggs, and whole-grain and enriched cereals
B_2 (riboflavin)	Carbohydrate metabolism Healthy eyes, skin, and mouth	Retarded growth Lesions at corner of mouth and on skin Cataract-like symptoms	Meat, eggs, and milk Whole-grain cereal Vegetables
B_{12}	Essential for normal blood formation Aids function of nerves Necessary for normal growth and maintenance	Pernicious anemia Nervous disturbance Retarded growth	Liver, kidney, and various seafoods
Niacin	Protein and carbohydrate metabolism Function of nerves Normal growth	Pellagra Dermatitis Gastrointestinal disturbance Nervous disturbance	Milk, liver, and meat Whole-grain cereal Peanut butter

APPENDIX J

Exchange list for menu planning

List 1. Milk exchange
Contains 12 g of carbohydrates; 8 g of protein; 10 g of fat.

Whole milk (plain or homogenized)	1 cup
Skim milk*	1 cup
Evaporated milk	½ cup
Powdered whole milk	¼ cup
Powdered skim milk*	¼ cup
Buttermilk (made with whole milk)	1 cup
Buttermilk (made with skim milk)*	1 cup

List 2. Vegetable exchange
Vegetables A
Contain little carbohydrate, protein, or fat; you may eat as much of these vegetables as you wish, except limit raw tomatoes to ½ cup; if cooked, use 1 cup for serving.

Asparagus	Greens	Lettuce
Broccoli	Beet	Mushroom
Brussels sprouts	Chard	Okra
Cabbage	Collard	Pepper
Cauliflower	Dandelion	Radishes
Celery	Kale	Sauerkraut
Chicory	Mustard	Stringbeans (young)
Cucumbers	Turnip	Summer squash
Escarole	Spinach	Tomatoes
Eggplant		Watercress

Vegetables B
Contains 7 grams of carbohydrate, 2 grams of protein; ½ cup is 1 exchange.

Beets	Pumpkin
Carrots	Rutabagas
Onions	Squash, winter
Peas, green	Turnips

List 3. Fruit exchange
Contains 10 g of carbohydrate; fruit may be fresh, dried, canned, or frozen as long as no sugar has been added.

Amounts to use		**Amounts to use**	
Apple (2-in diameter)	1 small	Grapes	12
Applesauce	½ cup	Grape juice	¼ cup
Apricot, fresh	2 medium	Honeydew melon	⅛ medium
Apricot, dried	4 halves	Mango	½ small
Banana	½ small	Orange	1 small
Blackberries	1 cup	Orange juice	½ cup
Raspberries	1 cup	Papaya	⅓ medium
Strawberries	1 cup	Peach	1 medium
Blueberries	⅔ cup	Pear	1 small
Cantaloupe (6-in diameter)	¼	Pineapple	½ cup
Cherries	10 large	Pineapple juice	⅓ cup
Dates	2	Plums	2 medium
Figs, fresh	2 large	Prunes, dried	2 medium
Figs, dried	1 small	Raisins	2 tablespoons
Grapefruit	½ small	Tangerine	1 large
Grapefruit juice	½ cup	Watermelon	1 cup

Based on material in *Meal planning with exchange lists,* prepared by Committees of the American Diabetes Association, and the American Dietetic Association in cooperation with the Chronic Disease Program, Public Health Service, US Department of Health and Human Services.
*Add 2 fat exchanges to meal when 1 cup is used.

Exchange list for menu planning—cont'd

List 4. Bread exchange
Contains 15 g of carbohydrates, 2 g of protein.

Amounts to use		Amounts to use	
Bread	1 slice	Flour	2½ tablespoons
Biscuit, roll (2-in diameter)	1	Vegetables	
Muffin (2-in diameter)	1	Beans, peas, dried and cooked	½ cup
Cornbread (1½-in cube)	1	Baked beans, no pork	¼ cup
Cereals, cooked	½ cup	Corn	⅓ cup
Dry, flake, and puffed types	¾ cup	Popcorn	1 cup
Rice, grits, cooked	½ cup	Parsnips	⅔ cup
Spaghetti, noodles, cooked	½ cup	Potatoes	
Macaroni, etc., cooked	½ cup	White	1 small
Crackers, graham (2-in square)	2	Mashed	½ cup
Crackers, oyster	20	Sweet	¼ cup
Saltines (2-in square)	5	Sponge cake, plain	1
Soda (2½-in square)	3	(1½-in cube)	
Round, thin (1½-in diameter)	6	Ice cream (omit 2 fat exchanges)	½ cup

List 5. Meat exchange
Contains 7 g of protein, 5 g of fat.

Meat and poultry (medium fat), e.g., beef, lamb, pork liver	1 ounce	Fish	
		Haddock, etc.	1 ounce
Cold cuts (4½-in × ⅛-in)	1 slice	Salmon, tuna, crab, lobster	¼ cup
Frankfurter, 8 to 9 per pound	1	Oysters	5 small
Egg	1	Sardines	3 medium
		Cheese	
		Cheddar type	1 ounce
		Cottage	¼ cup
		Peanut butter†	2 tablespoons

List 6. Fat exchange
Contains 5 g of fat.

Butter or margarine	1 teaspoon	French dressing	1 tablespoon
Bacon, crisp	1 slice	Mayonnaise	1 teaspoon
Cream, light	2 tablespoons	Oil or cooking fat	1 teaspoon
Cream, heavy	1 tablespoon	Nuts	6 small
Cream cheese	1 tablespoon	Olives	5 small
Avocado (4-in diameter)	⅛		

†Limit to 1 exchange.

APPENDIX **K**

STATE AND PROVINCIAL BOARDS OF PRACTICAL/VOCATIONAL NURSING*

STATE BOARDS OF NURSING

Alabama Board of Nursing
Suite 203, 500 Eastern Blvd
Montgomery, Alabama 36117
(205) 261-4060

Alaska Board of Nursing
Department of Commerce and Economic
   Development
Div of Occupational Licensing
The Frontier Building
1601 C Street, Suite 722
Anchorage, Alaska 99502-0333
(907) 561-2878

For exam information:
**Licensing Examiner, Board of
   Nursing**
Pouch D-LIC
Juneau, Alaska 99811
(907) 465-2544

**American Samoa Health Service
   Regulatory Board**
LBJ Tropical Medical Center
Pago Pago, American Samoa 96799
(684) 633-1222, ext 206
Telex no: #782-573-LBJ TMC

Arizona State Board of Nursing
5050 N 19th Avenue, Suite 103
Phoenix, Arizona 85015
(602) 255-5092

Arkansas State Board of Nursing
University Towers Bldg, Suite 800
Little Rock, Arkansas 72204
(501) 371-2751

**California Board of Vocational
   Nurses and Psychiatric Technical
   Examiners**
1020 N Street, Room 406
Sacramento, California 95814
(916) 323-2168

Colorado Board of Nursing
State Services Bldg, Room 132
1525 Sherman Street
Denver, Colorado 80203
(303) 894-2430

**Connecticut Board of Examiners for
   Nursing**
150 Washington Street
Hartford, Connecticut 06106
(203) 566-1032

Delaware Board of Nursing
Margaret O'Neill Building
PO Box 1401
Dover, Delaware 19901
(302) 739-4522

**District of Columbia Board of
   Nursing**
614 H Street, NW
Washington, DC 20001
(202) 727-7454

Florida Board of Nursing
111 Coastline Drive, East
Jacksonville, Florida 32202
(904) 359-6331

**Georgia State Board of Licensed
   Practical Nurses**
166 Pryor Street, SW
Atlanta, Georgia 30303
(404) 656-3921

Correspondence address:
Guam Board of Nurse Examiners
Dept of Public Health and Social
   Services
PO Box 2816
Agana, Guam 96910
(671) 734-2950
Telex no: RCA#6215

Hawaii Board of Nursing
PO Box 3469
Honolulu, Hawaii 96801
(808) 548-3086

Idaho Board of Nursing
500 S 10th Street
Suite 102
Boise, Idaho 83720
(208) 334-3110

**Illinois Department of Professional
   Regulation**
320 West Washington Street
3rd floor
Springfield, Illinois 62786
(217) 785-0800

Indiana State Board of Nursing
Health Professions Bureau
One American Square, Suite 1020
Box 82067
Indianapolis, Indiana 46282-0004
(317) 232-2960

Iowa Board of Nursing
Executive Hills East
1223 East Court
Des Moines, Iowa 50319
(515) 281-3256

Kansas Board of Nursing
Landon State Office Building
900 SW Jackson, Suite 551S
Topeka, Kansas 66612-1256
(913) 296-4929

Kentucky Board of Nursing
4010 Dupont Circle, Suite 430
Louisville, Kentucky 40207
(502) 897-5143

**Louisiana State Board of Practical
   Nurse Examiners**
Tidewater Place
1440 Canal Street, Suite 2010
New Orleans, Louisiana 70112
(504) 568-6480

Maine State Board of Nursing
295 Water Street
Augusta, Maine 04330
(207) 289-5324

**Maryland Board of Examiners of
   Nurses**
201 West Preston Street
Baltimore, Maryland 21201
(301) 764-4747

**Massachusetts Board of Registration
   in Nursing**
Leverett Saltonstall Building
100 Cambridge Street, Room 1519
Boston, Massachusetts 02202
(617) 727-7393

Michigan Board of Nursing
Dept of Licensing & Regulation
Ottawa Towers North
611 West Ottawa
PO Box 30018
Lansing, Michigan 48909
(517) 373-1600

Minnesota Board of Nursing
2700 University Ave West #108
St Paul, Minnesota 55114
(612) 642-0567

Mississippi Board of Nursing
135 Bounds Street, Suite 101
Jackson, Mississippi 39206-1311
(601) 354-7349

Missouri State Board of Nursing
PO Box 656
3523 N Ten Mile Drive
Jefferson City, Missouri 65102
(314) 751-2334, ext 141

Montana State Board of Nursing
Department of Commerce
Division of Business and Professional
   Licensing
1424 9th Avenue
Helena, Montana 59620-0407
(406) 444-4279

Nebraska Board of Nursing
Bureau of Examining Boards
Department of Health
PO Box 95007
Lincoln, Nebraska 68509
(402) 471-2001

Nevada State Board of Nursing
1281 Terminal Way, Suite 116
Reno, Nevada 89502
(702) 786-2778

New Hampshire Board of Nursing
Health & Welfare Building
6 Hazen Drive
Concord, New Hampshire 03301
(603) 271-2323

New Jersey Board of Nursing
1100 Raymond Blvd, Room 319
Newark, New Jersey 07102
(201) 648-2570

New Mexico Board of Nursing
4125 Carlisle, NE
Albuquerque, New Mexico 87107
(505) 841-6524, ext 28

New York State Board for Nursing
State Education Department
Cultural Education Center, Room 3013
Albany, New York 12230
(518) 474-3843/3845

For exam information:
**Division of Professional Licensing
Services**
State Education Department
Cultural Education Center
Albany, New York 12230
(518) 474-6591

North Carolina Board of Nursing
PO Box 2129
Raleigh, North Carolina 27602
(919) 733-5356

North Dakota Board for Nursing
Kirkwood Office Tower
Suite 504
7th Street South & Arbor Avenue
Bismarck, North Dakota 58501
(701) 224-2974

**North Mariana Islands
Commonwealth Board of Nurse
Examiners**
Public Health Center
PO Box 1458
Saipan, MP 96950
(670) 234-8950/8951/8952, ext 2018
or 2019

**Ohio Board of Nursing Education
and Nursing Registration**
65 South Front Street
Suite 509
Columbus, Ohio 43266-0316
(614) 466-3947

**Oklahoma Board of Nurse
Registration and Nursing
Education**
2915 N Classen Blvd
Suite 524
Oklahoma City, Oklahoma 73106
(405) 525-2076

Oregon State Board of Nursing
1400 SW 5th Avenue, Room 904
Portland, Oregon 97201
(503) 229-5653

Pennsylvania Board of Nursing
Department of State
PO Box 2649
Harrisburg, Pennsylvania 17105
(717) 787-7142

**Rhode Island Board of Nurse
Registration and Nursing
Education**
Cannon Health Building
75 Davis Street, Room 104
Providence, Rhode Island 02908-2488
(401) 277-2827

**South Carolina State Board of
Nursing**
1777 St Julian Pl, Suite 102
Columbia, South Carolina 29204-2488
(803) 737-6594

South Dakota Board of Nursing
304 S Phillips Avenue, Suite 205
Sioux Falls, South Dakota 57102
(605) 335-4973

Tennessee State Board of Nursing
283 Plus Park Blvd
Nashville, Tennessee 37217
(615) 367-6232

**Texas Board of Vocational Nurse
Examiners**
1300 East Anderson Lane
Building C, Suite 285
Austin, Texas 78752
(512) 835-2071

Utah State Board of Nursing
Division of Occupational & Professional
Licensing
Heber M Wells Bldg, 4th Floor
160 East 300 South
PO Box 45802
Salt Lake City, Utah 84145
(801) 530-6628

Vermont State Board of Nursing
Redstone Building
26 Terrace Street
Montpelier, Vermont 05602
(802) 828-2396

Virgin Islands Board of Nursing
Knud Hansen Complex
Charlotte Amalie
St Thomas, Virgin Islands 00801
(809) 774-9000, ext 132

Virginia State Board of Nursing
1601 Rolling Hills Drive
Richmond, Virginia 23229-5005
(804) 662-9909

**Washington State Board of Practical
Nursing**
PO Box 9649
Olympia, Washington 98504
(206) 586-1923

**West Virginia State Board of
Examiners for Practical Nurses**
922 Quarrier Street
Embleton Building, Suite 506
Charleston, West Virginia 25301
(304) 348-3572

**Wisconsin Bureau of Health
Professions**
1400 E Washington Avenue
PO Box 8935
Madison, Wisconsin 53708-8935
(608) 267-7222

Wyoming State Board of Nursing
Barrett Building, 4th Floor
2301 Central Avenue
Cheyenne, Wyoming 82002
(307) 777-7601

PROVINCIAL BOARDS OF NURSING

**Canadian Nurses Association/
Association Des Infirmieres Et
Infirmiers Du Canada**
50, The Driveway
Ottawa, Ontario
K2P 1E2
(613) 237-2133

**Nurses Association of New
Brunswick/Association Des
Infirmieres Et Infirmiers Du
Nouveau-Brunswick**
231 Saunders Street
Fredericton, New Brunswick
E3B 1N6

**Association of Nurses of Prince
Edward Island**
PO Box 1838, 17 Pownal Street
Charlottetown, Prince Edward Island
C1A 7N5

Yukon Nurses Society
PO Box 5371
Whitehorse, Yukon
Y1A 4Z2
(403) 668-1037

College of Nurses of Ontario
101 Davenport Road
Toronto, Ontario
M5R 3P1
(416) 928-0900

---

*Adapted from *Mosby's medical, nursing, & allied health dictionary,*
ed 3, St Louis, 1990, Mosby.

Comprehensive Examinations

COMPREHENSIVE EXAMINATION 1: PART 1

This examination contains individual questions, each containing a relevant clinical situation. Read all questions carefully. There is only *one best answer* for each question.

Test time allotment (Part 1): approximately 2 hours
Answers and rationales begin on p. 455.

1. Mrs. Winters is admitted to the hospital with bilateral cataracts. She is scheduled for removal of the right cataract. Your initial assessment must include:
   ① Type of lenses to be used after surgery
   ② Disability this problem has caused
   ③ Attitudes toward dependency
   ④ Degree of sight in the left eye

2. The nurse should suspect a secondary problem when her patient with cataracts states that she:
   ① Has painless hematuria
   ② Has occasional memory loss
   ③ Uses a hearing aid
   ④ Needs extra blankets at night

3. Postoperative care after removal of a cataract includes:
   ① Turning q2h
   ② Deep breathing q2h
   ③ Coughing q2h
   ④ Turning, coughing, and deep breathing q2h

4. After extraction of the cataract the nurse would anticipate the need for:
   ① Early ambulation
   ② IV fluids
   ③ Antiemetics
   ④ A visiting nurse

5. A patient with a detached retina will have the following problems:
   ① Halos around lights and headaches
   ② Flashes of light and blind spots
   ③ Blurred vision and pain
   ④ Pain and purulent exudate

6. Mrs. Franklin has been admitted with right upper quadrant pain and has been placed on a low-fat diet. Which of the following trays would be acceptable for her?
   ① Whole milk, veal, rice, and pastry
   ② Liver, fried potatoes, gelatin, and avocado
   ③ Skim milk, lean fish, tapioca pudding, and fruit
   ④ Ham, mashed potatoes, creamed peas, and gelatin

7. Mrs. Daniels is a 67-year-old woman with a diagnosis of congestive heart failure. She is on a 500-g sodium-restricted diet. Which tray would be most appropriate for her?
   ① Fresh beef, salt-free cottage cheese, one small sweet potato, and one large tangerine
   ② Smoked fish, prepared muffins, frozen lima beans, and an apple
   ③ Corned beef on rye sandwich, dill pickle, and pear
   ④ Ham and cheese on regular bread, unsalted hard-boiled egg, and an orange

8. Mrs. Foster has recently received a diagnosis of diabetes. Which of the following symptoms should the nurse include in explaining insulin shock to Mrs. Foster?
   ① Drowsiness, weakness, thirst, nausea and vomiting, dry skin, and flushed face
   ② Rapid pulse and respirations, restlessness, dizziness, headache, elevated temperature, and pain
   ③ Low blood pressure, rapid pulse, confusion, and pale, moist skin
   ④ Trembling, irritability, confusion, hunger, profuse perspiration, blurred or double vision, and poor concentration

9. The symptoms produced in insulin shock are caused by:
   ① Elevated blood sugar levels
   ② Abnormally low blood sugar levels
   ③ Insufficient insulin to metabolize glucose
   ④ Excessive food intake in relationship to insulin dose

10. You need to obtain a 24-hour urine specimen from Mr. Jenkins. Which of the following best describes the proper method for this procedure?
    ① Have him void at 8 AM: then have him void again at 8 AM the following day; send both specimens to the laboratory
    ② Have him void at 8 AM, discarding the specimen: then collect all urine for 24 hours; at 8 AM the following day have him empty his bladder, again discarding the specimen; send the collected urine to the laboratory
    ③ Have him empty his bladder at 8 AM, discarding the specimen; collect all urine for the next 24 hours; have him void again at 8 AM the following day, adding this specimen to the container; send urine to the laboratory
    ④ Have him void at 8 AM; include this specimen in the container: collect all urine for 24 hours; at 8 AM the following day have him void and add this specimen to the container; send to the laboratory

11. A nurse observing a 2-day-old, full-term infant girl in the nursery notices that her hands and feet are cyanotic but that her body and cheeks are pink. She has passed greenish black stool and has lost several ounces since birth. This baby is:
    ① Premature
    ② Immature
    ③ Normal
    ④ Slightly abnormal

12. Surgical severing of the vas deferens results in:
    ① Impotence
    ② Sterilization
    ③ Cryptorchidism
    ④ Epididymitis

13. Hypertrophy of the prostate gland in older men may cause:
    ① Difficulty in urinating
    ② Cryptorchidism
    ③ Failure to produce sperm
    ④ Failure to produce semen

14. Mrs. Jones has been treated with antibiotics for an upper respiratory tract infection for the past few months. She is now complaining of a white, cheesy vaginal discharge with severe itching. Mrs. Jones' symptoms are suggestive of:
    ① Trichomonas vaginitis
    ② Monilial vaginitis
    ③ Simple vaginitis
    ④ Gonorrhea

15. Usual treatment for a vaginal yeast infection would consist of:
    ① Alkaline douches
    ② Flagyl
    ③ Nystatin
    ④ Penicillin

16. You're on a camping trip with a friend. You've caught some trout, which your friend is cleaning with a sharp knife. You leave for a short time and return to find your friend unconscious and bleeding profusely from the left wrist. Your first nursing action would be to:
    ① Wrap a handkerchief tightly on the wrist
    ② Check for breathing
    ③ Elevate the wrist
    ④ Wash the wrist to examine it

17. It is important for the nurse to know that the type of shock resulting from hemorrhage is:
    ① Cardiogenic
    ② Hypovolemic
    ③ Neurogenic
    ④ Septic

18. Which of the following is a sign of shock?
    ① Elevated systolic blood pressure
    ② Increased urine output
    ③ Bounding pulse
    ④ Shallow, rapid respirations

19. To control bleeding from a slashed wrist, your immediate nursing action should be to:
    ① Apply a tourniquet above the wrist
    ② Apply direct pressure on the brachial artery
    ③ Apply direct pressure for at least 6 minutes
    ④ Apply a tourniquet on the wrist

20. Assuming that your first action to control bleeding from a slashed wrist was correct but unsuccessful, you should then:
    ① Apply a tourniquet
    ② Apply direct pressure for an additional 6 minutes
    ③ Apply pressure to the brachial artery
    ④ Apply pressure to the carotid artery

21. A tourniquet applied to a hemorrhaging extremity should be:
    ① Applied and removed at 15-minute intervals
    ② Removed immediately if the extremity feels numb
    ③ Removed as soon as the bleeding stops
    ④ Removed only by a physician

22. Alan, age 9, was admitted to the hospital in sickle cell anemia crisis. Symptoms of sickle cell crisis include all of the following *except:*
    ① Severe abdominal pain
    ② Elevated temperature
    ③ Joint pain
    ④ Elevated hemoglobin

23. Sickle cell disease is caused by a(n):
    ① Virus
    ② Abnormal hereditary trait
    ③ *Streptococcus* bacteria
    ④ Mismatched blood transfusion

24. Your patient is in the fourth grade at school. According to Erikson's theory of psychosocial development, the patient is in the stage of:
    ① Autonomy vs. guilt
    ② Industry vs. inferiority
    ③ Initiative vs. guilt
    ④ Trust vs. mistrust

25. Mr. Willis is a 42-year-old father of three children. He has been admitted to the hospital after an episode of vomiting "coffee ground" material. A diagnosis of peptic ulcer is made. Symptoms of peptic ulcer disease include the following:
    ① Nausea, vomiting, steatorrhea, and indigestion
    ② Nausea, vomiting, and gnawing pain in the epigastric area
    ③ Nausea, drowsiness, dizziness, and diaphoresis
    ④ Abdominal rigidity, rebound tenderness, and elevated temperature

26. Common complications associated with peptic ulcer disease include:
    ① Hemorrhage, perforation, and obstruction
    ② Perforation, peritonitis, and pancreatitis
    ③ Obstruction, jaundice, and anemia
    ④ Peritonitis, hepatitis, and cholecystitis

27. Based on findings of a gastric analysis, which of the following would best support a diagnosis of peptic ulcer disease?
    ① Increased gastric motility
    ② Decreased gastric motility
    ③ Decreased hydrochloric acid production
    ④ Increased hydrochloric acid production

28. In planning the care of a patient with a peptic ulcer, an important goal would be to:
    ① Emphasize the importance of returning to a vigorous activity level as soon as possible
    ② Instruct on the foods to avoid on a high-residue diet
    ③ Instruct on the importance of compliance to the prescribed regimen
    ④ Instructions on the use of sodium bicarbonate as an alternative to expensive antacids

29. A patient with a diagnosis of peptic ulcer disease develops symptoms of pain, abdominal distention, and projectile vomiting. These symptoms suggest which of the following situations?
    ① Cholecystitis
    ② Hemorrhage
    ③ Peritonitis
    ④ Obstruction

30. Mr. Evans has advanced cirrhosis of the liver. What type of food might you expect to find limited in his diet?
    ① Fruits
    ② Vegetables
    ③ Meats
    ④ Carbohydrates

31. Mrs. Gary has a duodenal ulcer. What foods would you suggest that she avoid?
    ① Refined cereals
    ② Protein foods
    ③ Raw foods
    ④ Broiled foods

32. Mrs. Paulino is a diabetic patient and uses the exchange lists to plan her menu. She does not like fish and would like to substitute something for 1 oz of fish at her afternoon meal. You tell her it is permissible to substitute:
    ① One piece of bacon
    ② One egg
    ③ ½ cup of pumpkin
    ④ 1 cup of whole milk

33. While changing Mrs. Johnson's sterile dressing, you spill normal saline solution on the sterile field. The area that becomes wet should:
    ① Be a good place to put the sterile sponges for cleaning the wound
    ② Be considered contaminated
    ③ Be dried before continuing the procedure
    ④ Be removed or covered with a dry towel

34. Mr. Peter's wound shows evidence of an inflammatory reaction. Indications of an inflammation include:
    ① Bleeding and pain
    ② Bruising and swelling
    ③ Coolness and limited motion
    ④ Redness and heat

35. Ms. Glass develops a wound infection and is placed in an isolation unit. You would explain to her that the purpose of isolation is to:
    ① Cure her infection
    ② Help prevent spread of microorganisms to others
    ③ Be sure that nursing personnel do not become infected
    ④ Protect her from further infection

36. Before leaving the isolation unit, the last thing you would do is:
    ① Reach into dirty linen hamper to push down the piled linen
    ② Remember to wash and sterilize the thermometer before taking the next patient's temperature
    ③ Remove the dietary tray from the bedside table
    ④ Remove the gown and gloves

37. Nosocomial refers to infections that:
    ① Are acquired in the hospital
    ② Are confined to a specific area
    ③ Have spread throughout the body
    ④ Have spread shock-causing toxins throughout the body

38. Which of the following may interfere with wound healing?
    ① Constricting bandages
    ② High-protein diet
    ③ Keeping surrounding area dry
    ④ Moderate activity

39. When assessing the apical-radial pulse, which of the following results would indicate an error in technique?
    ① Apical 100; radial 94
    ② Apical 110; radial 110
    ③ Apical 120; radial 130
    ④ Apical 128; radial 80

40. Your patient has bradycardia. You would expect the pulse rate to be in which range?
    ① 40 to 60 beats/min
    ② 60 to 80 beats/min
    ③ 80 to 100 beats/min
    ④ 100 to 120 beats/min

41. A manifestation of conflict that the nurse might observe is:
    ① Anxiety
    ② Homeostasis
    ③ Panic
    ④ Motivation

42. Communication techniques foster therapeutic relationships with patients. The most frequent type of communication used in psychiatric nursing is:
    ① Written
    ② Nonverbal
    ③ Oral
    ④ Proxemic

43. Defense mechanisms are:
    ① Pathologic
    ② Used by most people sometimes
    ③ Usually ineffective
    ④ Rewarding

44. The evaluation step in the nursing process:
    ① May lead to identifying new problems
    ② Is usually formal
    ③ Almost never involves family
    ④ Requires a nurse researcher

45. A necessary part of communication in mental health nursing is:
    ① The ability to argue logically
    ② To ask many questions
    ③ To allow feedback
    ④ To give advice

46. Personality is:
    ① Determined by heredity
    ② Determined by environment
    ③ Relatively fixed and consistent
    ④ Not consistent over time

47. The Freudian theory of personality holds that:
    ① Personality has three parts: id, ego, superego
    ② Stress is important in development
    ③ Personality mediates reality
    ④ Personality varies with time and place

48. "People who talk about suicide never do it." This is:
    ① A true statement about suicide
    ② True in approximately 50% of the cases
    ③ True in approximately 75% of the cases
    ④ A myth

49. Claudia is angry with her husband. When he comes home, she accuses him of being angry. This is an example of:
    ① Repression
    ② Projection
    ③ Displacement
    ④ Rationalization

50. A man who has a strong sexual desire but is married to a woman with less sexual interest begins painting nude models and sells these commercially. This is an example of:
    ① Projection
    ② Conversion
    ③ Intellectualization
    ④ Sublimation

51. Sally and Bob G, ages 26 and 28 years, respectively, have decided to have their second baby. Their first child is 4 years old. Sally has been on norethynodrel (Enovid) for the past several years. After Sally and Bob decided to expand their family, Sally stopped taking her Enovid and has been trying to conceive. She has not been successful. The probable cause for the delay in conception may be that:
    1. Their ages; especially Sally at 26
    2. It takes time for some individuals to adapt to the normal menstrual cycle after being on oral contraceptives
    3. They are both anxious to have another child and are therefore anxious and tense
    4. Four years is a long time to wait between babies, so the body does not respond quickly

52. Ms. P is pregnant for the second time and has a 4 year old at home. She would be considered a:
    1. Gravida I para 0
    2. Gravida II para I
    3. Gravida I para I
    4. Gravida II para II

53. Your patient's last menstrual period, which lasted 5 days, began April 24. Using Nägele's rule, when would her EDC (estimated date of confinement) be?
    1. January 17   3. February 17
    2. March 3   4. January 31

54. Four days before the EDC a patient's bag of waters ruptured spontaneously at 3:45 AM. Because she had a physician's appointment at 9 AM and did not experience any contractions, she kept the appointment. In the office she had several contractions 6 to 7 minutes apart. She was 65% effaced and 2 cm dilated. She was hospitalized, prepped, and placed on a fetal monitor. FHT is 146, strong, and regular. Strong contractions occur every 2 to 3 minutes. She is hungry and asks for lunch. Your answer would be:
    1. "I will make you some lunch if you will wait a few minutes."
    2. "You cannot eat anything, but I will ask the physician if I should start parenteral fluids."
    3. "Nothing by mouth, sorry."
    4. "Because you are in active labor, our policy is only liquids you can see through; however, perhaps you would prefer ice chips?"

55. If the bag of waters is to be ruptured by the physician, what is your responsibility as a nurse?
    1. Time and check contractions afterward and report
    2. Note time and instrument used and check FHT after procedure
    3. Note amount and characteristics of fluid, test with nitrazine, and report
    4. Note time and amount and place pad on perineum

56. Ms. C is in transition. What are the major signs and symptoms that will confirm she is indeed at that stage?
    1. Desire to push, slight bloody show, veins in neck bulging, 6 cm dilated
    2. Legs shaky, feels slightly nauseated, strong contractions, mood change, 8 cm dilated, needs reassurance, guidance
    3. Pressure on perineum, 10 cm, grunting, needs guidance, direction
    4. Titanic, pauseless contractions; use comfort measures, rub back, guide breathing; start oxytocin (Pitocin)

57. The newborn at rest should have a heart rate of:
    1. 100 to 110 beats/min
    2. 110 to 120 beats/min
    3. 120 to 140 beats/min
    4. 160 to 180 beats/min

58. To help a 4-year-old boy adjust to the newborn baby, the parents should be taught to:
    1. Make a plan to have him do simple chores around the house to increase his self-esteem and growing independence
    2. Buy him lots of presents too, since obviously the newborn will be getting presents
    3. Make him cuddle and kiss the baby to teach him the concept of love
    4. Include him in on the care of the baby and plan to spend some time with him alone

59. The health care team includes:
    1. The physician and nurse
    2. The patient and his family
    3. Social workers and physical therapists
    4. All of the above

60. One reason practical nursing evolved was to:
    1. Ease the shortage of nursing personnel
    2. Provide for better use of registered nurses
    3. Eliminate certain health care providers
    4. Ease the cost of nursing education

61. Seeking continuing education is the personal and professional responsibility of the LP/VN and may be accomplished by:
    1. Reading all health-related journals
    2. Attending hospital in-service programs
    3. Paying dues in professional organizations
    4. Attending courses in other disciplines

62. To encourage a professional relationship the nurse should:
    1. Call the patient by his or her first name
    2. Offer sympathy to the patient
    3. Identify self by name and title
    4. Explain all medical procedures

63. National accreditation recognizes high standards in practical nurse education. Schools of practical nursing may seek this accreditation through:
    1. NLN   3. NFLPN
    2. AMA   4. ANA

64. State boards of nursing are:
    1. Uniform in size
    2. Part of the Social Security Administration
    3. Responsible for approving schools of nursing
    4. Composed of only nurse members

65. Daniel Moore, age 20 years, has been admitted to the hospital with a diagnosis of hepatitis. To plan patient care, the nurse should be aware that the primary mode of transmission by which hepatitis A virus (HAV) is passed is:
    1. Contaminated needles
    2. Blood transfusions
    3. Fecal-oral route
    4. Misuse of drugs and chemicals

66. The primary purpose of instituting bed rest for a patient with hepatitis is to:
    1. Rest the liver by reducing the metabolic demands
    2. Control the spread of the disease
    3. Reduce the risk of developing cardiac problems
    4. Reduce the risk of hepatic coma

67. What special precaution will the nurse take in caring for a patient with hepatitis?
    ① Use gloves when removing the bedpan
    ② Wear a mask when entering the room
    ③ Prevent droplet spread of the infection
    ④ Sterilize equipment used in the room with a disinfecting agent

68. Drug addicts are at risk of acquiring which of the following types of hepatitis?
    ① HAV
    ② HBV
    ③ Non-HAV, non-HBV
    ④ Toxic hepatitis

69. The nurse is aware that the early symptoms of viral hepatitis, whether it be HAV or HBV, are similar. What are the early symptoms?
    ① Nausea, vomiting, belching, and right upper-quadrant pain
    ② Nausea, vomiting, fever, and epigastric pain that radiates to the back
    ③ Sternal pain, diaphoresis, dyspnea, and syncope
    ④ Coryza, fever, chills, and headache

70. When patients are receiving the beta-adrenergic blocking agent propranolol (Inderal), the nurse should monitor the patient's:
    ① Weight and diet
    ② Temperature and hematocrit
    ③ Blood pressure and pulse
    ④ Liver blood studies and urinalysis

71. Patients with pulmonary edema associated with congestive heart failure may benefit from the use of the alpha-adrenergic blocking agents because these drugs:
    ① Have a direct diuretic action on lung tissue
    ② Enhance the absorption of carbon monoxide
    ③ Lower elevated pulmonary arterial pressure
    ④ Achieve an indirect cardiotonic effect and thereby improve general circulation

72. While distributing medications, the nurse observes that a patient who has been taking digoxin has not touched any of his breakfast and that a partially filled emesis basin is on his bedside table. Acting on her knowledge of this drug, the nurse would be correct if she:
    ① Gives the drug if the radial pulse is above 60 and reports to the head nurse
    ② Omits the drug, checks the apical pulse, and reports to the head nurse
    ③ Postpones the administration of the drug until after lunch
    ④ Awaits the results of the daily ECG and then administers half the dose

73. Whenever a medication is ordered for its diuretic effect, the nurse should understand the importance of:
    ① Forcing fluids
    ② Placing the patient on bed rest
    ③ Measuring all fluid output
    ④ Daily urinalysis

74. The drug used on a daily maintenance dose to prevent recurrences of an acute manic-depressive episode is:
    ① Elavil
    ② Lithium
    ③ Marplan
    ④ Compazine

75. A nursing observation that would support evidence of the therapeutic effects of antianxiety drug therapy would be:
    ① Crying, facial grimaces, rigid posture
    ② Anger, aggressive behavior
    ③ Decrease in blood pressure, pulse, respirations
    ④ Verbal statements such as "more worried" or "resting poorly"

76. Mrs. Roberts has had progressive renal problems since childhood. Now, at 42 years of age, she is diagnosed as having end-stage renal disease. She is scheduled for hemodialysis. When preparing Mrs. Roberts for hemodialysis, the nurse will:
    ① Record her weight
    ② Restrict visitors
    ③ Keep her NPO until after the procedure
    ④ Monitor catheter drainage

77. To relieve pruritus from uremic frost you should:
    ① Add mineral oil to the bathwater
    ② Use no soap in bathing
    ③ Use hot water in bathing
    ④ Add a weak vinegar solution to the bathwater

78. In planning nursing care for a patient with end-stage renal disease, which goal would have priority?
    ① Providing rest
    ② Maintaining fluid balance
    ③ Preventing infection
    ④ Preventing contractures

79. Patients with end-stage renal disease have a tendency to bleed. When providing care the nurse would be sure to include:
    ① Mouth care q2h
    ② Maintaining complete rest
    ③ A high-protein diet
    ④ Administering medication by injection whenever possible

80. The nurse will assess for internal bleeding by observing:
    ① Sclera and nail beds
    ② Urine and stool
    ③ Temperature and weight
    ④ Posture and mobility

81. As a child, a patient had glomerulonephritis. The nurse knows that this would have occurred after:
    ① A wound infection
    ② Contamination after catheterization
    ③ A beta-hemolytic infection
    ④ Trauma in an automobile accident

82. Assessment of a child with acute glomerulonephritis would include assessing for:
    ① Pyuria, oliguria, and hypotension
    ③ Hematuria, hypotension, and headaches
    ② Polyuria, tachycardia, and hypertension
    ④ Orbital edema, hypertension, and albuminuria

83. Jack, 19 years old, is admitted to the hospital after briefly losing consciousness when he was tackled during the Thanksgiving Day football game. During the neurologic assessment the nurse is careful to note and report the following response by Jack:
    ① He did not know the name of the hospital
    ② He could not remember the name of the nurse
    ③ He said the month was June
    ④ He could not remember the incident on the football field

84. As you assess a patient for increased intracranial pressure, you would be concerned on observing:
    ① A change in level of consciousness
    ② Anorexia and thirst
    ③ Increased pulse and respiration rates
    ④ Blurred vision and halos around lights

85. A pneumoencephalogram is ordered for your patient. You explain that this procedure includes having x-ray films taken:
    ① And there will be no discomfort
    ② After an injection of dye into an artery
    ③ After an injection of a radioisotope
    ④ After an injection of air via a lumbar puncture

86. After a pneumoencephalogram, nursing care will include:
    ① NPO
    ② Low-sodium diet
    ③ Forcing fluids
    ④ Restricting fluids

87. Mr. Dorman, age 72, has bladder and bowel incontinence. At a nursing care planning conference the staff decides to proceed with a bowel-retraining program. Bowel retraining is initiated before bladder retraining because:
    ① Bowel retraining is easier than bladder retraining
    ② Bowel incontinence is more demoralizing to the patient
    ③ Bowel retraining may solve the patient's urinary incontinence
    ④ The patient is usually more cooperative

88. A bowel-retraining program requires suppository insertion. The most appropriate time for the nurse to initiate this action would be:
    ① One hour before breakfast
    ② One hour after breakfast
    ③ One half hour before lunch
    ④ One half hour before supper

89. A bowel-retraining program requires the nurse to do which of the following first:
    ① Assess the patient's bowel habits
    ② Obtain a bowel history
    ③ Implement the program at first sign of incontinence
    ④ Plan an individualized program

90. The most important factor for a successful bowel-retraining program is:
    ① Establishing regular day(s) and time to assist the patient to the toilet
    ② Making sure the patient understands the purpose of the program
    ③ Regular administration of a mild laxative
    ④ Skipping a day in the program if the patient has had more than one bowel movement the day before

91. Which of the following statements regarding glycerin suppository insertion is the nurse expected to know to be true?
    ① Glycerin suppositories should be warmed to room temperature before insertion
    ② It is not necessary to lubricate glycerin suppositories before insertion
    ③ Glycerin suppositories should be inserted into a bolus of stool
    ④ Glycerin suppositories should be inserted before an attempt is made to toilet a patient in a bowel-retraining program

92. Mrs. Edith Gram is a retired school teacher whose husband is on a low-cholesterol diet following a heart attack last June. She says she is totally confused about cholesterol and its importance. Which of the following statements about cholesterol is true?
    ① It is best to be totally eliminated from the diet
    ② It is a normal component of blood and all body cells
    ③ It is not necessary for normal body functions
    ④ It is found in increased amounts in grain products

93. Because respiratory embarrassment could occur following a subtotal thyroidectomy, it is advisable to:
    ① Have an IPPB machine in the room
    ② Place the patient in an oxygen tent for the first 48 hours
    ③ Keep a respiratory stimulant at the bedside
    ④ Keep a tracheostomy tray in the room until all danger has passed

94. The nurse notes that Mr. Jackson, who has a diagnosis of COPD, is more comfortable after:
    ① Being placed in low-Fowler's position
    ② Having postural drainage
    ③ Fluids are restricted
    ④ He has provided all his own care

95. The nurse knows that oral care is essential when a patient is receiving long-term Dilantin therapy because of:
    ① Formation of dental caries
    ② Gingival hypertrophy
    ③ Eroding of the tooth enamel
    ④ The possibility of xerostomia

96. Amyl nitrite is classified as a(n):
    ① Vasodilator
    ② Vasoconstrictor
    ③ Antispasmodic
    ④ Anticoagulant

97. Digitalis is classified as a:
    ① Depressant
    ② Heart tonic
    ③ Coagulant
    ④ Respiratory stimulant

98. The *major* adverse reaction associated with the use of sedatives-hypnotics is:
    ① Hypertension
    ② Respiratory depression
    ③ Anorexia
    ④ Urinary retention

99. The sympathetic stimulating drugs are also called:
    ① Adrenergic drugs
    ② Cholinergic drugs
    ③ Anticholinergic drugs
    ④ Anticholinesterase drugs

100. The principal use of alpha-adrenergic neuron blocking agents is in the management of:
    ① Hypertension
    ② Cardiac dysrhythmias
    ③ Obesity
    ④ Peripheral vascular disease

101. Mrs. Sara Lent has had insulin-dependent diabetes for 20 years. Now at age 68 she has begun to notice that her right foot and leg get numb and the skin is shiny. Last week she bumped her right leg while making her bed. The injured area has not healed and has worsened. During your initial assessment of Mrs. Lent you discover that she is wearing garters. It would be appropriate for you to:
    1. Make a note of this on Mrs. Lent's chart
    2. Notify the physician immediately
    3. Explain that garters retard circulation and should not be worn
    4. Explain that garters are better than girdles because they are not so restricting to circulation

102. Which of the following descriptions of an injured area on a diabetic patient's right leg would be most appropriate to chart?
    1. Large excoriated area on anterior aspect of the shinbone
    2. 50-cent size area on anterior aspect of lower leg with moderate amount of serous drainage
    3. 5-cm abraised lesion with small amount of serous drainage noted on right lower leg
    4. Severe injury with minimal amount of drainage noted on right lower leg

103. Your diabetic patient's right lower leg is taut and shiny. This is significant because:
    1. These symptoms indicate the diabetes is worsening
    2. This indicates the circulation to this extremity may be compromised
    3. Taut, shiny skin indicates edema of the extremity
    4. These symptoms are consistent with a positive Homans' sign

104. During admission your diabetic patient asks for assistance to the bathroom to void. You would:
    1. Assist her to use the bedpan; collect admission urinalysis (UA)
    2. Assist her to use the bedpan; collect admission BUN
    3. Call for help to walk the patient to the bathroom; collect admission UA
    4. Call for help to walk the patient to the bathroom; collect admission BUN

105. You would notify the physician immediately if which of the following findings were noted on a diabetic patient?:
    1. Right pedal pulse was bounding; admission FBS, 168 mg/dl
    2. Right femoral pulse was difficult to palpate; right foot cooler than left foot
    3. Right pedal pulse was not palpated; FBS, 320 mg/dl
    4. Right pedal pulse was thready; right foot cooler than left foot

106. To protect the diabetic patient's affected extremity from further injury you would:
    1. Promote mobility and apply antiembolism stockings
    2. Administer anticoagulants and apply warm, moist compresses
    3. Wrap the leg tightly with an elastic bandage and administer antibiotics
    4. Apply a bed cradle and heel protectors

107. Symptoms of diabetic ketoacidosis are:
    1. Hypotension, hypoglycemia, and thirst
    2. FBS, 400 mg/dl; Kussmaul's respirations; fruity odor on breath
    3. Tremors, sweating, tachycardia
    4. Hypertension, convulsions, and diaphoresis

108. Before withdrawing insulin preparations, which are suspensions, it is important to:
    1. Shake the vial
    2. Rotate the vial
    3. Chill the vial
    4. Heat the vial

109. Factors that may increase insulin requirements for a diabetic patient include:
    1. Decreased caloric intake, renal insufficiency
    2. Increased physical activity, hyperthyroidism
    3. Pregnancy, acute infections
    4. Weight reduction, recovery from acute infections

110. Which of the following types of insulin acts most rapidly?
    1. Ultralente
    2. Regular
    3. NPH
    4. Globin

111. Insulin is administered subcutaneously rather than orally because:
    1. Intestinal absorption is impaired in the diabetic patient
    2. Insulin is inactivated by the gastric juice
    3. Parenteral administration produces a more rapid effect
    4. Hormones tend to be irritating to mucous membranes

112. Your patient is receiving 30 units of NPH insulin every morning at 7:30 AM. You might expect a hypoglycemic reaction at:
    1. 1 PM
    2. 4 PM
    3. 11 PM
    4. 3 AM

113. The injured area on your diabetic patient's leg worsens. Objective data to support this conclusion would be:
    1. FBS, 420 mg/dl; polyuria; and BUN, 16 mg/dl
    2. Purulent drainage, cool right foot, and temperature of 101.6° F (38.7° C) orally
    3. Polyuria, polydipsia, and polyphagia
    4. Ability to dorsiflex *both* feet and FBS, 300 mg/dl

114. Diabetes is a predisposing factor to peripheral vascular disorders because diabetes is a(n):
    1. Mendelian recessive trait common to persons with poor venous integrity
    2. Endocrine disorder that stimulates the kidneys to raise the blood pressure
    3. Metabolic disorder of carbohydrate (CHO) metabolism in which accelerated fat metabolism leads to changes in arterial walls
    4. Disorder in which the administration of insulin causes inhibition of blood supply to the lower extremities

115. The physician tells his patient that he has decided to perform an above-the-knee amputation (AKA). After the physician leaves the patient's room, she turns her head away from you and begins to cry. You would:
    ① Leave the room quietly and allow her to cry without embarrassment
    ② Stay and encourage her to talk about postoperative coughing and deep breathing
    ③ Leave the room and call her husband to come to the hospital to console her
    ④ Stay with her while quietly holding her hand

116. Your patient is taken to OR for above-the-knee amputation; you begin preparing the area for her return. Equipment most appropriate to obtain would be:
    ① IV pole, tourniquet, and extra pillows
    ② Bed boards, Buck's extension equipment, and emergency drug box
    ③ Sandbags, extra pillows, and emesis basin
    ④ Booklet explaining phantom limb pain, IV pole, and extra elastic bandages

117. Symptoms exhibited immediately postoperatively on an AKA that would necessitate emergency action would be:
    ① BP, 100/70; pulse rate, 110 beats/min; respirations, 26/min; and large amount of red drainage on posterior aspect of dressing
    ② Continued flexion of the hip and urine output of 100 ml 2 hours postoperatively
    ③ BP, 150/90; pulse rate, 86 beats/min; and moderate amount of red drainage on anterior aspect of dressing
    ④ Hemoglobin level, 12.6 g/dl; BP, 140/90; and complaints of pain

118. To prevent hip contractures postoperatively on an AKA, you would position the residual limb:
    ① Flexed on a pillow
    ② Extended
    ③ Externally rotated using pilows
    ④ Internally rotated using a trochanter roll

119. As a result of surgery a patient's insulin requirements would be:
    ① Increased
    ② Decreased
    ③ Given intravenously
    ④ Unchanged

120. Since surgery you notice your patient has become increasingly demanding. Today you enter her room, and she yells at you, "Get out of my room. Can't you see I am sleeping?" Your response would be:
    ① "Sorry, but I have to get the baths done before noon."
    ② "Are you having trouble sleeping at night?"
    ③ "You seem angry. Would you like to talk?"
    ④ "Oh, excuse me. I'll come back later."

121. To prepare the residual limb for a prosthetic device you should encourage:
    ① Gluteal setting exercises and straight leg raises and wrapping the residual limb with elastic bandages
    ② Upper extremity push-ups and active ROM exercises
    ③ Massaging of the residual limb and irrigation of the suture line with Betadine solution
    ④ Placing the residual limb in a dependent position constantly to promote blood supply to the area

122. Considering the length of the hospital stay for a diabetic patient with an amputation, it would be most appropriate for you to:
    ① Review diabetic foot care before discharge
    ② Send patient to a nursing home
    ③ Teach patient to administer own insulin
    ④ Ask the family to assist with the housekeeping chores

123. One day your patient asks if she may have beets on her diabetic diet. Your response would be:
    ① "No, they contain too much natural sugar."
    ② "Yes, they are on the diabetic exchange list."
    ③ "Yes, you could. I'll call the dietitian, and you two can review the exchange list."
    ④ "I don't know. Ask your physician. Your diet is too important in your treatment to change very much."

124. Physical signs of alcohol withdrawal include:
    ① Increased blood pressure, increased pulse rate
    ② Low body temperature
    ③ Menorrhagia
    ④ Low blood pressure

125. A patient receiving chlorpromazine (Thorazine) should be advised to:
    ① Avoid certain foods containing tyramine
    ② Use a sunscreen when outdoors
    ③ Take medication with milk
    ④ Use prophylactic antacid

COMPREHENSIVE EXAMINATION 1: PART 2

This examination contains individual questions, each containing a relevant clinical situation. Read all questions, carefully. There is only *one best answer* for each question.

Test time allotment (Part 2): approximately 2 hours
Answers and rationales begin on p. 460.

1. Mandy, age 5, is admitted to the hospital with a possible diagnosis of acute glomerulonephritis. Symptoms of acute glomerulonephritis include which of the following?
   1. Severe edema, proteinuria, fever
   2. Distended abdomen, decreased serum protein
   3. Hematuria, fever, elevated BUN level
   4. Respiratory distress, oliguria, malnutrition

2. A patient's diagnosis of acute glomerulonephritis was most likely preceded by:
   1. A streptococcal infection
   2. *H. influenzae* meningitis
   3. An injury to one or both kidneys
   4. An allergic reaction to a food or medication

3. Treatment measures for a patient with acute glomerulonephritis include all of the following *except:*
   1. Bed rest for 2 to 4 weeks
   2. Antibiotics as ordered
   3. Corticosteroids to reduce edema
   4. Urine testing for protein and specific gravity

4. A patient is ordered to receive ampicillin 250 mg q6h IVPB. The ampicillin is mixed and diluted in 50 ml D5W. The IV tubing delivers 20 gtt/ml. In order to administer the ampicillin over 30 minutes, you would set the drip rate at:
   1. 20 gtt/min
   2. 33 gtt/min
   3. 44 gtt/min
   4. 50 gtt/min

5. An important nursing assessment for an ambulatory patient receiving care for congestive heart failure would include monitoring for:
   1. Ankle edema when sitting upright
   2. Sacral edema when sitting upright
   3. Swelling of the hands and face
   4. Abdominal distention and diarrhea

6. To obtain a urine culture and sensitivity from an indwelling catheter, you:
   1. Attach a sterile drainage bag and obtain the specimen from the outlet spout
   2. Protect the end of the drainage tubing while letting urine drip from the catheter into a sterile specimen tube
   3. Use a needle and syringe, inserting the needle directly into the catheter
   4. Use a needle and syringe, inserting the needle into the port

7. Johnny is out in the yard with his 10-year-old friend Greg practicing for the Little League game. Greg runs into the house and tells you that Johnny is hurt and to come quick. Your *priority* action should be to:
   1. Call EMS immediately, then bring Johnny into the house
   2. Tell Greg to stay in the house and go outside to Johnny
   3. Take Greg with you and go outside to attend to Johnny
   4. Send Greg outside to stay with Johnny while you call EMS

8. You observe that a patient has sustained a contusion to the left eye from a recent fall. Your *initial* nursing intervention should be to:
   1. Apply a sterile patch immediately
   2. Apply an ice pack immediately
   3. Apply warm compresses immediately
   4. Irrigate the eye with saline solution

9. Following initial emergency nursing intervention for a child who has sustained an eye injury, your next priority would be to:
   1. Have the patient lie down in a darkened room
   2. Take the patient to the local emergency room
   3. Call your pediatrician for the name of an optician
   4. Monitor the patient's level of consciousness

10. Following emergency medical treatment, your patient is released and you are told to observe for intraocular hemorrhage. You know to notify the physician at once if you observe signs of:
    1. Nausea and vomiting
    2. Sudden, sharp eye pain
    3. Radiating neck pain
    4. Blurred vision in the right eye

11. A patient expresses concern that his friends will laugh at his black eye. You can *best* hasten absorption of the ecchymosis by applying:
    1. Cold compresses
    2. Warm compresses
    3. Cosmetic foundation
    4. Clay face mask

12. Mental health and mental illness are defined:
    1. In scientific studies
    2. In cultural settings
    3. By behavior
    4. By feelings

13. Historically the treatment of the mentally ill:
    1. Was usually humane
    2. Included exorcism
    3. Was in general hospitals
    4. Was based on scientific principles

14. The development of tranquilizing drugs in the 1950's led to:
    1. Great reductions in the incidence of mental illness
    2. Many patients becoming amenable to other forms of therapy
    3. Closing of mental health facilities
    4. Numerous untoward reactions to medications

15. In community mental health programs, patients are:
    1. Not hospitalized
    2. Hospitalized near their homes
    3. Treated in large mental hospitals
    4. Hospitalized for more than 6 months

16. Mr. Fellows has a diagnosis of hypothyroidism. He is placed on a thyroid replacement drug called Synthroid and will return to the clinic in 2 weeks for follow-up laboratory studies. Which of the following classic symptoms of hypothyroidism might the nurse anticipate Mr. Fellows displaying?
    ① Hirsutism, buffalo hump between the shoulder blades, hypertension
    ② Thirst, dry skin, urinary frequency
    ③ Fatigue, hypotension, urinary frequency
    ④ Muscle cramping, weakness, slow response time

17. Your new patient needs instructions regarding the proper administration of Synthroid. Patient teaching should include:
    ① Withholding medication if pulse rate is below 60 beats/min
    ② Taking the medication at bedtime
    ③ Discontinuing drug therapy when all symptoms have subsided
    ④ Withholding medication and calling the physician if the pulse rate is over 100 beats/min

18. Mrs. Hernandez, 34 years of age, is complaining of infertility, metrorrhagia, and dyspareunia. Examination reveals endometrial-like cells growing elsewhere in her pelvic cavity. This condition is known as:
    ① Endometriosis
    ② Endometritis
    ③ Pelvic inflammatory disease
    ④ Paraphimosis

19. Mr. Knight underwent surgery for a suprapubic prostatectomy. Three days after surgery the cystotomy tube was removed. A specific nursing responsibility at this time is to:
    ① Force fluids
    ② Keep dressing dry
    ③ Encourage ambulation
    ④ Monitor fluid balance

20. Following a transurethral resection of the prostate (TURP) the most common postoperative complication the nurse would assess for is:
    ① Hemorrhage
    ② Pneumonia
    ③ Thrombophlebitis
    ④ Fluid imbalance

21. Considering the symptoms of cancer of the prostate, the nurse's responsibilities include:
    ① Encouraging examination of sexual partners
    ② Making daily assessments for changes
    ③ Encouraging rectal examination for men over 40 years of age
    ④ Maintaining asepsis in all care

22. Lung cancer accounts for the highest cancer mortality in both men and women. How can the nurse best address this issue during routine health promotion?
    ① Emphasize early detection
    ② Emphasize the importance of a well-balanced diet
    ③ Strongly urge to not smoke
    ④ Teach the seven warning signs of cancer

23. Mr. Higgins is a 58-year-old man who has been experiencing intermittent anginal pain during the past 5 months. The pain is more evident during periods of exertion and is relieved with sublingual nitroglycerin and rest. In developing a teaching plan for Mr. Higgins, the nurse is aware that angina pectoris may be precipitated by which of the following situations?
    ① Exercise, emotions, exposure to cold, or eating
    ② Exercise, smoking, exposure to heat, or overeating
    ③ Exposure to heat, smoking, ingestion of caffeine, or anxiety
    ④ Anxiety, overeating, lying supine for long periods, or exposure to cold

24. The symptoms of angina pectoris are caused by which of the following situations?
    ① Increased blood flow to the myocardium
    ② Increased blood flow through the coronary arteries
    ③ Decreased oxygen to the coronary arteries
    ④ Decreased oxygen to the myocardium

25. A patient with a diagnosis of angina asks, "How does the nitroglycerin relieve my chest pain?" The *best* response by the nurse is:
    ① "It improves the pumping action of the heart."
    ② "It increases cardiac output."
    ③ "It constricts coronary vessels."
    ④ "It dilates the coronary arteries."

26. Mr. G experiences headaches after taking nitroglycerin. During a clinic visit he mentions this to the nurse. The nurse's best reply would be:
    ① "I'll mention this to the physician. You may need to take a different drug."
    ② "This is a common effect of this drug. In time the symptom should go away."
    ③ "The physician may need to reduce the dosage of your medicine."
    ④ "You might try taking two aspirins to relieve the symptom."

27. Mr. Johnson, age 62 years, is admitted to the hospital complaining of fatigue, malaise, and sore, stiff joints. His wife informed the physician that at home he had been running low-grade fevers and was definitely losing weight. Admission diagnosis was possible rheumatoid arthritis. In addition to the signs and symptoms given, you would expect Mr. Johnson to have:
    ① Enlarged lymph nodes
    ② Tophi in cartilage of ears, hands, and feet
    ③ Dysphagia
    ④ Hematuria

28. A patient recently admitted to your unit had two diagnostic tests performed: WBC count and erythrocyte sedimentation rate (ESR). In an individual with rheumatoid arthritis you would expect the results to be:
    ① Within normal range
    ② Below normal
    ③ Elevated
    ④ Absent

29. A patient with rheumatoid arthritis is started on a treatment plan that includes all the following *except*:
    ① Antiinflammatory agents or analgesics
    ② Corticosteroids
    ③ Immunosuppressive drugs
    ④ Uricosuric drugs

30. The nurse must stress which of the following when caring for a patient with rheumatoid arthritis?
    ① Continuous activity during the day
    ② Self-performance activities
    ③ Use of the semifirm mattress for greater comfort
    ④ ROM exercises beyond limits of pain tolerance

31. Successful treatment of a person with addiction disorders usually includes:
    ① Electroconvulsive therapy
    ② Tranquilizing drugs
    ③ Dance therapy
    ④ AA-type organization

32. Ms. Jones, a staff nurse on the psychiatric unit, insists that her patient be up and bathed by 9:00 AM. The patient has difficulty complying, saying that she becomes flustered and nervous. This violates which of the following principles?
    ① Be aware of your own resources and limitations
    ② Respect the patient as a person; take time to listen to what is being said
    ③ Be honest
    ④ Help reduce anxiety by making few demands on the patient

33. Special legal consideration is given to the relationship between psychiatric nurses and their patients. This is called:
    ① Privileged communication
    ② Habeas corpus
    ③ Malpractice
    ④ Locus tenems

34. A deprivation particular to the elderly is:
    ① Nutritional diet
    ② Touch
    ③ Intellectual stimulation
    ④ Olfaction

35. When caring for a patient who has just completed an electroconvulsive therapy treatment, an important nursing action is to:
    ① Obtain consent
    ② Give a complete bed bath
    ③ Keep accurate input and output data
    ④ Provide patient with orienting data on awakening because memory may be disturbed

36. The first organization to disseminate materials on birth control in the United States was:
    ① Sheppard Towner (Congress of the United States)
    ② Planned Parenthood Organization
    ③ Margaret Sanger Research Bureau
    ④ The Children's Bureau (United States governmental agency)

37. According to the history of maternity care in the United States the single greatest deterrent to maternal complications, particularly pregnancy induced hypertension (PIH), has been:
    ① Discovery and use of antihypertensive drugs
    ② Good prenatal care
    ③ The advocation of salt-free diet
    ④ The age of the mother

38. In the prenatal clinic you observe Mrs. Edwards being examined by Dr. Jones. He says, "Hmm, your uterus is at the level of your umbilicus." After the examination, Mrs. Edwards asks you what the physician meant by that statement. Your best answer would be:
    ① "It means you have just passed your first trimester of the pregnancy."
    ② "You are approximately in your sixth month of pregnancy."
    ③ "You should be feeling your baby drop soon."
    ④ "You are about 6 weeks from delivery now."

39. Rochelle Brown contracted AIDS from sharing contaminated needles with her husband, Willie. They have one child Jason, 15 months, whom her mother is taking care of. She has just discovered that she is 5 months pregnant. To guide and help Rochelle and her husband, what should you know about AIDS?
    ① It is a highly contagious disease so patients must be isolated
    ② It is likely that her unborn child will be infected with the HIV virus and may have a shortened life expectancy
    ③ It is unlikely that her unborn child will be infected and may expect to enjoy a normal life
    ④ Read all you can about the etiology of the disease

40. As a nurse in the labor and delivery room, you should be familiar with the AIDS protective procedures outlined by the Centers for Disease Control. What precautions would you implement in your nursing care of an active labor patient with a diagnosis of AIDS?
    ① Mask and gloves with blood and body fluid precautions for caring for the newborn and the mother
    ② Gloves with blood and body fluid precautions for caring for the mother and baby
    ③ Gown, mask, and gloves with blood and body fluid precautions during labor and delivery
    ④ Reverse isolation techniques when caring for AIDS-infected patients

41. If you are pregnant and work in the labor and delivery room, what should you know about your vulnerability to the AIDS virus?
    ① You are at a greater risk of contracting the HIV virus
    ② Nurses are not known to be at greater risk of contracting the HIV infection
    ③ Strict adherence to precautions will not protect you from contracting the infection
    ④ An HIV infection during pregnancy will put the infant at risk, so do not care for AIDS patients

42. Ms. Booth, an 86-year-old retired school nurse, is admitted to a nursing home following hospitalization for a fractured left wrist sustained from a fall in her garden. Her medical diagnoses are chronic brain syndrome, arteriosclerotic heart disease, and status post left wrist fracture. The nurse observes Ms. Booth to be withdrawn, frequently nonresponsive to conversation directed to her, complaining that everyone mumbles, and believing that others are talking about her. The nurse should suspect that Ms. Booth is experiencing:
    ① Psychosis
    ② Presbycusis
    ③ Presbyopia
    ④ Presbyophrenia

43. Mr. Z, who has a diagnosis of chronic brain syndrome, approaches the nurse's station and says to the nurse, "Could you please show me where I can get the bus home to Poughkeepsie?" Which response by the nurse would be most therapeutic?
    ① "Go straight down the hall and turn right."
    ② "Do you have money for the bus?"
    ③ "The last bus to Poughkeepsie left 10 minutes ago; you'll have to come back tomorrow."
    ④ "You don't live in Poughkeepsie anymore, Mr. Z. You live here with us in New City."

44. The nutritional status of the institutionalized elderly requires regular monitoring. Ms. Charles is 86 years old; it's important for the nurse to know that her:
    ① Caloric requirements are greater than when she was younger
    ② Caloric requirements are less than when she was younger
    ③ Caloric requirements are the same as when she was younger
    ④ Nutritional requirements are greater now that she's advancing in age

45. Ann Harris is a 30-year-old mother of Adam, 8 months old, whom she is breast-feeding. What would you suggest as an appropriate source of high-quality iron for Adam?
    ① Raisins
    ② Carrots
    ③ Egg yolks
    ④ Yogurt

46. What physical evidence might suggest that an infant's diet is deficient in vitamin A?
    ① Dry skin and mucous membranes
    ② Malformed teeth
    ③ Anemia
    ④ Numerous bruised areas

47. Sammy, age 4 years, has become a "picky eater," a fact that is a constant concern to his mother. What might be suggested as acceptable ways to increase the nutritional content of his diet?
    ① Large servings that make him feel older
    ② Coaxing him to eat by offering after-dinner rewards
    ③ Offering "finger foods" such as celery sticks with peanut butter as snacks
    ④ Making sure that he finishes everything on his plate

48. How should a mother, who is breast-feeding, adjust her diet to meet the nutritional demands of breast-feeding?
    ① Higher in iron and lower in fluids
    ② Lower in fats and sodium
    ③ Lower in cellulose and carbohydrates
    ④ Higher in calories and proteins

49. If an infant's diet consists of nothing more than breast milk, what nutrient would most be lacking?
    ① Iron
    ② Calcium
    ③ Protein
    ④ Vitamin C

50. The absorption of iron is aided and enhanced by what vitamin?
    ① Vitamin D
    ② Vitamin C
    ③ Vitamin B_6
    ④ Vitamin E

51. Your 17-year-old patient has just received the diagnosis of chickenpox. You should place your patient in which category-specific isolation?
    ① Drainage/secretion
    ② Respiratory
    ③ Strict
    ④ Universal blood and body fluid

52. Your patient's care plan indicates he has orthopnea; your nursing intervention will include:
    ① Keeping the bed in high-Fowler's position
    ② Maintaining oxygen at 40% by Venturi mask
    ③ Taking vital signs q2h
    ④ Using log-rolling technique to turn him to his side

53. While obtaining a throat culture, the structure to *avoid* touching with the swab is the:
    ① Nasal turbinate
    ② Posterior pharynx
    ③ Tonsil
    ④ Uvula

54. Mr. Raymond Jenner, 59 years old, is brought to the emergency room after collapsing at work. A friend reports that he complained of a severe headache and then fell to the floor. Mr. Jenner exhibits right-sided weakness that includes drooping of the mouth on the right side. His vital signs are as follows: BP, 200/120; pulse rate, 118 beats/min; respirations, 16/min; and temperature, 99.6°F (37.5°C). Initial diagnosis: cerebral vascular accident (CVA). Emergency nursing care of a patient with a possible CVA includes:
    ① Placing the patient on the unaffected side to prevent aspiration while maintaining a flat position
    ② Elevating the head slightly to promote venous drainage while turning to the affected side
    ③ Encouraging the patient to talk to maintain level of consciousness
    ④ Lowering the head to increase circulation to the brain

55. Physical examination reveals that your patient is suffering from systemic hypertension. Possible causes of hypertension include:
    ① Loss of fluid and electrolytes
    ② Overstimulation of the sympathetic nervous system
    ③ Decreased elasticity of the arterioles
    ④ Decreased blood volume

56. Normal blood pressure for a man 55 to 60 years of age would be:
    ① 100/40
    ② 140/90
    ③ 160/100
    ④ 200/120

57. Rehabilitation of the CVA patient must begin on the day of admission. The *immediate* nursing goal in addition to lifesaving efforts during the acute stage is to:
    ① Retrain the paralyzed side
    ② Ambulate with assistance
    ③ Encourage PO fluid intake
    ④ Prevent deformities and complications

58. CVA patients with expressive aphasia will benefit *most* if you:
    ① Speak more slowly and louder
    ② Use gestures and facial expressions
    ③ Provide the patients with a tablet and pencil
    ④ Remove unnecessary items from the environment

59. In caring for a CVA patient who has exhibited dysphagia, it is most important that you *first:*
    1. Gear verbal communication techniques to compensate for the patient's deficits
    2. Assess the gag reflex
    3. Use simple pictures to retrain the patient in the identification of objects
    4. Offer small sips of water and progress as tolerated

60. When positioning a CVA patient on his back, the lower arm and hand of the affected side should be placed:
    1. Across the chest
    2. Parallel with the body, with the elbow extended
    3. Elevated on a pillow beside his chest and trunk
    4. Extended above the head

61. To promote retraining of the affected side and a faster return to independence, CVA patients should be encouraged to:
    1. Comb their hair; wash their face; brush their teeth
    2. Participate actively in physical therapy
    3. Perform daily push-ups
    4. Use a pen with the affected hand

62. Mr. Todd was admitted 2 days ago with a diagnosis of CVA. His wife tells you, "Every time I go into the room he cries. I am afraid I have done something to upset him." The best response is:
    1. "He is trying to get your sympathy. You must ignore the crying and talk about other things."
    2. "He has no control over his crying. It is a symptom of his illness and does not mean that he is unhappy."
    3. "He needs some time alone to sort out his feelings. You should consider staying away for a few days."
    4. "He might benefit from a psychiatric consultation. Perhaps you could talk to your physician."

63. To prevent constipation in your CVA patients, you should encourage them to:
    1. Take daily enemas
    2. Use a daily laxative
    3. Increase fruits and fluids in their diet
    4. Plan a bowel movement for early morning

64. To avoid urinary complications associated with decreased mobility you should encourage patients to:
    1. Increase intake of citrus fruits
    2. Decrease intake of fluids
    3. Decrease intake of dairy products
    4. Increase urine acidity

65. To *best* assist Mr. A, who has been on bedrest, to prepare for ambulation you should:
    1. Dangle the patient's legs and swing them back and forth daily
    2. Have him push his popliteal space against the bed to the count of five, several times daily
    3. Perform passive range of motion exercises three times daily
    4. Have him perform push-ups and use the bed trapeze bar as much as possible

66. Sarah, age 32, in her last trimester, was admitted for induction of labor. She complains of feeling faint, particularly in a prone position, during labor. You know that the failure of venous return of blood from the legs and pelvis may be caused by compression of the inferior vena cava by the uterus, so you would:
    1. Take her blood pressure stat
    2. Place her in Trendelenburg's position
    3. Turn her on her left side
    4. Start suction machine; have intubation equipment ready

67. Patients receiving oxytocin (Pitocin) to induce labor must be carefully observed for:
    1. Hypotension
    2. Hyperstimulation of the uterus
    3. Prolapse of the umbilical cord
    4. Maternal exhaustion

68. If a patient is to have a forceps delivery, the physician would be sure that the bag of waters has ruptured and that the head is engaged. The nursing responsibility would be to check that:
    1. Sterile forceps are available
    2. Forceps are well lubricated
    3. The bladder is empty; catheterize if necessary
    4. The fetal heart tones are regular

69. On admission, Mr. Katz's wife reports that her husband has complained of headaches and has had three blackout spells in the past 6 months. He has complained of numbness and tingling on his right side at intervals but has refused to see his physician since the symptoms have subsided. Previous symptoms experienced by Mr. Katz indicate transient ischemic attacks (TIAs), which are caused by a:
    1. Complete obstruction in oxygen supply to the brain, resulting in necrosis
    2. Decreased amount of circulating oxygen
    3. Complete obstruction in the afferent nerve tracts
    4. Temporary lack of oxygen to an area of the brain

70. Coumadin is a possible drug of choice in the treatment of TIAs. Patients taking Coumadin should be instructed to:
    1. Increase their intake of vitamin K
    2. Use razors and sharp instruments with care
    3. Massage and exercise their legs daily
    4. Take aspirin four times daily

71. The effects of Coumadin on the patient can best be assessed by monitoring the:
    1. Lee-White clotting time
    2. Prothrombin time
    3. Platelet count
    4. Partial thromboplastin time

72. In caring for patients taking Coumadin it is important to:
    1. Change the IV site every 48 hours
    2. Record intake, output, and daily weight
    3. Observe mucous membranes, urine, and stools
    4. Observe skin texture and turgor

73. A patient who complains of tinnitus is describing a symptom that is:
    1. Functional
    2. Diagnostic
    3. Objective
    4. Subjective

74. During preoperative teaching the nurse explains why a local anesthetic will be given for removal of a cataract. The correct explanation is:
    1. This is an individual physician's preference
    2. Recovery time is shorter with local anesthesia
    3. Local anesthetic lessens postoperative bleeding
    4. General anesthetic frequently causes vomiting, which puts stress on the sutures in the eye

75. The nurse is bathing Mary Thomas, 37 years old, who was admitted for observation after sustaining a head injury in an automobile accident. The nurse is concerned when Mary:
    1. Vomits her breakfast
    2. Insists on giving self care
    3. Refuses to take any medications
    4. Cries after talking on the phone with her children

76. The nurse observes Mr. DeMarco, who has multiple sclerosis and is experiencing diplopia. He has worn his eye patch over his right eye since admission 3 days ago. The nurse should explain the necessity of:
    1. Using a new sterile eye patch daily
    2. Washing eye with saline daily
    3. Alternating the patch between the 2 eyes
    4. Wearing the patch only at night

77. A patient's BUN (blood urea nitrogen) level is markedly elevated. The nurse understands that a priority in care is:
    1. Forcing fluids
    2. Skin care
    3. Mouth care
    4. Keeping the side rails up

78. Positioning of an unconscious patient includes:
    1. Elevating the head slightly to promote venous return
    2. Elevating the feet to promote circulation to the brain
    3. Placing the patient on his or her side to prevent aspiration
    4. Placing the patient flat to allow the diaphragm to expand

79. Fluids and electrolytes are carefully monitored in patients with renal disease. A priority concern would be an elevation of:
    1. Sodium
    2. Potassium
    3. Chloride
    4. Calcium

80. During a class, a student nurse observes that a classmate has fallen to the floor and appears to have lost consciousness. The classmate is having spastic movements of her extremities. During this grand mal seizure, the student nurse acts to prevent injury. Appropriate action at this time includes:
    1. Removing all furniture from the area
    2. Holding the classmate's arms
    3. Returning the classmate to the chair
    4. Getting assistance to move classmate to a rest area

81. Tammy Pride, a 14-year-old girl, had a spina bifida repaired at birth. She has since developed a marked scoliosis and is now admitted to the hospital for spinal fusion and instrumentation. During Tammy's admission procedure the primary goal is to provide:
    1. Privacy
    2. Orientation to ward
    3. Her mother's presence
    4. Introduction to her roommates

82. Your teenage patient, Paula, is scheduled for spinal fusion and instrumentation in the morning. The evening before surgery she comes to the nursing station making demands. You understand this behavior is primarily a result of:
    1. Maladjustment to hospitalization
    2. Stress of pending surgery
    3. Past hospital experiences
    4. Inadequate preparation for surgery

83. Your preoperative patient continually interrupts activities at the nursing station until late in the evening. To help alleviate this behavior, your best nursing action would be to:
    1. Continue to ignore her behavior
    2. Provide opportunity for conversation
    3. Allow her to make phone calls
    4. Insist that she return to her room

84. The morning of surgery your patient asks you for a drink. You understand that the patient must be kept NPO because:
    1. This is routine for all surgery
    2. The risk of aspiration is present
    3. The IV will provide adequate hydration
    4. PO fluids may cause edema

85. Susan returns to her room from the ICU where she was nursed for 24 hours postoperatively. She is allowed to eat but must have a high-protein intake. Which of these foods is highest in protein content?
    1. Dried beans and peas
    2. Eggs and cheese
    3. Fresh vegetables
    4. Cooked cereals

86. Pam, 15 years old, becomes embarrassed when you attempt to do her perineal care 2 days after her surgery for a spinal fusion. You can best handle this situation by:
    1. Telling her you will do it today and she can do it next time
    2. Postponing it until her mother comes in so she can do it
    3. Allowing her to participate while you assist
    4. Leaving the room so she can do it without embarrassment

87. Lee, age 13, asks you how much longer before she can go home. She says she doesn't like it here with all the "calling out and noises at night." Your best response would be:
    1. "Would you prefer to be in a room by yourself?"
    2. "I can stay with you now for a while if you'd like."
    3. "You have to ask the physician because we have no say in those matters."
    4. "You must stay at least 2 weeks when you have this kind of surgery."

88. Your patient has been fitted with a lumbar brace but complains that it rubs and doesn't fit well. Your first reaction should be to:
    1. Reassure her it takes time to adjust
    2. Remove brace and return for adjustments
    3. Notify nurse and physician of faulty brace
    4. Inspect the brace for correct application

89. Seth, a 15-year-old boy who was recently fitted with a full back brace, asks you "May I leave off this brace for school parties?" Your best response would be:
    1. "Every now and then as long as your back doesn't bother you."
    2. "Your brace shouldn't be off at all, only when bathing."
    3. "It is most important for you to have it on when taking long walks."
    4. "After a couple of weeks you should be able to wean yourself from the brace."

90. Mr. Polanski is a 55-year-old male with a 10-year history of gout as well as a history of osteoarthritis. He is also overweight. Gout can be caused by which of the following?
    1. Obesity
    2. Trauma
    3. Bacterial organism
    4. Disturbance in purine metabolism

91. Your patient's uric acid levels are high. The physician orders a medication that interferes with the conversion of purine to uric acid. This medication is known as:
    1. Solganal
    2. Urised
    3. Motrin
    4. Zyloprim

92. Conservative therapy is instituted for a patient with a diagnosis of gout. Nursing care may include all of the following *except:*
    1. Limiting fluids
    2. Instituting a weight management program
    3. Encouraging a diet low in meat protein and high in fruits and vegetables
    4. Monitoring the status of the presenting symptoms

93. Mrs. Break is a 75-year-old female who slipped and fell while working in her yard. Her diagnosis is subcapital fracture of the right hip. She is scheduled for surgery tomorrow morning. The nurse is aware that until the time of surgery, the fracture must be reduced. The nurse will anticipate using which of the following devices?
    1. Buck's extension
    2. Bryant's traction
    3. Hodgen splint
    4. Thomas splint with a Pearson attachment

94. All of the following are nursing considerations when assessing a patient's traction device *except:*
    1. Cord should be strung through the pulleys
    2. Assess for the correct poundage
    3. Be sure that bed linen is not wrapped around the cord or pulley
    4. Be sure the weights rest squarely against the floor

95. Ms. E has a total hip replacement. The postoperative orders include aspirin, grains 5, PO, daily. The nurse is aware that the rationale for this treatment is to:
    1. Prevent joint inflammation
    2. Produce a mild anticoagulant effect
    3. Provide better pain-control
    4. Maintain normal body temperature

96. In reviewing discharge instructions for your patient who had a total hip replacement, you would advise the patient and family of all the following instructions *except:*
    1. Do not flex hips more than 30 degrees
    2. Do not bend at the waist more than 90 degrees
    3. Do not sit in low chairs
    4. Do not cross the legs

97. Mr. Chung has had an above-the-knee amputation (AKA) because of complications stemming from long-standing, uncontrolled diabetes mellitus. Following an amputation, the *immediate,* most serious postoperative complication(s) is(are):
    1. Infection
    2. Hemorrhage
    3. Contractures
    4. Pneumonia

98. In caring for a patient who has undergone a midthigh amputation, the nurse should *not* elevate the residual limb after the first 24 hours. The purpose of this precaution is to prevent:
    1. Phantom limb pain
    2. Circulatory embarrassment
    3. A hip flexion contracture
    4. Damage to the peroneal nerve

99. Mr. Horn, who recently had a below-the-knee amputation (BKA), tells the nurse that he feels a burning sensation in the toes of the leg that was amputated. In developing a reply to his statement, the nurse should consider which of the following?
    1. He is probably imagining the sensation as a result of all the medication he has received
    2. He is probably trying to deny having had the surgery by thinking that the leg was not removed
    3. The complaint is a common one in persons developing a flexion contracture
    4. The sensation is probably valid and is known to develop following an amputation

100. Bob Marken is 37 years old. Two days ago, he was admitted with shortness of breath and a temperature of 104°F (40°C). Bob lives in a nearby city. On admission he stated he was a homosexual and lives with Ralph Sargent, who has been his partner for over 4 years. The physician thinks that Bob may have AIDS and places him on isolation precautions. The reasoning for this is that:
    1. All homosexuals are at high risk for AIDS
    2. Respiratory problems are usually the first observed in patients with AIDS
    3. All patients with pneumonia must be isolated
    4. All patients must be isolated until AIDS has been ruled out

101. Nursing assessment must be accurately documented. The charted observation states that a patient had "tachypnea." The nurse knows that respirations were:
    1. Increased in rate and depth
    2. Slow and regular in rate
    3. Deep and fast, then shallower and slower with apneic periods
    4. Increased in rate and decreased in depth

102. Your patient has returned to his room after a bronchoscopy. A priority in care would be for the nurse to:
① Explain that bed rest is necessary
② Observe for allergic reaction
③ Test gag reflex before giving oral food or fluids
④ Force fluids to loosen secretions

103. The diagnosis of AIDS is confirmed on Mr. M and isolation precautions must be taken. You understand how the disease is transmitted and as his nurse you explain that he will require:
① Complete isolation precautions
② Reverse isolation and room restriction
③ Room restriction and restriction of visitors
④ Body fluids and respiratory isolation

104. A supportive nurse must recognize that a patient's first reaction to a diagnosis of AIDS will be:
① Anger
② Bargaining
③ Denial
④ Depression

105. Persons who have had sexual contact with someone who has AIDS will be tested for the AIDS virus. The nurse lessens their anxiety by explaining:
① AIDS is rarely transmitted in monogamous relationships
② Infection with HIV does not always result in the AIDS disease
③ Many people have a natural immunity to AIDS
④ Measures can be taken to prevent the disease in someone recently exposed to the virus

106. In caring for an AIDS patient with pneumonia, you note his pneumonia is responding to antibiotics. However, he continues to be weak and anorexic. One morning you note large, purple, raised marks on his legs. You record and report it immediately because this could be:
① An allergic reaction to the antibiotic
② A sign of internal bleeding
③ Kaposi's sarcoma
④ A suicide attempt

107. A 37-year-old AIDS patient who is homosexual has increased susceptibility to disease because of:
① Immune suppression
② His age
③ His sexual preference
④ Side effects of medication

108. When discussing an AIDS patient's decreasing resistance to infection, the nurse explains:
① The need to remain in the hospital indefinitely
② How the patient will be of great danger to those with whom he or she comes in contact
③ The expense of being maintained on antibiotics
④ That the patient will have to take measures to avoid exposure to new organisms

109. Gerri F. is your postpartum patient. This is her third day following delivery, and she complains that her left leg aches. You feel that it is warm. What should you do while awaiting the arrival of the physician?
① Apply ice bags to the leg
② Apply heat to the leg
③ Exercise the leg vigorously
④ Elevate the leg on pillows

110. How would you explain natural childbirth education to parents?
① "It is a method free from the use of drugs during labor and delivery."
② "Basically, it is preparation for labor and delivery by teaching relaxation exercises and breathing exercises to be used during pregnancy, labor, delivery, and postpartum."
③ "It prepares young couples to be good parents by teaching about newborns, nutrition, exercises, labor and delivery, and child care."
④ "It is preparing to have your baby in as natural a setting as you can, free from noise, in a quiet environment with soft music."

111. Classes in psychoprophylactic or Lamaze method of natural childbirth education are usually begun:
① As soon as the pregnancy is diagnosed
② Shortly after quickening
③ After lightening
④ 8 to 10 weeks before EDC (expected date of confinement)

112. Fred and Amy Haase wish to have children. They have been married 5 years and have no demonstrable physical impairments. Amy has read that all IUDs are dangerous and are being recalled. She says she knows several friends who are using them and wonders if she should alert them. Your best response would be:
① "IUDs often cause pelvic inflammatory disease."
② "Only the Dalkon shield has been recalled; other types of IUDs are still used with an 80% or higher success rate. However, other options are available. Would you like me to tell you about them?"
③ "There are other alternatives to IUDs. Would you like me to explore them with you?"
④ "It is none of your business what other people use."

113. You work in an obstetrics clinic, and your patient and her husband wish to know about rhythm or safe method of contraception, even though their problem is fertility and not family planning per se. You would teach them that:
① Investigations by the woman and her husband to determine the time of ovulation are necessary
② Abstinence from coitus for 10 days before and after the calculated date of ovulation is imperative
③ A record of her menstrual cycle for at least 3 months is necessary before initiating the method
④ Regular 30-day menstrual cycles are necessary for the method to be useful

114. While bathing Mr. Seth, you notice a reddened area on his right hip. The appropriate nursing action is to:
① Massage the area every 2 hours and keep him off his right side
② Clean with alcohol and apply a sterile dressing
③ Apply warm, moist compresses intermittently
④ Apply lotion and powder before turning him on the right side

115. Ms. Poi cannot close her left eye completely because of a recent injury. Nursing measures to protect her eye include:
① Irrigating the eye daily with sterile water
② Keeping the lights dim in the room
③ Instilling artificial tears and covering eye with a patch
④ Applying an antibiotic ointment to the lower eyelid

116. After being stuck with a contaminated needle, you receive a dose of gamma globulin. This injection provides:
    ① Acquired active immunity
    ② Natural active immunity
    ③ Acquired passive immunity
    ④ Natural passive immunity

117. Kevin O'Brian, 4 weeks old, is admitted to your unit for a cleft lip repair. He has a bilateral cleft lip and palate. His mother states he has been a problem to feed, and she found an Asepto syringe to be best. She says the baby has had the sniffles. Kevin's vital signs are temperature 100.8° F (38.2° C), pulse rate 90 beats/min, respirations 36/min, BP 70/35. The nurse should know that a common complication in children with Kevin's diagnosis is:
    ① UTI
    ② URI
    ③ PIO
    ④ SOB

118. Sid, 6 weeks old, is admitted for surgical repair of a cleft lip. Vital signs are temperature 100.8°F (38.2°C), pulse rate 90 beats/min, respirations 36/min, BP 70/35. Which vital sign is abnormal and what would you do about it?
    ① Respirations: call anesthesia
    ② Pulse rate: notify anesthesia
    ③ Temperature: notify admitting physician
    ④ Blood pressure: notify admitting physician

119. Your patient's mother wishes to bathe her baby. While caring for her baby, you should:
    ① Support the mother emotionally
    ② Clean the utility room
    ③ Take a break
    ④ Prepare chart for the OR

120. Paul goes to the OR for repair of a bilateral cleft lip and cleft palate. On his return he has a Logan bar in place to support his lip. He is cranky and trying to suck on his fists. To keep his fists out of his mouth, you should:
    ① Tie his hands to the bed
    ② Apply elbow restraints
    ③ Apply mummy restraint
    ④ Not worry about this

121. On return from the recovery room your infant patient (4 weeks old) appears to be hungry. The order reads, "Return to diet for age when fully awake." What would you give the infant first?
    ① Formula
    ② Cereal
    ③ Fruit
    ④ Water

122. Tom, a 10-month-old infant, refuses his diet from you while you are caring for him. You should:
    ① Get an order for NG feedings
    ② Have his mom try to feed him
    ③ Get another nurse to try
    ④ Wait; when he gets hungry he'll eat

123. After several failed attempts to feed your infant patient with a rubber-tipped Asepto syringe, a nasogastric tube is inserted. Before each feeding, you must:
    ① Check the placement
    ② Heat the formula
    ③ Burp the baby
    ④ Hold the baby

124. Asepto syringe feedings are to be resumed on Pete, a 6-week-old infant. You are instructed to pull the NG tube after he tolerates Asepto feedings. You should:
    ① Feed him with the Asepto syringe while the NG tube is still in place
    ② Remove the NG tube and give him his feeding
    ③ Wait 2 hours after Asepto feeding and pull the tube
    ④ Both 1 and 3

125. Which of the following would be the most suitable toy for an infant with wrist restraints?
    ① Stuffed animal
    ② Rattle
    ③ Mobile
    ④ Radio

COMPREHENSIVE EXAMINATION 2: PART 1

This examination contains individual questions, each containing a relevant clinical situation. Read all questions carefully. There is only *one best answer* for each question.

Test time allotment (Part 1): approximately 2 hours
Answers and rationales begin on p. 466.

1. A small southern town has been devastated by a hurricane that has blown out to sea. You're part of a volunteer rescue team searching for local missing persons. The team splits up; you're alone and you find a man lying on his back moaning. Rapid assessment reveals a questionable back injury. Which of the following nursing actions should have the highest priority?
   ① Keeping the victim in supine position
   ② Positioning the victim in a side-lying position
   ③ Permitting the victim to assume the most comfortable position
   ④ Sitting the victim up to properly assess his pulmonary status

2. Driving to work one morning you stop at the scene of a motor vehicle accident. You note the victim's lower extremities are paralyzed. As a nurse you should immediately suspect:
   ① Quadriplegia
   ② S-1 injury
   ③ Paraplegia
   ④ Injury to C6-7

3. Which of the following nursing interventions should have the highest priority in an emergency situation?
   ① Immobilization
   ② Pain control
   ③ Control of hemorrhage
   ④ Treatment of shock

4. Mrs. Baxter is a 62-year-old retired teacher who has come to the emergency room with a complaint of coughing, ankle edema, and difficulty breathing when in a supine position. A diagnosis of congestive heart failure (CHF) is made. In evaluating nursing actions, the nurse is aware that CHF results from which of the following conditions?
   ① The inability of the heart to pump out as much blood as is received
   ② The left ventricle empties more rapidly than the right ventricle
   ③ There is incomplete emptying of the right atrium
   ④ Pooling of blood in the heart because of hypovolemia

5. In implementing the plan of care for a patient with CHF, the nurse should anticipate administering what cardiac drug to relieve the CHF?
   ① Lidocaine
   ② Lanoxin
   ③ Levophed
   ④ Nitroglycerin

6. In planning the nursing care of a patient with acute CHF, the nurse should consider which of the following?
   ① Provide a high-calorie diet; prevent deformities; provide exercise
   ② Prevent infection; force fluids; encourage exercise and activity
   ③ Provide gradual return to activity; maintain skin integrity; provide a sodium-restricted diet
   ④ Provide bed rest during hospitalization; force fluids; provide a high-calorie, nutritious diet

7. Ms. C, a patient with CHF, is placed in a high-Fowler's position. What is the rationale for placing the patient in this position?
   ① To reduce the volume of blood returning to the heart
   ② To increase the volume of blood returning to the heart
   ③ To increase cardiac output and stroke volume
   ④ To reduce ankle edema and prevent dysrhythmias

8. Pulmonary edema is a complication of CHF. Which of the following findings suggests pulmonary edema?
   ① Angina, nausea, vomiting, and dyspnea on exertion
   ② Confusion, diaphoresis, bradycardia, and hypotension
   ③ Angina, cough, bradycardia, and cyanosis
   ④ Restlessness; frothy, pink-tinged sputum; and dyspnea

9. Your license as a practical nurse permits you to:
   ① Give first aid to those in your neighborhood
   ② Recommend particular physicians when asked
   ③ Supervise patient care in a long-term care facility
   ④ Render nursing service to the public

10. The function of the state board of nursing is to:
    ① Establish specific nursing procedures in the state
    ② Legislate and execute laws pertaining to nursing
    ③ Operate schools of nursing in the state
    ④ Establish in-service programs in the state

11. The primary purpose of states' requiring nurses to be licensed to practice nursing is to:
    ① Protect the LP/VN employer and nurse
    ② Protect the patient and nursing practice
    ③ Protect the patient and employee
    ④ Protect the LP/VN from malpractice

12. If a patient is dissatisfied with his or her physician, the LP/VN may:
    ① Report the matter to the head nurse or team leader
    ② Suggest three other physicians to the patient
    ③ Report the matter to the medical director
    ④ Report the matter to the patient's family

13. The patient has the right to:
    ① Refuse treatment
    ② Choose own physician
    ③ Receive a proper standard of care
    ④ All of the above

14. Lamaze-instructed mother, Mrs. David, primipara, is now telling you she feels like pushing. The physician examines her and says she is 10 cm dilated, 100% effaced, with the fetal head at station 0. She has had a lot more bloody show in the last hour, and she states she wants to use the bedpan. Your nursing care would be:
    ① Getting her ready to be transferred to the delivery room stat
    ② Assisting her to bear down correctly during contractions until a quarter-size part of the caput is showing
    ③ Preparing to catheterize her since she feels like using the bedpan
    ④ To tell her to relax; the baby will be born in 5 minutes

15. The husband of your patient in labor is worried that the increased bloody show is a warning of an impending hemorrhage. Your best nursing action would be:
    ① To reassure the father by reviewing how bloody show develops (since he has been Lamaze trained) and the normal sequence of progress
    ② Call the physician immediately to examine the mother once more for possible abruptio placentae
    ③ Take blood pressure and report any changes
    ④ Apply extra perineal pads to the perineum

16. Ms. F is a 34-year-old patient who was admitted to the hospital with a diagnosis of sarcoidosis. She has a history of smoking half a pack of cigarettes a day and social drinking. Ms. F has symptoms of tiring easily, breathlessness, and having a cold that will not go away. She also complains of swollen glands. Before developing the nursing care plan for Ms. F, the nurse should:
    ① Read the physician's orders for medications
    ② Research the diagnosis
    ③ Talk with the family
    ④ List the close patient contacts

17. The nursing care plan for a patient with sarcoidosis should include:
    ① Respiratory isolation precautions
    ② Complete bed rest with bathroom privileges only
    ③ A daily visit outside for sunshine
    ④ Activity as tolerated

18. A patient with a diagnosis of sarcoidosis wants to know why the physician is planning to perform a biopsy of the lymph node. The nurse's most appropriate reply is:
    ① "He wants to see how far the sarcoidosis has spread."
    ② "Has the physician explained the procedure to you?"
    ③ "That is the way to definitely diagnose this disease."
    ④ "He can find out why your glands are swollen."

19. In providing health education to a patient with sarcoidosis, the nurse should most appropriately include:
    ① Ways to determine if the pulmonary system is getting more involved
    ② Agencies and methods to use to quit smoking
    ③ Methods to self-test for mediastinal node involvement
    ④ Symptoms of fibrosis of the advanced stage of disease

20. You are in the delivery room with Mr. and Mrs. Robbit, and they have a fine, healthy little girl weighing 8 lb (3600 g). Parents first touch the child with their fingertips, then palm, then body contact. The baby receives routine delivery room care followed by routine nursery care. It is important that the parents get to hold their newborn:
    ① Within 24 hours
    ② After the first hour
    ③ As soon as possible
    ④ After the baby is weighed

21. You have been assigned to care for Mr. Jenkins, a 42-year-old man with pneumonia. Your patient's 24-hour urine collection ends at 2 PM. At 2 PM you have the patient:
    ① Drink a large amount of fluid so he can void soon
    ② Stop collecting any more urine
    ③ Void and discard the specimen
    ④ Void and include the specimen in the collection container

22. In assessing a patient with pneumonia, which of the following observations takes immediate priority?
    ① Rectal temperature 100° F
    ② Skin pale, moist
    ③ Urinal is full
    ④ Weight gain of 1 lb since yesterday

23. You read in a patient's chart that he has orthopnea. This term means that he:
    ① Can breathe best only when sitting in an upright position
    ② Has periods during which his breathing stops
    ③ Has very noisy respiratory sounds
    ④ Is breathing very rapidly

24. For which of the following stool tests must the specimen still be warm when it reaches the laboratory?
    ① Culture and sensitivity
    ② Guaiac
    ③ Hematest
    ④ Ova and parasites

25. The best time to obtain a sputum specimen from a patient with pneumonia is:
    ① After patient brushes his teeth at bedtime
    ② In the morning before breakfast
    ③ Just before lunch
    ④ When patient begins a coughing spell

26. To evaluate nursing care you must determine if:
    ① All assigned nursing measures were completed
    ② Goals are being accomplished
    ③ Patient feels better
    ④ Patient is happy with the quality of care

27. Suction apparatus is placed at your patient's bedside in case it is needed. You remember that in nasopharyngeal suctioning you:
    ① Suction only when introducing the catheter
    ② Suction continuously for 15 to 30 seconds followed by a 10-second rest period
    ③ Slowly withdraw suction catheter using rotating motion while suction continues
    ④ Use only medical asepsis

28. Mr. T's breathing is less labored when oxygen is administered by cannula at 3L/min. Safety precautions when oxygen is in use include:
    ① Avoiding use of friction-producing toys or equipment
    ② Using only gases that mix with oxygen to prevent explosions
    ③ Making sure the room is airtight
    ④ Making sure the room has a self-contained ventilation system

29. The physician tells you that the patient should start ambulating today. Your first step would be to:
    ① Check the written order
    ② Have the patient dangle legs for 5 minutes
    ③ Have the patient sit in the chair in the morning, walk in the afternoon
    ④ Take the patient's vital signs

30. A patient's rectal temperature is 100° F. This is considered to be:
    ① An error if taken with an electronic thermometer
    ② An indication to retake temperature
    ③ Febrile
    ④ Normal

31. Your patient's chart reveals hypokalemia. The patient should be assessed for:
    1. Bleeding tendency
    2. Cardiac dysrhythmias
    3. Nausea and vomiting
    4. Thirst

32. Your patient has tachycardia. You would expect the pulse rate to be in which range?
    1. 40 to 60 beats/min
    2. 60 to 80 beats/min
    3. 80 to 100 beats/min
    4. 100 to 120 beats/min

33. When assessing the apical-radial pulse, all of the following results are possible *except*:
    1. Apical 100; radial 94
    2. Apical 110; radial 110
    3. Apical 100; radial 120
    4. Apical 128; radial 80

34. Kyle, age 4, has develped small, reddish blisters on his face and trunk. He has a headache, a slight fever, and complains of itching. These symptoms suggest:
    1. Measles
    2. Chickenpox
    3. Scarlet fever
    4. Rubella

35. Lindsay, age 3, has a possible diagnosis of pinworms. The pediatrician has ordered the "cellophane tape test" to attempt to capture the eggs around the anal area. The best time for you to perform this test is:
    1. After breakfast
    2. Before her nap
    3. After a bowel movement
    4. During the early morning hours

36. Tinea capitis is a fungal infection on the:
    1. Scalp
    2. Arms
    3. Trunk
    4. Feet

37. A group of disorders caused by a malfunction of the motor centers of the brain is known as:
    1. Cystic fibrosis
    2. Muscular dystrophy
    3. Cerebral palsy
    4. Crohn's disease

38. Erikson's theory of child development is based on:
    1. The child's psychosexual development
    2. Intellectual (cognitive) development
    3. Psychosocial development as a series of developmental tasks
    4. The child's sensorimotor development

39. Freud's theory of child development states that infants are in the:
    1. Anal stage
    2. Oedipal stage
    3. Genital stage
    4. Oral stage

40. David is 3 weeks old. His mother states that he has not been taking his formula well, and is listless and unresponsive when she holds and cuddles him. He has lost 5 oz since birth. He is otherwise healthy and has no congenital defects. The pediatrician diagnoses David's condition as:
    1. Celiac disease
    2. Failure to thrive
    3. Hirschsprung's disease
    4. Pyloric stenosis

41. Impetigo is:
    1. A streptococcal or staphylococcal infection of the skin
    2. The same as pinworms
    3. Dermatitis caused by an allergic reaction
    4. Infestation of lice on scalp

42. The cause of sudden infant death syndrome (SIDS) is:
    1. A respiratory viral infection
    2. Obstruction of the airway by a small foreign body
    3. Hypertrophy of the larynx
    4. Unknown

43. Nathan, age 4, is admitted with a diagnosis of nephrotic syndrome. Nephrotic syndrome is caused by:
    1. Injury to the kidney
    2. Frequent bladder infections
    3. Septicemia and streptococcal throat infections
    4. Damage to the glomeruli of the kidney

44. A patient with nephrotic syndrome is most likely to exhibit symptoms of:
    1. Dehydration
    2. Constipation
    3. Edema
    4. Harsh cough

45. Treatment for a toddler with nephrotic syndrome will include:
    1. High-Fowler's position
    2. Regular diet
    3. Diuretics as ordered
    4. Sodium and potassium supplements

46. Janice, age 18, is admitted to the hospital with a diagnosis of anorexia nervosa. Her symptoms would most likely include which of the following?
    1. Dysmenorrhea
    2. Periods of hyperactivity
    3. Tachycardia
    4. Diarrhea

47. Treatment and nursing interventions for a patient with anorexia include all the following *except*:
    1. Reinforcement of her present self-image
    2. Identification of the psychologic cause
    3. Correction of malnutrition
    4. Use of behavior modification techniques

48. Connie has stopped at the scene of a motor vehicle accident and has administered the necessary emergency care to the driver of the vehicle. The victim is unresponsive with spontaneous respirations and does not exhibit signs of any spinal trauma. In which of the following positions should Connie place the victim?
    1. Supine with a pillow under the head
    2. Supine with hips and legs elevated
    3. Prone with head turned to the side
    4. Recovery position (side-lying position)

49. Which of the following rates for rescue breathing would the nurse be correct in administering to a child?
    1. 1 breath every 2 seconds
    2. 1 breath every 3 seconds
    3. 1 breath every 4 seconds
    4. 1 breath every 5 seconds

50. John has been receiving antipsychotic drugs; he reports that he has a dry mouth, tight throat, and mouth movements. The nurse should consider that:
    1. These may be somatic delusions
    2. John is probably manipulating for more medication
    3. These are transitory reactions that will disappear
    4. These may be extrapyramidal reactions that require intervention

51. Psychiatric nursing is a field in which:
    1. Nurses are not sued because patients are not legally competent
    2. Suits may be brought by patients who believe they have not been actively treated
    3. Nurses are not called on to testify in legal cases because there is no "hands-on" care
    4. Few cases are tried because patients lose their civil rights

52. Which of the following statements is true about human sexuality:
    1. Children are essentially asexual
    2. There are sexual needs throughout life
    3. Homosexuality is a treatable illness
    4. Minor sexual dysfunctions are difficult to treat

53. Physical signs of alcohol withdrawal include:
    1. Increased blood pressure, increased pulse rate
    2. Low body temperature
    3. Menorrhagia
    4. Low blood pressure

54. Barry is working in the newborn nursery, when a baby that one of his colleagues is feeding begins to choke on the formula. Immediately Barry assesses the situation and begins the procedure for obstructed airway on a *conscious infant*. To perform the procedure correctly, Barry knows that he has to administer:
    1. eight back blows and eight chest thrusts
    2. six back blows and six chest thrusts
    3. five back blows and five chest thrusts
    4. four back blows and four chest thrusts

55. Sylvia is treated with imipramine (Tofranil). Before starting the medication, which of the following should be completed?
    1. Electrocardiogram
    2. Urinalysis
    3. IQ testing
    4. Chest x-ray examination

56. Cathy Mills, the elder of two girls in a family, recently went away to college. The younger sister Carol is still at home. Mrs. Mills has grown increasingly anxious and depressed saying that she can't manage the large house and all its problems. Carol, a typical teenager, is frequently upset over demands made by her mother that she considers unfair. Mr. Mills finally brings them to the clinic because he is fed up with all the wrangling. An appropriate intervention strategy might be:
    1. Get Mrs. Mills some temporary housekeeping help
    2. Suggest that Carol, as the problem focus, enter long-term therapy
    3. Suggest that the physician start Mrs. Mills on tranquilizers
    4. Since Mr. Mills asked for help, suggest he enter therapy

57. When performing cardiopulmonary resuscitation (CPR) it is necessary to administer chest compressions in addition to ventilations. Which of the following statements is correct regarding rate of compressions?
    1. For an infant the rate administered is 120 compressions/min
    2. For an adult the rate administered is 100 compressions/min
    3. For a child the rate administered is 80 compressions/min
    4. For an infant and a child the rate administered is 100 compressions/min

58. Gerry is on her way to work at a nearby hospital when she spots a child lying on the side of the road. No one appears to be nearby. Gerry calls out for help and proceeds to assess the child, who appears to be about 6 years old. Gerry determines that the child is unresponsive, is not breathing, and does not have a pulse. She then proceeds to:
    1. Perform one minute of cardiopulmonary resuscitation (CPR) only
    2. Activate the emergency medical system (EMS) only
    3. Perform one minute of CPR, then activate the EMS
    4. Activate the EMS, then perform one minute of CPR

59. John H arrives in the emergency room seeking help. When asked the date, he says it is April 1886. He also speaks rapidly and changes the topic frequently. John is best described as:
    1. Oriented × 3
    2. Not oriented in time
    3. Confused
    4. Dishonest

60. Your patient's rapid speech pattern might be called:
    1. Unintelligible
    2. Disorganized
    3. Variable
    4. Pressured

61. The nurse might infer that a patient's thought processes were scattered based on:
    1. Frequent changes of topic
    2. The rapidity of speech
    3. Physical appearance
    4. Recent history

62. You have volunteered to teach a class on nutrition at the local community church. Your students range from mothers with young children to retired senior citizens. All are extremely interested in what constitutes good nutrition and ask a variety of questions on the subject. Mrs. Nancy Adams states that she is taking a diuretic, and her physician said that she should increase her intake of potassium. You would state that which of the following are good sources of potassium?
    1. Whole grain breads, oranges, and bananas
    2. Egg yolk, green leafy vegetables, and raisins
    3. Citrus fruits, strawberries, and green peppers
    4. Sunshine, fortified milk, and fish liver oils

63. Sandy Altman is a young mother of two. Her question concerns botulism. Which of the following statements is true of botulism?
    1. Caused by a *staphylococcus* bacteria quite resistant to heat
    2. Prevented by keeping hot foods over 140° F
    3. Prevented by keeping cold foods below 40° F
    4. Often caused by home-canned, low-acid foods

64. For which of the following patients might you see a low-carbohydrate diet prescribed?
    1. Mrs. Adams with dumping syndrome
    2. Mrs. Zee with hyperthyroidism
    3. Mr. Tackas with liver disease
    4. Mr. Dodd with kidney disease

65. Mrs. Jones asks a question about the Recommended Dietary Allowances (RDA) that she sees listed on packaging. You respond that:
    1. They are used as requirements for individuals with specific nutritional deficiencies
    2. They consist of four basic food groups
    3. They were developed by the U.S. Department of Agriculture to discourage excesses in the diet
    4. They are suggested levels of essential nutrients to meet the nutritional needs of most healthy individuals

66. Mrs. Foster, a 25-year-old mother of three children, was admitted to the hospital complaining of fatigue, weakness, and an infected toe. Her symptoms are suggestive of diabetes mellitus, so the following orders were written by the physician: fasting blood sugar (FBS) and CBC in AM. The nurse gave Mrs. Foster the following instructions regarding the FBS: you will have a sample of blood drawn in the morning and:
    ① You may drink fluids but do not eat any food from 8 PM until the blood is drawn
    ② Do not eat or drink anything from 8 PM until the blood is drawn in the morning
    ③ Do not eat or drink for 2 hours after you eat breakfast
    ④ You will have a liquid breakfast before the blood is drawn

67. Your patient's FBS level was 300 mg/dl, which indicates she had:
    ① Nothing to eat for 12 hours
    ② Too little glucose in her blood
    ③ Too much insulin in her blood
    ④ Difficulty using the glucose in her blood properly

68. The nurse's instructions to her patient concerning a glucose tolerance test (GTT) should be that she will be NPO from 12 midnight until the test is over in the morning and that she will have:
    ① One blood sample drawn and a urine specimen collected, after which she will receive a loading dose of glucose solution to drink; then four blood samples and urine specimens will be collected 30 to 60 minutes apart
    ② A blood sample drawn and a 24-hour urine sample collected
    ③ A blood sample drawn 2 hours after each meal and at bedtime with a urine sample collected at the same time
    ④ A loading dose of glucose solution to drink and blood and urine samples taken 2 hours later

69. The GTT measures:
    ① Effectiveness of insulin dose the patient is receiving
    ② Effectiveness of glucose metabolism after a loading dose of glucose is administered
    ③ How well the patient tolerates a loading dose of glucose
    ④ Relative ketone level after administration of a loading dose of glucose

70. Mr. Jennings has recently arrived on your unit. He is 82 years old, heavyset, and unconscious. He is breathing normally with occasional snoring. His right cheek puffs out with each expiration. His preliminary diagnosis is left-sided CVA. Neurologic assessments necessary to obtain a Glasgow Coma Scale score include:
    ① Vital signs and pupil response
    ② Facial symmetry and motor responses
    ③ Eye opening, verbal responses, and motor responses
    ④ Handgrip and pupil response

71. Which would be the most beneficial intervention in dealing with your patient's mobility impairment while unconscious?
    ① Get the patient out of bed to a chair for 2 hours
    ② Turn and reposition patient q2h
    ③ Give passive range-of-motion exercises twice each shift
    ④ Place the patient in Fowler's position once each shift

72. Your patient has regained consciousness and has right-sided hemiplegia. In assisting him to get dressed, how would you help him to put on his shirt?
    ① Over the head first, then both arms together
    ② Right arm first
    ③ Left arm first
    ④ However he is used to doing it

73. Now that your patient is conscious, you assess that he understands but has difficulty speaking. You record this observation as:
    ① Expressive aphasia
    ② Receptive aphasia
    ③ Dysphagia
    ④ Hemiphasia

74. Mr. Bart has recently suffered a CVA. In assisting him to improve cognitive skills, the nurse would:
    ① Provide memory aids and stimuli
    ② Provide range-of-motion exercises
    ③ Initiate bowel and bladder training
    ④ Provide leisurely, recreational activities so he doesn't have to think

75. Mrs. Davis is an alert 90 year old who came to the hospital after falling at home and scraping her elbow. She has a history of slight vertigo for which she takes meclizine and benzodiazepine. The physician notes a cardiac murmur and orders digoxin and propranolol. Before developing the nursing care plan for Mrs. Davis, the nurse should obtain:
    ① A history of her activities of daily living at home
    ② A family history of diabetes mellitus
    ③ A list of nursing homes that will accept Mrs. Davis
    ④ The address of her children for an emergency

76. Adverse reactions to digitalis preparations include:
    ① Hypernatremia, nausea, dehydration
    ② Anorexia, nausea, yellow vision
    ③ Urinary retention, constipation, edema
    ④ Hypertension, dyspnea, hypokalemia

77. The diuretic action of cardiac glycosides is produced because of the ability of the drug to:
    ① Pull edematous fluid from the tissues
    ② Make the patient thirsty and increase fluid intake
    ③ Relax the arteries in the kidney
    ④ Improve the general circulation

78. The usual range of a maintenance dose of digoxin is:
    ① 0.125 to 0.5 mg daily
    ② 0.1 to 0.3 mg daily
    ③ 0.5 to 1 g daily
    ④ 0.75 to 1 g daily

79. While preparing to administer digitalis, the nurse counted an apical pulse rate of 52 beats/min. She would be correct if she:
    ① Gave the drug as usual
    ② Omitted the drug and reported it to the physician
    ③ Gave the patient half the dosage
    ④ Gave the drug but with twice as much water as usual

80. Three days after admission, your patient becomes confused. The nurse's care plan should recommend:
    ① Ambulation and maintaining mobility by ROM exercises
    ② Moving the patient to the psychiatric ward
    ③ Reviewing the medication regimen with the physician
    ④ Obtaining an order for medication to decrease confusion

81. At lunch time your patient appears to have difficulty swallowing and appears to choke. The nurse should:
    1. Feed the patient at a slower rate
    2. Note the episode on the chart
    3. Suction the secretions as needed
    4. Perform the abdominal thrust maneuver

82. After discontinuing the cardiac medication and the benzodiazepine, Ms. Ellie's confusion clears and she asks why she could not remember. The nurse's best reply would be:
    1. "That was a side effect of the medicine for your heart."
    2. "That was a side effect of the medicine for your vertigo."
    3. "You were very ill and that happens sometimes."
    4. "Sometimes one medicine does not combine well with another medicine."

83. Mark, a 22 year old, is seen in the emergency room. He appears disheveled and has strong body odor, stating that there are "Mafia hit men" out to harm him. The ER nurse begins her interview with Mark by saying, "The Mafia rarely miss their targets; how have you been able to escape them?" This illustrates which *nontherapeutic technique?*
    1. Accept the patient as a person
    2. Reflective questioning
    3. Challenging the patient's statement
    4. Probing

84. Ben reports that he has been using "crack" (a form of cocaine) for the last 3 days, has slept very little, and is afraid "they are out to get him." The nurse may conclude:
    1. His paranoid thoughts are probably psychotic delusions
    2. He may be in realistic danger from drug dealers
    3. Crack users are rarely functionally psychotic
    4. Drug use must be reported to legal authorities

85. Carla Nowell is a 30-year-old female, who has a history of waking up at midnight with severe pain in the epigastrium. Her skin has a slight yellow cast. She reports noticing a darkening of her urine over the past few weeks. She also reports experiencing intermittent nausea, vomiting, and some moderate epigastric pain over the past 3 months. Carla is hospitalized for evaluation of the gallbladder. If Carla's pain is of gallbladder origin, the pain would probably be precipitated by:
    1. Excessive exercise
    2. Emotional stress
    3. Ingestion of protein
    4. High fatty diet

86. If a patient's problem was related to blockage of the bile duct by a stone, the nurse could anticipate the stool to appear:
    1. Tarry
    2. Very watery
    3. Clay colored
    4. Full of mucus

87. Your patient undergoes a cholecystectomy and duct exploration. She returns to the floor with an IV, nasogastric tube to low suction, and a T-tube in place. The purpose of the T-tube is to:
    1. Remove serous fluid from the abdominal cavity
    2. Provide an access to irrigate the operative area
    3. Remove excessive bile from the intestines
    4. Promote bile duct patency until edema subsides

88. Mr. Evans is a 59-year-old truck driver who came to the emergency room with a right leg that is reddened, warm, and tender. A diagnosis of thrombophlebitis is made. Thrombophlebitis can be precipitated by which of the following conditions?
    1. Early ambulation following surgery
    2. The use of elastic stockings after surgery
    3. Prolonged standing or sitting
    4. Range-of-motion exercises during periods of bed rest

89. Initial treatments that the nurse may anticipate for a patient with thrombophlebitis include:
    1. Warm, moist heat applications to the affected extremity
    2. Exercise to the affected leg four times daily
    3. Keeping the affected leg lower than the rest of the body
    4. Administering Coumadin to help dissolve the clot

90. Mr. Hayes is discharged on a regimen of Coumadin. He is to wear antiembolism stockings and avoid situations that hamper circulation. What instructions will the nurse include in the teaching plan concerning the drug Coumadin?
    1. If pain should develop, aspirin may be taken
    2. The stockings should be taken off for bathing and reapplied in a sitting position
    3. Instruct the patient to carry a medical identification tag while on anticoagulants
    4. There will be no restrictions regarding activity

91. Kathy has a cesarean section and delivers a 5 lb (2200 g) baby girl. Kathy has just learned that her baby is in the Isolette. Kathy had planned to breast-feed, and she asks, "What will I do now?" As the nursery nurse you would answer:
    1. "You will not be able to breast-feed, but don't worry, the nurses will be feeding her formula."
    2. "As soon as you are able, probably in a day or so, you may go to the nursery and breast-feed in a special area, as the baby will tolerate only short periods out of the incubator."
    3. "Perhaps you can ask your physician."
    4. "You will probably be able to breast-feed when the baby goes home; don't worry."

92. Your patient had a cesarean section, and she and her husband want to know why their baby must be kept in the Isolette, whereas her roommate's baby (who was also 5 lb) was never kept in an Isolette. You would tell them:
    1. "Section babies are always immature and therefore must be kept in an Isolette for observation."
    2. "Section babies are always observed for respiratory distress, and keeping them in an incubator in a controlled environment is a precautionary measure."
    3. "Vaginally delivered babies never have respiratory distress symptoms, but cesarean babies do."
    4. "Section babies often suffer from a cephalohematoma, so it is important to watch for central nervous system symptoms."

93. Ann asks you whether her lochia will be heavier because of her cesarean section. Your best answer would be:
    ① "Lochia after a cesarean section will be bright red longer and will be more copious than after a vaginal delivery."
    ② "The characteristics will be the same except that the flow will be for a longer duration than the flow after vaginal delivery."
    ③ "The amount, duration, and characteristics of the lochia are the same for a cesarean section as for a vaginal delivery."
    ④ "The flow will be of a much shorter duration because the vaginal tract was not used."

94. One important complication to avoid after a cesarean section is a pelvic thrombosis; thus your nursing care plan would include:
    ① Teaching good perineal care
    ② Encouraging early ambulation
    ③ Splinting the lower abdomen when coughing
    ④ Keeping the urinary and bowel tracts emptied by forcing fluids and offering stool softeners

95. Mrs. Willis, age 56, has been admitted to the hospital with a diagnosis of arteriosclerosis obliterans and hypertension. She has been treated for the last 5 years for hypertension. Vital signs on admission: BP 150/94, temperature 99° F (37.2° C), pulse rate 90 beats/min, respirations 22/min. In performing an assessment of the lower extremities, what *objective* findings might the nurse anticipate?
    ① Cramping, bounding pulses, ankle edema
    ② Pallor, coldness, diminished pulse rate
    ③ Warmth, moist skin, regular pulse rate
    ④ Tenderness, edema, palpation of hardened veins

96. In planning care for a patient with arteriosclerosis obliterans, the nurse would consider which of the following?
    ① Direct application of heat to improve circulation to the affected area
    ② Give instructions in avoiding injury and maintaining circulation
    ③ Elevate the foot of the bed to increase arterial circulation
    ④ Massage the extremities several times a day to improve circulation

97. The alpha-adrenergic blocking agents are useful in the treatment of peripheral vascular disease because they:
    ① Promote the development of collateral circulation
    ② Produce vasodilation and increase blood flow to the involved areas
    ③ Cause reflex stimulation of skeletal muscles to aid in venous blood return
    ④ Inhibit the sensory nerve endings to the area, thereby reducing pain

98. A significant nursing action in the administration of antihypertensive agents is to:
    ① Check blood pressure before each dose
    ② Check apical pulse rate before each dose
    ③ Weigh patient each day
    ④ Monitor patient's blood pressure daily

99. An adrenergic, neuron-blocking agent that inhibits the release of norepinephrine and that is used in the treatment of hypertension is:
    ① Serpasil
    ② Priscoline
    ③ Pro-Banthine
    ④ Inderal

100. If the nurse is instructing the patient on factors that predispose someone to hypertension, which of the following would be identified in the teaching plan?
    ① Obesity, heavy salt intake
    ② Smoking, heavy calcium intake
    ③ Age, intake of polyunsaturated fat
    ④ Age, passive personality

101. While the Diamonds were driving to the park for a family picnic, they were hit from behind by a speeding car. The resulting explosion and fire killed both parents of 3-year-old Bill. Bill sustained a fractured left femur and second- and third-degree burns over 43% of his body. The emergency medical technician communicated to the hospital that Bill was burned on both anterior and posterior aspects of his torso, arms, and hands. As part of the emergency team, you would help prepare for Bill's arrival by obtaining a:
    ① Tracheostomy tray
    ② Stretcher with sterile sheets
    ③ Cardiac difibrillator
    ④ Sterile dressing tray

102. On arrival to the emergency room, the 3-year-old burn patient is semiconscious, whining, and calling for his mother. Once he has been transferred to the trauma room, you begin to obtain baseline data. His radial pulse rate, 160 beats/min; respirations, 32/min; and BP, 60/30. Based on the initial data, you would report vital signs to the physician and assist as ordered in initiation of:
    ① Removal of clothing
    ② Central venous line
    ③ IV fluids
    ④ Antibiotics

103. Immediate physical observations of a burn patient would most importantly include:
    ① Physical development
    ② Head circumference
    ③ Height and weight
    ④ Quality of respirations

104. The physician chooses the closed method of dressing the burned areas. On the pediatric ward, your patient's room would be set up to provide which type of isolation?
    ① Enteric
    ② Strict
    ③ Reverse
    ④ Respiratory

105. During the first 24 hours of treating a patient for burns, you can assist in assessing fluid replacement needs by monitoring hourly:
    ① Urine specific gravity
    ② IV fluid rate
    ③ Vital signs
    ④ IV fluid intake

106. On the second day of hospitalization, your 3-year-old patient becomes more fretful and cries continuously for his mother. To provide emotional support, you would:
    ① Plan care so that you can spend as much time in his room as possible
    ② Frequently administer phenobarbital elixir as ordered
    ③ Tell him not to cry because "brave boys don't cry"
    ④ Explain to him that his grandmother is coming to stay after supper

107. Your patient has been placed in Russell traction and keeps tugging at the pulley ropes. To help him cope with being immobilized, you can:
    ① Play Chinese checkers with him as a diversional activity
    ② Apply Russell traction to his favorite teddy bear
    ③ Place mitten restraints on his hands
    ④ Retie the pulley ropes out of his reach

108. Frequent assessment of a patient with a fractured leg would include maintaining proper alignment and:
    ① Checking sensation and circulation in the leg
    ② Increasing the weight of traction as necessary to maintain countertraction
    ③ Taking the apical pulse every 2 hours
    ④ Checking temperature and range of motion in his right leg

109. When changing the burn dressing, you would help a young patient control his feelings of fear and pain by:
    ① Having another nurse restrain the patient until the treatment is over
    ② Explaining firmly what is to be done and how he can help
    ③ Allowing the patient to cry until he is tired and less combative
    ④ Repeating administration of the prescribed pain medication

110. Normal nutritional requirements of a preschooler include food from the four basic food groups. As a result of severe burns, your 3-year-old patient would need a diet:
    ① High in proteins, carbohydrates, and calories
    ② High in proteins, iron, and calcium
    ③ Low in sodium and cholesterol
    ④ Low in calcium and high in carbohydrates

111. Normally preschoolers have little interest in eating and the anorexia associated with burns presents a problem of nutrition. Your 3-year-old patient would most likely eat better if:
    ① Other children ate with him
    ② His grandmother ate with him
    ③ You would feed him
    ④ Tube feedings were given when he did not eat

112. Your patient has not had a bowel movement in 3 days. You can promote elimination by encouraging him to eat:
    ① Eggs and cheese toast
    ② Popsicles and oranges
    ③ Apples and carrot sticks
    ④ Chicken and whole grain cereal

113. Several weeks following a patient's discharge from the hospital, his grandmother calls the unit. She is concerned about him because for the first time since the accident that killed his parents, he is asking for them. You would suggest the grandmother respond as follows:
    ① "What do you think happened to Mommy and Daddy?"
    ② "Come here. Let me tell you a story about what happened to Mommy and Daddy."
    ③ "What do you remember about the accident that you were in with Mommy and Daddy?"
    ④ "Do you remember when Aunt Jessie died?"

114. Your young patient begins to cry when his grandmother talks about the accident. The best response to his crying is to:
    ① Leave him alone in the room to cry
    ② Continue discussing the accident
    ③ Hold him closely while he cries
    ④ Tell him not to cry and that everything will be all right

115. James Wetherbee is a 45-year-old executive for a major computer firm. He has been hospitalized for the past 2 weeks with the diagnosis of myocardial infarction (MI). For the first week following his MI, Mr. Wetherbee was on a soft diet. For what reason did his physician probably order this diet?
    ① To reduce the caloric intake of his diet because Mr. Wetherbee is overweight
    ② To increase the amount of high-protein foods necessary for tissue repair
    ③ For easy digestion to rest the heart as much as possible
    ④ To promote the healing of the gastric mucosa

116. In addition to the cholesterol restriction, a patient with cardiac disease questions you about the sodium restriction. He asks, "What, other than table salt, contains large amounts of sodium?" You would reply:
    ① Meats and milk products
    ② Fruits
    ③ Vegetables
    ④ Legumes and root products (carrots)

117. Following the acute phase of hospitalization for a myocardial infarction, your patient is placed on a low-sodium, low-cholesterol diet. He asks you what foods are especially high in cholesterol. You would respond:
    ① Fortified milk and cheese
    ② Citrus fruits, broccoli, and green peppers
    ③ Oranges, bananas, and apricots
    ④ Liver, egg yolks, and shellfish

118. Your patient is confused about saturated and unsaturated fats and their relationship to heart disease. Of the following statements, which would be most accurate?
    ① Saturated fats are usually from plant sources and are recommended to reduce blood lipid levels
    ② Polyunsaturated fats are usually solid at room temperature and contribute to the development of atherosclerosis
    ③ Polyunsaturated fats are usually liquid at room temperature and are recommended for reducing blood lipid levels
    ④ Saturated fats are from animal sources and are recommended for lowering blood lipid levels

119. Of the following menus, which selection indicates that the patient has a good understanding of what is included on a low-sodium, low-cholesterol diet?
    1. Smoked sausage, french fries, and milk
    2. Roast beef (lean), boiled potatoes, and iced tea
    3. Liver and onions, mashed potatoes and gravy, and coffee
    4. Cheese and egg casserole, salad, and milk
120. Which statement is true of water-soluble vitamins?
    1. They require sufficient fat in the diet to carry them
    2. They are stored in the body so deficiencies are slow to appear
    3. They are fairly stable in cooking and storage
    4. They have to be resupplied each day because the body excretes what it does not need
121. Which statement is applicable to thiamine?
    1. Good sources include green pepper, cantaloupe, and potatoes
    2. It aids in absorption of iron
    3. One of its functions is the formation and maintenance of capillary walls and collagen formation
    4. Maintains muscle and nerve functioning
122. Your neighbor is surprised that after exposure to rubella, her 6-week-old son did not get the disease. You explain that the baby has:
    1. Active acquired immunity
    2. Active natural immunity
    3. Passive acquired immunity
    4. Passive natural immunity
123. The practical nurse observes a co-worker using the following techniques in caring for a patient on respiratory isolation. Which technique is in error?
    1. Leaving the glass thermometer in the patient's room
    2. Washing hands before entering the patient's room
    3. Wearing a mask while applying TED stockings
    4. Wearing a gown while obtaining a sputum specimen
124. While assessing your patient's ankle edema, in addition to inspection, which other technique would you use?
    1. Auscultation
    2. Evaluation
    3. Palpation
    4. Percussion
125. You and another team member have just taken an apical-radial pulse. The results were apical 76; radial 82. Your next action should be to:
    1. Place the patient flat in bed
    2. Repeat the procedure
    3. Report results to the nurse in charge
    4. Report results to the physician

COMPREHENSIVE EXAMINATION 2: PART 2

This examination contains individual questions, each containing a relevant clinical situation. Read all questions carefully. There is only *one best answer* for each question.

Test time allotment (Part 2): approximately 2 hours
Answers and rationales begin on p. 472.

1. Mary needs to see her dentist, but is very frightened. She finally makes an appointment and writes it in her calendar. On the day of the appointment, she looks at the wrong day in her calendar and misses the appointment. This is an example of:
   ① Repression ③ Displacement
   ② Projection ④ Rationalization

2. Ms. Smith interacts with a patient who persistently moves his leg in a tapping motion. The psychiatric principle that applies here is:
   ① Be honest
   ② The nurse-patient relationship is professional and realistic
   ③ The staff is viewed as role models
   ④ There is a reason for all behavior

3. According to the theorist Eric Erikson, the first stage of development is focused on:
   ① Autonomy vs. shame and doubt
   ② Pleasure principle
   ③ Anal gratification
   ④ Trust vs. mistrust

4. In reviewing the plan of care for John, a 24-year-old schizophrenic with regressive behavior, you see the following outcome (goal): patient will complete all ADL and be neatly groomed within 2 days. You may conclude:
   ① The goal is appropriate
   ② The goal is too broad
   ③ The goal is unrealistic
   ④ It is a long-term goal

5. According to Maslow's hierarchy, which basic needs must be met first?
   ① Esteem
   ② Love and belonging
   ③ Physiologic
   ④ Safety and security

6. While bathing a patient with skin markings left by the radiotherapy department you:
   ① Avoid cleansing the body region where the marks are located
   ② Carefully cleanse so that markings remain
   ③ Rub the markings with lotion so they disappear before the next therapy treatment
   ④ Use only soap and water to completely remove the markings

7. In which of the following situations would taking a rectal temperature be contraindicated?
   ① First day postoperative hemorrhoidectomy
   ② Newly admitted 6 month old
   ③ Toddler following tonsillectomy
   ④ Unconscious, elderly adult

8. Immunity develops:
   ① After having an inflammatory illness
   ② On exposure to a contagious disease
   ③ When antibodies are present
   ④ When resistance is low

9. To calculate urine output when emptying the drainage container of a patient with a continuous bladder irrigation you would:
   ① Measure the total drainage and total irrigant used, recording both
   ② Send the total drainage to the laboratory for an accurate analysis
   ③ Subtract amount of solution used from amount of drainage
   ④ Subtract total drainage from amount of solution used

10. Which type of barrier technique is used for patients with AIDS?
    ① Blood/body fluids
    ② Enteric
    ③ Respiratory
    ④ Strict

11. Which of these may indicate that death is approaching?
    ① Decreased body temperature
    ② Deep, slow respirations
    ③ Dry, cool skin
    ④ Dull, glazed eyes

12. Bill Jones, 14 years old, dove into a shallow pond while on a camping expedition. Friends rescued him from drowning when they saw he was in difficulty. When the emergency team arrived, they placed Bill on a stretcher, being especially careful *not* to:
    ① Move his extremities unnecessarily
    ② Flex his head
    ③ Put pressure on his diaphragm
    ④ Strap him to the stretcher too tightly

13. Diagnosis of spinal cord injury is most often made as soon as possible by x-ray studies on arrival at the hospital. The reason for this is to:
    ① Detect the presence of edema around the cord
    ② Lessen movement of the spinal column at a critical period
    ③ Detect spinal shock
    ④ Check for hemorrhage into the spinal cavity

14. The most critical level for a spinal cord injury to occur is at the:
    ① Sacral level
    ② Cervical level
    ③ Lumbar level
    ④ Thoracic level

15. Following cervical spinal cord injury the patient almost always requires immediate:
    ① Relief from excruciating pain
    ② Respiratory assistance
    ③ Crisis intervention
    ④ Immobilization

16. A common type of stabilization maneuver used in injuries to the cervical spinal cord is:
    ① Steinmann's pins
    ② Crutchfield tongs
    ③ Kirschner wires
    ④ Harrington rod

17. Care must be taken to ensure that skeletal traction is put to its intended use. Which of the following actions is appropriate for the nurse to consider in ensuring the effectiveness of such traction?
    1. Elevate the head of the bed 45 degrees
    2. Place sandbags above the patient's shoulders
    3. Make certain that weights barely touch the floor
    4. Allow for rest by releasing traction periodically

18. When first feeding patients in hyperextension who are lying on their back, you should:
    1. Use suction on the patients first
    2. Offer sips of liquid to prepare them for solid food
    3. Raise the head of the bed to facilitate swallowing
    4. Offer soft food

19. Mrs. Kate Murphy, age 40, is admitted to the hospital after several episodes of right upper-quadrant abdominal pain and intolerance to fatty and gas-forming foods. She also reports episodes of light-colored stools and slight jaundice with the more acute episodes of her pain. A diagnosis of biliary colic is made. The ingestion of fatty foods will precipitate the pain of biliary colic because:
    1. Increased fat in the stomach increases peristalsis
    2. Fat in the duodenum initiates contraction of the gallbladder
    3. Fat in the duodenum increases abdominal distention
    4. Increased fat intake may result in a gallbladder obstruction

20. Diet instructions for a patient with a diagnosis of biliary colic should encourage the restriction of:
    1. Breads, cereals, and pasta
    2. Poultry, rice, and skim milk
    3. Lima beans, cabbage, and onions
    4. Cooked fruits, lean meats, and caffeine

21. Following insertion of a nasogastric tube before surgery you ascertain that the tube is properly placed by:
    1. Placing the end of the tube in a glass of water to make sure bubbles appear in the water on expiration
    2. Injecting 10 ml of air into the tube and palpating for abdominal distention
    3. Listening for the sound in the stomach with a stethoscope as 5 ml of air is injected into the tube
    4. Feeling the end of the tube for the passage of air from the stomach

22. As a preoperative medication, 75 mg of Demerol is to be given intramuscularly. Demerol injection contains 50 mg/ml. How much of the solution should be administered?
    1. 0.5 ml
    2. 0.75 ml
    3. 1 ml
    4. 1.5 ml

23. You are to give $1/100$ gr of atropine intramuscularly. Atropine injection contains 1 mg/ml. How much should be injected?
    1. 0.01 ml
    2. 0.4 ml
    3. 0.6 ml
    4. 1 ml

24. Following a cholecystectomy, your patient returns to her room from recovery in stable condition. Fluids are being given intravenously. She has a T-tube to bedside drainage, a Foley catheter to bedside drainage, and a nasogastric tube to low suction. Once settled in her bed, she complains of nausea and looks like she is gagging. Your initial response in this situation is to:
    1. Administer ordered antiemetic
    2. Check the nasogastric tube for patency
    3. Check the wound for bleeding or dehiscence
    4. See whether the T-tube has been dislodged

25. Use of a Penrose drain following a cholecystectomy is for:
    1. Rerouting bile flow to the reconstructed bile duct
    2. Draining bile while the common duct is edematous
    3. Removing bile and blood from the operative area
    4. Preventing bile from causing contamination and infection of the cystic duct

26. To prevent the most common complication following a cholecystectomy, it would be most important for the nurse to assist the patient to:
    1. Have the abdominal dressing changed prn for heavy drainage
    2. Increase fluid intake and decrease fat intake
    3. Receive prn pain medication at intervals ordered
    4. Cough and deep breathe every 2 hours and fully expand her lungs

27. Following the first postoperative dressing change the physician's order is to change the abdominal dressing every 8 hours and prn. In changing your patient's dressing following a cholecystectomy, it is particularly important to place sterile 4 × 4s around the Penrose drain because:
    1. Leakage of bile from the Penrose can cause severe skin irritation
    2. The evacuated bile is normally high in bacteria and should not contact the abdominal incision
    3. Absorption of bile by 4 × 4s aids in accurate measurement
    4. The suture line must be protected from moisture

28. Your patient is to receive 1000 ml of IV fluids every 8 hours. The IV set delivers 10 gtt/ml. The drip rate should be set at
    1. 10 gtt/ml
    2. 21 gtt/ml
    3. 36 gtt/ml
    4. 42 gtt/ml

29. In administering an IM analgesic, you should insert the needle at a:
    1. 15-degree angle
    2. 45-degree angle
    3. 60-degree angle
    4. 90-degree angle

30. Ms. Charles' abdomen feels distended, and she complains of nausea. Her nasogastric tube appears to be in place. Your first action would be to:
    1. Notify the physician
    2. Administer the prescribed antiemetic
    3. Irrigate the tube with 10 ml of sterile normal saline, if ordered
    4. Inject 50 ml of air into the tube to check for patency

31. A patient complains of tenderness at her IV puncture site. On assessment you note redness and swelling. You should first:
    1. Stop the flow of the IV fluids, and report this to your head nurse
    2. Notify the physician, and fill out an incident report
    3. Elevate the arm, and apply warm compresses to the puncture site
    4. Change the dressing over the puncture site using sterile technique

32. While changing your patient's abdominal dressing it is most important for you to:
    1. Use forceps
    2. Touch sterile articles with sterile articles only
    3. Replace all unused 4 × 4s in their package
    4. Apply ice packs to the incision to decrease swelling

33. A postoperative symptom that should be reported to the physician immediately is:
    1. A temperature of 101° F (38.3° C)
    2. An incisional pain
    3. A productive cough
    4. Audible bowel sounds

34. Following a cholecystectomy, your patient asks you, "Will I have to stay on a fat-free diet for the rest of my life?" The *best* response would be:
    1. "You need to talk to your physician about that."
    2. "A fat-free diet will always be necessary if you wish to stay well."
    3. "After you have completely recovered you will probably be able to eat a normal diet without excessive fat."
    4. "Complications of this type of surgery might cause you to have to abstain from all fats."

35. The purpose of Good Samaritan laws is to:
    1. Mandate nurses and physicians to stop and render care at accident sites
    2. Encourage emergency aid at accident sites
    3. Prevent any liability arising from care rendered at accident sites
    4. Have universal laws mandating emergency aid at accident sites

36. Consent for special procedures shall include full information of procedure and signature of patient or guardian *except:*
    1. Routine operating-room cases
    2. Extreme emergency where failure to treat may be considered negligence
    3. Intravenous pyelogram (IVP) with injection of dye
    4. Family gave verbal consent

37. The nurse practice act legally defines the scope of practice for the LP/VN. Which of the following is *not* correct?
    1. Nursing laws are passed by the state's legislature
    2. Nursing laws are uniform in all states
    3. Standards of care are part of the laws
    4. Nursing laws address licensure and renewal of license

38. LP/VN Smith's assignment today included Mrs. Burns, a 2-day postoperative patient. Mrs. Burns requested to remain in bed and stated she felt dizzy. Ms. Smith said, "Oh, you'll feel better if you sit in the chair a while." When getting out of bed, Mrs. Burns slipped and fractured her wrist. Ms. Smith can be charged with:
    1. Assault and battery
    2. Accountability
    3. Negligence
    4. Causation

39. The evening shift nurse is administering the 10 PM medications. Carol is to receive Nembutal 15 mg at bedtime. When the nurse enters her room, she is talking on the telephone. The nurse should:
    1. Leave the medication at her bedside for her to take when she is finished with her phone conversation
    2. Omit the drug because Carol appears relaxed talking on the phone and won't need a sedative to sleep
    3. Leave the medication at her bedside and tell her to let the night shift nurse know that she took the medication
    4. Instruct her to call for the medication when she is finished with her conversation

40. Sedatives are those drugs capable of:
    1. Inducing sleep
    2. Promoting amnesia
    3. Producing relaxation; decreasing anxiety
    4. Preventing muscular tension

41. The principal difference between hypnotics and sedatives is:
    1. Only sedatives can produce drug dependency
    2. Hypnotics produce fewer adverse effects
    3. A difference of degree and depends largely on dosage
    4. Hypnotic drugs cause excitement of the central nervous system

42. Mr. Gonzales is a 45 year old with recent onset of chest pain. He came to the clinic after experiencing a second episode of chest pain. He has been experiencing short episodes of what he describes as "skipping heart beats," accompanied by "trouble catching my breath." To evaluate Mr. Gonzales, the nurse might anticipate assisting the patient with a diagnostic test that evaluates the heart rate and rhythm over a 24-hour period. Such a study is known as:
    1. An electrocardiogram
    2. An electroencephalogram
    3. A cardiac catheterization
    4. Holter monitoring

43. One of the underlying causes of chest pain is arteriosclerosis. What physiologic changes are associated with this condition?
    1. Blood vessels dilate, flooding an organ with blood
    2. Plaque formation reduces blood vessel size and blood flow
    3. A diminished supply of blood to the lungs reduces tissue oxygen availability
    4. Thickened blood vessel walls cause ballooning of blood vessels and pooling of blood, making blood unavailable to tissues

44. It is common for chest pain to be precipitated by:
    1. Sleep
    2. Allergies
    3. Exertion
    4. Diarrhea

45. In assessing a patient's chest pain, the nurse should note which of the following characteristics?
    ① Elevation of temperature
    ② Respiratory rate
    ③ Presence of incontinence
    ④ Radiation of pain to the jaw or arm

46. Mrs. Harjo has a diagnosis of primary dysfunction of the adrenal cortex. The physician has ordered replacement therapy. Which of the following is an important point to stress in patient teaching?
    ① The hormones will have to be taken for the rest of her life
    ② The hormones must be taken until the body's stores have been replenished
    ③ The hormones will only need to be taken during periods of stress
    ④ Daily visits to the physician will be necessary as the dose will be adjusted daily

47. Mrs. Anderson is on a clear liquid diet. Which of the following groups of foods would be allowed on a clear liquid diet?
    ① Cream of tomato soup, jello, and tea
    ② Cherry-flavored ice, beef boullion, and apple juice
    ③ Strained cooked cereal, sherbet, and coffee
    ④ Ginger ale, custard, and cocoa

48. The nutritional requirements of a diabetic patient:
    ① Are the same as for a nondiabetic patient
    ② Will be lower in calories than for a nondiabetic patient
    ③ Will be lower in carbohydrates than for a nondiabetic patient
    ④ Will be higher in protein than for a nondiabetic patient

49. Of the following foods, which would you recommend as good sources of potassium?
    ① Milk, cheese, and kale
    ② Liver, egg yolks, and spinach
    ③ Tomatoes, green peppers, and broccoli
    ④ Oranges, bananas, and dried apricots

50. You work in an internist's office. Morning office hours are from 8:30 AM to 11:30 AM. The physician always arrives promptly at 7:45 AM and lives two blocks from the office. At 7:30 AM a patient presents symptoms of lower right-sided chest pain, pallor, and slight shortness of breath. Your *priority* nursing action would be to:
    ① Tell the patient the physician will be in shortly
    ② Start nasal oxygen immediately
    ③ Telephone the physician at home
    ④ Place the patient in high-Fowler's position

51. The nurse's immediate intervention with a victim of sexual assault should be to ensure:
    ① The victim is examined and treated as quickly as possible
    ② The victim is left alone to seek medical care when desired
    ③ Privacy and solitude are rapidly provided the victim
    ④ Accommodations for bathing and douching are offered promptly

52. You come across a motor vehicle accident (MVA). Your decision whether to help any injured persons should be based on the:
    ① Civil Defense Laws
    ② State nurse practice act
    ③ ANA Code for Nurses
    ④ Good Samaritan Act of state

53. Your neighbor Ms. Stephens runs into your yard screaming hysterically and you see that her bathrobe is on fire. The *immediate* nursing action you should take is to:
    ① Instruct Ms. Stephens to remove her bathrobe
    ② Call the fire department
    ③ Roll her in a blanket
    ④ Tell her to lie down

54. Ms. Glass has burns on the front and back of both her legs and her right arm. What percent of her body would you estimate has been involved?
    ① 45%   ③ 72%
    ② 54%   ④ 18%

55. Within the first few hours after treating a severe burn patient, the nurse should observe for which of the following?
    ① Laryngeal and tracheal edema
    ② Eschar formation
    ③ Absence of pain
    ④ Leathery appearance to skin

56. John and Sally have been camping for the past week. John has been complaining of indigestion for the past few days, but has refused to see the camp physician. This morning they both set out for a day of hiking in the mountains. At about 10 AM John decides to rest for awhile and sits down under the nearest shade tree. Sally looks around the area and returns to find John slumped over and unresponsive. Because Sally is a nurse, she knows that her first priority is to:
    ① Perform one minute of cardiopulmonary resuscitaion (CPR), then activate the emergency medical service (EMS)
    ② Activate the EMS first, then return to the victim and perform CPR
    ③ Call for help and perform CPR until someone responds to assist
    ④ Perform CPR for two minutes and then look for someone who may help

57. When performing cardiopulmonary resuscitation (CPR), ventilations should be given over a period of:
    ① 1 to 1½ seconds
    ② 1½ to 2 seconds
    ③ 2 to 2½ seconds
    ④ 2 to 3 seconds

58. Lisa Newby is a gravida 1, para 0, admitted to the labor unit in beginning labor. She is accompanied by her husband who appears to be very excited about the upcoming delivery. He tells you that they have been attending Lamaze classes in preparation for childbirth. True labor is best characterized by which of the following?
    ① Braxton Hicks contractions and pinkish vaginal discharge
    ② Regular, forceful contractions and cervical dilation
    ③ Spontaneous rupture of the amniotic membrane (sac) and abdominal pain
    ④ Descent of the presenting part into the pelvis

59. Ms. Poi is having contractions 2 minutes apart, of 45 seconds duration, and of moderate intensity. Fetal heart tones at this time should be monitored:
    ① During contractions
    ② Simultaneously with the mother's vital signs
    ③ Between contractions, every 30 minutes
    ④ Immediately following each contraction

60. Ms. D's physician informs you that she is completely dilated and effaced. The fetal heart tones and maternal vital signs are within safe limits. She says she feels the urge to push with contractions. The most important nursing action to perform at this time is to:
    ① Prepare the delivery room and equipment
    ② Increase frequency of monitoring fetal heart tones and maternal vital signs
    ③ Place Ms. D's legs in stirrups and apply wrist restraints
    ④ Assist the physician to gown and glove

61. The newborn is considered to be premature when he or she:
    ① Is large for gestational age
    ② Has a gestational age of 37 weeks or less
    ③ Weighs under 5½ pounds at birth
    ④ Has a deficiency of surfactant in alveolar spaces

62. The most important sign of possible hemolytic disease of the newborn that is noted on assessment by the nurse is:
    ① Difficult, grunting respirations
    ② Appearance of jaundice at birth or soon after
    ③ Persistent watery or frequent greenish stools
    ④ Lethargy or hyperirritability

63. When assessing the premature newborn, which of the following characteristics would you *not* expect to see?
    ① Shallow, irregular respirations
    ② Thin, transparent skin
    ③ Flaccid movements and poor muscle tone
    ④ Thick eyelashes and eyebrows

64. Oxygen therapy for the newborn must be administered with caution to prevent:
    ① Ophthalmia neonatorum
    ② ABO incompatibility
    ③ Respiratory distress syndrome
    ④ Retrolental fibroplasia

65. Sandi Jenkins is a 30-year-old school teacher who has had Type I diabetes since she was 12 years old. Sandi complains of many symptoms. Symptoms characterizing diabetes that is out of control include all of the following *except*:
    ① Polyuria
    ② Polydipsia
    ③ Polyphagia
    ④ Polymorphic

66. In reviewing home care with a patient who has newly diagnosed diabetes, the nurse cautions against exercising to extremes without taking the proper precautions. Exercise:
    ① Can rapidly lower the blood sugar
    ② Increases the need for insulin
    ③ Causes weakness and fatigue
    ④ Prevents muscle cells from using glucose

67. In reviewing the complications of diabetes with a patient, the nurse is aware that all of the following are possible complications of uncontrolled diabetes, *except:*
    ① Blindness
    ② Neuropathy
    ③ Osteoporosis
    ④ Nephropathy

68. The physician orders a sliding scale insulin for his patient based on the results of her finger sticks (Accu-check, Chemstrip, Dextro-stix). What insulin is given by sliding scale?
    ① NPH
    ② Lente
    ③ Regular
    ④ Semi-lente

69. An important nursing goal in caring for the newborn with a myelomeningocele is to:
    ① Maintain the newborn in a prone position
    ② Observe the lower extremities for movement
    ③ Promote wound healing
    ④ Prevent infection and harm to the meningocele sac

70. To keep the meningocele sac moist, you would expect the physician to order which of the following?
    ① Placing the newborn in an Isolette in high humidity
    ② Pouring sterile normal saline over the sac every 2 hours
    ③ Applying sterile gauze soaked with an antibacterial solution
    ④ Keeping a diaper, wet with sterile water, over area

71. Following repair of a myelomeningocele, you would observe daily for signs of hydrocephalus by:
    ① Palpating anterior and posterior fontanelles
    ② Maintaining strict intake and output
    ③ Weighing newborn each morning
    ④ Measuring head circumference

72. During the postoperative period following repair of a myelomeningocele, signs of increased intracranial pressure you observe for are:
    ① Increased blood pressure and pulse and decreased pulse pressure
    ② Bulging fontanelles, high-pitched cry, and separated cranial sutures
    ③ Cheyne-Stokes respirations, hypotension, and increased pulse pressure
    ④ Decreased reflexes, bulging fontanelles, weak cry, and hypotension

73. You find an elderly man with heat exhaustion. Which of the following are signs and symptoms the nurse might expect the victim to manifest related to his diagnosis?
    ① Marked diaphoresis; cool, pale, damp skin; possible temperature elevation
    ② Cessation of sweating; flushed, hot, dry skin; elevated temperature
    ③ Red, blistering skin with wet appearance and edema
    ④ Hyperemic skin with blister formation and edema

74. The patient who is immobilized because of spinal cord injuries should have a diet high in:
    ① Calories
    ② Carbohydrates
    ③ Fats
    ④ Proteins

75. The best means of preventing a urinary tract infection is:
    ① High fluid intake and clean, intermittent catheterizations
    ② High fluid intake and continuous bladder irrigations
    ③ Lower fluid intake and indwelling catheterizations
    ④ Lower fluid intake and continuous bladder irrigations

76. Regardless of the level of the injury, the patient with a spinal cord injury must begin early mobilization. This can begin with:
    ① Active or passive turning movements and ROM
    ② Wheelchair or bracing exercises
    ③ Resistive exercises
    ④ Turning every hour

77. Long-term nursing measures for the patient with a cervical cord injury include:
    ① Meticulous skin care
    ② Weekly exercise programs
    ③ Taking vital signs every 2 hours
    ④ Daily catheter care

78. Psychologically, the patient experiencing a spinal cord injury has a loss that he or she mourns. It is not uncommon for the patient to experience shock, denial, anger, and depression before adjustment. One morning as you enter your patient Sal's room, you note that he is crying. He turns his head away from you and says, "Get out, leave me alone! I don't need anybody!" Your initial response might be:
    ① "Okay, Sal, cut this out. You're just feeling sorry for yourself."
    ② "Sure, Sal. But I'll be back in a few minutes."
    ③ "Would you like to talk, Sal?"
    ④ "I'll give you something to calm you down."

79. A patient with spinal cord injury has a sudden extreme elevation in blood pressure, a throbbing headache, nasal stuffiness, sweating and flushing, and chills and pallor. These symptoms indicate:
    ① Urinary tract infection
    ② Autonomic dysreflexia
    ③ Transient ischemic attack
    ④ Septicemia

80. When a patient is on bed rest and unable to exercise, the muscles tend to:
    ① Atrophy
    ② Elongate
    ③ Hypertrophy
    ④ Twitch

81. A person who has suffered damage to the cerebellum would most likely experience problems with:
    ① Breathing
    ② Hearing
    ③ Coordination of muscular activities
    ④ Visual and hearing disturbance

82. Regulation of appetite is a function of the:
    ① Medulla
    ② Hypothalamus
    ③ Cerebellum
    ④ Cerebral cortex

83. The cranial nerve that functions in regard to swallowing, speaking, and peristalsis is the:
    ① Trigeminal
    ② Hypoglossal
    ③ Vagus
    ④ Glossopharyngeal

84. Laura, age 11, has an order for prochlorperazine (Compazine) 4 mg IM. On hand, you have Compazine 10mg/ml. You give Laura:
    ① 0.2 ml
    ② 0.4 ml
    ③ 0.8 ml
    ④ 1.2 ml

85. Using Young's rule, answer the following problem:
    Child's age: 5
    Average adult dose: 500 mg
    What is the child's dose?

    $$\text{Young's rule: } \frac{\text{Child's age}}{\text{Age} + 12} \times \text{Average adult dose}$$

    ① 147 to 148 mg
    ② 174 to 175 mg
    ③ 199 to 200 mg
    ④ 224 to 225 mg

86. Using Clark's rule, answer the following problem:
    Child's weight: 30 lb
    Average adult dose: 10 mg
    What is the child's dose?

    $$\text{Clark's rule: } \frac{\text{Weight in pounds} \times \text{Adult dose}}{150}$$

    ① 1 mg
    ② 2 mg
    ③ 2.5 mg
    ④ 3 mg

87. Brian, age 4 weeks, is admitted to the hospital with a diagnosis of pyloric stenosis. A classic symptom of pyloric stenosis is:
    ① Projectile vomiting
    ② Diarrhea
    ③ Sharp, colicky abdominal pain
    ④ Distended abdomen

88. Baby Jill has surgery to correct the defect of pyloric stenosis. Postoperative nursing care measures will include:
    ① Positioning her on her back
    ② Nasogastric (NG) tube to low suction
    ③ Feeding her small amounts of glucose water q2h
    ④ Maintaining NPO status for 24 hours

89. You come across a number of injured people. You have to determine the care priorities and know that civilian triage gives care priority to those whose life is threatened. The victims who need immediate care are those with:
    ① Sucking chest wounds
    ② Closed or simple fractures
    ③ First-degree burns of 25% of the body
    ④ Concussions

90. A patient is receiving the anticoagulant, Coumadin, and the physician orders the antidote. The nurse prepares to give:
    ① Protamine sulfate
    ② Vitamin K
    ③ Heparin
    ④ Embolex

91. Mr. Jacks has a diagnosis of leukemia. Tylenol 650 mg is ordered prn. For which of these reasons is Tylenol ordered rather than aspirin?
    ① Aspirin is less effective than Tylenol in relieving pain that caused this disease
    ② Tylenol is absorbed in the stomach more rapidly than aspirin
    ③ Aspirin preparations interfere with prothrombin formation
    ④ Aspirin preparations have a long therapeutic effect

92. Mr. Frank is to receive Lanoxin 0.125 mg PO qid. Available is 0.25 mg tablets. How many tablets do you give?
    ① 0.5
    ② 5
    ③ 2
    ④ 1

93. A patient is to receive Prednisone 15 mg PO qd. The label reads: 5 mg tablets. How many tablets would you give?
    ① 1
    ② 2
    ③ 2.5
    ④ 3

94. Before administering an antibiotic to a patient with a severe wound infection, the nurse knows the usual procedure is to:
    ① First obtain a culture of the wound
    ② Hold the medication and recheck to order
    ③ First check the patient's vital signs
    ④ Wait 30 minutes after the patient has eaten

95. The patient is to receive ASA 600 mg. The label reads gr V. How many tablets should be given?
    ① 1.5
    ② 2
    ③ 2.5
    ④ 3

96. Ryan Carlton is a 32-year-old construction worker hospitalized for the past 4 weeks with a compound fracture of the distal tibia. His physician anticipates that Ryan will be immobilized for another month while the fracture mends. Extended periods of immobility can create many complications, including constipation. To prevent constipation, a diet containing adequate cellulose is recommended. Cellulose is found primarily in:
    ① Refined cereals
    ② Milk products
    ③ Lean tender meats
    ④ Raw fruits and vegetables

97. Janet Goldberg, age 21, has recurrent ulcerative colitis. She is admitted to your unit because of increasing frequency of her diarrheic stools. She is to graduate from college in 2 months. Because Janet's chief complaint is frequent diarrheic stools you would include which of the following in your initial assessment?
    ① Symptoms of fluid and electrolyte imbalance
    ② Urinalysis for presence of urobilinogen
    ③ Pupil check
    ④ Clinitest and Acetest

98. Which of the following symptoms would indicate that a patient with ulcerative colitis suffers from electrolyte imbalance secondary to diarrhea?
    ① Serum potassium level of 3 mEq/L and muscle weakness
    ② Serum sodium level of 135 mEq/L and convulsions
    ③ Serum potassium level of 3.8 mEq/L and diarrhea
    ④ Serum sodium level of 120 mEq/L and edema of feet

99. Placenta previa is characterized by which of the following problems?
    ① Painless vaginal bleeding and boardlike rigidity over the abdomen
    ② Vaginal bleeding and fetal distress
    ③ Severe, sudden abdominal pain and shock
    ④ Hidden or vaginal bleeding and severe abdominal pain

100. Protein is necessary for tissue repair and is especially important in Dee's diet while she is recovering from a fracture of the left femur. Good sources of protein are:
    ① Dark yellow vegetables
    ② Meats, fish, and poultry
    ③ Cereals and cereal products
    ④ Green leafy vegetables

101. The absorption of calcium and phosphorus is aided by a fat-soluble vitamin found in significant amounts in:
    ① Dark yellow fruits and vegetables
    ② Wheat germ and vegetable oils
    ③ Sunshine and fortified milk
    ④ Citrus fruits and green peppers

102. Also important in preventing complications of immobility would be a diet high in:
    ① Fluids
    ② Calcium
    ③ Fats
    ④ Sodium

103. Mr. Dorman, confused and disoriented, is unable to remember the location of his room and is constantly approaching nursing staff members and asking, "Where do I live?" The most appropriate nursing approach to this problem is:
    ① Color coding
    ② Reminiscence therapy
    ③ Reality orientation
    ④ Remotivation therapy

104. Scoliosis is best defined as a(n):
    ① Inflammation of the cartilage between the vertebrae
    ② Arthritic changes in the intervertebral disks
    ③ Lateral curvature of the spine
    ④ Severance of the nerves along the spinal pathway

105. Which of the following will aid in early detection of scoliosis?
    ① Complete blood count
    ② Screening programs
    ③ Pneumography tests
    ④ Bone marrow aspirations

106. In preparing Mrs. Stuart for surgery, which of the following laboratory values would concern you enough to call the physician?
    ① WBC, 10,000
    ② Hemoglobin level, 9 g/dl
    ③ Urine pH, 8.5
    ④ Hematocrit, 42%

107. To obtain a urine specimen from an infant, you would:
    ① Clean and dry genitalia, perineum, and skin; apply a self-adhesive plastic bag (urine strap)
    ② Clean and dry perineum; catheterize infant with sterile infant feeding tube
    ③ Apply disposable diaper; aspirate urine from diaper with needle and syringe
    ④ Place infant on small fracture pan, pour urine into specimen container

108. When taking MAO inhibitors, foods with a high tyramine content should be avoided. Which of the following groups of foods should you caution your patient to avoid most?
    ① Fish, baked potato, yogurt
    ② Chicken, mashed potato, beer
    ③ Liver, asparagus, oranges
    ④ Cheese, wine, ice cream

109. A wound caused by a needle stick is an example of which of the following:
    1. Contusion
    2. Incision
    3. Laceration
    4. Puncture

110. A common portal of exit for microorganisms is the:
    1. Mouth
    2. Skin
    3. Urethra
    4. Vagina

111. Sickle cell anemia is a disease produced by:
    1. Chemical agents
    2. Congenital factors
    3. Hereditary factors
    4. Physical agents

112. Mrs. Adams awakens in the recovery room following a right-sided mastectomy, grabbing at the operative site and moaning, "It's gone. It's all over." She pleads with you to "let me die." Even though Mrs. Adams was prepared by the surgeon for the possible removal of her breast, you must be aware that it is common to react with anger, withdrawal, depression, or other emotions. The next day when Mrs. Adams cries during her morning care, you say:
    1. "Don't cry. You're not going to help yourself by doing this."
    2. "Go ahead and cry. Get it all out. You'll feel better afterward."
    3. "It must be very upsetting for you right now. Let me get your husband."
    4. "It must be very upsetting for you right now. Would you like me to stay with you awhile?"

113. Postoperative exercises for the mastectomy patient are done primarily to:
    1. Aid in healing of the wound
    2. Help prevent shoulder motion limitation and impairments
    3. Aid in recovering sufficiently to resume homemaking activities
    4. Help her assume self-care

114. Breast irradiation often produces which of the following side effects?
    1. Pain
    2. Dysphagia
    3. Alopecia
    4. Pyrexia

115. The single most valuable procedure in the early detection of breast cancer is routine:
    1. Mammography
    2. Xeromammography
    3. Individual breast self-examination
    4. Thermography

116. In performing breast self-examination the most effective pattern to follow is to begin in the:
    1. Lower inner quadrant
    2. Lower outer quadrant
    3. Upper outer quadrant
    4. Upper inner quadrant

117. Breast self-examination should:
    1. Be done once a month, just before the menstrual period
    2. Be done once a month, just after the menstrual period
    3. Be done every 6 months
    4. Not necessary after menopause

118. Instructions to prepare a postmastectomy patient for going home would include cautioning her against:
    1. Wearing loose rubber gloves when washing dishes
    2. Allowing blood to be drawn from the arm of her operative side
    3. Wearing a thimble when sewing
    4. Allowing pulse to be taken in affected area

119. Reach to Recovery volunteers can be especially helpful to mastectomy patients because they are:
    1. Nurses trained to deal with crisis situations
    2. Women who have had successful recoveries from mastectomies themselves
    3. Volunteers who have undergone a 6-month training course
    4. Women trained to fit patients with a prosthesis

120. Causes of mental illness are generally considered to be:
    1. Purely biochemical
    2. Essentially unresolved conflicts of early childhood
    3. Culturally influenced
    4. Interaction among biologic, psychologic, and cultural influences

121. Marie, a 22-year-old woman, has a medical diagnosis of anorexia nervosa. One element of her care plan would include:
    1. Weighing patient daily at the same time dressed in pajamas without shoes
    2. Offering frequent snacks
    3. Offering large meals and firmly suggest she eat them
    4. Offering prn medications before mealtimes

122. Freud's understanding of human behavior is based on:
    1. Nine stages of ego development
    2. Sexuality and aggression
    3. Cultural and environmental factors
    4. Interpersonal conflict

123. John, a 28-year-old stockbroker, claims that he is the richest man in Michigan and a genius. He may be exhibiting:
    1. Tactile hallucinations
    2. Flight of ideas
    3. Delusions of grandeur
    4. Neurosis

124. Jim, a 42-year-old black man, has ingested 18 Valium (diazepam) tablets and 18 unidentified capsules. He is in the ER and is now alert after gastric lavage. He is calling his son to come and take him home. He is exhibiting which of the following defenses:
    1. Sublimation
    2. Projection
    3. Denial
    4. Regression

125. Ruth, an 18-year-old Hispanic woman, states, "It's such a beautiful day; will my new dog learn to sit up; give me some fruit." She is exhibiting:
    1. Confusion
    2. Flight of ideas
    3. Delusions
    4. Hallucinations

Answers and Rationales for Chapter Review Questions

All questions have been classified by cognitive level, nursing process, client need, and level of difficulty; these classifications follow the question number. The first word signifies the cognitive level of the question: knowledge, comprehension, or application. The second word indicates the phase of the nursing process: assessment, planning, implementation, or evaluation. The third word indicates the type of client need and is abbreviated as follows: environment = safe, effective, care environment; physiologic = physiologic integrity; psychosocial = psychosocial integrity; health = health promotion/maintenance.

The letters in parentheses indicate the difficulty of the question. The letter *a* signifies that more than 75% of students should answer the question correctly; *b* signifies that between 50% and 75% should answer correctly; and *c* signifies that between 25% and 50% should answer correctly.

Rationales for all four answer choices for each question are provided. The rationale for the correct answer is listed first, followed by the other rationales.

Chapter 2: Basic Nursing Concepts and the Nursing Process

1. Comprehension, assessment, environment (a)
   3 Older adults vary greatly in their levels of functioning.
   1, 2, 4 Because of the variations in levels of functioning and of health, no assumptions can be made. Careful assessment reveals problems.
2. Comprehension, assessment, environment (a)
   3 Cultural beliefs and practices influence many aspects of illness and health.
   1 The body uses these methods to defend itself (e.g., sneezing). They are not influenced by cultural background.
   2 Natural immunity could not be influenced; acquired immunity could only be influenced if the culture refused immunization.
   4 People of all cultural backgrounds are found at all socioeconomic levels.
3. Application, assessment, environment (b)
   3 Other staff members may have an approach that elicits the patient's cooperation.
   1, 2 Would not be appropriate before consulting with the nursing staff.
   4 Would not be appropriate before consulting with the nursing staff and then the physician.
4. Application, planning, environment (b)
   4 Whenever possible, patient's requests are honored in planning individualized care.
   1 This response reflects the nurse's opinion rather than helping to plan individualized care.
   2, 3 Hospital routines and staffing rarely dictate that all bathing be done in the morning.

5. Comprehension, implementation, physiologic (a)
   4 Humidity reduces drying of nasal passages.
   1, 2, 3 Not true.
6. Application, implementation, environment (a)
   1 In the absence of an emergency, a physician's order is required.
   2 The application of restraints often increases a patient's stress and anxiety.
   3 Restraints are tied to the bed frame rather than to side rails to prevent injury when rails are raised or lowered.
   4 Restraints are applied securely enough to protect yet permit good circulation.
7. Comprehension, assessment, physiologic (a)
   3 Indicates finger edema.
   1, 2, 4 Associated with fluid deficit.
8. Knowledge, implementation, environment (a)
   2 An order for oxygen must include the method of administration and the rate of flow or concentration.
   1 Not the next action in this situation.
   3 Not until an order indicates which equipment to obtain.
   4 Nurse's note is written *after* an event has occurred.
9. Application, assessment, psychosocial (a)
   1 Assessing the reasons for Mrs. Jackson's sadness must be done to plan appropriate interventions.
   2, 3 Not appropriate until patient has had an opportunity to express her thoughts and feelings.
   4 This may not be true.
10. Application, implementation, physiologic (a)
    4 Relieves pressure on the area.
    1 Useful when patient is lying on sacrum, but pressure must be relieved completely by turning patient off sacrum q2h.
    2 Sheepskin reduces abrasions but pressure must be relieved q2h.
    3 Exercises joints but does not help in relieving pressure from sacrum.
11. Knowledge, implementation, physiologic (a)
    4 Reduces trauma to nasal passages and pharynx.
    1 Rotating motion is used while *withdrawing* catheter to suction secretions from all surfaces.
    2 10 to 15 seconds. Suctioning removes oxygen the patient is inhaling as well as secretions.
    3 Surgical asepsis is usually required to prevent introduction of microorganisms.
12. Knowledge, implementation, physiologic (b)
    1 Maintains good alignment.
    2 Narrow base of support; easy to lose balance.
    3 Back and arms would do most of the work.
    4 Need to stand close to the object being moved.
13. Application, planning, physiologic (b)
    3 Soap tends to dry skin.
    1 Requires a physician's order; this situation indicates need for basic nursing interventions.
    2 Bathing would still be necessary to meet patient's need for hygiene.
    4 Not required for this situation; may be required if basic nursing interventions are ineffective.

14. Comprehension, implementation, environment (b)
    2 The nurse's response is judgemental and offers false re-assurance.
    1 Instead of fostering a helping relationship, this response indicates the patient needs no help.
    3 The response has indicated the patient's feeling is not worthy of further discussion.
    4 Continuing assessment would require further communication. This response would tend to end communication.

15. Knowledge, assessment, physiologic (b)
    3 Impacted hardened stool allows only liquid feces from the upper colon to pass through the rectum.
    1 Diarrhea is the frequent passage of loose watery stools.
    2 Flatulence is an accumulation of gas in the intestines.
    4 Incontinence is the inability to control passage of feces.

16. Knowledge, assessment, environment (a)
    1 Hemocult is a test for occult (hidden) blood.
    2 Stool is not tested for the presence of malignant cells.
    3, 4 Examined in stool for ova and parasites.

17. Knowledge, assessment, environment (a)
    4 Redness can be observed by another person.
    1, 2, 3 Experienced by the patient; cannot be observed by another person.

18. Comprehension, implementation, physiologic (c)
    2 Moving joints through each of their possible motions on a regular basis minimizes loss of joint function.
    1, 3 Maintaining tone and size of muscles requires contraction and actual use of the muscles.
    4 Bone strength is maintained by weight bearing.

19. Application, implementation, physiologic (b)
    4 Blanket rolls secured next to the thighs from hip to popliteal space prevent the natural external hip rotation that occurs in the supine position.
    1, 2 These positions are only used for examinations, procedures, and childbirth.
    3 In Sims' position there is no external hip rotation.

20. Application, implementation, physiologic (b)
    4 As soon as the site is cleansed, the puncture is made.
    1, 3 Measures to enhance blood flow to the puncture site are performed before cleansing the site.
    2 Explanations are given before beginning the procedure.

21. Application, implementation, physiologic (b)
    4 Sitting next to the patient enhances a sense of trust and caring.
    1 Assessing the reason for the crying is made easier by sitting next to her.
    2 The patient is the primary source of data.
    3 This would indicate disapproval of her crying.

22. Knowledge, assessment, physiologic (a)
    3 Closed wound, bruise; caused by blunt force.
    1 Rubbed or scraped-off skin or mucous membrane.
    2 An immediate and temporary loss of brain function as a result of a blow to the head.
    4 A tear or rip leaving jagged edges.

23. Comprehension, implementation, physiologic (b)
    1 Teaching during the preoperative period generally results in better learning.
    2, 3, 4 This information should be given by the surgeon.

24. Application, implementation, physiologic (b)
    2 Skin, mucous membranes, and nail beds are assessed for level of oxygenation and circulation.
    1, 3, 4 These are not considerations.

25. Knowledge, implementation, physiologic (b)
    2 Clothing other than the hospital gown could become lost or stained and could interfere with positioning and draping for surgery.
    1 The physician would order manner of dress other than the hospital gown and only in rare instances.
    3, 4 Warmth is provided by blankets.

26. Comprehension, implementation, physiologic (b)
    1 During the transfer from the recovery room, saliva may have pooled in the throat causing an obstruction; the airway is always a priority.
    2, 3, 4 All of these are important and are assessed after determining that the airway is patent.

27. Application, assessment, physiologic (b)
    3 Restlessness is an early indication of hypoxia.
    1 This is within normal limits.
    2 This is an expected response.
    4 This is normal.

28. Comprehension, assessment, physiologic (b)
    3 Prevents entry of microorganisms.
    1 The physician generally changes the initial dressing.
    2 This amount of drainage would not necessitate notification of the physician.
    4 Removing the dressing unnecessarily allows entry of microorganisms.

29. Knowledge, implementation, physiologic (b)
    2 Voluntary control over bladder function often requires 6 to 8 hours for the effects of the anesthesia to wear off.
    1 See rationale for statement 2.
    3, 4 Waiting this long may allow the bladder to become overdistended.

30. Comprehension, assessment, physiologic (a)
    4 Indicates return of peristalsis.
    1, 3 Does not indicate peristaltic functioning.
    2 May indicate that peristalsis has not returned.

31. Application, implementation, physiologic (b)
    4 Activity stimulates the return of peristalsis.
    1 Only appropriate if distension or constipation occurs; requires a physician's order.
    2 Coughing and deep breathing are not related to stimulation of peristalsis.
    3 Does not stimulate peristalsis.

32. Comprehension, assessment, physiologic (b)
    4 The body attempts to compensate for reduced circulating volume by constricting blood vessels and increasing the heart rate.
    1, 3 In hypovolemic shock there is constriction of peripheral blood vessels resulting in pale, cool skin.
    2 In hypovolemic shock the body attempts to better circulate oxygen by increasing the respiratory rate.

33. Comprehension, assessment, physiologic (b)
    4 Prolonged pressure deprives an area of tissue of its circulation so that adequate nourishment cannot be brought to the area and accumulated blood and wastes cannot leave the area, resulting in redness.
    1 Lice do not become embedded under the skin and would not be likely to affect the coccyx area.
    2 If moved properly, without friction and shearing of the skin, redness would not occur.
    3 Although adequate nourishment, especially of proteins and ascorbic acid, is necessary for maintenance and repair of tissue, a reddened coccyx is more likely caused by prolonged pressure.

34. Application, implementation, physiologic (a)
    3 If a thrombus is present in the legs, massaging could dislodge it and allow it to travel (embolus).
    1 Bending the knee would have no adverse effect on this patient.
    2 Bath water needs to be changed when it becomes soapy.
    4 To reduce discomfort of tickling, use long, firm, smooth strokes.

35. Application, assessment, physiologic (b)
    4 Temperature, integrity, and overall condition are terms that include all aspects of skin assessment.
    1, 2, 3 Does not include all aspects of skin assessment.

36. Application, implementation, environment (b)
    4 Adequate rest and sleep enhance the body's ability to defend itself against invading organisms.
    1 Assessment of vital signs does not increase resistance to disease.
    2 Bathing frequently with soap may dry and crack the skin, thus increasing susceptibility.
    3 Street clothes do not provide a defense against infection.

37. Application, implementation, environment (c)
    4 Starting with bent knees while lifting allows the long, strong muscles of the legs to bear most of the weight.
    1 When lifting, you must stand close to the object being lifted.
    2 Lifting under the patient's strong side keeps him from assisting.
    3 Straight arms and legs cannot be levers.

38. Comprehension, implementation, psychosocial (b)
    3 Using the bedpan at frequent intervals may reduce soiling of linen and reduce embarrassment.
    1 Mr. McGinnis does not have diarrhea.
    2 Would not reduce soiling.
    4 Would not reduce his emotional stress. Stress may be increased because of the idea of being diapered.

39. Application, assessment, psychosocial (a)
    3 Each person has the right to pursue or refuse a visit by the clergy.
    1 When the patient is capable of making decisions, he or she should be consulted.
    2 Assessing the patient's feelings about the clergy visiting would precede discussing communion.
    4 Spiritual needs should be assessed before the patient becomes gravely ill.

40. Knowledge, planning, psychosocial (b)
    4 Observe Sabbath from sundown Friday to sundown Saturday.
    1, 2, 3 Observe Sabbath on Sunday.

41. Knowledge, implementation, environment (c)
    3 This distance approximates distance from nares to stomach.
    1, 2, 4 Does not approximate distance from nares to stomach.

42. Knowledge, implementation, physiologic (a)
    1 To lessen the chance of aspiration if the patient should regurgitate the feeding.
    2, 3, 4 Feeding could be aspirated if patient regurgitated.

43. Application, implementation, environment (a)
    2 Solution entering the trachea would trigger the cough reflex and obstruct the flow of oxygen.
    1 Introducing solution too quickly may cause nausea or cramping.
    3 Introducing cold solution may cause chilling of the patient.
    4 Too thick a solution may obstruct the nasogastric tube.

44. Comprehension, implementation, physiologic (b)
    2 If the feeding is administered too rapidly, the stomach does not have time to accommodate the fluid; thus it empties too rapidly.
    1 Air entering the stomach may cause cramping but not diarrhea.
    3 Too much water introduced after the feeding may result in the stomach not emptying completely but not in diarrhea.
    4 Other than by x-ray examination, there is no way of determining exactly where in the stomach the tube is located. As long as the tube is in the stomach, its exact location should have no effect on tolerance of the feeding.

45. Application, implementation, physiologic (b)
    1 Patient needs to lie flat until the body replaces the removed spinal fluid. Lying flat usually prevents headaches after the lumbar puncture.
    2 Not a part of the aftercare following a lumbar puncture.
    3,4 Not necessary after a lumbar puncture.

46. Knowledge, implementation, environment (a)
    4 Ten minutes is required for the body's temperature to return to its previous level.
    1, 2, 3 Insufficient time.

47. Knowledge, implementation, environment (b)
    2 In the event that the nurse made an error in counting the first time.
    1, 3, 4 Only after counting the pulse again.

48. Comprehension, implementation, psychosocial (b)
    3 Therapeutic indicates helping. In the nurse-patient relationship, therapeutic communication is directed toward the patient: determining and meeting needs.
    1 Therapeutic communication may not be easily understood and may need frequent clarification and repetition.
    2 Therapeutic communication determines much more than just attitudes.
    4 Most people are accustomed to conversational communication rather than therapeutic.

49. Comprehension, implementation, environment (b)
    2 Lithotomy position allows for visualization and examination of the female genitals.
    1 Knee-chest position would not allow best visualization possible.
    3 Prone position would not allow good visualization.
    4 Sims' position would not allow good visualization.

50. Comprehension, implementation, environment (b)
    1 Clean dentures over a towel or basin of water so that if they are dropped they would be less likely to break.
    2 Dentures should be held with gauze or cloth to provide a good grip so there is less likelihood of dropping; tissues would dissolve under running water.
    3 There is no reason to soak dentures before cleansing.
    4 Very hot water may cause dentures to warp or crack.

51. Application, implementation, psychosocial (a)
    2 Apologize when appropriate; accept the patient's feelings.
    1 This response disregards the patient's feelings at the moment and may be offering unwarranted reassurance.
    3 A defensive response.
    4 Disregards patient's feelings.

52. Analysis, assessment, psychosocial (a)
    1 Anxiety may cause hostility and fear of being alone.
    2 Stereotyping the patient as a particular kind of person disregards needs and feelings that need to be dealt with.
    3, 4 Stereotyping disregards patient's needs and feelings.

53. Knowledge, implementation, environment (a)
    2 Correct method in a legal document.
    1 Entries in a legal document cannot be obliterated.
    3 Entries in a legal document cannot be erased.
    4 In a legal document you cannot write another nurse's note nor write another nurse's signature.

54. Comprehension, assessment, environment (b)
    1 Habits influencing health practices are most often a result of cultural background.
    2 Genetic background has little effect on patterns of health practices.
    3 Economic status has less effect on habits than has cultural background.
    4 Social status has less effect on habits than has cultural background.

55. Application, implementation, physiologic (a)
    2 Reducing tension and anxiety often helps reduce pain.
    1 Cool sponge baths are not associated with pain reduction.
    3 Although speaking to the physician may reduce tension and anxiety, he or she is often not available during all the times pain is present.
    4 Not associated with pain reduction.
56. Comprehension, implementation, environment (a)
    3 Washing hands thoroughly and frequently is the most effective way to help prevent spread of organisms.
    1 Effective, but only in situations in which linens are involved.
    2 Necessary only when enteric infections exist.
    4 Protects only the nurse, not other patients.
57. Knowledge, implementation, environment (a)
    2 Good posture and body mechanics contribute to effective and efficient use of muscles.
    1 The nurse cannot avoid lifting heavy objects; girdle may provide support.
    3 Use of back muscles only may cause injury.
    4 Would be helpful, but bed making is only one aspect of nursing activity.
58. Application, assessment, physiologic (c)
    3 Goal is specific, patient centered, and measurable.
    1 Goal is not specific or measurable.
    2 Goal is specific but not patient centered.
    4 Goal is not specific or measurable.
59. Application, implementation, physiologic (a)
    4 A clean and comfortable bed helps promote rest and sleep.
    1 Unless the television is part of the patient's sleep routine, it may provide too much stimulation for relaxation to occur.
    2 Reading the newspaper to the patient may provide too much stimulation for relaxation to occur.
    3 May provide too much stimulation.
60. Comprehension, implementation, physiologic (b)
    2 Counting for 1 full minute, preferably apically, allows for a more accurate count and assessment of the pattern of irregularity.
    1 Applying less pressure on the artery may result in missing some beats of the heart.
    3 An apical-radial pulse would be necessary only if determination of the pulse deficit was required.
    4 Taking the carotid pulse would be necessary if the radial site was unavailable or not palpable.
61. Knowledge, assessment, environment (a)
    2 Must be assessed.
    1 Not a part of IV assessment.
    3 Peripheral venous pressure is not included in IV assessment.
    4 Rate of flow must be included in IV assessment.
62. Analysis, implementation, physiologic (b)
    1 Range-of-motion exercises can be initiated on all patients unless specifically contraindicated.
    2 The type of diet given to the patient requires a physician's order.
    3 Application of elastic bandages requires a physician's order.
    4 The administration of medications requires a physician's order.
63. Knowledge, implementation, physiologic (a)
    3 Custard is made up largely of measurable quantities of milk, thus is measured as intake in most facilities.
    1 Although vegetables contain a large percentage of water, it is unmeasurable.
    2 Although fruits contain a large percentage of water, it is unmeasurable.
    4 Although the components of a stew contain a large percentage of water, it is unmeasurable.

64. Application, implementation, physiologic (c)
    4 Monitoring daily weights is the best way of measuring fluid gains or loss since normal body weight varies little from day to day.
    1 Although medication dosages are often based on a person's weight, changes in dosage are rarely made on a daily basis according to weight changes.
    2 There is no indication that she is on a low-calorie diet. Weight changes as a result of reduced calories vary only slightly on a daily basis.
    3 This is not true.
65. Application, implementation, physiologic (b)
    1 Encouraging patients to help serve themselves helps preserve and promote their feelings of independence and control.
    2 This may make the patient feel even more dependent and helpless.
    3 Unless contraindicated, activity should be encouraged to maintain and/or strengthen muscle tone.
    4 Although feeding patients yourself is often easier and faster than allowing them to help, it does not promote their feelings of independence and control.
66. Knowledge, implementation, environment (b)
    4 Donning the sterile gloves is done as soon as the package is opened.
    1 Sterile drapes must be arranged with sterile gloves on.
    2 The meatus is cleansed with sterile gloves on.
    3 The procedure is explained before opening the sterile package.
67. Knowlege, implementation, physiologic (a)
    2 Usually far enough to ensure entrance to the bladder.
    1 May not reach to the bladder.
    3, 4 Does not need to be inserted so far.
68. Comprehension, implementation, health (c)
    4 Passive natural immunity is received by the fetus from the mother; it lasts about 6 months.
    1 Active acquired immunity results from administration of live or killed vaccines or toxoids.
    2 Active natural immunity results from having had a specific disease.
    3 Passive acquired immunity results from administration of immune serum or gamma globulin.
69. Application, assessment, physiologic (b)
    4 Touching the uvula causes the patient to gag or vomit.
    1 The nasal turbinates are located in the nasal passages, not in the throat.
    2, 3 The posterior pharynx and tonsils are areas where throat microorganisms are located.
70. Comprehension, assessment, physiologic (b)
    2 An error has been made. The number of heart beats felt at the radial site cannot be greater than the number of beats heard at the apex.
    1 The patient needs no care—an error has been made.
    3, 4 An error has been made—results should not be reported.
71. Comprehension, assessment, environment (b)
    3 Palpation reveals the amount of pitting involved.
    1 No sounds are produced by ankle edema.
    2 Evaluation is a step in the nursing process.
    4 Percussion is used to assess masses, organs, and body cavities.
72. Comprehension, assessment, environment (c)
    4 The port on drainage tubing is specifically designed for obtaining specimens.
    1 Attaching a new drainage bag requires opening the closed system, which is to be avoided.
    2 This would require opening the closed system, which is to be avoided.
    3 On most catheters, inserting the needle would leave a hole that would leak urine.

73. Knowledge, implementation, physiologic (a)
    1 High-Fowler's position allows better lung expansion, thus promoting better oxygenation.
    2 Oxygen therapy would require a physician's order.
    3 Vital sign frequency is determined by a complete assessment of the patient.
    4 Log-rolling technique is used to turn a patient whose back cannot be flexed.
74. Knowledge, implementation, environment (c)
    3 Strict isolation is used for diseases that are transmitted through the air, such as chickenpox.
    1 Drainage/secretion isolation is used only to prevent contact with infected drainage.
    2 Respiratory isolation is used for diseases spread by air droplets.
    4 Universal blood and body fluid isolation is used to prevent contact with infected body fluids or blood.
75. Application, implementation, environment (b)
    4 Respiratory isolation prevents transmission of disease through air droplets; a gown would not be required.
    1 The glass thermometer should be left in the room to prevent its use by any other patient.
    2 Hands should be washed before caring for any patient.
    3 A mask is always worn while caring for any patient in respiratory isolation.

Chapter 3: Anatomy and Physiology

1. Knowledge (a)
   4 Platelets stick together and form a plug that seals the wound. They release chemicals that eventually result in formation of clot.
   1 Antibodies are produced in response to a specific antigen.
   2 Leukocytes are WBCs, which destroys pathogens.
   3 Erythrocytes are RBCs, which carry oxygen from lungs to tissues.
2. Knowledge (a)
   1 The body is constantly stabilizing and equalizing its environment to prevent any sudden or severe change.
   2 Diffusion is the process of dissolved particles being distributed evenly throughout a fluid.
   3 Osmosis is the movement of water through a permeable membrane.
   4 Filtration is the movement of water and solutes through a membrane because of a greater pushing force on one side of the membrane.
3. Knowledge (a)
   4 The DNA molecules in the nucleus of a cell duplicate themselves, and the cell divides, forming two cells.
   1 Osmosis is the movement of water through a permeable membrane.
   2 Crenation is the shrinking of red cells placed in a hypertonic salt solution.
   3 Lyse is the swelling of red cells placed in a hypotonic salt solution.
4. Knowledge (a)
   3 In acquiring passive immunity the body of the recipient plays no active part in response to an antigen.
   1 In active immunity the resistance to a disease results from the development of antibodies within the body.
   2 Autoimmune immunity occurs by the body's producing antibodies to its own tissue.
   4 Newborn babies receive a short-term immunity as a result of the antibodies of their mother.

5. Knowledge (a)
   2 The functional unit is suspended near the center of the cell and has the property of division.
   1 Cytoplasm is the portion of the protoplasm of a cell outside the nucleus.
   3 Protoplasm is a thick, viscous substance that exists only in cells.
   4 The cytoplasmic membrane encloses the cytoplasm.
6. Knowledge (a)
   3 Produced by the thyroid gland, thyroxin controls the rate glucose is burned and converts it to heat and energy.
   1 Oxytocin initiates and maintains labor.
   2 Aldosterone promotes sodium and water retention in the kidney.
   4 Cortisone assists the body to respond to stress and reduces inflammation.
7. Knowledge (a)
   3 Estrogen and progesterone promote development of the female sex characteristics and sex organs and regulate menstruation for the purpose of reproduction.
   1, 2 Testosterone is produced in the testes.
   4 Prolactin is produced in the pituitary gland.
8. Comprehension (b)
   2 Dilation of the blood vessels brings more blood to the surface so that heat can be dissipated.
   1 Contraction slows the amount of blood in the veins and serves to protect the skin and deeper tissue from excess heat loss.
   3 The production of sweat is increased by dilation of blood vessels but is not the primary cause of loss of body heat.
   4 An increase in blood supply constricts muscles rather than relaxing them.
9. Knowledge (a)
   1 The area is located slightly below the center of each breast and contains slightly raised areas (glands of Montgomery).
   2 Bartholin's glands lie on each side of the vaginal outlet.
   3 Cowper's glands are located on either side of the urethra and just below the prostate gland in the male.
   4 Urochrome gives urine its color.
10. Knowledge (a)
    3 The male sex glands produce the hormone that regulates male sex characteristics.
    1 Progesterone is produced by the ovaries.
    2 Estrogen is produced by the ovaries.
    4 Aldosterone is produced by the adrenal cortex.
11. Knowledge (a)
    1 The connective tissue is made of dense fibrous tissue in the shape of a cord and has great strength.
    2 Ligaments attach bones to bones.
    3 Cartilage makes a slick surface for rotation and absorbs shock.
    4 Osseous is commonly called bony tissue.
12. Knowledge (b)
    3 The lymphatic system drains excess fluids through a series of filters, lymph nodes, where bacteria and foreign bodies are trapped and destroyed.
    1 The lymphatic system destroys bacteria.
    2 Erythrocytes are manufactured primarily in long bones.
    4 Clotting of blood is aided by platelets.
13. Comprehension (c)
    4 Iron is an essential mineral in the formation of hemoglobin.
    1 Copper assists in the use of iron.
    2 Magnesium is essential in general metabolism.
    3 Calcium is essential in bone and tooth formation.

14. Knowledge (b)
    2 Fat globules must be broken down into very small particles, emulsified, to be digested. Bile is the enzyme that emulsifies fat.
    1 Bile does not act on protein, which is a part of meat fiber. Pepsin and hydrochloric acid break down protein.
    3 Bile does not assist in the breakdown of sugar, only fats.
    4 The liver cells convert complex sugar, glycogen, to glucose.

15. Comprehension (a)
    3 Epithelial tissue has many forms—flat and irregular, square, long and narrow—that are arranged in single or many layers to form a protective covering and lining.
    1 Periosteum is a connective tissue covering the bone.
    2 Pericardium is a fibrous sac lined with serous membrane that surrounds the heart.
    4 Connective tissue supports and connects other tissues and parts of the body.

16. Comprehension (a)
    1 The cardiac sphincter separates the esophagus from the stomach region close to the heart.
    2 Rugae are the folds in the stomach lining.
    3 Chyme is a semiliquid mixture of gastric juices and food.
    4 The pyloric sphincter is located between the distal end of the stomach and the proximal end of the small intestine and determines how long food stays in the stomach.

17. Comprehension (a)
    3 The small intestine secretes enzymes that digest proteins and carbohydrates, and most of the digestive process, absorption, occurs in the small intestine.
    1 The liver has many functions, such as storing glucose and manufacturing bile.
    2 The stomach serves as a storage pouch and a digestive organ.
    4 The large intestine stores and eliminates waste and reabsorbs water.

18. Knowledge (a)
    2 Circular muscles contract when stimulated, closing an opening.
    1 Adduction is movement toward the body.
    3 Extensors cause the angle of the joint to become larger.
    4 Flexors cause the angle of the joint to become smaller.

19. Knowledge (a)
    4 A small opening into the nose at the inner corner of the eye allows the fluid to drain through.
    1 The ciliary body is a smooth muscle structure to which the lens is attached.
    2 The lacrimal gland releases tears into the anterior surface of the eyeball.
    3 The eustachian tube connects the middle ear chambers with the throat.

20. Knowledge (a)
    3 Incisors are the four top and bottom front teeth.
    1 Eye teeth, or canines, appear later in the baby.
    2 Molars are the last to appear, usually by 2 to 2½ years.
    4 Canines are another name for eye teeth and appear after the incisors.

21. Knowledge (a)
    3 Many gray matter areas that form the cranial nerves are located in the medulla and are involved in the control of vital activities.
    1 The cerebellum controls muscle tone, coordination, and equilibrium.
    2 The cerebrum controls the highest level of functioning, sensation, memory, reasoning, and intelligence.
    4 The pons carries messages between the cerebrum and the medulla.

22. Knowledge (a)
    2 As peristalsis moves content along, water is absorbed through the walls into the circulation, and the remaining cellulose passes on to the rectum.
    1 Absorption of food occurs in the small intestine.
    3 Enzymes are produced in the mouth, stomach, pancreas, and small intestine.
    4 Enzymes are secreted from the mouth, stomach, pancreas, and small intestine.

23. Knowledge (a)
    4 The progressive, wavelike movement that occurs involuntarily forces food forward.
    1 Pylorospasm is a spasm of the pyloric sphincter.
    2 Rugae are large folds of mucous membrane.
    3 Mastication is chewing.

24. Comprehension (b)
    1 Gastric and intestinal enzymes gradually break down the protein molecule into its separate amino acids.
    2 Ptyalin is an enzyme found in saliva.
    3 Hydrochloric acid is an enzyme found in the stomach.
    4 Glucose is the breakdown product of carbohydrates.

25. Knowledge (a)
    3 The process of digestion is accelerated, and as the food moves through the loops of the intestine, it is digested and absorbed by the villi into the blood and lymph capillaries.
    1 The large intestine absorbs water after digestion is completed.
    2 The process of digestion continues in the stomach.
    4 Sigmoid is a part of the large intestine.

26. Comprehension (b)
    1 Bile is produced in the liver but is not an enzyme.
    2, 3, 4 Is a function of the liver.

27. Comprehension (b)
    4 Iodine is an element that aids in the formation of thyroxin, which is a hormone produced in the thyroid.
    1 Calcium aids in the formation of bones and teeth.
    2 Phosphorus aids in the calcification of bones and teeth.
    3 Iron is essential in the formation of hemoglobin.

28. Comprehension (a)
    1 Capillaries connect arterioles with venules and function as exchange vessels.
    2 Veins transport the blood back to the heart.
    3 Arterioles carry blood to capillaries.
    4 Venules carry blood from capillaries to veins.

29. Comprehension (a)
    1 Deoxygenated blood returns from body tissues through the superior and inferior vena cava into the right atrium.
    2 Left atrium receives oxygenated blood.
    3 Right ventricle receives deoxygenated blood from the right atrium.
    4 Left ventricle receives oxygenated blood from the left atrium.

30. Knowledge (a)
    3 Epinephrine is a hormone manufactured in the adrenal medulla and increases blood pressure and heart rate.
    1 Insulin is manufactured in the pancreas and decreases blood sugar levels.
    2 Aldosterone is produced in the adrenal cortex and aids in regulating electrolytes and water balance.
    4 Testosterone is produced by the testes and stimulates growth and development of sex organs.

31. Comprehension (c)
    3 Antidiuretic hormone (ADH) produced in the posterior pituitary promotes reabsorption.
    1 Oxytocin produced in the posterior pituitary causes uterine muscles to contract.
    2 Calcitonin is produced in the thyroid and assists in decreasing calcium level in blood.
    4 Prolactin is produced in the anterior pituitary and promotes growth of all body tissues.

32. Comprehension (a)
    2 The diffusion of gas occurs across the thin, squamous epithelium lining of the alveoli.
    1 The bronchi carry air to the right and left lung.
    3 Bronchioles are the smallest branches of the bronchi.
    4 Venules collect blood from capillaries.
33. Knowledge (a)
    4 SA node, located in the right atrium, starts each heart beat.
    1 AV node receives the impulse from SA node.
    2 Bundle of His receives the impulse from AV node.
    3 Purkinje fibers receive impulses from bundle of His, resulting in the contraction of the ventricles.
34. Comprehension (a)
    1 The pulmonary artery carries deoxygenated blood from the heart.
    2 Aorta carries oxygenated blood from the heart.
    3 Coronary carries oxygenated blood to the heart.
    4 Carotid carries oxygenated blood to the brain.
35. Comprehension (a)
    2 T-cells are lymphocytes that are produced by the thymus and produce an immunity.
    1 The thyroid influences cell metabolism.
    3 The pineal secretes melatonin, which may regulate sexual development.
    4 The pituitary produces many hormones that affect growth and development, protects the body in stressful situations, promotes reabsorption of water, etc.
36. Comprehension (b)
    3 The greater trochanter is the ball-like head, which articulates with the hip bone.
    1 Acetabulum is the deep socket in the hip bone.
    2 Acromion is the highest point of the shoulder.
    4 Olecranon process is the upper end of the elbow; forms point of elbow.
37. Comprehension (a)
    3 Periosteum is a strong fibrous membrane that covers the bone and provides growth, nutrition, and repair.
    1 Red blood cells are formed in red marrow of bone.
    2 Yellow bone marrow is a fatty material found inside the long bone.
    4 Adipose tissue is stored in the diaphysis or shaft.
38. Comprehension (a)
    2 Perineum is the external region between vulva and anus in a female or between scrotum and anus in the male and forms the pelvic floor.
    1 Peritoneum lines the abdominal cavity and folds over abdominal organs.
    3 Mons pubis is the fatty rounded area overlying the pubic symphysis.
    4 Rectus abdominus is an abdominal muscle.
39. Comprehension (b)
    3 The integumentary system includes the skin and appendages. Rashes, bruises, and decubitus are noted on the skin.
    1 Blood pressure and pulse are considered part of the respiratory and cardiovascular system.
    2 Blood sugar levels would be an assessment of the endocrine system, pancreas.
    4 Although rashes and bruises are considered assessment of the integumentary system, blood sugar levels are assessed with the endocrine system.
40. Comprehension (b)
    3 Sebaceous glands produce an oily secretion for lubrication. Blackheads are a mixture of dirt and sebum and collect at the openings of the sebaceous glands.
    1 Ceruminous glands or wax glands are in the ear.
    2 Lacrimal glands produce tears, which keep the conjunctiva of the eye moist.
    4 Sudoriferous glands are sweat glands that regulate body temperature.

41. Comprehension (b)
    4 Normal urine has a low specific gravity.
    1 Urine is a clear, amber liquid.
    2 Urine is composed of nitrogenous waste products.
    3 Urine is slightly aromatic.
42. Comprehension (b)
    3 The upper surfaces of the dermis have raised and depressed areas that are unique to each individual and thus a means of identification.
    1 Elastic connective tissue is found in the subcutaneous layer.
    2 The subcutaneous layer is below the dermis.
    4 Upper surface of the epidermis consists of the outermost cells that are constantly lost to wear and tear.
43. Comprehension (c)
    2 Aldosterone is released by the adrenal cortex in response to decreased blood volume, decreased blood sodium ions, or increased potassium ions.
    1 ADH prevents excess water loss in the urine.
    3 Parathormone regulates calcium-ion homeostasis of the blood.
    4 Oxytocin stimulates uterine muscles during birth.
44. Knowledge (b)
    4 Oxygen prevents the accumulation of lactic acid, which can cause muscle fatigue, and the glycogen is a source of food.
    1 Acetylcholine is important in the transmission of nerve impulses and synapses.
    2 Lactic acid is a waste product and causes muscle fatigue.
    3 Acetylcholine is important in the transmission of nerve impulses and synapses.
45. Comprehension (b)
    1 The left motor control center in the brain controls the right side of the body because of the crossing of the nerve tracts within the brain.
    2 The left side of the body is controlled by the right side of the brain.
    3 Only one side of the body is affected if an injury is to only one side of the brain.
    4 Only one arm would be affected, depending on which side of the brain was injured.
46. Comprehension (a)
    3 The diaphragm separates the abdomen from the thoracic cavity. It contracts with inspiration and relaxes with expiration.
    1 The latissimus dorsi is located in the middle lower back.
    2 The sternocleidomastoid is located alongside the neck.
    4 Gastrocnemius is located in the calf of the leg.
47. Comprehension (c)
    4 The parasympathetic division of the autonomic nervous system maintains homeostasis by regulating digestion and circulation.
    1 Sensory neurons carry impulses toward the CNS.
    2 Interneurons (connecting) conduct impulses from the sensory neurons to the motor neurons.
    3 The sympathetic nervous system controls the "fight or flight" response.
48. Comprehension (a)
    2 The hypothalamus is an important autonomic nervous system center and controls body temperature.
    1 Medulla controls heart rate, blood pressure, breathing, and swallowing.
    3 Cerebral cortex is the outer layer of the cerebrum.
    4 Cerebellum controls muscle tone and coordination and coordinates action of the voluntary muscles.
49. Comprehension (b)
    2 The snail-like cochlea is the organ of Corti and contains hearing receptors.
    1 Tympanic membrane is the eardrum.
    3 Semicircular canal controls equilibrium.
    4 Malleus is part of the middle ear.

50. Comprehension (c)
    1 The eustachian tube connects the middle ear with the throat; swallowing or yawning equalizes the pressure, which allows the eardrum to vibrate easily.
    2 The labyrinth is the internal ear.
    3 Sound waves are passed through the oval window to the internal ear.
    4 Ossicles are the three tiny bones in the middle ear.
51. Comprehension (c)
    2 When water intake is excessive, the kidneys excrete generous amounts of urine; if water intake is lost, they produce less urine; the process is regulated by hormones.
    1 The bladder is the reservoir for urine.
    3 Islets of Langerhans produce insulin.
    4 Gonads are the sex glands.
52. Comprehension (a)
    3 The islets of Langerhans are located in the pancreas and produce insulin.
    1 Pineal gland is found in the brain and atrophies at an early age.
    2 Insulin is released into the duodenum, a division of the small intestine.
    4 The liver produces bile.
53. Comprehension (a)
    2 Gluteus medius is a deep muscle located in the upper outer-quadrant of the hip and buttocks.
    1 Gluteus maximus is the fleshy, large part of the hip and buttocks.
    3 Iliopsoas crosses the front of hip joint to the femur.
    4 Sartorius winds down the thigh, ileum to the tibia.
54. Comprehension (b)
    2 Primary function is to act against most bacteria, viruses, tumor cells, and foreign organs.
    1 B-cells are responsible for humeral immunity.
    3 T-cells do clone into helpers and suppressors to carry out primary function, but statement 2 is most explicit.
    4 B-cells clone antibody-producing plasma cells.
55. Knowledge (a)
    1 Abduction moves part away from midline.
    2 Adduction moves part toward midline.
    3 Flexion makes angle at a joint smaller.
    4 Pronation rotates a part to face downward.
56. Knowledge (b)
    4 The aqueous humor, a watery fluid that fills muscle of the eyeball, maintains the slight forward curve of the cornea.
    1 Dilation of the pupil is regulated by the involuntary iris muscle.
    2 The lacrimal gland produces tears.
    3 The thickness of the lens is regulated by the contraction of the ciliary body.

Chapter 4: Pharmacology

1. Application, implementation, environment (a)
    2 Regulation of Controlled Substances Act.
    1, 3, 4 Not applicable.
2. Knowledge, assessment, environment (a)
    4 Definition of the law.
    1 Replaced by Controlled Substances Act.
    2 No such act.
    3 Regulates distribution of narcotics and other drugs of abuse.
3. Knowledge, assessment, environment (a)
    2 Study of drugs.
    1 Study of the processes a drug undergoes in the body.
    3 Place where drugs are stored and dispensed.
    4 Study of movement of drugs in the body.
4. Knowledge, assessment, environment (a)
    4 Definition.
    1 Name as listed in official publications.
    2 Name given by developer of drug.
    3 Chemical composition of drug.
5. Knowledge, assessment, environment (a)
    3 Proper data collection.
    1 Limiting.
    2 Not necessary.
    4 Limiting.
6. Knowledge, assessment, physiologic (a)
    2 Definition.
    1 Released a small amount at a time over relatively long period of time.
    3 Circular or oblong disks.
    4 Outer portion dissolves in stomach; inner pill dissolves in intestine.
7. Knowledge, assessment, environment (a)
    3 May cause harmful effect.
    1, 2, 4 Not applicable.
8. Knowledge, implementation, physiologic (a)
    3 Muscle tissue has a greater blood supply.
    1, 2 Slow absorption.
    4 Not applicable.
9. Knowledge, assessment, environment (a)
    1 Adverse reaction.
    2, 3, 4 Not applicable.
10. Knowledge, implementation, environment (a)
    2 When removing the container, while measuring the drug, and before returning or discarding the container.
    1, 3, 4 Not applicable.
11. Knowledge, implementation, environment (a)
    4 Most accurate method.
    1, 2, 3 Unreliable method.
12. Application, implementation, environment (a)
    4 To promote safety and prevent errors.
    1, 2, 3 Not applicable.
13. Knowledge, implementation, environment (a)
    1 Straightens the canal and promotes maximum contact between tissue and drug.
    2 Proper procedure for children.
    3, 4 Not applicable.
14. Knowledge, implementation, environment (b)
    3 Correct calculation.
    1, 2, 4 Incorrect.
15. Application, implementation, environment (a)
    3 Proper procedure.
    1, 2, 4 Not applicable.
16. Knowledge, implementation, environment (a)
    2 Best anatomic position.
    1, 3, 4 Not applicable.
17. Knowledge, implementation, environment (a)
    3 Correct calculation.
    1, 2, 4 Incorrect.
18. Comprehension, assessment, environment (a)
    4 Tinnitis is the most common side effect of salicylate toxicity.
    1, 2, 3 Not applicable.
19. Knowledge, evaluation, environment (a)
    3 Definition.
    1, 2 Undesired effect of drug.
    4 Unusual or unexpected effect.
20. Knowledge, implementation, environment (b)
    3 Correct calculation.
    1, 2, 4 Incorrect.

21. Knowledge, assessment, environment (a)
    1 Definition.
    2 Unusual or unexpected effect.
    3 Two drugs taken together produce greater effect than each taken alone.
    4 Decreased results.
22. Knowledge, assessment, environment (a)
    3 Definition.
    1 Inactivation of drug in body.
    2 Elimination of drug from body.
    4 Adverse reaction of drug.
23. Knowledge, implementation, environment (b)
    3 Correct calculation.
    1, 2, 4 Incorrect.
24. Knowledge, planning, physiologic (a)
    2 Most promising; other drugs are being tested.
    1, 3, 4 Not applicable in this situation.
25. Application, evaluation, physiologic (a)
    1 Drug action
    2, 3, 4 Not applicable in this situation.
26. Knowledge, assessment, physiologic (a)
    3 Definition.
    1 Time drug enters the body and time it enters bloodstream.
    2 Transport of drugs in body.
    4 Elimination of drugs from body.
27. Knowledge, assessment, physiologic (a)
    1 Definition.
    2 Transport of drug molecules in the body.
    3 Inactivation of drugs in the body.
    4 Elimination of drug from the body.
28. Knowledge, implementation, environment (a)
    2 Correct equivalent.
    1, 3, 4 Not applicable.
29. Knowledge, implementation, environment (a)
    4 Accepted equivalent.
    1, 2, 3 Not applicable.
30. Knowledge, implementation, environment (a)
    1 Accepted equivalent.
    2, 3, 4 Not applicable.
31. Knowledge, implementation, environment (a)
    2 Accepted equivalent.
    1, 3, 4 Not applicable.
32. Knowledge, implementation, environment (a)
    2 Accepted equivalent.
    1, 3, 4 Not applicable.
33. Knowledge, planning, environment (a)
    4 Correct measurements.
    1, 2, 3 Not applicable.
34. Application, implementation, environment (a)
    4 According to state nurse practice acts, the nurse who draws up the medication is responsible for giving the drug.
    1, 2, 3 Not a responsible action for this situation.
35. Application, implementation, environment (a)
    3 Could lead to adverse reactions.
    1, 2, 4 Not applicable.
36. Knowledge, assessment, physiologic (b)
    2 Hypokalemia can increase risk of toxicity.
    1, 3, 4 Not applicable.
37. Knowledge, implementation, environment (a)
    2 Large muscles are rich in nerves and blood vessels.
    1, 3, 4 Not applicable.
38. Knowledge, assessment, physiologic (a)
    1 Definition.
    2 Act at site of application.
    3 Relieve symptoms.
    4 Cure disease.

39. Application, evaluation, environment (a)
    2 Early sign.
    1, 3, 4 Not applicable.
40. Application, implementation, environment (a)
    3 To allow for diuresis during patient's normal waking hours.
    1, 2, 4 Not applicable.
41. Application, implementation, environment (b)
    1 Can produce drug-diet interactions.
    2, 3, 4 Not applicable.
42. Knowledge, assessment, physiologic (a)
    1 Given intravenously to control seizures.
    2, 3, 4 Not applicable.
43. Knowledge, assessment, psychosocial (a)
    2 Antidepressant.
    1, 3, 4 Not applicable.
44. Application, analysis, environment (a)
    2 Correct procedure.
    1, 3, 4 Not applicable.
45. Knowledge, assessment, environment (a)
    3 Depresses the medulla oblongata.
    1, 2, 4 No significant effect.
46. Application, assessment, physiologic (b)
    3 Decreases physiologic manifestations.
    1 Signs of anxiety.
    2 Paradoxical reaction.
    4 Signs of anxiety.
47. Application, implementation, environment (a)
    3 Safety precautions.
    1, 2, 4 Not applicable.
48. Knowledge, assessment, physiologic (a)
    3 Action of the drug.
    1 Antitussive action.
    2 Analgesic action.
    4 Adverse reaction.
49. Knowledge, assessment, environment (a)
    2 One brand name.
    1, 3, 4 Not applicable.
50. Knowledge, assessment, physiologic (a)
    3 Used in addiction management.
    1, 2, 4 Not applicable.
51. Knowledge, assessment, environment (a)
    1 Common side effects.
    2, 3, 4 Not applicable.
52. Application, evaluation, physiologic (a)
    4 Expected outcome.
    1, 2, 3 Adverse reaction.
53. Knowledge, assessment, physiologic (a)
    1 Peaks in 2 to 4 hours.
    2, 3, 4 Not applicable.
54. Application, evaluation, physiologic (b)
    2 Effective against *Neissera gonorrhoeae*, which can cause blindness in infants. Erythromycin also protects against *Chlamydia.*
    1, 3, 4 Not applicable.
55. Application, evaluation, environment (a)
    3 Major adverse reaction.
    1, 2, 4 Not applicable.
56. Knowledge, assessment, physiologic (a)
    2 Dosage individualized according to blood coagulation tests.
    1, 3, 4 Not applicable.
57. Knowledge, evaluation, environment (a)
    3 Caused by abnormal fat deposits.
    1, 2, 4 Not applicable.
58. Knowledge, implementation, environment (a)
    2 Considered to be ulcerogenic.
    1, 3, 4 Not applicable.

59. Application, assessment, environment (b)
    1 Stimulates uterine contractions.
    2, 3, 4 Not applicable.
60. Application, implementation, environment (b)
    3 Rotating injection sites enhances absorption of the drug and prevents hardening of the tissue at the site of injection.
    1, 2, 4 Not applicable.
61. Knowledge, assessment, physiologic (a)
    3 Peaks in 10 to 16 hours.
    1, 2, 4 Not applicable
62. Knowledge, assessment, physiologic (a)
    3 Rapid onset of action.
    1, 2, 4 Not applicable.
63. Knowledge, assessment, physiologic (a)
    4 Peaks in 14 to 24 hours.
    1, 2, 3 Not applicable.
64. Application, implementation, health (a)
    1 Correct procedure.
    2, 3, 4 Not applicable.
65. Knowledge, assessment, physiologic (a)
    1 Glucose reverses too much insulin.
    2, 3, 4 Not applicable.
66. Application, assessment, health (a)
    3 Early signs of hyperinsulinism.
    1, 2, 4 Not applicable.
67. Knowledge, implementation, environment (a)
    3 To prevent possible obstruction as a result of thickening and expansion of the drug.
    1, 2, 4 Not applicable.
68. Knowledge, evaluation, physiologic (a)
    1 Therapeutic effect.
    2, 3, 4 Not applicable.
69. Knowledge, assessment, physiologic (a)
    1 Sedation is part of therapy.
    2, 3, 4 Not applicable.
70. Application, implementation, environment (b)
    1 Allows peak drug activity during daytime hours.
    2, 3, 4 Not applicable.
71. Knowledge, implementation, environment (a)
    3 Inhibits daytime and nocturnal gastric acid secretion as well as gastric acid stimulated by food.
    1, 2, 4 Not applicable.
72. Application, evaluation, physiologic (a)
    2 Therapeutic effect.
    1, 3, 4 Not applicable.
73. Knowledge, implementation, environment (a)
    3 Proper procedure.
    1, 2, 4 Not applicable.
74. Application, evaluation, physiologic (c)
    3 Small doses of these drugs can cause toxic levels.
    1, 2, 4 Not applicable.
75. Knowledge, evaluation, environment (a)
    1 Major adverse reaction.
    2, 3, 4 Not applicable.
76. Comprehension, implementation, health (b)
    2 Compliance to the drug regime is essential because of the survival nature of the causative microorganism.
    1, 3, 4 Not applicable.
77. Comprehension, assessment, environment (a)
    2 Adverse reaction.
    1, 3, 4 Not applicable.
78. Comprehension, assessment, environment (b)
    4 Elderly metabolize drugs slower because of declining body functions.
    1, 2, 3 Not applicable.
79. Application, assessment, environment (a)
    3 Mydriatic action.
    1 Antiinfective action.
    2 Miotic action.
    4 Osmotic action.

80. Knowledge, implementation, health (a)
    2 Appropriate behavior.
    1, 3, 4 Not applicable.
81. Knowledge, assessment, physiologic (a)
    3 Relieve pain perception.
    1 Produce relaxation and decrease anxiety.
    2 Produce sleep.
    4 Reduce fever.
82. Knowledge, implementation, environment (b)
    1 Correct procedure.
    2, 3, 4 Not applicable.
83. Knowledge, assessment, environment (b)
    1 Common side effects.
    2, 3, 4 Not applicable.
84. Knowledge, assessment, environment (a)
    2 Allows for optimal absorption.
    1, 3, 4 Not applicable.
85. Comprehension, implementation, health (b)
    3 Adverse reaction.
    1, 2, 4 Not applicable.
86. Knowledge, assessment, environment (a)
    1 Common side effect.
    2, 3, 4 Not applicable.
87. Knowledge, assessment, environment (b)
    4 Can increase intraocular pressure.
    1, 2, 3 Not applicable.
88. Comprehension, evaluation, environment (a)
    2 Can increase heart rate.
    1, 3, 4 Not applicable.
89. Comprehension, implementation, environment (a)
    3 Could cause patient injury.
    1, 2, 4 Not applicable.
90. Comprehension, planning, environment (b)
    1 Correct calculation.
    2, 3, 4 Incorrect calculation.
91. Comprehension, planning, physiologic (a)
    3 Drug is irritating to the GI tract; administering the drug with food decreases the irritation.
    1, 2, 4 Not applicable.
92. Knowledge, assessment, environment (a)
    1 Dilates the pupil and increases intraocular pressure.
    2, 3, 4 Not applicable.
93. Comprehension, evaluation, physiologic (c)
    3 Aminophylline is a bronchodilator and relaxes the smooth muscles of the bronchi.
    1, 2, 4 Not applicable.
94. Comprehension, assessment, environment (a)
    1 Life-threatening level.
    2, 3, 4 Not applicable.
95. Knowledge, implementation, physiologic (a)
    2 Correct procedure.
    1, 3, 4 Not applicable.
96. Application, implementation, environment (b)
    2 Essential to know that tube is in stomach and *not* in the lungs.
    1, 3, 4 Not applicable.
97. Application, evaluation, environment (b)
    4 Demerol is a CNS depressant, thereby depressing respirations.
    1, 2, 3 Not applicable.
98. Application, assessment, physiologic (b)
    1 Action of the drug.
    2, 3, 4 Not applicable.
99. Application, implementation, physiologic (b)
    2 Increases gastrointestinal muscle tone and motility.
    1, 3, 4 Not applicable.
100. Application, assessment, health (b)
    3 Identifying the location and intensity of the pain ensures the problem is not a complication; provides information maintaining quality of care.
    1, 2, 4 Not applicable.

Chapter 5: Nutrition

1. Knowledge, planning, health (a)
   1 A low-fat diet is recommended to avoid aggravating gall-bladder disease. These items are all acceptable on a low-fat diet.
   2 Ice cream would not be allowed on a low-fat diet.
   3 All these are high-fat foods.
   4 Avocado and chocolate milk are not allowed on a low-fat diet.

2. Comprehension, planning, physiologic (b)
   2 Fat-soluble vitamins are carried by fats. In a low-fat diet fat-soluble vitamins (such as these with vitamin A) may be deficient.
   1 Good sources of vitamin C, a water-soluble vitamin.
   3 Good sources of potassium, a mineral.
   4 Good sources of iron, a mineral.

3. Application, assessment, health (b)
   3 Rumbling stomach indicates return of bowel sounds, which means peristalsis has started; hence, oral feedings can resume.
   1 Hunger does not necessarily mean bowel sounds have returned.
   2 Distention could indicate lack of peristalsis.
   4 Although she may be able to tolerate food, this does not indicate return of peristalsis.

4. Comprehension, planning, physiologic (b)
   4 Contains foods liquid at room or body temperature, also many milk-based foods.
   1 Cottage cheese is on a soft diet.
   2 Pureed sweet potatoes and ground beef would be on a soft diet.
   3 Bananas and baked squash would also be on a soft diet.

5. Comprehension, planning, physiologic (b)
   4 The tomato sauce, mashed potatoes, and strawberries are all good sources of vitamin C—the vitamin especially needed for tissue healing.
   1 No good source of vitamin C. Peaches are a source of vitamin A.
   2 Although mashed potatoes supply vitamin C, there are other, better choices. Carrots are a source of vitamin A.
   3 Squash is a source of vitamin A but none is a good source of vitamin C.

6. Knowledge, implementation, health (b)
   4 Practices such as storing vitamin C foods cut up rather than whole, storing unwrapped, and overcooking in large amounts of water will significantly decrease the amount of vitamin C in a substance.
   1 Vitamin C is a water-soluble vitamin that needs to be replenished each day.
   2 Current research indicates vitamin C has a minor effect on reducing the number and severity of cold symptoms.
   3 Symptoms of vitamin A deficiency, not vitamin C.

7. Knowledge, implementation, physiologic (b)
   1 A high-fiber diet is recommended for diverticulosis because it helps prevent the development of high pressure segments and increases the volume and weight of fecal material in the colon.
   2 Bland diets are sometimes recommended following gastric surgery or in peptic ulcer disease.
   3 Low-fiber diets may be ordered in diverticulitis (inflammatory stage), ulcerative colitis, or before and after bowel surgery.
   4 Low-fat diets may be used in gallbladder disease, cardiovascular disease, or obesity.

8. Knowledge, planning, physiologic (a)
   1 All three are high in potassium.
   2 Good sources of vitamin D but not potassium.
   3 Good sources of vitamin C but not potassium.
   4 Good sources of calcium and phosphorus but not potassium.

9. Knowledge, planning, health (b)
   4 Table salt contains a great amount of sodium. Substituting other flavorings for salt can make it easier to cut down on the amount of salt used.
   1 Canned and processed meats are high in salt.
   2 Dairy products contain much salt.
   3 Fresh fruits and vegetables are low in salt and can be used freely on a sodium-restricted diet.

10. Knowledge, planning, health (a)
    2 Lactose intolerance refers to the inability to digest milk sugar (lactose) because of a deficiency of the enzyme, lactose.
    1 Contains no milk so would not interfere with digestion.
    3 Contains no lactose such as in milk products.
    4 Contains no lactose.

11. Knowledge, assessment, health (a)
    1 Many nutrients are lost in the cooking process.
    2 There is no correlation between a meal's price and its nutritive value.
    3 Grading of canned goods is related to appearance rather than nutritive value.
    4 Refined products have many of the nutrients removed, whereas those fortified have had additional nutrients added.

12. Comprehension, assessment, health (b)
    3 Meat and dairy products are the main source of protein in our diets.
    1 Green, leafy vegetables and dried fruits can be good sources of iron.
    2 Bread and cereal group can supply many B complex vitamins.
    4 Many fruit and vegetables can be good sources of vitamins A, D, C, and K.

13. Knowledge, assessment, health (a)
    4 Metabolism slows down in the older person; therefore, fewer calories are needed.
    1 Frequently less tolerance to fat and harder to digest.
    2 Vitamin and mineral intake should be maintained, and perhaps increased, to account for decreased absorption.
    3 Fluid intake should be increased to help eliminate waste products.

14. Comprehension, evaluation, physiologic (b)
    3 Cardiac arrhythmias are a serious consequence of potassium deficiency. Hypokalemia is frequently associated with diuretic therapy.
    1 Indicate a deficiency of riboflavin.
    2 Deficiency of vitamin C.
    4 Deficiency of B complex vitamins or niacin.

15. Knowledge, planning, health (b)
    1 Mineral oil is indigestible and, if taken with meals, carries fat-soluble vitamins with it as it leaves the body.
    2 Because it is indigestible, mineral oil doesn't add calories; but it can't be considered a good idea to use it routinely because of its action on fat-soluble vitamins and as a laxative.
    3 Not irritating but not a good idea.
    4 Mineral oil adds no calories because it isn't digested.

16. Comprehension, implementation, physiologic (a)
    4 Foods included in a bland diet are mild flavored and nonirritating. They reduce peristalsis and excessive flow of gastric juices.
    1 Roast beef, tomatoes, and coffee are not allowed on a bland diet; they are too irritating to the digestive tract.
    2 Fried foods and carbonated beverages are not allowed on a bland diet.
    3 Iced beverages and raw vegetables are not allowed on a bland diet.

17. Knowledge, planning, health (c)
    2 Honey contains botulism spores, which could be a problem for very young babies (older children and adults are not affected by the spores).
    1 Current advice from the American Academy of Pediatrics suggests not beginning solid food until 3 months of age.
    3 It is better not to get the baby used to the taste of additives, such as sugar and salt, that have no significant nutritional value.
    4 Most allergies to eggs are caused by the white, not the yolk.

18. Knowledge, planning, health (b)
    4 Of the choices provided, rice cereal causes the fewest allergic reactions in children.
    1 Eggs, especially the egg white, causes many cases of food allergies.
    2 Cow's milk is known to cause allergic reactions in certain children.
    3 Wheat, oats, and barley cereals cause more allergic reactions than does rice cereal.

19. Knowledge, planning, health (a)
    1 Eating high-carbohydrate foods such as dry toast or crackers on awakening is a common suggestion for alleviating morning sickness.
    2 Fluids should be ingested between meals.
    3 High-fat foods are a common cause of nausea and should be avoided.
    4 High-carbohydrate foods may help alleviate the nausea.

20. Knowledge, planning, physiologic (a)
    4 Dried fruits are excellent alternative sources of iron.
    1 Good sources of vitamin A, not iron.
    2 Milk and other dairy products contain very little iron.
    3 Refined cereals have had much of the valuable nutrients removed.

21. Comprehension, planning, physiologic (b)
    3 Iron absorption is enhanced when given with vitamin C. Citrus juices are excellent sources of vitamin C.
    1 Milk and dairy products contain no vitamin C.
    2 Fish liver oils contain vitamins A and D, not C.
    4 Green, leafy vegetables contain vitamins A, E, and K, not C.

22. Knowledge, assessment, health (a)
    2 The exchange system is based on the fact that each food within an exchange is equivalent in nutrients to every other one. Therefore substituting one food for another within an exchange does not significantly alter the diet.
    1 One advantage of using the exchange system is that specialized foods are not needed.
    3 Food exchanges are important to space nutrient ingestion over the entire day so the body is able to metabolize each.
    4 The recommended number of exchanges is usually set up by a dietitian, but substitution is easily done by the diabetic patient.

23. Application, planning, physiologic (a)
    2 All fruits and fruit juices are on the fruit exchange and so can be substituted for blackberries.
    1 Milk is on the milk exchange.
    3 Cheese is on the meat exchange (protein foods).
    4 Pecans are on the fat exchange.

24. Application, implementation, physiologic (b)
    4 An egg, because it is protein, is on the meat exchange, the biscuit on the bread exchange, and the 2 teaspoons of butter are two fat exchanges.
    1 No milk, one bread, and two fat exchanges.
    2 No milk or fruit exchange and two fats.
    3 No vegetable exchange and two fats (1 teaspoon = one exchange).

25. Comprehension, evaluation, health (a)
    2 Oranges and orange juice are readily digestible and absorbed carbohydrate.
    1 Crackers are a starchy carbohydrate and take longer to be digested and absorbed.
    3 Bread and butter (starch and fat) both take longer to be absorbed.
    4 Cereal is also a starch and takes longer to be absorbed.

26. Application, planning, physiologic (b)
    1 Low protein provided by this diet limits end products of protein metabolism—an important consideration in kidney disease.
    2 Steak and milk provide more protein than is desirable for this patient.
    3 Hamburger and milk provide protein not desirable in this case.
    4 Liver, cottage cheese, eggs, and cream provide a high-protein diet.

27. Knowledge, planning, physiologic (a)
    3 Clear liquids, nonresidue, nonirritating, and non–gas forming.
    1 Cream-based soups are considered full liquids.
    2 Sherbet is a full liquid.
    4 Orange juice is a full liquid.

28. Knowledge, planning, physiologic (a)
    1 A diet low in residue to avoid irritating the colon, but high in vitamins and proteins to replace nutrients that are frequently lost in ulcerative colitis and provide for tissue repair.
    2 High residue may further irritate the already irritated colon.
    3 Patients with colitis frequently need increased amounts of calories.
    4 No reason for low-sodium or low-carbohydrate diet.

29. Knowledge, implementation, physiologic (b)
    4 Soft diets are easier to digest, thereby reducing the workload of the heart.
    1 Unless the patient is overweight, no specific reason to reduce calories.
    2 Not the primary reason for the soft diet in this situation.
    3 Decreasing irritation to the digestive tract would be a consideration in certain gastrointestinal disorders, not cardiovascular.

30. Application, planning, physiologic (b)
    2 A high-fiber diet provides the bulk that stimulates peristalsis, thereby decreasing constipation.
    1 Very little residue provided by this diet.
    3 All foods on this diet provide very little residue.
    4 Again, very little residue the way these foods are prepared.

31. Knowledge, assessment, health (b)
    4 Fats, especially saturated fats, are prime contributors to high blood cholesterol levels and atherosclerotic heart disease.
    1 Total calories only need to be reduced if the individual is overweight.
    2 Carbohydrates should constitute approximately 50% to 60% of total caloric intake.
    3 Polyunsaturated fats should replace saturated fats in dietary considerations.

32. Knowledge, assessment, health (a)
    2 Milk and milk products are excellent sources of calcium and protein.
    1 Milk and milk products are poor sources of vitamin C.
    3 Milk is a poor source of iron.
    4 Milk is a poor source of B complex vitamins.

33. Knowledge, assessment, health (b)
    1 Currently, medical experts think that the severe restrictions of the past are not warranted and that a diet of omitting only what irritates is healthier.
    2 Milk increases the secretion of gastric acid more than it buffers it.
    3 Caffeine, chocolate, and alcohol are strong stimulants of gastric acid.
    4 Use of the bland diet has decreased because there is no evidence that such a restrictive diet helps the healing process.
34. Knowledge, planning, health (a)
    4 Including high-fiber foods in menu planning lowers blood glucose and blood cholesterol levels.
    1 The best carbohydrates are unrefined, high-fiber, complex carbohydrates.
    2 Although it should be taken with food and in limited amounts, a moderate amount of alcohol (1 to 2 oz once or twice a week) can be consumed.
    3 The exchange list system of menu planning allows a wide variety of food choices.
35. Knowledge, planning, health (a)
    2 The two primary sources of cholesterol are the diet and that which is synthesized by the body. Diet is the primary controllable factor.
    1 The recommendation is that blood cholesterol levels be maintained at below 200 mg/dl.
    3 LDL is considered to be "bad cholesterol" and should be lowered in relation to HDL.
    4 Dietary treatment is the primary treatment for high blood cholesterol. Medications are added only if dietary measures fail to bring cholesterol levels down to targeted levels.
36. Knowledge, assessment, environment (c)
    2 The pyramidal shape graphically places those foods to be eaten the most (breads, cereals, and pasta) at the broad base, followed upward by lesser foods to the tip, which illustrates that fats, oils, and sweets are to be eaten sparingly.
    1 Breads, cereals, and pasta are at the base then followed by fruits and vegetables.
    3 Only 2 to 3 servings of meats, poultry, fish and eggs are needed as compared with 6 to 11 servings of cereal and pasta.
    4 Fats, oils, and sweets are at the top of the pyramid, indicating they are to be eaten sparingly.

Chapter 6: Medical-Surgical Nursing

1. Knowledge, assessment, physiologic (a)
   4 Disorder tends to progress, and involvement of other systems is common with advancement of the disorder.
   1 This is more characteristic of osteoarthritis.
   2 Rheumatoid arthritis that appears in early childhood may run its course and dissipate in later years, but this is not true in the majority of cases.
   3 RH is a disease of joints as well as supportive structures.
2. Knowledge, assessment, environment (a)
   3 Salicylates reduce the inflammatory process.
   1, 2 Not a first-line drug of choice.
   4 Not classically used in management of RH.

3. Comprehension, implementation, health (a)
   2 Reduces gastric irritation.
   1 Does cause an appreciable change in mentation or awareness.
   3 CNS effects are not commonly associated with this group of drugs.
   4 Gastric irritation will occur on an empty stomach and may lead to nausea, vomiting.
4. Knowledge, assessment, physiologic (b)
   4 This is important—skin color, warmth, sensation, and pulses should be checked frequently.
   1 Diet should be high in protein and vitamins to promote healing.
   2 Fluid intake should be increased to 2000 to 3000 ml/day to prevent such complications as constipation, renal calculi, and urinary tract infections.
   3 Isometric and ROM exercises are encouraged.
5. Knowledge, assessment, physiologic (b)
   3 Frequently the first signs.
   1 There is no pain.
   2 Respirations increase and are rapid and shallow.
   4 Kussmaul's respirations are not associated with COPD; see rationale for statement 2.
6. Application, planning, physiologic (a)
   1 Increased oral or parenteral fluids will yield more watery pulmonary secretions, which are easier to remove through coughing or suctioning.
   2, 3, 4 See rationale for statement 1.
7. Knowledge, implementation, environment (b)
   1 The respiratory center in the brain responds to increased oxygen; respirations may decrease or stop if too much oxygen is given.
   2, 3, 4 See rationale for statement 1.
8. Knowledge, assessment, physiologic (c)
   3 The alveoli rupture, and the capillary beds are destroyed. Gas exchange is not possible.
   1 This would be a secondary infection.
   2, 4 Related to asthma, which may lead to COPD.
9. Knowledge, planning, environment (a)
   2 Caused by the organisms *Mycobacterium tuberculosis, M. bovis,* or *M. avium.*
   1 Idiopathic is defined as occurring without known cause.
   3 Genetic is defined as inherited.
   4 Congenital is defined as present at birth.
10. Application, planning, health (b)
    1 Medication must be continued and not stopped until ordered by physician, usually 2 years.
    2 Some changes might be needed because fatigue must be avoided.
    3 Not indicated; copious secretions that are difficult to cough up are not characteristic of TB.
    4 Not necessary when medication therapy is in progress.
11. Knowledge, assessment, health (b)
    1 A positive test results in all people who at any time have been infected or have had contact with the tubercle bacillus; does not reveal if active disease is present.
    2, 3, 4 See rationale for statement 1.
12. Comprehension, evaluation, physiologic (a)
    2 This position facilitates breathing since patient is in a sitting position.
    1, 4 Patient is lying flat on back so has greater difficulty with breathing.
    3 Here also patient is lying flat; only this time on either left or right side, which in no way facilitates breathing.
13. Comprehension, assessment, physiologic (b)
    2 Classic symptoms.
    1 Symptoms of neurocirculatory impairment.
    3 May indicate embolism.
    4 Symptoms of neurologic impairment.

14. Application, implementation, physiologic (b)
    3 When pain is severe, evaluate the neurologic and circulatory status first; initial presentation of complications may be that of severe pain.
    1 Evaluate the patient's status first; then give ordered medication; be suspicious of pain unrelieved by medication.
    2 Provide supportive care.
    4 Elevation reduces edema; leg rotation is not usually a standard measure.

15. Comprehension, assessment, physiologic (b)
    4 Fever indicates infection; a "hot spot" indicates an inflammatory process beneath a cast.
    1 Indicates a neurologic problem such as a tight cast.
    2 A normal finding.
    3 Indicates a neurologic problem, possibly caused by the swelling.

16. Comprehension, implementation, physiologic (b)
    1 The air is in the pleural space that surrounds the lungs.
    2 Although a correct statement, a nasal tube would not help the problem; see rationale for statement 1.
    3 Never a correct response; avoids the patient's concerns.
    4 This is the treatment of choice; pneumothorax with lung collapse is always an emergency.

17. Application, implementation, environment (b)
    3 This strips clots from the lumen of the tube and promotes drainage.
    1 The nurse changes the dressing only when there is a specific physician's order.
    2 Should ambulate, turn, and exercise unless contraindicated.
    4 Water-sealed bottles never lifted above patient's chest.

18. Application, planning, environment (c)
    4 A clamp must be available and visible; if there is a break in the system, the chest tube should be clamped immediately as close to the chest wall as possible.
    1, 2, 3 Any break in the system is a hazard; air can enter and be drawn into the pleural space.

19. Comprehension, implementation, environment (b)
    3 To avoid backflow of drainage into the pleural space.
    1 Chest tubes are never clamped until prepared for removal.
    2, 4 Activity should not cause pain or difficulty breathing.

20. Comprehension, planning, environment (c)
    2 Prevents reentry of air that might recollapse lung.
    1, 3, 4 Not possible; not recommended; see rationale for statement 2.

21. Comprehension, evaluation, physiologic (b)
    1 Sharp chest pain would be an indication that the lungs had recollapsed or that there was air in the pleural space.
    2 Assists in lung expansion; should be encouraged.
    3, 4 It is essential to have moderate exercise.

22. Knowledge, assessment, physiologic (b)
    3 Priority assessment postoperatively; check for increasing drainage.
    1 Not a complication, but can occur during the postoperative period because of the change in body image.
    2 A complication in any major surgery; most patients undergoing amputation are mobilized early on.
    4 Not necessarily classified as a complication; patient may still sense the presence of the amputated limb.

23. Comprehension, planning, physiologic (a)
    1 A goal of therapy to restore oxygen to a damaged myocardium.
    2 A goal of overall management.
    3 High anxiety levels may increase oxygen demand.
    4 Oxygen does not prevent shock.

24. Comprehension, assessment, physiologic (a)
    3 Classic symptoms of cardiogenic shock.
    1, 2, 4 Not classic symptoms of this type of shock.

25. Analysis, assessment, physiologic (c)
    4 As the heart fails, circulating blood backs up into the pulmonary tree; a sign of congestion is rales (crackles) in lung bases.
    1, 2, 3 Not associated with manifestation of pulmonary congestion related to heart failure.

26. Comprehension, planning, physiologic (b)
    4 Reduces risk of constipation and straining, which may put a strain on damaged myocardium.
    1 Not a standard of care in MI.
    2 Prolonged bed rest is no longer advocated.
    3 Not a standard of care in MI.

27. Analysis, assessment, physiologic (b)
    1 Common manifestation of heart failure.
    2, 3, 4 Not associated with heart failure.

28. Knowledge, assessment, physiologic (a)
    4 Classic symptoms of thrombophlebitis.
    1 More of a neurologic manifestation.
    2, 3 Symptoms are arterial in nature.

29. Knowledge, assessment, physiologic (a)
    2 Commonly affected by hypertension.
    1 Not associated with complications related to hypertension.
    3 See rationale for statement 1.
    4 Brain may be affected, but the blood and bladder are not associated with hypertensive complications.

30. Knowledge, assessment, physiologic (a)
    4 Common manifestations.
    1 Increased urination is not commonly associated with hypertension.
    2 Nausea and vomiting are not common manifestations.
    3 Not common manifestations.

31. Knowledge, planning, physiologic (a)
    4 Diuretic.
    1 Supresses gastric acid secretion.
    2 Antiinflammatory.
    3 Cardiotonic.

32. Comprehension, implementation, health (a)
    3 Many diuretics cause excretion of both sodium and potassium; it is important to maintain adequate potassium levels for proper heart function.
    1 Not an aspect of teaching in diuretic therapy.
    2, 4 See rationale for statement 1.

33. Knowledge, assessment, physiologic (a)
    3 Classic symptoms of hyperthyroidism.
    1 Typical of hypothyroidism.
    2 Not a classic symptom of thyroid dysfunction.
    4 Typical of hypothyroidism.

34. Comprehension, implementation, physiologic (b)
    1 Keeps the eyes (cornea) from drying out.
    2 Dilate eyes; do not lubricate.
    3 Do not lubricate eyes.
    4 Increases risk of corneal abrasion and eye problems.

35. Application, planning, physiologic (b)
    2 Diet should supply calories, protein, and carbohydrates caused by the increased metabolic demands imposed by the disease.
    1 Calories are insufficient; restriction of purine is not necessary.
    3 Will not meet the metabolic demands of the body.
    4 Sodium restrictions are not usually indicated.

36. Comprehension, planning, psychosocial (a)
    1 Calm environment is of importance; these patients are usually in a hyperexcitable state.
    2 Visitors may need to be limited to avoid overtaxing the patient's energies.
    3 Private room ensures better control over the environment.
    4 Provide a supportive environment; do not overtax the patient.

37. Comprehension, assessment, physiologic (b)
    3 Classic symptoms of carpopedal spasm and facial twitch.
    1, 2, 4 Not classic symptoms of tetany.
38. Comprehension, assessment, physiologic (a)
    1 Increasing hoarseness will occur.
    2 Does not occur with laryngeal nerve damage.
    3 Indicates tetany.
    4 May indicate hemorrhage.
39. Comprehension, assessment, physiologic (b)
    2 Increased hydrostatic pressure in the portal system causes fluid to collect in the peritoneal space.
    1 Decreased albumin level is associated with ascites.
    3 Ammonia levels may be elevated but do not cause cirrhosis.
    4 Does not cause ascites.
40. Knowledge, assessment, physiologic (a)
    3 Damaged parenchymal cells are unable to metabolize bilirubin, which gives the stool its normal color; bilirubin in the circulation causes jaundice, pruritus, and dark urine.
    1 Stools are clay colored because of the liver's inability to metabolize bilirubin.
    2 Urine is dark in liver dysfunction.
    4 Stools are clay colored, and urine is dark.
41. Knowledge, implementation, physiologic (a)
    2 Usually 1000 to 1500 ml is removed or enough to relieve symptoms; larger amounts place the patient at risk of developing hypovolemic shock; color is an indicator of infection and bleeding.
    1 High-Fowler's is the preferred position.
    3 The abdomen is always prepared aseptically.
    4 A sterile pressure dressing is applied to prevent leakage.
42. Comprehension, implementation, physiologic (a)
    2 The tube is a triple-lumen tube with an esophageal balloon to control bleeding of varices; one lumen is for lavage, and one is for suction.
    1 Iced saline solution is used.
    3 Vasodilators do not control bleeding.
    4 Platelets need not be replaced; refrigerated blood lacks prothrombin and coagulation factors needed for clotting.
43. Comprehension, implementation, physiologic (a)
    2 Conversion of protein produces ammonia; ammonia affects the brain tissue.
    1 Carbohydrates are tolerated by a diseased liver.
    3 Cation-exchange enemas remove toxic wastes.
    4 Will not decrease ammonia levels.
44. Application, implementation, environment (a)
    1 The sense of hearing is frequently present when the patient is unresponsive.
    2 See rationale for statement 1.
    3 Rest periods must be provided.
    4 A restful, quiet environment is therapeutic.
45. Application, assessment, environment (a)
    3 Hypostatic pneumonia is a complication of immobility.
    1 Unresponsive patients are NPO.
    2 This specimen is not indicated.
    4 Chest pain would be a sign of pulmonary disease, not difficulty removing secretions.
46. Application, planning, environment (a)
    4 Position of choice; sputum or vomitus cannot be swallowed by patient in coma.
    1 Head should be elevated, patient on side.
    2 Patient should be turned side to side.
    3 Pillow may help block airway—should support head and shoulders.
47. Comprehension, implementation, physiologic (a)
    2 An independent nursing action to be done qid for joint mobility.
    1, 3, 4 All are necessary in care; statement 2 takes precedence, as it is solely a nursing responsibility.

48. Application, implementation, health (b)
    2 Corneal ulceration is the result of neglect of eye care when the patient is unconscious or has corneal anesthesia.
    1 An infection.
    3 Drooping of eyelid from paralysis; nursing care cannot prevent this.
    4 Lack of tearing is a problem nursing care should be concerned with; the nurse cannot prevent this.
49. Comprehension, planning, health (a)
    4 These frequent complications of immobility must be included in the nursing care plan.
    1 Convulsions should be anticipated; the nurse cannot prevent them.
    2 Anxiety for a patient in coma cannot be assessed, nor can intervention be evaluated.
    3 These are problems needing intervention; they cannot be prevented by nursing care.
50. Comprehension, evaluation, psychosocial (a)
    4 Patients who are unable to speak and form words can frequently write their thoughts.
    1, 3 Is not complete communication, although it may be used.
    2 Speech therapy may take time to produce obvious results.
51. Knowledge, assessment, environment (b)
    1 The sounds of speech do not correspond to sounds the person has known.
    2 While this may be a possibility, it will be caused by additional problems.
    3 May or may not have difficulty communicating.
    4 There are always verbal and nonverbal communication skills to be used with a patient.
52. Knowledge, assessment, physiologic (a)
    3 Allows maximal access to all areas to be auscultated: front, back, and sides.
    1, 2, 4 All of these allow minimal access, minimal chest expansion.
53. Knowledge, assessment, physiologic (a)
    1 Allows better resonance—easier to hear and identify adventitious sounds.
    2, 3, 4 Incorrect procedure; these methods do not allow for maximal sound transmission.
54. Knowledge, assessment, physiologic (b)
    2 Early morning specimen is best; this procedure usually gets results.
    1, 3 Incorrect procedure; best specimen obtained in early AM.
    4 Only as a last resort, if patient is unable to expectorate sputum on his own.
55. Knowledge, implementation, physiologic (a)
    1 Correct procedure, facilitates expectoration of blood.
    2, 4 Incorrect, this will promote swallowing of blood.
    3 Incorrect, will not promote proper drainage nor allow proper nursing care to be given.
56. Knowledge, planning, physiologic (a)
    4 Suction tracheostomy to facilitate breathing.
    1, 2, 3 All important, but not more important than 4.
57. Application, implementation, psychosocial (b)
    4 Best intervention to solve problem; very effective for patient to interact with someone who has faced and conquered problem.
    1 Shows lack of understanding.
    2 Part of implementation; however, nurse does not need to take total control away from patient.
    3 Passing the buck, ignoring the problem.

58. Comprehension, implementation, physiologic (c)
   1 Pneumonia infection interferes with O_2-CO_2 exchange in alveoli, resulting in reduced O_2 in blood.
   2 Indirectly, but not the best answer.
   3 Oxygen does not kill bacteria.
   4 Oxygen has no effect on adventitious lung sounds.
59. Comprehension, implementation, psychosocial (c)
   4 Teaching is needed so patient understands her symptoms; progressive activity is important.
   1 Ignores patient's problem.
   2 This statement usually is said to relieve nurse's anxiety when she doesn't know what to say.
   3 This statement shows the nurse does not understand pathology nor treatment plan.
60. Comprehension, evaluation, health (c)
   1 Shows patient knows to never smoke again.
   2 Theophylline preparations may cause these symptoms; do not discontinue but notify physician.
   3 Dependence on bronchodilators, especially beta agonists, may have adverse effects on disease.
   4 Patient thinks he is now an invalid; inappropriate plan of care.
61. Knowledge, assessment, physiologic (a)
   2 Cardinal symptoms.
   1 Hypertension is not a common symptom; some patients with high ketone levels have reported headaches.
   3, 4 Not cardinal symptoms.
62. Comprehension, implementation, physiologic (a)
   1 Most fast-acting insulins peak in 2 to 4 hours following administration.
   2, 3, 4 Not standard peak times for fast-acting insulins.
63. Comprehension, implementation, physiologic (b)
   1 Should raise blood glucose level.
   2 Diet drinks will not help in raising the blood glucose level.
   3 May raise glucose to a higher level than required.
   4 Insufficient amount to raise glucose level; will take several sugar cubes.
64. Application, implementation, physiologic (c)
   4 Commercial glucose concentrates can be absorbed between the buccal mucosa and gum; when patient fully awakens, give a fast-acting carbohydrate by mouth.
   1 Insulin lowers glucose levels; patient's blood glucose level needs to be elevated in hypoglycemia.
   2, 3 These actions will place patient at risk of aspiration; should not attempt getting patient to swallow unless she is fully conscious.
65. Application, implementation, physiologic (b)
   3 Fluids are important in resolving a urinary tract infection.
   1 Inappropriate, unrelated to problem.
   2 Physician's order, not nursing intervention.
   4 Physician's order, inappropriate.
66. Comprehension, assessment, environment (a)
   4 This is the purpose of culture and sensitivity; contamination would make diagnosis invalid; uncontaminated cultures must be grown in laboratory and then treated with antibiotics.
   1 Obscure.
   2 True, but not the primary question.
   3 Too vague, means nothing.
67. Application, implementation, physiologic (a)
   1 Most appropriate intervention for acute pain.
   2 Secondary, true, but will not relieve his current pain.
   3 Not applicable to pain.
   4 May be inappropriate.
68. Application, assessment, physiologic (b)
   2 Classic symptom; usually less than 30 ml/hr.
   1, 3, 4 May be present, but on their own do not indicate renal failure.

69. Application, implementation, physiologic (a)
   4 Monitoring drainage frequently helps to ensure continuous flow and allows for assessing normalcy of drainage.
   1 Inappropriate action; drainage is normal.
   2 Not necessary unless ordered and flow is restricted.
   3 Totally wrong; drainage needs a clear path to leave the body; clamping catheter is contraindicated.
70. Comprehension, evaluation, physiologic (b)
   1 Recovery and discharge depend on these improvements.
   2, 3, 4 Less important, not immediately essential to discharge.
71. Comprehension, assessment, environment (a)
   2 This pain is characteristic of ruptured disk.
   1 Walking is usually painful.
   3 A problem with some spinal cord injuries; does not occur with injuries in the lumbar region or with a ruptured disk.
   4 There is pain and difficulty using bedpan; incontinence is not a problem.
72. Comprehension, implementation, physiologic (b)
   1 Causes relaxation and decompression of tissues of the lumbar region.
   2, 3 Bed rest is usually ordered; movement increases pain.
   4 Pillow under popliteal space is always contraindicated.
73. Application, implementation, environment (b)
   4 Patient remains flat, frequently in body cast; recovery time is long to allow for bone graft union to take place.
   1, 2, 3 Contraindicated; see rationale for statement 1.
74. Knowledge, assessment, environment (b)
   3 Characteristic problems.
   1 Problems with detached retina.
   2 Problems with infection.
   4 Problems with cataract.
75. Application, planning, physiologic (b)
   2 Essential to prevent progression of this chronic disease.
   1 Not visually impaired if treatment is maintained.
   3 This is diagnostic; patient has glaucoma and will need more frequent medical supervision.
   4 See rationale for statement 1.
76. Comprehension, assessment, physiologic (c)
   3 Varies with each patient and at different times for the same patient because of the remissions and exacerbations.
   1, 2 Unrelated to disease.
   4 Problem for patient is ataxia, loss of muscle tone, tremor, and spastic weakness, not paralysis.
77. Comprehension, assessment, physiologic (a)
   2 The disease is progressive; however, there are periods of remission, and every effort should be made to keep the patient from becoming dependent.
   1 Patient will become dependent.
   3 This is not an infectious disease.
   4 A high-calorie, high-protein diet is indicated.
78. Knowledge, assessment, environment (b)
   1 Frequent problem.
   2 Elimination problems are retention and incontinence.
   3 Unrelated to multiple sclerosis. These are signs and symptoms of ear problems. Patients with multiple sclerosis frequently have visual problems.
   4 The patient may have emotional problems; mental ability is not altered.
79. Knowledge, assessment, physiologic (a)
   4 Characteristic of this disease.
   1, 2, 3 There is no medication effective in controlling or curing multiple sclerosis.

80. Application, assessment, physiologic (a)
    2 Establishing a routine for elimination is essential for bowel training.
    1 Fluids should be encouraged to prevent constipation.
    3 A high-roughage diet is essential for proper bowel elimination.
    4 Elimination should be as natural as possible for patient to maintain independence.

81. Knowledge, assessment, psychosocial (c)
    1 Usually observed in patients with multiple sclerosis.
    2, 3, 4 Not related to multiple sclerosis.

82. Application, implementation, health (b)
    4 This attitude is obsolete.
    1, 2, 3 All true.

83. Application, evaluation, health (b)
    4 Shows learning of principles.
    1, 2, 3 Show no learning.

84. Application, implementation, health (b)
    3 Family history is important for heightened awareness.
    1, 2, 4 All true.

85. Knowledge, assessment, physiologic (a)
    4 Correct definition of words describing lesions.
    1, 2, 3 Incorrect definitions of macula (red) papular (raised) vesicles (fluid-filled sac).

86. Application, planning, environment (a)
    3 Promotes independence.
    1 Not applicable to independence.
    2 Inappropriate to promote independence.
    4 Reading too much into question; not applicable to independence.

87. Knowledge, implementation, physiologic (c)
    2 Correct, usually administered in eyedrop form.
    1 Contraindicated, dilates the pupil.
    3 Not administered in eyedrop form.
    4 Not an indicated drug in glaucoma.

88. Knowledge, assessment, physiologic (c)
    1 Correct procedure. Pupil size is observed *before* shining light on them.
    2 As soon as light shines on the eye, pupil constricts. Nurse must measure and report pupil size *before* constriction.
    3 Inappropriate. Pupils may have constricted and started to dilate again. Reading now gives incorrect assessment.
    4 Rapidly passing flashlight over eyes will cause pupil constriction, as stated in rationale 2. Incorrect assessment technique.

89. Application, implementation, environment (b)
    4 Appropriate for this patient.
    1 Usually not necessary with mild impairment.
    2 Usually not necessary to speak loudly with mild impairment.
    3 Never touch first before getting patient's attention.

90. Application, implementation, health (a)
    1 Discarding the urine at 9 AM and collecting all urine produced between that time and the last voided specimen at exactly 9 AM the next day will avoid including any urine produced before or after the 24-hour testing period.
    2, 3, 4 All have chance of error.

91. Comprehension, implementation, physiologic (b)
    2 In peritoneal dialysis, the dialysis takes place across the peritoneal membrane. Blood does not leave the body.
    1 Peritoneal dialysis takes longer.
    3 Fluids and solids removed are controlled in each procedure.
    4 Results of each method are observed immediately.

92. Comprehension, assessment, physiologic (a)
    2 Peritonitis is the most common complication. Cloudy dialysate drainage would be an indication of this infection.
    1 A complication that may be related to a new catheter or from the small amounts of heparin added to the inflow solution to prevent the catheter from becoming clogged. Not related to infection.
    3 Blood pressure must be monitored every 15 minutes because there may be excessive fluid loss. Changes in vital signs may indicate impending shock over hydration. Not related to infection.
    4 Kidneys are not producing urine; the bladder should remain empty.

93. Application, implementation, environment (a)
    2 Avoids the sharp edge of a razor blade, which might cut the patient and cause bleeding.
    1 Would be irritating and could cause bleeding. A soft bristle toothbrush is indicated.
    3 Nausea and vomiting are frequent problems with end-stage renal disease. Antiemetics should be given as indicated to prevent possible gastric bleeding.
    4 Aspirin is contraindicated for patients with a bleeding tendency. This order should be questioned and discussed with the physician.

94. Application, implementation, environment (a)
    4 Documented as the best method of preventing the transmission of organisms.
    1 Not indicated, antibiotics not given routinely.
    2 Not indicated.
    3 Cannot prevent invasion of microbes.

95. Comprehension, implementation, physiologic (a)
    1 The signs and symptoms of the disease progress as the pressure increases.
    2 Contraindicated.
    3 Conservative medical management for a detached retina.
    4 Unrelated to infection.

96. Knowledge, assessment, physiologic (b)
    1 There is a gradual loss of peripheral vision in untreated glaucoma.
    2 A symptom of detached retina.
    3 Seen in conjunctivitis.
    4 Usually related to a vitamin A deficiency.

97. Knowledge, assessment, environment (c)
    1 Correct.
    2 Found in cataracts.
    3 Found in detached retina.
    4 Found in head injury.

98. Knowledge, assessment, physiologic (b)
    1 Seen in untreated glaucoma.
    2 Unrelated to glaucoma.
    3 Peripheral vision is lost.
    4 No alteration in color perception.

99. Comprehension, assessment, physiologic (b)
    2 Correct.
    1, 4 Not appropriate.
    3 Contraindicated.

100. Comprehension, assessment, health (b)
    4 A medication must never be omitted. A medical identification tag would instruct anyone giving assistance in case of emergency involving a patient unable to communicate.
    1 Appropriate for a diabetic patient.
    2, 3 Glasses not indicated.

101. Knowledge, planning, physiologic (c)
    3 Correct.
    1, 2 Miotic drugs will cause the pupil to contract and the iris to draw away from the cornea and allow the aqueous humor to drain.
    4 Oral glycerin acts to reduce osmotic pressure.

102. Comprehension, planning, environment (a)
    3 Current use of assistive devices is important in planning care and for safety considerations.
    1 Excessive use of alcohol is a consideration in any patient; tobacco use does not play a role in priority planning in this case.
    2 Significant for planning of diversional activity if hospitalization is prolonged.
    4 May be significant if patient is not eating properly.

103. Knowledge, assessment, physiologic (b)
    1 Classic finding.
    2, 3, 4 More common in rheumatoid arthritis.

104. Comprehension, implementation, environment (a)
    4 Obesity increases strain on weight-bearing joints; reduction of weight minimizes some of the presenting symptoms.
    1 Does not reduce joint strain, but maintains existing range of motion.
    2 Does not control strain in joints.
    3 Provides comfort in strained joints.

105. Comprehension, implementation, physiologic (a)
    4 For severe disease, accompanied by pain and loss of ROM; reconstruction of one or both articulating joint surfaces may be needed.
    1 Stabilizes joint by restricting ROM.
    2 Not performed on joints.
    3 Diagnostic aid used to visualize the inside of a joint.

106. Application, assessment, physiologic (b)
    2 Changes in the neurologic or circulatory status of the involved extremity indicate a complication.
    1 Is not associated with serious sequelae.
    3, 4 Not a postoperative complication.

107. Comprehension, assessment, environment (b)
    4 Nurse must be alert for these symptoms of TIA.
    1, 2, 3 Symptoms not specific to TIAs.

108. Knowledge, implementation, physiologic (a)
    1 No special preparation required for CT scan without contrast medium.
    2 Unrelated to diagnostic test.
    3 Unnecessary.
    4 For CT scan with contrast medium only.

109. Knowledge, implementation, physiologic (a)
    2 Allows for maximal fluid absorption back into venous system while not promoting fluid stasis in head.
    1 Uncomfortable for the patient.
    3, 4 Might promote stasis or increase of fluid in head (increased intracranial pressure).

110. Comprehension, implementation, health (b)
    1 Usually indicated in treatment of TIAs—best answer.
    2 Unrelated to TIAs.
    3 Muscle relaxants unrelated to TIA treatment; antihypertensives may be indicated if hypertension exists.
    4 Unrelated to TIA treatment.

111. Knowledge, assessment, physiologic (a)
    1 Phenomenon that warns the patient of an impending seizure; may be visual, olfactory, or some other sensory experience.
    2 Tonic muscle spasm, which is associated with low calcium levels.
    3 Motor disturbance seen in liver disease.
    4 Refers to the absence of sweating.

112. Application, implementation, environment (a)
    1 Restraining may actually result in injuries to bones or soft tissue.
    2, 3, 4 All are appropriate in various situations involving seizures.

113. Knowledge, planning, environment (a)
    2 Anticonvulsant; raises the seizure threshold.
    1 Thyroid replacement hormone.
    3 Osmotic diuretic.
    4 Corticosteroid.

114. Comprehension, implementation, health (a)
    2 Usually the medication is lifelong. Patients have the misconception that they can get by without taking their medication or that they have outgrown their seizures.
    1, 3 Treatment is usually long term.
    4 Has little bearing on the medication regimen.

115. Comprehension, planning, health (b)
    3 Common side effect in long-term therapy.
    1, 2, 4 Are not characteristic side effects.

116. Comprehension, assessment, physiologic (b)
    4 Nocturia: waking during the night to void; hesitancy: waiting before being able to have a forceful stream; urgency: a strong desire to void.
    1, 2, 3 These terms to not describe the patient problems as discussed.

117. Comprehension, planning, environment (c)
    2 With increased toxicity the patient becomes confused.
    1 Nursing care measures will not prevent edema caused by decreased renal function.
    3 Fluids may be restricted.
    4 Not related to increased BUN level.

118. Comprehension, assessment, physiologic (a)
    1 Allergic reactions can occur after the administration of the contrast medium; prompt recognition and treatment may be lifesaving.
    2, 3, 4 Not related to IVP.

119. Application, implementation, physiologic (a)
    3 Fluids are forced to 3000 ml a day unless contraindicated.
    1 See rationale for statement 3.
    2 Assessment will not meet patient's needs.
    4 Oral intake should meet desired amount.

120. Application, implementation, physiologic (c)
    4 Slow decompression is used to reduce the degree of postobstructive hematuria; hemorrhage is a potential complication.
    1 Catheters are irrigated only when indicated.
    2 This would not be an indwelling catheter.
    3 Only when there is a medical order.

Chapter 7: Mental Health Nursing

1. Comprehension, assessment, psychosocial (b)
    3 Uses repression in part to rid self of unacceptable feelings, while conscious effort is made to express opposite type of feelings.
    1 A blocking of painful or unacceptable feelings.
    2 Giving of or assigning of unacceptable feelings to someone else.
    4 Explaining away, via logical construction, of unacceptable thoughts, feelings, or acts.

2. Comprehension, assessment, psychosocial (b)
    3 Apprehension level; anxiety is related to a concrete future event.
    1 Panic includes loss of control.
    2 Free-floating has no specific object or event.
    4 Alertness level is less severe, only vague symptoms.

3. Comprehension, planning, psychosocial (b)
   1 Correct because nurse diagnose and treat human responses to illness, behaviors, or problems related to their probable causes.
   2 Nurses diagnose responses and not disease entities.
   3 The medical diagnosis may or may not be related to the nursing diagnosis.
   4 Nursing diagnosis is useful in many diverse settings.
4. Comprehension, assessment, environment (b)
   4 Most authorities agree that as depression lifts the patient is at greatest risk of committing suicide.
   1 The attention of the patient being admitted is diverted and focused on the admission, and he or she is not likely to commit suicide during the admission process.
   2 Discharge will *not* occur if the patient is actively suicidal.
   3 As the depression deepens, it is less and less likely that suicide will occur, because the patient is experiencing decreasing physical functioning.
5. Comprehension, assessment, psychosocial (a)
   4 By definition, the ideas are flying by; hence flight of ideas.
   1 Word salad is a mixture of *just* words.
   2 Ambivalence is "I hate you, I love you"—opposite feelings within the same thought.
   3 Confabulation is filling in a memory lapse with untrue statements.
6. Comprehension, assessment, psychosocial (c)
   4 Anxiousness is characterized by accelerated behavior and activity, hence depression will *least likely* be observed; depression is not exhibited by high levels of activity.
   1 Fear may represent the cause for anxiety.
   2 Phobias always have an anxiety component.
   3 Hostility may be seen in the anxious patient.
7. Comprehension, assessment, psychosocial (c)
   1 Persecutory delusion; the television does not curse Mary; she feels persecuted by it.
   2 Not visual hallucination.
   3 Not incoherent, but structured.
   4 Not flight of ideas.
8. Comprehension, implementation, psychosocial (c)
   4 Accepts reality of Mary's experience and suggests self-control.
   1 Denies reality of Mary's experience.
   2 Enters into the delusion.
   3 Denies reality of Mary's experience.
9. Comprehension, implementation, physiologic (b)
   2 Gives a clear message; helps organize patient.
   1 May lead to a power struggle.
   3 Not true; she should be encouraged to begin routine self-care as soon as possible.
   4 Moralizing does not help patient.
10. Knowledge, planning, environment (b)
    3 Chlorpromazine is the generic name for Thorazine.
    1 Fluphenazine is the generic name for Prolixin.
    2 Mesoridazine is the generic name for Serentil.
    4 Compazine is the trade name for prochlorperazine.
11. Comprehension, assessment, psychosocial (b)
    2 Suspicion and jealousy are the predominant thoughts of the paranoid patient.
    1 Paranoid patients are so preoccupied with suspicion and jealousy that these are not substantial possibilities.
    3 Self-pity and self-centeredness are more closely associated with the depressed patient who is trying to blame self or relieve feelings of guilt.
    4 This is the definition of ambivalence.
12. Comprehension, assessment, psychosocial (b)
    4 These are the two that satisfy the condition of examples.
    1 Poverty is an economic condition.
    2 See rationale for statement 1.
    3 Poisoning is not an example of paranoia.

13. Knowledge, assessment, physiologic (a)
    3 Symptoms occur on stopping the drug.
    1 Tolerance means increasing doses to achieve effects.
    2 To abstain is not to drink.
    4 Dementia is unrelated.
14. Knowledge, implementation, physiologic (a)
    4 Tyramine.
    1 Not correct.
    2,3 An amino acid, but not correct.
15. Comprehension, implementation, physiologic (b)
    3 The least restrictive means is always the rule. If the patient is destroying the milieu, herself, or others, then physical restraining would be necessary. Aggression and hyperactivity would best be handled by offering diversional activities.
    1 Will be appropriate if destruction is occurring.
    2 Unless the behavior is destructive, seclusion would be used.
    4 Depending on the cause of the aggression/hyperactivity, the patient may not be able to control the behavior. It would be more appropriate to say, "You seem really aggressive, can you tell me why?"
16. Comprehension, assessment, psychosocial (a)
    1 Denial is the chief defense mechanism in that the addict can always find a reason to drink.
    2 The addiction is the weakness and has an underlying cause that is uncompensated.
    3 Underlying feelings of guilt, sadness, etc. are relieved by the addiction, but these feelings return once the drug wears off. The addiction isn't the expression of an opposite attitude; it is relief from the underlying feelings.
    4 Sublimation does not fit in the discussion of addiction.
17. Comprehension, implementation, psychosocial (c)
    4 Lithium is the medication of choice in the treatment of bipolar disorders.
    1 Chlorpromazine (Thorazine) is an antipsychotic. Not used in bipolar disorder.
    2 Perphenazine (Trilafon) is an antipsychotic-neuroleptic.
    3 Imipramine (Tofranil) is an antidepressant of the tricyclic group.
18. Comprehension, assessment, psychosocial (b)
    4 Assurance and willingness to listen are keys to good therapeutic relationships.
    1 You should not acknowledge that you have knowledge and want to know more about "them." Avoid "buying into" the delusion or hallucination.
    2 Avoid denial of what the patient is seeing or doing. Remember to be nonjudgmental and nonthreatening.
    3 See rationale for statement 1.
19. Comprehension, assessment, psychosocial (b)
    3 Classical symptoms of borderline personality disorder.
    1 No delusions or hallucinations reported.
    2,4 Not relevant.
20. Comprehension, assessment, physiologic (a)
    1 Poor impulse control; superficial wrist-cutting is impulsive behavior.
    2 Regressive is not correct; situation does not indicate earlier, more comfortable behavior.
    3 May be manipulative, but situation does not indicate this.
    4 Probably not depressive; situation does not include this.
21. Comprehension, planning, physiologic (b)
    2 Clearly a goal that is attainable and appropriate.
    1, 3, 4 Unrealistic.
22. Comprehension, implementation, environment (b)
    2 This is a realistic, feasible approach.
    1 Blanket approval is unrealistic.
    3 Gwen should begin to learn to tolerate separation.
    4 Unrealistic; leads to mistrust.

23. Comprehension, assessment, physiologic (b)
    2 Vomiting is the end result of serious physiologic changes occurring as a result of detoxification. Of these answers, it has the most serious consequences and requires measuring the physiologic parameters. The vomiting is uncontrollable and interferes with nutritional and liquid intake. Whatever the patient ingests is vomited within minutes. The offer of an antiemetic would be appropriate *after* blood pressure, pulse, respiration, and temperature are taken.
    1 Usually the "shaking" are internal feelings, not outward signs. Medication is routinely ordered to control this feeling.
    3 No need to measure vital signs unless there are other accompanying complaints.
    4 This response is irrelevant.
24. Comprehension, assessment, environment (b)
    4 Manipulate and control are key features.
    1 They manage to get by, but tend to cause avoidant behavior among those who know them.
    2 They never seem to learn from previous mistakes. Rather, they repeat them time and time again.
    3 Delusions maybe, but never hallucinations unless a problem coexists with the borderline personality.
25. Comprehension, planning, environment (b)
    2 Identify the plan, then intervene.
    1 "Tell me more" may not identify the plan.
    3 Although this is true, it does not address the plan.
    4 Incorrect. If anyone approaches you with statements like the ones in this question, find out if they have a plan.
26. Knowledge, implementation, health (a)
    3 Of the choices here, this is the most correct one.
    1 Not true. Psychotics can think; it is disorganized.
    2 Psychotics are rarely depressed; mostly they cannot operate in reality.
    4 These statements are reversed. The psychotic isn't in reality; the neurotic is in reality, but reality may be distorted.
27. Comprehension, assessment, physiologic (c)
    1 This is the correct answer. The patient may be experiencing the beginning effect called EPS (extrapyramidal symptoms). These symptoms are associated with the administration of antipsychotic medications. Incidentally, there will probably be an anti-EPS medication ordered to reverse the EPS effects.
    2,3 Not appropriate as a *first* response.
    4 Not a first response, but may be required at some point in the event.
28. Knowledge, assessment, physiologic (a)
    2 Basis of theory.
    1 Usually resolve in some fashion without long-term damage.
    3 False statement.
    4 Usually resolve in a few weeks.
29. Knowledge, implementation, environment (a)
    3 Often a new observer is helpful in sorting out complexities and offering useful solutions.
    1 Not a goal.
    2 Treatment is always time limited.
    4 Old ties are often strengthened.
30. Comprehension, assessment, psychosocial (b)
    2 Affective disorder characterized by depressed mood, low energy, and somatic delusions.
    1,3 Not indicated in situation.
    4 Unknown from data given; may or may not be.
31. Knowledge, assessment, psychosocial (b)
    3 Psychomotor retardation characterizes low motor activity based on psychologic factors.
    1, 2 Irrelevant.
    4 Not in situation.

32. Comprehension, assessment, psychosocial (a)
    2 The behavioral changes indicate mania.
    1 May not be true; diagnosis was accurate for the presenting symptoms.
    3 Not true; change too rapid and extreme.
    4 Unrelated.
33. Knowledge, assessment, psychosocial (b)
    3 These are the four As of schizophrenia.
    1 Poverty is an economic state; hence this answer is incorrect.
    2 Schizophrenic patients may have hallucinations and delusions, but the other parts of the answer are not correct.
    4 Apathy is not one of the four As.
34. Knowledge, assessment, psychosocial (a)
    2 Mood swings are the characteristics of bipolar disorder. Manic (elation) to depression are two phases.
    1 Paranoid disorders generally do not involve mood swings at all.
    3 Schizophrenia is characterized by disorganized thinking.
    4 Persons with eating disorders do not suffer from mood swings.
35. Comprehension, implementation, psychosocial (b)
    2 Patient should be alerted before being touched.
    1 The delusion is very real to patient.
    3 Agreeing may or may not be helpful.
    4 Placebo may or may not be helpful.
36. Comprehension, assessment, environment (c)
    1 High risk: mood change may signal behavior change.
    2 The nurse should not assume crisis has passed.
    3 This is a medical diagnosis, not a nursing assessment.
    4 Not necessarily true.
37. Knowledge, assessment, environment (b)
    2 Concrete, lethal plan is a very high-risk factor.
    1 Treatment duration is usually unrelated.
    3 Past attempt is high risk but not for reason stated.
    4 Unrelated.
38. Knowledge, assessment, psychosocial (a)
    3 Orderliness is the single feature of the obsessive-compulsive disorder; usually done in ritual format.
    1 The obsessive-compulsive patient is so busy thinking and doing, there would be no time for seclusion.
    2 Aggression is not an obsessive-compulsive characteristic.
    4 Instant gratification is related to poor impulse control. The obsessive-compulsive patient has an overwhelming need to perform activities that release the underlying feelings.
39. Knowledge, assessment, health (a)
    4 Marijuana is a cannabinol.
    1 It is not highly addictive; however, a psychologic dependency can develop.
    2 Amphetamine is a class of psychoactive substance that is a cerebral stimulant.
    3 Marijuana causes impaired brain function, but it is generally not known to generate hallucinations.
40. Knowledge, assessment, psychosocial (a)
    1 These are exact definitions of the respective terms.
    2 See rationale for statement 1.
    3 Delusions are always false, as are hallucinations.
    4 See rationale for statement 3.
41. Comprehension, assessment, environment (c)
    4 The more details contained in the plan of self-destruction, the more likely it is to occur.
    1 Suicide is not 100% preventable. Many previous accidental deaths have proven to be suicides. Surviving suicide is increasingly difficult as the instances of attempts increase.
    2 Not a true statement.
    3 Most suicides occur after ample warnings have been offered.

42. Application, implementation, psychosocial (a)

3 Open-ended question, with ample time to listen, is the best therapeutic technique in this situation.

1 You should indicate an interest in what the patient has said. Saying nothing is the wrong activity.

2 The pressing issue is death of parents; diversion of discussion is not appropriate.

4 Inappropriate, and it is a put-down.

43. Comprehension, assessment, environment (b)

2 Verbal intervention is always the first course of action.

1 This action may be required later, depending on the ability to verbally deescalate the situation.

3 Go for the underlying feeling *first*.

4 Not until it is necessary.

44. Comprehension, assessment, psychosocial (c)

4 Always go for the underlying feeling.

1 A good second-choice answer.

2 Not true. This is imprisonment.

3 This is viewed as punitive for asking a question and has no foundation in fact for such an action.

45. Knowledge, planning, psychosocial (a)

4 This is true. Patients have the right to view their own medical records.

1 Not everyone has access to the medical record.

2 Mental health workers from all disciplines may view the records.

3 Mental health workers from all disciplines may make entries into the medical record, provided they are caring for the patient.

46. Comprehension, planning, psychosocial (b)

4 The depressed patient may become overwhelmed if too much is offered too soon. They should be engaged in structured, goal directed activities.

1 Could lead to withdrawal or seclusive behavior.

2 Overwhelming to the patient at the beginning of treatment.

3 Feelings cannot be restructured, but they can be dealt with if the patient will allow.

47. Knowledge, assessment, psychosocial (b)

4 A key indicator of depression.

1, 2 Not consistent with depression.

3 The most distant feeling from depression.

48. Comprehension, assessment, physiologic (a)

3 Disulfiram (Antabuse) causes violent nausea and vomiting if taken within 24 hours of consuming alcohol.

1 Is a major antipsychotic.

2, 4 Is an antipsychotic.

49. Comprehension, implementation, psychosocial (b)

2 This is most therapeutic.

1 This will have a negative effect.

3 Previous unacceptable behavior should be challenged and integrated into current behavioral activities.

4 This is not therapeutic.

50. Comprehension, assessment, environment (a)

2 The most therapeutic in providing safety from self-destruction.

1 Not true.

3 Inappropriate response.

4 Irrelevant and inappropriate.

Chapter 8: Obstetric Nursing

1. Comprehension, assessment, health (b)

4 This is another term for an ultrasonography, which can outline the embryo, the placenta, and fetal parts as early as 4 weeks; this is a positive sign of pregnancy.

1 Not a positive sign. The human chorionic gonadotropin (HCG) used in pregnancy tests may also emanate from a hydated mole or other nonpregnant sources. This is a probable sign.

2 This is also a probable sign noted by an examiner. It is a softening of the lower segment of the uterus.

3 This is a presumptive sign, which the mother realizes after she has missed a period. Various occurrences from emotional stress to physical stress could cause amenorrhea, so this is not a correct answer.

2. Knowledge, implementation, psychosocial (c)

4 Still considered the most effective method of birth control with very little side effects. This is the best answer.

1 Incorrect. Intrauterine devices are still controversial. These are devices placed in the uterus to prevent pregnancy; however, there have been cases of extreme irritability to the uterus resulting in excessive bleeding and possible contamination. The jury is still undecided on the efficacy of this insertion method. It is invasive.

2 Incorrect. Sperm can escape into the vagina if ejaculation is not carefully controlled. Very tenuous method subject to psychosocial factors as well.

3 Sheath that prevents sperm from entering the cervix. Must be placed effectively, and must be reliable—made from material that will not tear. Psychosocial factors influence this method. This is the recommended method to prevent spread of AIDS, but for the prevention of pregnancy, not 100% effective.

3. Comprehension, assessment, environment (b)

3 Correct answer. Early, frequent, and continual testing of urine and blood pressure would signal early signs that could be addressed rapidly and appropriately.

1 This is usually a third-trimester complication and would not be considered a preventable condition.

2 This is not exactly preventable but can be helped by easing discomfort, teaching, and advising on care.

4 Abortions—spontaneous ones might have some early signs and symptoms that alert pending conditions, but this is not the best answer.

4. Knowledge, evaluation, physiologic (a)

4 Correct answer. This is a digestive system change that occurs after an episode of morning sickness, which is a particular digestive system change.

1 This belongs to the nervous system changes.

2 This is caused by the activity of the lactiferous ducts, which are not a part of the digestive system, and the traces of sugar in the urine are a direct result of the activity of the ducts on the urinary system.

3 This is a "mask of pregnancy" and is an integumentary system change.

5. Comprehension, planning, physiologic (a)
   2 Correct answer. Elevated levels of AFP indicate up to 5% to 10% of a neural defect, but must be followed by two consecutive AFP tests, ultrasound readings, and an amniocentesis.
   1 Fetal maturity is tested by an L/S ratio that determines lung maturity by measuring the ratio of the two components of surfactant (lecithin and sphingomyelin). An amniocentesis done after the 35th week of pregnancy should show an increase in the amount of lecithin and a decrease in sphingomyelin.
   3 Genetic work-up, including family history and a series of blood tests, can evaluate risk of disease in offspring.
   4 Respiratory distress syndrome is most likely to occur in low-birth-weight babies, premature babies, or babies known to be at risk for immature lung development.

6. Knowledge, assessment, physiologic (a)
   3 Correct answer. Without this, the embryo and fetus could not survive. This hormone changes the walls of the endometrium to prepare to accept a fertilized ovum.
   1 Stimulates endometrium to thicken; a "preparation" hormone to thicken uterine lining.
   2 Controls ovarian function.
   4 This is secreted by the fertilized ovum and helps the corpus luteum to produce progesterone for the first trimester. This hormone affects pregnancy testing, and without it there would be no positive test results.

7. Knowledge, comprehension, physiologic (a)
   3 Correct answer.
   1 This is ballottement or locating of fetal parts. It is not a part of a nonstress test.
   2 Sex of an infant may be seen on a screen during a sonogram, but not by a fetal monitoring device that only measures fetal heart tones—strength of contractions and fetal movements through the FHT response.
   4 Wrong. The mother is given orange juice for a nonstress test; for the stress test she is given oxytocin intravenously.

8. Knowledge, planning, health (b)
   3 Correct answer. In seminars by the March of Dimes the single abuse most negatively affecting the pregnant woman is crack and cocaine; alcohol abuse is also important.
   1 Economic and ethnic status does not necessarily affect mother or child negatively. It does affect nutrition and other physical deprivations, but there are social workers, related programs such as WIC, food stamps, and entitlement programs that may help.
   2 These are routine questions included in taking history and are rarely omitted in interviewing.
   4 This is also included in the initial interviews but not in interviewing techniques. It may affect the ability to learn baby care and self-care. Important, but not current.

9. Comprehension, evaluation, physiologic (c)
   2 DTRs are absent; respiratory effort may quickly be impaired.
   1 BP is not affected by the drug.
   3 It is being given to decrease the DTRs.
   4 Should use good nursing judgment if DTRs are absent.

10. Knowledge, implementation, environment (b)
    3   100 ml in 1 hr
        $\times 15$ gtt ml
        1500 gtt in 1 hr
        1500 gtt divided by 60 min = 25 gtt/min
    1, 2, 4 Incorrect calculation.

11. Knowledge, implementation, physiologic (b)
    1 When the patient becomes eclamptic, she has a seizure.
    2, 3 BP should be watched but is an indication of preeclampsia.
    4 You should watch all pregnant patients for labor. This does not cause eclamptic conditions.

12. Comprehension, implementation, physiologic (c)
    4 Within 72 hours, danger of seizure passes.
    1, 2 Danger of seizure lasts longer. Normal recovery may be 1 to 2 hours or more.
    3 Danger of seizure lasts longer than 24 hours.

13. Comprehension, planning, physiologic (b)
    2 Correct answer. Teenage nutritional patterns are poor whether the patient is rich, middle class, or poor.
    1 Incorrect answer. Although this is very important, psychosocial standards vary. A poor teenager brought up by a single, unmarried mother may view her situation as being able to have something (someone) whom she can love and will love her. The nurse must know her patient's psychosocial background to counsel effectively.
    3 Incorrect answer. It is true that many very young pregnant patients have underdeveloped pelvic bones and immature physiologic boney development, but this includes only a certain age group. Teenagers vary greatly in developmental maturity.
    4 Incorrect answer. It is not relevant only to pregnant teenage patients. It is important, but not the major concern.

14. Comprehension, planning, physiologic (a)
    2 Milk is high in calcium, and natural sources are absorbed more fully.
    1 Only a small portion of calcium is absorbed from a supplement, compared with a natural source.
    3 Greens have less calcium than milk.
    4 Only a small portion of calcium is absorbed from a supplement, compared with a natural source.

15. Knowledge, implementation, physiologic (a)
    4 This is the correct hormone.
    1 Levels significant toward end of pregnancy.
    2 Levels gradually increase to "hold" pregnancy.
    3 Hormone that lowers peristalsis of the stomach and slows metabolism during pregnancy.

16. Knowledge, comprehension, health (a)
    3 Correct and direct answer to Elisabeth's question.
    1 Correct statement, but irrelevant to the question.
    2 Incorrect information.
    4 Wrong. This is a partial explanation of fetal circulation.

17. Knowledge, assessment, health (b)
    1 Heart beating during embryonic period—correct.
    2 Incorrect.
    3 Is third month; heart and cardiovascular system would have had to been working long before.
    4 Placenta begins to form shortly after implantation and continues to form for 16 to 20 weeks into gestation, so this answer is wrong.

18. Knowledge, comprehension, physiologic (b)
    4 Correct answer.
    1 All true, but not a good answer to a pregnant mother.
    2 Also true, but not the best answer.
    3 Too vague; not the best answer.

19. Knowledge, assessment, physiologic (b)
    2 Because Elisabeth delivered a boy and a girl, they must be fraternal or unidentical. If they had been the same sex, the placenta and sacs would have to be identified.
    1 Monozygotic twins are always the same sex.
    3 Blood tests are not the *best* answer; as a nurse you should know the status by identifying the placenta and sacs.
    4 DNA tests are not the *best* answer; as a nurse you should know the status by identifying the placenta and sacs.

20. Comprehension, assessment, physiologic (a)
    3 Scientifically established.
    1 Unlikely; has probably had nutritional counseling for both pregnancies.
    2 Further testing needed to confirm this as gestational diabetes.
    4 False statement.

21. Comprehension, assessment, environment (a)
    3 Pregnant twice, one child. Correct.
    1 Pregnant once, one child. Incorrect.
    2 Pregnant twice, two children. Incorrect.
    4 Twice pregnant, no children. Incorrect.

22. Comprehension, assessment, physiologic (a)
    1 Two negatives are compatible.
    2 A negative and a positive are not compatible.
    3 Her son has nothing to do with the pregnancy.
    4 RhoGAM prevents problems when given either prenatally or within 72 hours of delivery.

23. Comprehension, planning, environment (a)
    2 According to Nägele's formula this is correct.
    1 Wrong according to Nägele's formula.
    3 Incorrect.
    4 Do not use the last day of the LMP.

24. Knowledge, assessment, physiologic (c)
    2 Correct answer. Signs and symptoms are bright red clots first, then light, painless bleeding.
    1 In abruptio placentae, there is pain, and there may or may not be bleeding. If there is bleeding, it is dark red and usually not clotted.
    3 Bright red in variable amounts with pain.
    4 Painless vaginal bleeding with bloody amniotic fluid.

25. Knowledge, implementation, physiologic (b)
    3 Correct. Simply relieving pressure by changing positions.
    1 The symptoms are pallor, light-headedness, dizziness, and slight nausea—rubbing the legs does not correct the syndrome.
    2 Incorrect. It is caused by the heavy uterus exerting pressure on the aorta and hampering good circulation. Determine the cause and effect first, then plan the intervention.
    4 Know cause and effect. Because patient is dizzy, you would not recommend walking.

26. Application, implementation, physiologic (b)
    3 Correct information and advice.
    1 This does not alleviate leg cramps.
    2 This is for relief from the discomfort of varicose veins.
    4 Not incorrect but not best answer.

27. Application, implementation, physiologic (b)
    3 Best answer.
    1 Relieve perineal discomfort.
    2 Temporary relief at best.
    4 Improper advice.

28. Comprehension, assessment, physiologic (b)
    2 Correct statement and correct answer.
    1 You would consider doing follow-up tests to determine precise findings, and the physician would consider what medical treatment is needed.
    3 False assumption.
    4 Not a part of the nursing process to make this kind of determination.

29. Knowledge, implementation, physiologic (a)
    3 Correct instructions.
    1 This is acceptable for a routine urinalysis.
    2 Pregnancy tests do not require a sterile specimen.
    4 Untrue.

30. Comprehension, planning, health (a)
    1 Reportable signs and symptoms which should be taught to the patient.
    2 Usual signs and symptoms and are normal.
    3 Nonemergency signs and symptoms, which can be addressed during regular visits.
    4 Later signs and symptoms; nonemergency.

31. Comprehension, planning, physiologic (b)
    4 Usually estriol levels are tested for placental functioning in the third trimester; a level of 12 mg is good, but below 12 mg in 24 hours may place the fetus in jeopardy.
    1 Fetal age is determined by uterine height, calculation of EDC.
    2 Amniocentesis procedure may reveal surfactant lecithin/sphingomyelin ratio and help determine lung maturity.
    3 Human gonadotropin hormonal levels in the urine are tested early on in pregnancy, but the words *uterine nomenclature* are not related to the question.

32. Knowledge, assessment, health (a)
    2 German measles have a devastating effect on fetal growth: physical abnormalities, mental retardation, hearing impairment or deafness, blindness.
    1 Chickenpox may have a more severe action on the mother, but will not cause fetal physiologic defects or problems.
    3 Synonym for chickenpox.
    4 Regular measles; does not affect the unborn.

33. Knowledge, planning, environment (c)
    3 Third-trimester bleeding conditions, particularly because it includes no vaginal/rectal examinations.
    1 The bleeding, pain, or contractions would not be as acute.
    2 The pregnancy in itself would not necessitate these nursing measures unless the mother had symptoms.
    4 Postpartum hemorrhage most likely would occur in recovery or within an hour or so after delivery. Because the baby is born, there would be no fetal monitoring.

34. Application, evaluation, environment (a)
    2 Correct. Responsible nursing procedure.
    1 Done as part of the routine responsibility, but statement 2 is specific to procedure accomplished.
    3 Incomplete recording.
    4 Part of the routine nursing care and not specific to this question.

35. Comprehension, implementation, physiologic (a)
    4 As the fetal presenting part descends down the birth canal, a full bladder will create an impediment to descent.
    1, 2, 3 Possible but unlikely.

36. Comprehension, planning, physiologic (a)
    1 Correct answer.
    2 Incorrect answer. These are nursing responsibilities for the second stage of labor.
    3 Incorrect answer. These are major nursing interventions for the third stage of labor.
    4 Incorrect. These are nursing care measures for the fourth stage of labor, or 1 hour after delivery, usually in the recovery room.

37. Knowledge, implementation, environment (a)
    2 Fear is a major threat to women in labor.
    1 Whatever progress is made, the fear of facing labor alone is worse.
    3 That statement is of no help if the physician is not beside her.
    4 It is during labor she needs support.

APGAR SCORING CHART

Sign	0	1	2
HEART RATE	Absent	Slow (below 100)	Over 100
RESPIRATORY EFFORT	Absent	Weak cry, hypoventilation	Good strong cry
MUSCLE TONE	Limp	Some flexion of extremities	Well flexed
REFLEX RESPONSE 1. Response to catheter in nostril (tested after oro-pharynx is clear)	No response	Grimace	Cough or sneeze
2. Tangential foot slap	No response	Grimace	Cry and withdrawal of foot
COLOR	Blue, pale	Body pink, extremities blue	Completely pink

The Apgar scoring chart (From Philips CR: Family-centered maternity/newborn care: a basic text, ed 2, St Louis, 1987, Mosby).

38. Knowledge, assessment, environment (b)
    2 Correct answer. The LOP position means the bony back of the head presses against the spine, causing lower back pain because it presents bone against bone. The head must turn until the face is against the spine; this may happen spontaneously or by artificial means (maneuvers by the physician). Usually a slow and painful process of descent
    1 This is a more normal descent and does not present itself to dystocia and pain.
    3 Almost an impossible vaginal delivery position or lie; most certainly a cesarean section elective.
    4 Does not describe a presentation.
39. Knowledge, planning, physiologic (b)
    1 See text; this is the correct answer.
    2 Does not explain the physiologic dynamics.
    3 Pitocin is an oxytocic acting on the uterus.
    4 Does not explain the physiologic dynamics of immediate postpartum phenomenon.
40. Comprehension, assessment, physiologic (a)
    2 Correct answer. Apgar score is 6. (See chart above.)
    Heart rate = 1
    Respiratory effort = 1
    Muscle tone = 1
    Reflex response = 2
    Color = 1
    1, 3, 4 Incorrect.
41. Comprehension, evaluation, physiologic (a)
    3 Correct answer. Birth injury—occurs when the upper arm has been injured in such a way that the nerves of the brachial plexus are severed or injured, resulting in a paralysis.
    1, 2 These are normal.
    4 Normal cranial deviations resulting from normal vaginal delivery; these conditions occur as the caput descends through the birth canal
42. Comprehension, assessment, physiologic (a)
    3 Symptoms indicative of abruptio placentae.
    1 This would give rise to painless bleeding.
    2 Onset gradual, accompanied by nausea, possibly vomiting, and gradual shock; abdomen tender but not board-like.
    4 Not a rigid, boardlike abdomen.

43. Comprehension, implementation, psychosocial (a)
    2 Attempts to teach, reassure, and describe condition.
    1 Alarming, senseless, and incorrect response; insensitive as well.
    3 Inappropriate, incorrect answer.
    4 Does not reassure or answer George's concern.
44. Application, planning, psychosocial (c)
    3 Explaining procedure, giving reassurance.
    1 Rude, curt; did not answer question.
    2 The physician was in the room, but he asked you.
    4 Answer creates unnecessary anxiety with no explanation.
45. Knowledge, implementation, environment (b)
    3 In abruptio placentae this is standard practice.
    1 If bleeding subsides or stops, vaginal delivery is preferable.
    2 Should bleeding continue, a vaginal delivery places both mother and fetus in jeopardy.
    4 Unlikely; emergency delivery tray items limited.
46. Comprehension, evaluation, physiologic (a)
    1 True statement. Physician and nurse should check to determine location of tear.
    2 Calcification indicates age, not a tear.
    3 An abruptio does not preclude size or weight.
    4 Unlikely. Confirmation by physician sufficient.
47. Comprehension, implementation, physiologic (b)
    2 First priority is to establish patent airway so baby can breathe, cry, and fill her lungs with oxygen.
    1 Not first priority.
    3 Umbilical cord can be left attached; there is no danger in delaying the cutting of the cord while tasks with a higher priority are performed.
    4 The delivery of the placenta may take anywhere from 5 to 20 minutes, since it must separate itself from the walls of the uterus; therefore this too is not top priority.
48. Comprehension, assessment, physiologic (b)
    2 The suddenness of precipitous delivery always predisposes the patient to possible hemorrhage.
    1 Not top priority; usual checking of IV and administration of any drug.
    3 Many women experience this after delivery.
    4 Precipitous delivery does not of itself cause massive infection.

49. Comprehension, planning, environment (b)
    2 Regulations for NSB clearly outlined in hospital policy.
    1 Depends on policy and will be determined by nursery supervisor.
    3 Varied policies, that is, nursery nurse may be responsible for these procedures.
    4 Administration of medication may be ordered and given on admission (to nursery).

50. Comprehension, planning, physiologic (b)
    2 Interpreting what is happening to Mary, the best assistance would be to prepare for medical interventions and anticipate what nursing actions you will implement.
    1 You will anticipate this, but you will have the necessary equipment ready.
    3 You would not intervene unless requested to do so by the physician.
    4 With massive bleeding, your patient is probably in shock and needs nursing and medical intervention stat.

51. Comprehension, assessment, psychosocial (b)
    2 Explain procedure.
    1 She wants to know what is going to happen to her, nothing else.
    3 This is an unnecessary anxiety-causing statement, irrelevant at this time.
    4 Not a comforting statement; implies stupidity.

52. Comprehension, implementation, physiologic (b)
    1 Your analysis and plan of action are correct.
    2 It is a positive test for trouble, and waiting for the pattern to change may compromise the fetus.
    3 Together with the head nurse you may proceed to this.
    4 There is nothing in this situation that tells you of an imminent delivery.

53. Knowledge, assessment, physiologic (a)
    2 From your textbook readings you know this to be true.
    1 Though Gwen may indeed have a normal pregnancy and delivery, she is in a high-risk group.
    3 The question asked for "classification."
    4 This "gran" refers to pregnancy and children not "age."

54. Application, planning, psychosocial (a)
    1 Reassurance and explanation.
    2 Levels of perception of pain differ, so do not promise there will be "no pain."
    3 This test takes from 20 minutes to over an hour.
    4 Untrue. Most women will never need this test.

55. Knowledge, planning, health (a)
    2 From your readings you know this is true so you will plan your nursing care accordingly.
    1 These are genetic anomalies not caused by overdue date.
    3 An overdue baby may be larger than normal but will not necessarily have meconium-stained fluid.
    4 See rationale for statement 2.

56. Application, planning, environment (a)
    2 Best response: preparation is started, so if the procedure is ordered, time is not lost.
    1 Responsibility is not assumed until order is given by physician.
    3 Unless there is a standing order, this would not be appropriate.
    4 Alarming family without proper teaching or preparation is inadvisable.

57. Comprehension, implementation, environment (a)
    3 Prevent convulsions; be able to respond stat.
    1 A severely eclamptic mother should not be in a semi-private room, and certainly not in a sunny room with visitors.
    2 Must be quiet with absolutely no visitors.
    4 Bright sunshine will aggravate the central nervous system, and being far from the nurses' station will hamper emergency nursing care.

58. Knowledge, assessment, environment (b)
    2 Significant symptom of an impending convulsion.
    1 Sign of change in blood pressure, preeclampsia.
    3 Eye changes would not be noticed by the mother.
    4 Not necessarily a sign of impending convulsions; rather of fluid retention.

59. Application, implementation, health (a)
    1 To reduce perineal swelling and edema.
    2 Normal location of the fundus a few hours after delivery.
    3 Natural reaction is to be happy over an apparently successful birthing experience.
    4 One pad saturated with red lochia several hours after delivery is normal and not a sign of hemorrhage.

60. Knowledge, evaluation, environment (b)
    2 Correct answer by definition, usually born of patients with gestational diabetes mellitus (GDM).
    1 *Macro* is large; *micro* is small.
    3 Milia are small white visible papules on the face of the newborn and have nothing to do with infant size.
    4 Large babies are screened and tested for diabetes, but this does not necessarily mean that they are or will become insulin-dependent diabetics.

61. Comprehension, implementation, environment (b)
    3 Correct answer.
    1 Incorrect. This is still a procedure used in some nurseries, however, more and more hospitals are using universal precaution protocol.
    2 Incorrect. It is not the responsibility for a nurse to report to the Centers for Disease Control. The nurse is responsible to the supervisor (or equivalent).
    4 The mask, gloves, and a gown at all times is not correct because most HIV-positive patients are not necessarily ill with the signs and symptoms of active AIDS. This precaution is for the patient whose immune system places him or her at risk or whose body fluid symptoms are positive.

62. Comprehension, planning, health (c)
    1 Correct answer. The sooner the mother is seen and evaluated, the better.
    2 If the opportunity to see the high-risk mother was not before this time (20 to 24 weeks' gestation), by all means see her. It is never too late.
    3 Although scheduled evaluation should be even before, it is never too late to schedule continuing evaluations.
    4 Evaluation scheduling should have been started as early as possible and continue at appropriate times throughout pregnancy.

63. Knowledge, planning, health (b)
    1 Correct answer. Most patients with pregnancy-induced diabetes or gestational diabetes mellitus (GDM) will return to normal by the 6-week checkup with the obstetrician.
    2 Not a good statement for health teaching. This is a scare tactic and not accurate. Some studies indicate that women who have successive large babies, and gain considerable weight, or are grossly overweight before and after pregnancy may experience some problems, but good follow-up teaching with emphasis on weight and nutritonal care should help in maintaining sugar-free urine, etc.
    3 There is no indication that a blanket number ensures against diabetes. There is considerable evidence to support the claim that excess weight is detrimental to health.
    4 Unfounded statement. In education of pregnancy-induced diabetes or GDM, teaching mothers to follow up after each pregnancy is a good idea.

64. Comprehension, planning, psychosocial (b)
    1 Correct answer. To prevent FAS, the woman who drinks should have early and continuous counseling to prevent FAS and to maintain her psychosocial integrity needs. Record her family history, immediate family circumstances, and social activities.
    2 Fetal damage has already begun.
    3 Never too late to try, but by the second trimester counseling aims to curb consumption to limit fetal damage.
    4 Continued counseling; planned care to confront and assist in lowering alcohol dependency.

65. Comprehension, evaluation, psychosocial (c)
    1 Correct answer. Because all newborns have an immature liver, putting a drug into the system jeopardizes the infant.
    2 Prolonged use of a drug by the mother just before conception does not necessarily cause newborn addiction unless the mother continues the habit from conception throughout pregnancy to term.
    3 This answer in itself is not correct. Usage must be continued during pregnancy.
    4 Drugs may affect uterine growth because the addictive mother seldom has good nutritional habits, but if carried through term, the infant does not necessarily have RDS.

Chapter 9: Pediatric Nursing

1. Knowledge, assessment, environment (b)
    4 A Wilms' tumor is found only in the kidney and kidney area.
    1 It is not found in the brain.
    2 It is not found in the small intestine.
    3 It is not found in the colon.

2. Knowledge, assessment, psychosocial (b)
    3 This is the period of life known as infancy.
    1 Birth to 4 weeks is the newborn period; birth to 6 weeks includes newborn and part of infancy.
    2 Birth to 4 weeks is the newborn period and is not considered part of the infancy period.
    4 After 1 year of age until 3 years of age is considered the toddler period.

3. Application, implementation, environment (b)
    2 Demerol: $DD = 20$ mg
    $\qquad\qquad DH = 50$ mg
    $\qquad\qquad V\ = 1$ ml
    $$\frac{DD}{DH} = \frac{20 \text{ mg}}{50 \text{ mg}} \times 1 \text{ ml} = 0.4 \text{ ml}$$
    Atropine: $DD = 0.08$ mg
    $\qquad\qquad DH = 0.2$ mg
    $\qquad\qquad V\ = 1$ ml
    $$\frac{DD}{DH} = \frac{0.08 \text{ mg}}{0.2 \text{ mg}} \times 1 \text{ ml} = 0.4 \text{ ml}$$
    0.4 ml $+ 0.4$ ml $= 0.8$ ml
    1, 3, 4 This is not the correct amount.

4. Comprehension, assessment, environment (c)
    2 These are symptoms of rubeola.
    1 Symptoms of chickenpox include a clear, vesicular rash, fever, irritability, and pruritus.
    3 Symptoms of rubella do not include a high fever or white spots at the back of the throat.
    4 Symptoms of mumps include enlarged parotid glands and fever, with no rash.

5. Application, implementation, environment (a)
    4 This equipment may be necessary if the enlarged epiglottis completely obstructs the airway.
    1 Any examination of the throat could lead to laryngospasm.
    2 The child with epiglottitis has difficulty swallowing.
    3 Warm steam is not a method of treatment in epiglottitis.

6. Application, implementation, psychosocial (b)
    2 This is the most important goal for a nurse taking care of a child with a respiratory problem.
    1 This must also be done, but it is not the most important concern of the nurse.
    3 This is not the most important concern of the nurse.
    4 Karen may be NPO, or she may be on clear fluids; however, this is not the most important concern of the nurse.

7. Application, implementation, physiologic (b)
    2 This is the most honest, helpful answer the nurse can give.
    1 This is a lie.
    3 At 5 years of age she is not really a "big girl"; she is a child and should be allowed to act like one.
    4 She should be allowed to cry if the blood test hurts. Telling her not to cry only gives her something else to worry about.

8. Comprehension, assessment, environment (b)
    1 *H. influenzae* is the responsible organism in most cases of epiglottitis.
    2 The trachea and esophagus are not affected.
    3 This is not the cause.
    4 Although the child may have other symptoms of URI, the cause is bacterial, not viral.

9. Application, implementation, environment (b)
    3 $DD = 750$ mg
    $\quad DH = 0.5$ g (500 mg)
    $\quad V\ = 5$ ml
    $$\frac{DD}{DH} = \frac{750 \text{ mg}}{500 \text{ mg}} \times 5 \text{ ml} = 7.5 \text{ ml} = 1\frac{1}{2} \text{ tsp.}$$
    1, 2, 4 This is not the correct amount.

10. Comprehension, assessment, health (b)
    3 This is when adolescence is considered to begin in each child's life.
    1 This occurs more than once in childhood.
    2 Developing a self-image is part of adolescence, but it may be positive or negative during the teenage years.
    4 Adolescent boys are often attracted to adolescent girls at an earlier age than the girls are attracted to the boys.

11. Knowledge, assessment, physiologic (a)
    1 Adolescents are at the stage where they are constantly struggling to develop a positive self-image and their own identity and independence.
    2 These are the developmental skills developed during infancy and toddlerhood.
    3, 4 This occurs during the preschool stage.

12. Knowledge, assessment, physiologic (a)
    4 Preschoolers are at the stage where they are learning how to interact with other people, as well as proper behavior; this helps them develop a sense of initiative and accomplishment.
    1 This is the stage of infants.
    2 This is the stage of school-age children.
    3 This is the stage of toddlers.

13. Comprehension, implementation, psychosocial (a)
    2 The parents will deal best with a nurse who is open and honest with them.
    1 This will put a strain on the relationship between the parents and the nurse.
    3 The nurse should answer as many questions as possible and only refer questions that she cannot answer to the physician.
    4 The parents should be involved as much as possible in their child's care and recovery, and this should be encouraged by the nurse.

14. Knowledge, assessment, environment (b)
    4 Rheumatic fever is a chronic disease caused by a streptococcal infection.
    1 It is not caused by a fungus.
    2 It is not caused by *staphylococcus* bacteria.
    3 It is not caused by a virus.
15. Comprehension, assessment, environment (c)
    1 This is the most common, serious complication of rheumatic fever; the endocardium and valves become inflamed and often are permanently damaged.
    2 This is not a common complication of rheumatic fever.
    3 Arthritis is a symptom of rheumatic fever but not the most serious complication.
    4 This is not a complication of rhematic fever.
16. Knowledge, assessment, environment (a)
    4 Although there is no cure for AIDS, acyclovir has been effective in reducing overwhelming viral infections.
    1 Cimetadine (Tagamet) is used in the treatment of gastritis.
    2 Penicillin has no effect on the AIDS virus or viral infections.
    3 Neostigmine is a cholinesterase inhibitor.
17. Comprehension, assessment, environment (a)
    3 Large amounts of abnormally thick mucus are produced in the lungs, as well as the pancreas and liver. The mucus from the lungs leads to airway obstruction.
    1 This does not occur in cystic fibrosis.
    2 This occurs in epiglottitis.
    4 This does not occur in cystic fibrosis.
18. Knowledge, assessment, environment (a)
    3 Pancreatic enzymes are given regularly with food to improve the digestion and absorption of proteins and fats in the small intestine.
    1 Pancreatic enzymes do not directly affect vitamin absorption.
    2 Pancreatic enzymes do not affect carbohydrate metabolism.
    4 Although sodium levels are a problem in the child with cystic fibrosis, pancreatic enzymes do not affect them.
19. Knowledge, assessment, environment (a)
    2 The main function of aerosolized bronchodilators and chest physiotherapy is to dilate the bronchioles and loosen and move secretions out of the lungs.
    1 Nothing has been shown to be effective in decreasing mucus production.
    3 Efficiency of the diaphragm is not a problem in cystic fibrosis.
    4 Although chest physiotherapy may stimulate coughing to some degree, it is not done to increase oxygen consumption.
20. Comprehension, assessment, environment (a)
    2 This is a classic sign seen in children diagnosed with Down's syndrome.
    1 These children are hypotonic.
    3 These children have hyperflexibility of the joints.
    4 This is a symptom seen in bacterial endocarditis.
21. Comprehension, assessment, environment (a)
    1 Some form of congenital heart defect is often seen in children with Down's syndrome.
    2, 3, 4 This is not frequently seen in children with Down's syndrome.

22. Application, implementation, physiologic (a)
    2 The nurse should always be honest with the child when giving medicine; medicine should never be called "candy."
    1 Using juice or a food to cover unpleasant tastes of medicines makes the child more willing to take the medicine.
    3 It is important not to lie to children when a shot or procedure is going to hurt. Allowing them to decide whether to get the shot "now, or in 5 minutes" gives them some control in the situation.
    4 As for adults, the child's arm band should be checked before any medications are administered.
23. Knowledge, implementation, psychosocial (b)
    2 This is the best developed muscle in infants and therefore is the safest for IM injections.
    1 This muscle is not well developed in infants, toddlers, or young children.
    3, 4 This muscle is not well developed in infants and toddlers.
24. Knowledge, assessment, environment (a)
    4 Celiac disease is a basic defect of metabolism, leading to impaired fat absorption.
    1 Celiac disease does not affect absorption of proteins.
    2 Celiac disease does not affect absorption of carbohydrates.
    3 Celiac disease does not affect absorption of vitamins.
25. Knowledge, assessment, environment (b)
    4 These are all common symptoms of celiac disease.
    1 Constipation is not a symptom of celiac disease.
    2 An appetite for sweets is not a symptom of celiac disease.
    3 Constipation is not a symptom of celiac disease.
26. Comprehension, planning, environment (a)
    1 Rice cereal is digested properly in the infant with celiac disease.
    2 Because of the defect in metabolism in the child with celiac disease, ingestion of wheat leads to impaired fat absorption.
    3 Ingestion of oats leads to impaired fat absorption.
    4 Ingestion of barley leads to impaired fat absorption.
27. Knowledge, assessment, psychosocial (a)
    3 The cellophane tape test is used in diagnosing pinworms.
    1 The child's history and symptoms are not enough to definitely diagnose pinworms; a stool culture will not diagnose pinworms.
    2 A blood culture would not be helpful in diagnosing pinworms.
    4 A stool culture will not diagnose pinworms.
28. Comprehension, assessment, environment (a)
    4 These symptoms of leukemia result directly from changes in the bone marrow.
    1 These symptoms are caused by leukemic effects on the nervous system that lead to increased intracranial pressure.
    2 These symptoms result from the body's increasing need to meet the metabolic needs of the leukemic cells.
    3 These are not symptoms of leukemia.
29. Comprehension, assessment, environment (b)
    4 Bryant's traction is the usual method of treatment for an infant with a fractured femur.
    1 This is more extensive treatment than is usually needed.
    2 Skeletal traction is not usually used for infants with fractured femurs; often used in older children.
    3 Traction is usually necessary before casting can be done if the fracture is to heal properly.

30. Knowledge, assessment, environment (a)
    1 Scoliosis of the spine often occurs because of rapid growth; seen most often in girls.
    2 Nephrosis is a disease of the kidneys, causing edema and proteinuria.
    3 Lordosis is a concave curvature of the spine; called swayback.
    4 Kyphosis is a convex curvature of the spine; called hunchback.
31. Knowledge, assessment, environment (b)
    4 The CSF of a child with meningitis is cloudy because of the increased WBC count.
    1 Meningitis causes an increased protein level.
    2 Meningitis causes a decreased glucose level.
    3 There is an increase in the CSF pressure in meningitis.
32. Comprehension, assessment, environment (b)
    2 These signs are the most notable because these symptoms are caused by increased intracranial pressure, a serious complication in meningitis.
    1 The child's cry would be shrill and high pitched.
    3, 4 These are not signs seen in meningitis.
33. Application, implementation, environment (b)
    3 Observing the length and type of seizure is important, as is preventing the child from injuring himself.
    1 This could injure the child's mouth.
    2 Suctioning may be needed, but would not be feasible until the seizure was over.
    4 Restraints could lead to severe injury.
34. Comprehension, assessment, environment (a)
    4 The eustachian tubes are shorter and wider in the young child than in the older child, which allows for easier introduction of bacteria.
    1 The shape and position of the esophagus do not affect otitis media.
    2 The shape and position of the tympanic membranes do not affect otitis media.
    3 The external ear canals are basically the same shape and in the same position in young and older children.
35. Application, planning, psychosocial (b)
    3 Having a parent assist in procedures often helps to calm the child, making it much easier to perform the procedure.
    1 Sedation is only used as a last resort when absolutely necessary.
    2 Restraints may be needed if assistance by a parent or by another nurse has not been effective.
    4 Bringing in another nurse may frighten a small child; strange faces may upset the child instead of help calm him or her.
36. Knowledge, assessment, environment (a)
    2 This is the classic symptom of asthma, caused by trapping of air in the alveoli.
    1, 3, 4 This is not a symptom of asthma.
37. Comprehension, assessment, environment (b)
    2 These changes in the respiratory system lead to narrowing of the child's airway.
    1, 3, 4 This does not occur in asthma.
38. Knowledge, assessment, environment (a)
    1 Epinephrine is used in acute asthma because it is a fast-acting bronchodilator.
    2 Corticosteroids are not used in the acute stages of asthma.
    3 Ephedrine is not used in acute asthma.
    4 Cough syrup with codeine is not used in acute asthma.
39. Application, implementation, environment (b)
    2 25 lb = 11.3 kg
    100 mg × 11.3 kg/day = 1130 mg/day
    $$\frac{1130 \text{ mg}}{4 \text{ doses}} = 282 \text{ mg}$$
    Appropriate order = 250 mg qid.
    1, 3, 4 This is not an appropriate order for this infant.
40. Application, implementation, environment (b)
    3 DD = 300 mg
    DH = 500 mg
    V = 2 ml
    $$\frac{DD}{DH} = \frac{300 \text{ mg}}{500 \text{ mg}} \times 2 \text{ ml} = 1.2 \text{ ml}$$
    1, 2, 4 This is not the correct amount.
41. Knowledge, assessment, environment (a)
    2 "Binge" eating followed by induced vomiting is the classic symptom of bulimia.
    1 This is a symptom of anorexia nervosa.
    3, 4 This is not a symptom of bulimia.
42. Comprehension, assessment, environment (a)
    4 The Jones criteria are used only to diagnose rheumatic fever.
    1 This is a viral disease diagnosed by the symptoms and the Monospot test.
    2, 3 This is a hereditary disease.
43. Comprehension, assessment, environment (a)
    4 The infant with bronchiolitis needs oxygen to relieve his extreme dyspnea and resultant hypoxemia.
    1 Oxygen would not reduce a fever.
    2 This is not the primary reason for oxygen therapy.
    3 Oxygen would not liquefy secretions.
44. Comprehension, assessment, environment (b)
    1 Severe tachypnea seen in bronchiolitis is a contraindication for oral feedings.
    2 Bronchiolitis normally causes tachycardia.
    3, 4 This is not a contraindication for oral fluids.
45. Knowledge, assessment, physiologic (b)
    2 Toddlers use parallel play when playing with other children.
    1 Infants usually play alone or with an adult.
    3 Preschoolers use associative play.
    4 School-age children use associative play.
46. Comprehension, assessment, environment (b)
    4 Cerebral palsy is a disorder that affects the motor centers of the brain; it is usually caused by birth trauma or head trauma.
    1 This is a chromosomal abnormality.
    2 This is an S-shaped lateral curvature of the spine.
    3 This is an infection of the bone.
47. Comprehension, assessment, psychosocial (a)
    1 This statement about children's pain is true.
    2 Recovery from a painful experience does not occur faster in children.
    3 Narcotics are both safe and often necessary in the management of children's pain.
    4 Children do not have increased pain thresholds.
48. Knowledge, assessment, physiologic (a)
    3 The posterior fontanel closes by this age.
    1 This develops at 6 to 7 months of age.
    2 This develops at 8 to 9 months of age.
    4 This occurs at 7 to 8 months of age.
49. Knowledge, assessment, psychosocial (a)
    3 Although some SIDS occur later, most occur by 6 months of age.
    1, 2, 4 This is not true of SIDS.
50. Knowledge, assessment, health (a)
    4 These are the only two immunizations given at 2 months of age.
    1 The OPV is also given.
    2 The PPD is not given.
    3 The HbCV vaccine is not given.
51. Comprehension, assessment, health (b)
    3 Accidents of all types are the leading cause of death in this age level.
    1 Meningitis is seldom fatal.
    2 Leukemia occurs less often than accidents.
    4 Polio occurs only rarely.

52. Knowledge, assessment, physiologic (a)
    3 Hydrocephalus occurs when there is an obstruction of the cerebrospinal fluid drainage pathways.
    1 Opisthotonos is a sign of increased intracranial pressure.
    2 It does not cause the formation of a Wilms' tumor.
    4 It does not cause meningitis.
53. Knowledge, assessment, environment (a)
    3 The infant with FTT is very listless and floppy in posture.
    1, 2, 4 This is a characteristic of an infant with FTT.
54. Knowledge, assessment, environment (b)
    1 Gastroesophageal reflux is an organic (physical) cause of FTT.
    2 Nonorganic FTT is usually caused by psychosocial factors.
    3 Idiopathic FTT has no explainable cause.
    4 There is no classification with this name.
55. Comprehension, implementation, environment (b)
    4 This may indicate nerve damage at the fracture site or pressure from the cast and should be reported immediately.
    1, 2 This is a normal finding.
    3 This is usually a normal finding; any sudden increase in pain or severe muscle spasms should be reported to the physician.
56. Knowledge, assessment, psychosocial (b)
    4 In cases of child abuse, the history given by the caregiver does not fit with the severity or type of injury.
    1 This may occur with other types of injury as well as child abuse.
    2 This is not an indication of abuse; the child may not have been home at the time of the abuse or injury.
    3 This is not an indication of abuse.
57. Application, implementation, health (b)
    3 Introducing new foods one at a time helps to determine the infant's likes, dislikes, and possible allergies to certain foods.
    1 Mixing the food with formula does not allow the infant to taste the new food.
    2 Mixing the food with other foods does not allow the infant to taste the new food.
    4 New foods should be introduced one at a time for 2 to 3 days to determine possible allergies the infant might have.
58. Knowledge, assessment, physiologic (a)
    2 School-age children are in the stage of industry vs. inferiority.
    1 This is the developmental task in the preschooler.
    3 This is the developmental task in the adolescent.
    4 This is the developmental task in the young adult.
59. Knowledge, assessment, physiologic (b)
    3 Toddlers (age 1 to 3 years) are in the stage of autonomy vs. shame and doubt.
    1 Infants are in the stage of trust vs. mistrust.
    2 Preschoolers are in the stage of initiative vs. guilt.
    4 School-age children are in the stage of industry vs. inferiority.
60. Comprehension, assessment, environment (b)
    2 These are classic symptoms of an infant with pyloric stenosis.
    1 These are not symptoms of Hirschsprung's disease.
    3 These are not symptoms of esophageal atresia.
    4 These are not symptoms of intussusception.
61. Knowledge, assessment, environment (a)
    2 A child in sickle cell crisis often experiences abdominal pain, swollen, painful joints, and fever.
    1 Seizures and coma do not occur in sickle cell crisis.
    3 Polycythemia is not a symptom of sickle cell crisis.
    4 Severe itching is not a symptom of sickle cell crisis.

62. Knowledge, implementation, environment (b)
    2 Oxygen therapy to prevent tissue deoxygenation is of primary importance in sickle cell crisis.
    1 This is part of the treatment for children with chronic sickle cell disease.
    3 This may be part of the treatment in chronic sickle cell disease.
    4 Hydration is important in treating sickle cell crisis; however, oxygen therapy ranks first in order of importance.
63. Comprehension, assessment, environment (b)
    2 The Denis Browne splint is often used for the treatment of congenital clubfoot.
    1 It is not used to treat scoliosis.
    3 It is not used to treat DDH.
    4 It is not used to treat a fractured femur.
64. Application, planning, health (b)
    2 The child should not be told to "be brave"; child should be allowed to cry if something hurts.
    1, 3, 4 Should be covered during preoperative preparation of the child.
65. Knowledge, implementation, environment (b)
    3 This is the correct rate of infusion.
    1, 2 This rate is too slow.
    4 This rate is too fast.

Chapter 10: Gerontologic Nursing

1. Comprehension, assessment, environment (a)
   1 Pain and limited motion occur as the disease progresses. Extent of the knee flexion and extension is essential baseline data to provide a clear understanding of the patient's health status. Your nursing decisions and interventions will be based on this data.
   2, 3, 4 Important data, but not initially the most important.
2. Application, planning, environment (a)
   2 Continuous passive motion (CPM) device is used postoperatively to facilitate joint range-of-motion. Equipment to be used postoperatively should be introduced, demonstrated, and made familiar to the patient preoperatively.
   1 Not appropriate, enhances fracture healing.
   3 Not appropriate; skin traction is used for hip injuries before surgery.
   4 Not appropriate, used for tibia fractures.
3. Application, implementation, physiologic (a)
   1 Routine postoperative total knee replacement (TKR) care to control edema and bleeding.
   2 Not appropriate, used with postoperative total hip replacements (THR) to prevent acute hip flexion.
   3 Not appropriate, used with postoperative hip replacements.
   4 Not appropriate, used with postoperative hip replacements to keep hip in abduction.
4. Application, assessment, physiologic (a)
   3 Vasoconstriction will control bleeding and edema.
   1 CPM device is used to increase circulation and movement.
   2 Good infection-control measures will reduce the chance of infection.
   4 Wound suction drain will remove joint fluid accumulation.

5. Knowledge, assessment, environment (a)
   1 Fever (pyrexia) would be the earliest indication of pathogen invasion.
   2 Although pain is a symptom of inflammation, there will be some postoperative pain that would not necessarily indicate infection.
   3 Purulent drainage would indicate infection but usually is a later sign.
   4 Swelling, although a symptom of inflammation, would be expected postoperatively and by itself would not necessarily indicate infection.

6. Comprehension, planning, environment (a)
   3 Weight-bearing limits are always determined by the physician and depend on the surgical technique used, the patient's postoperative condition, and the type of prosthesis.
   1, 2, 4 Incorrect, because a physician's order is required for postoperative weight-bearing limits.

7. Comprehension, evaluation, health (a)
   3 5.1 fiber g/100 g
   1 0.3 fiber g/100 g
   2 2.1 fiber g/100 g
   4 0.8 fiber g/100 g

8. Application, planning, physiologic (a)
   4 Head of bed should be elevated to prevent movement of the hernia by gravity and passive reflux.
   1 Management includes frequent small feedings that can readily pass through the esophagus.
   2 Low-fat diets are usually less irritating and more readily digested, reducing discomfort and reflux.
   3 Patients should sit up for at least 1 hour after eating to prevent hernial movement and reflux.

9. Knowledge, assessment, physiologic (a)
   3 Alzheimer's disease is diagnosed by exclusion and confirmed only by autopsy.
   1, 2 CT and PET may refute or support a diagnosis, but they are not conclusive.
   4 Serial neuropsychologic testing will reveal progressive cognitive impairment but is not specific to Alzheimer's disease nor in any way diagnostically conclusive.

10. Application, implementation, environment (a)
    3 Distraction is facilitated by short-term memory loss and the least anxiety provoking.
    1 Security department presence implies force and will only increase the patient's anxiety and place him at risk for dysfunctional behavior.
    2 Although this may on occasion be an acceptable intervention, it is not the most appropriate.
    4 Again, force increases the patient's anxiety and places the patient's physical safety at risk.

11. Application, implementation, environment (b)
    3 Restlessness and agitation are best reduced by an active intervention such as walking.
    1, 2, 4 All are passive interventions that will not reduce the agitation and restlessness and produce the required calming effect.

12. Application, planning, environment (b)
    1 Hoeing is a repetitive action that does not require planning or decision making and therefore is the most appropriate activity.
    2, 3, 4 All require either planning and/or decision making and are not the most appropriate.

13. Comprehension, planning, environment (b)
    1 Excess environmental stimuli increase anxiety, are upsetting to the patient, and frequently precipitate a combative state.
    2, 4 These maintain cognitive function.
    3 Promotes physical safety.

14. Knowledge, assessment, environment (b)
    3 Drug toxicity is the only reversible state listed.
    1, 2, 4 All characterized by progression and are irreversible.

15. Application, implementation, environment (b)
    3 Pictures reduce environmental confusion and are good memory aids for the cognitively impaired.
    1 Unrealistic and does not promote independence in self-care activities.
    2 This would add to the patient's confusion.
    4 Never threaten a patient.

16. Application, implementation, physiologic (b)
    4 Convenient method for ensuring nutritional intake when the patient will not sit and eat a meal.
    1 Restraints are totally inappropriate and are used for patient safety only.
    2 This does not promote independence in self-care activities.
    3 Appropriate on a day-to-day basis but not the most appropriate when the patient won't stay seated.

17. Application, planning, environment (b)
    4 Short-term memory loss is characteristic of impaired cognition. If short sentences are used, it is easier for the patient to remember.
    1 Too much information for the patient to remember.
    2 This does not support the patient's cognitive function.
    3 Again, too much information for the patient to absorb and remember. Patient would also have difficulty remembering to look at the schedule.

18. Comprehension, planning, environment (b)
    3 This is the only answer choice that is accurate and demonstrates knowledge of agitated behavior.
    1 "All agitated patients" is an inappropriate generalization.
    2 Properly applied restraints released in accordance with facility policy along with other appropriate nursing measures will prevent decubiti.
    4 The use of restraints does not cause incontinence.

19. Application, assessment, psychosocial (a)
    4 This is the only response that demonstrates respect and courtesy.
    1, 2, 3 All inappropriate responses that fail to demonstrate compassion and understanding.

20. Application, implementation, psychosocial (b)
    1 This is the only response that does not chastise and humiliate the patient and that demonstrates an understanding of the situation.
    2, 3, 4 All inappropriate responses that fail to demonstrate compassion and understanding.

21. Knowledge, implementation, physiologic (a)
    1 The patient's daughter is asking the reason the drug is being given to her father. This is the only response that answers her question.
    2, 3, 4 Inappropriate: they do not acknowledge what the daughter has said, and they turn off communication.

22. Knowledge, assessment, physiologic (c)
    3 Toxic effects of Sinemet.
    1, 2, 4 These are symptoms of Parkinson's disease.

23. Comprehension, implementation, physiologic (b)
    2 This is accurate information and directly addresses the daughter's communication.
    1 Not necessary.
    3 Threatening response that turns off communication.
    4 Not necessary and inappropriate.

24. Application, implementation, physiologic (a)
    1 Administering medication before meals decreases gastric upset.
    2 Administering the medication on a full stomach will alter its absorption rate.
    3 Medications should never be mixed with a patient's food. Medications that are distasteful will turn the patient off to the food.
    4 The level of effectiveness of a medication is recorded and reported to the physician. Physicians prescribe and adjust dosage.
25. Comprehension, evaluation, environment (b)
    3 This is the only appropriate description.
    1, 2 Huntington's disease.
    4 Creutzfeldt-Jakob disease.
26. Application, implementation, physiologic (b)
    3 It's not imperative that Mrs. Jacobs take a once a day medication at exactly 9 AM. This type of person has mood alterations and often attempts to exert control by refusing medications and treatments and might well take it later if offered.
    1 A person with paranoid behavior would be threatened by this inappropriate action and might feel that the staff is trying to harm her.
    2 Appropriate to do this eventually but not until the individual has again been offered the medication.
    4 The nurse might have to do this ultimately, but not before the medication has again been offered.
27. Knowledge, assessment, environment (a)
    1 Hallucinations are not usually characteristic of paranoid behavior in the elderly.
    2, 3, 4 All are expected characteristics of paranoid behavior in the elderly.
28. Application, implementation, environment (b)
    2 Demonstrates therapeutic calmness and provides an atmosphere of acceptance of Mrs. Jacobs but not of her behavior.
    1 Not appropriate to reinforce unacceptable behavior.
    3 Reinforce beliefs of persecution or mistreatment by staff.
    4 Does not accept or acknowledge Mrs. Jacobs' problem and reinforces beliefs of persecution or mistreatment by staff.
29. Application, implementation, psychosocial (b)
    3 Refusal is not uncommon as Mrs. Jacobs struggles with feelings of powerlessness and unacceptable impulses.
    1, 2 Inappropriate, as you are assuming that Mrs. Jacobs doesn't like the food.
    4 Inappropriate, as sufficient time is not being provided for Mrs. Jacobs to use a more appropriate coping mechanism for whatever is bothering her.
30. Comprehension, evaluation, environment (a)
    3 Characteristically expressed feelings of being taken advantage of or plotted against.
    1, 2, 4 Mrs. Jacobs really isn't exhibiting any of these behaviors but rather is displaying subjective data of paranoia.
31. Knowledge, planning, psychosocial (a)
    1 Allows Mrs. Jacobs to function independently in an area where she can be successful.
    2, 3, 4 Would not be able to be successful with these activities because of debilitated state of her hands, and such activities would most likely increase her paranoia.
32. Comprehension, assessment, psychosocial (a)
    4 Moving at this time would threaten Mr. Fiore's feelings of safety and security, contributing further to his losses.
    1 Situation does not indicate paranoid behavior.
    2 Situation does not indicate eccentric behavior.
    3 Situation does not indicate that he's afraid to move but rather that he chooses not to experience additional losses.

33. Application, implementation, psychosocial (b)
    1 Informing the family of Mr. Fiore's concern should be sufficient to activate an appropriate plan of action in this case.
    2 Inappropriate response because it ignores Mr. Fiore's concern.
    3 It is inappropriate to suggest he experience another loss.
    4 Inappropriate nurse-patient relationship.
34. Knowledge, assessment, physiologic (a)
    4 The situation as presented does not indicate the cause.
    1, 2, 3 All are possible causes but inappropriate responses. Thorough assessment is required.
35. Comprehension, assessment, environment (a)
    1 Easier to digest and conserve energy.
    2 No indication in the situation for blenderized foods.
    3 No indication in the situation for warm liquids.
    4 Rolls do not stimulate the appetite.
36. Knowledge, assessment, environment (b)
    2 Impairment in orientation to time, place, and person is disorientation.
    1, 3, 4 These are signs of chronic brain syndrome, and the situation specifies a time impairment.
37. Application, implementation, physiologic (a)
    4 This is the only nursing intervention that meets the patient's needs and that is appropriate.
    1, 2 These actions reinforce guilt, shame, and embarrassment, which should never be done.
    3 If the patient has just voided, it's unlikely he would have to void again so soon—not the most appropriate response.
38. Comprehension, assessment, physiologic (a)
    4 This is a common cause of constipation in the elderly.
    1 Too much fiber in the diet does not cause constipation.
    2 Too much bulk in the diet does not cause constipation.
    3 Daily laxatives are a common cause of constipation in the elderly.
39. Comprehension, assessment, psychosocial (c)
    2 Hoarding is a manifestation of insecurity.
    1 Decreased self-esteem is associated with role losses and is not related to hoarding.
    3, 4 Increased confusion and disorientation are symptoms of organic brain syndrome and are not related to hoarding.
40. Comprehension, planning, environment (b)
    1 Characteristic of the aging process.
    2 Thorough assessment should be done before medication is given.
    3 Sleep time does not necessarily change in the elderly but rather the quality and continuity of sleep patterns change.
    4 This would not be compatible with the rest needs of the patient.

Chapter 11: Emergency Nursing

1. Comprehension, assessment, physiologic (c)
   4 General symptoms of unstable fractures of the pelvic ring include ecchymosis, deformity, edema, pain in weight bearing, and tenderness over the celiac crest, anterior disk spines, sacrum, coccyx, or symphysis pubis.
   1 Bowel sounds are monitored in patients with a fractured sacrum.
   2 External rotation of the leg is a clinical manifestation of a hip fracture.
   3 Pain on defecation and sitting are characteristic of coccyx fractures.

2. Comprehension, implementation, physiologic (a)
   1 Hemorrhage is a serious, life-threatening complication of pelvic fractures, and the physician should be notified immediately of the observation.
   2 Although the physician may order a stool guaiac reaction test, the priority is to notify the physician of the observation.
   3 Not a priority in a life-threatening situation.
   4 To wait for the next stool specimen would be a highly inappropriate delay in essential medical care.

3. Application, implementation, physiologic (c)
   1 The priority is always A, B, C: airway, breathing, and circulation.
   2 Although important, not the priority.
   3 Necessary and important, but not the priority.
   4 A person cannot breathe unless the airway is patent.

4. Application, planning, environment (b)
   3 CDC recommends using universal precautions at all times.
   1 In emergency situations, patients are often not able to provide accurate information.
   2 Highly impractical.
   4 Inappropriate to rely on only the obvious.

5. Comprehension, assessment, psychosocial (b)
   2 Acute disorganization that characteristically follows sexual assault is either verbally expressed or hidden. Regardless of the manner of expression, the survivor experiences feelings of shock, anger, guilt, humiliation, and even fear.
   1, 3 Usually follows acute disorganization and precedes reorganization.
   4 Reorganization indicates that the survivor has put the event in perspective and moves toward some degree of recovery.

6. Comprehension, planning, psychosocial (c)
   2 The only appropriately written short-term goals: patient centered, realistic, reachable, time oriented.
   1, 3, 4 Long-term goals.

7. Application, implementation, physiologic (b)
   3 With an unconscious victim the priority is airway. To open the airway the victim first has to be properly positioned.
   1, 2, 4 Appropriate, but not done first.

8. Application, implementation, physiologic (a)
   2 With an unconscious victim the priority is always airway, breathing, and circulation.
   1 This assumes that Mr. Meshel is in insulin shock.
   3 This assumes that Mr. Meshel is in diabetic coma.
   4 Mouth-to-mouth resuscitation cannot be given until a patent airway has been established.

9. Application, implementation, physiologic (a)
   4 Always continue breathing until help arrives or victim spontaneously resumes breathing.
   1 You do not compress the sternum in the presence of a pulse.
   2 The victim must be in a supine position.
   3 This measure is performed in the presence of an upper airway obstruction only.

10. Application, evaluation, physiologic (a)
    1 Reassessment is done every minute until spontaneous resumption of breathing.
    2 This measure is performed immediately after establishing an airway.
    3 Sharp blow to the chest is not performed at all during CPR.
    4 This measure is performed as part of the procedure for clearing an upper airway obstruction.

11. Knowledge, planning, physiologic (a)
    1 Standard CPR procedure calls for a 15:2 count for 60 seconds providing 80 compressions in one-rescuer CPR.
    2, 3, 4 Inadequate compression.

12. Knowledge, implementation, environment (b)
    3 This distance prevents damage to ribs and internal structures while providing adequate cardiac output.
    1 May cause lower rib damage and low cardiac output.
    2 May cause internal organ damage and no cardiac output.
    4 May cause left lower rib damage.

13. Knowledge, planning, physiologic (a)
    4 In two-rescuer CPR the standard ratio of compression to breaths is 5:1.
    1 15:2 is correct for one-rescuer CPR.
    2 Overventilation.
    3 Too many compressions for two-rescuer CPR.

14. Knowledge, planning, physiologic (b)
    4 Standard rescue breathing procedure.
    1 Breaths should be full but at 1½ to 2 seconds per breath, allowing the lungs to deflate between breaths.
    2 Breaths should be given at the lowest possible pressure to avoid gastric distention.
    3 Not standard rescue breathing procedure.

15. Application, implementation, physiologic (a)
    1 Do not interfere if he can cough, speak, or breathe. To determine if a person is choking, ask him.
    2, 3 Need not indicated in the situation.
    4 Back blows are not administered to a person who may be choking.

16. Application, assessment, physiologic (b)
    4 Very young and the elderly are at greatest risk.
    1, 2, 3 Neither very young nor elderly.

17. Application, implementation, physiologic (a)
    2 Victim is displaying signs of respiratory distress. Airway and breathing are the priorities.
    1, 3, 4 Are interventions for shock that follow establishment of airway, breathing, and circulation.

18. Comprehension, assessment, physiologic (a)
    1 Body itching is the only systemic sign listed.
    2, 3, 4 Identified as localized signs.

19. Comprehension, evaluation, physiologic (a)
    2 Epinephrine's therapeutic effects are bronchodilation, cardiac stimulation, vasoconstriction, and reversing the symptoms of an anaphylactic reaction.
    1 Epinephrine does not have a sedative effect.
    3 Not an effect of Epinephrine. Antihistamines and steroids are given to reduce recurrence of symptoms.
    4 Epinephrine is not an antianxiety medication.

20. Application, implementation, physiologic (a)
    1 Radial artery can be sufficiently damaged in a crush injury so that it won't be palpable. Whenever a pulse cannot be palpated, move on to the next major artery to check circulation.
    2, 3 No indication of need in the situation.
    4 Take care of airway, breathing, and circulation first; send another person to activate EMS if you can.

21. Comprehension, implementation, physiologic (a)
    1 All are correct interventions for hemorrhage, but the priority is to stop or control the bleeding.
    2 Appropriate intervention after bleeding is under control.
    3 After applying pressure the affected body part should be elevated to aid in control of hemorrhage.
    4 Movement stimulates circulation; immobilization will aid in controlling hemorrhage.

22. Comprehension, assessment, physiologic (b)
    3 Emergency nursing calls for a rapid clinical assessment with emphasis on airway, breathing, circulation, establishing priorities, and then the instituting of lifesaving measures.
    1 Although calling for help is important, it is not the priority.
    2 Not the priority.
    4 Good Samaritan law should be known before traveling out of home state.
23. Application, implementation, physiologic (c)
    4 Priority is always airway, breathing, and circulation.
    1, 2, 3 Appropriate, but not the highest priority.
24. Comprehension, implementation, physiologic (b)
    2 Priority is always airway, breathing, and circulation.
    1 Appropriate, but not the immediate priority.
    3 The lower extremities are elevated to treat shock.
    4 Shock has already been established.
25. Knowledge, implementation, physiologic (a)
    1 The first step in treating hemorrhage is to apply pressure for at least 6 minutes.
    2 Application of ice is not an emergency measure.
    3 Elevating the affected part aids in controlling the bleeding but would not stop it.
    4 This action will not stop occipital bleeding.
26. Knowledge, implementation, physiologic (b)
    2 These are appropriate assessments of circulation.
    1, 3 This may cause further damage to the ulna.
    4 Prevention is not part of assessment.
27. Application, implementation, environment (b)
    1 Victim requires immediate medical care.
    2 Appropriate but not the first priority.
    3 Inappropriate, as victim needs immediate medical care.
    4 Referring a victim to a physician does not put you at legal risk. Not referring a victim to a physician could result in legal action being initiated against you.
28. Knowledge, assessment, environment (a)
    1 The very young and the elderly are especially at risk.
    2, 3, 4 Not at risk, as are neither very young or elderly.
29. Knowledge, assessment, physiologic (a)
    3 Prevents edema, facilitates vasoconstriction, increases blood viscosity, and acts as a local anesthetic.
    1 Treatment of a strain.
    2, 4 Treatment of a fracture.
30. Application, planning, physiologic (a)
    1 Oxygenation is compromised, and airway is always the priority.
    2 Oxygenation will be compromised if the hemorrhaging is not controlled or stopped.
    3 No immediate problem with airway, breathing, and circulation.
    4 Fractures are suspected at multiple trauma scenes. The priorities are always airway, breathing, and circulation—in that order.
31. Application, implementation, physiologic (a)
    3 The hemodynamic instability following burn injury must be stopped to proceed with airway, breathing, and circulation and prevent further trauma to the victim.
    1 Situation does not indicate that CPR is necessary.
    2, 4 Appropriate, but not the priority.
32. Application, implementation, physiologic (a)
    3 Bleach is a corrosive substance, which should be diluted only if the victim is conscious.
    1, 2 Do not do anything besides call the poison control center if you are not absolutely sure of the antidote.
    4 Do not induce vomiting. This could cause burning of the esophagus, throat, and mouth.

33. Application, implementation, physiologic (a)
    2 The chemical will continue to burn the victim as long as it is on the skin.
    1 Ice or ice water should not be used in burns because the burn has decreased the body's ability to retain heat. Overcooling will further increase metabolic demands.
    3 Appropriate, but not the priority.
    4 Stop the burning first, then proceed with airway, breathing, and circulation.
34. Comprehension, implementation, physiologic (a)
    4 These products seal in the heat, causing further trauma to the victim.
    1 Burns left open place the victim at further risk for infection.
    2 Ice should not be applied because it causes body heat loss, thereby placing the victim at further risk.
    3 Blisters should not be broken. Intact skin prevents infection.
35. Application, implementation, physiologic (b)
    4 This is the only position that will prevent the victim from swallowing blood and being at risk for aspiration.
    1, 2, 3 Victim at risk for aspiration.

Chapter 12: Current Trends in Nursing and Health Care in the United States and Canada

1. Knowledge (a)
   4 Each state's board of nursing approves nursing programs.
   1, 2, 3 NAPNES, the NLN, and the federal government have no role in approving nursing programs.
2. Knowledge (a)
   2 Voluntary accreditation may be sought by nursing programs through the NLN.
   1, 3, 4 NAPNES, the federal government, and state boards of nursing have no role in accreditation.
3. Comprehension (a)
   1 Each individual has a responsibility to professional growth and accountability.
   2 Continuing education can be obtained through the employer, publications, nursing organizations, and private providers.
   3 Continuing education is required by *some* states.
   4 The NLN has no requirements regarding individuals' continuing education.
4. Comprehension (a)
   3 Hospitalized psychiatric patients are generally considered unstable. Therefore the LP/VN would assist in the patient's care—not be in charge on night shift.
   1, 2, 4 Under the supervision of a registered nurse or physician, these are all accepted roles of the LP/VN.
5. Knowledge (a)
   4 Each state's nurse practice act determines the LP/VNs' functions in that state.
   1, 2, 3 The ANA, NCSBN, and the NLN have no legal role in determining the role of LP/VNs.
6. Knowledge (a)
   4 The medical record is the property of the hospital and the contents the property of the patient.
   1 The medical record is confidential information and only authorized personnel may have access to it. Patient must give permission for others to view.
   2 Legal document that must be safeguarded by hospital after discharge.
   3 See rationale for statement 2.

7. Comprehension (a)
   2 In the functional method, each person is assigned specific tasks or functions.
   1 The district method of providing nursing care is the same as the team method but usually in a smaller geographic area.
   3 In the primary method, the registered nurse has total responsibility for specific patients.
   4 In team nursing a group of patients is cared for by a team of nursing personnel.

8. Knowledge (a)
   1 Trust must be established at the beginning of the nurse-patient relationship.
   2 There is no interim phase in the nurse-patient relationship.
   3 The working phase begins when trust has been established.
   4 The termination phase is the period of time preceding separation.

9. Comprehension (a)
   2 To develop a relationship the nurse must first understand self including attitudes, values, and beliefs.
   1 Part of the initiation phase.
   3 Not necessary to know at the beginning of the relationship.
   4 Not necessary to build the relationship.

10. Knowledge (a)
    2 Role of LP/VN is to give nursing care to patients whose condition is stable.
    1 Critical care nursing may have LP/VN on team but not usual position for LP/VN.
    3, 4 RN assumes responsibility for care of patients in complex situation.

11. Knowledge (a)
    2 Each LP/VN has the responsibility to practice professionally and ethically.
    1, 3, 4 Various nursing organizations may establish standards of practice and codes of ethics, but the individual LP/VN must uphold them.

12. Comprehension (b)
    2 This is negligence—a tort.
    1 Assault is a threat or attempt to do harm.
    3 Battery is making contact with a patient without the patient's permission.
    4 Acting unwisely or without caution; not a legal charge.

13. Knowledge (a)
    4 WHO definition of health.
    1 There is more to health than physical aspects.
    2 Lack of evidence of chronic or acute illness does not constitute wellness.
    3 Lack of evidence of disability does not constitute wellness.

14. Knowledge (a)
    3 Emphasis is on prevention of illness and maintenance of health.
    1 Previous focus; technical advances have decreased communicable diseases in the United States.
    2 Chronic illness does not necessarily require hospitalization.
    4 DRGs are promoting shorter hospitalization.

15. Comprehension (b)
    2 Secondary care includes early diagnosis and treatment of disease.
    1 Primary care implies health promotion and disease prevention.
    3 Restoration of health is a goal but not one of the three levels of health care delivery.
    4 Tertiary care involves returning a patient to maximum functioning.

16. Comprehension (b)
    3 Primary health care is the promotion of health and prevention of disease.
    1 Tertiary care.
    2 Tertiary health care with rehabilitation measures.
    4 Secondary health care.

17. Knowledge (a)
    4 This is tertiary care—returning a patient to maximum functioning.
    1 Primary care involves health promotion and disease prevention.
    2 Secondary care involves early diagnosis and treatment of disease.
    3 Restoration of health is a goal but not one of the three levels of health care delivery.

18. Comprehension (b)
    4 High-level wellness is functioning at one's best.
    1 Level of wellness depends on mental as well as physical factors.
    2 Individual ability to adapt to factors.
    3 Level of wellness is continually changing.

19. Knowledge (a)
    1 The unnecessary restriction of the freedom of another.
    2, 4 Not a legal term.
    3 Restraints must be ordered by a physician.

20. Knowledge (a)
    1 Most practical method of rendering effective and efficient patient care, because nursing personnel work to the maximum of their ability.
    2 Nurses are accountable to give good nursing care no matter what type of care system the hospital utilizes.
    3 Student nurses are under the direction of a registered nurse instructor, who may use method for student to gain leadership skills.
    4 Assigning team members to tasks best suited for their individual capabilities provides quality care for patient.

21. Comprehension (a)
    3 Hospitals are legally responsible for reporting suspected cases of child abuse to the designated law enforcement or health and welfare agency.
    1 A subjective sign, but child may be shy and may not be able to communicate rationales for bruises.
    2 Subjective sign, mother's comment may or may not be factual.
    4 Objective sign, which the nurse is in key position to observe.

22. Knowledge (a)
    1 Patient's Bill of Rights is a statement of what the patient can expect from the institution, which includes the staff.
    2 Recreation activities: recreation therapy and volunteer departments.
    3 Choices can only be within diet orders from physician.
    4 American Medical Association affiliation not concern of Patient's Bill of Rights.

23. Knowledge (b)
    2 A beneficiary of a will is not permitted to serve as a witness to the signing of a will.
    1 Not necessary to serve as a witness to signing.
    3 Not necessary.
    4 Not legally necessary; may be an agency policy.

24. Knowledge (a)
    2 Organized to promote the development of practical/vocational nursing education and recognition of the LP/VN as a member of the health team; first national organization to accredit practical nursing schools.
    1 Organized in 1912 and major interest was registered nursing schools. In 1949 established practical nurse council.
    3 Organized in 1949 to foster standard in practical nursing and practical nurse education.
    4 National organization and official organization for RNs.

25. Comprehension (b)
    2 Invasion of privacy is the unauthorized disclosure about a patient even if the information is true.
    1 Defamation is an attack on another through false and malicious statements to a third person.
    3 Libel is written, false and malicious statements to a third person.
    4 Slander is oral, false and malicious statements to a third person.
26. Comprehension (b)
    2 Advocate acts on behalf of another person.
    1 Advocate supports patient with his decision.
    3 May arrange to have someone from billing department to advise.
    4 May act on behalf, via social services department.
27. Comprehension (b)
    2 Good Samaritan laws provide legal protection only during an actual emergency in a noninstitutional setting.
    1 Not necessary.
    3 Care rendered must not be carried out recklessly.
    4 Good Samaritan laws cover care rendered; statements could be invasions of privacy or defamation.
28. Knowledge (b)
    1 Insurance provided by an employer generally only covers the employee while on duty.
    2, 3 Most malpractice insurance policies cover all but fraud and purposeful injury.
    4 Unless the situation was an actual emergency, it would not be covered by a Good Samaritan law.
29. Knowledge (a)
    1 Organizations sponsor seminars and conventions; magazines contain valuable information.
    2 State boards do not require membership in a nursing organization.
    3 Membership in an organization is not required for licensure renewal.
    4 Although organizations may offer reduced premium insurance, merely belonging to an organization does not reduce premiums.
30. Knowledge (b)
    3 Membership in the NFLPN is open only to LP/VNs and student P/VNs.
    1 Membership in NAPNES is open to LP/VNs, RNs, agency administrators, and interested laypersons.
    2 Only state boards of nursing belong to the NCSBN.
    4 Membership in the NLN is open to anyone interested in nursing.
31. Knowledge (a)
    3 Most malpractice insurance companies will advise and recommend course of action.
    1 Expected, but not necessary.
    2 Not necessary.
    4 Not an interested party.

32. Knowledge (a)
    2 The ANA publishes the *AJN.*
    1 The AHA does not publish a nursing journal.
    3 NAPNES publishes the *Journal of Practical Nursing.*
    4 The NFLPN does not publish a journal.
33. Knowledge (a)
    2 Hospital admissions divided into diagnosis-related groups (DRGs) and payment will be made based on the average cost of each category.
    1, 3, 4 Not applicable.
34. Knowledge (a)
    4 Voluntary agencies such as the American Cancer Society receive donations from the public and make no profit.
    1, 2, 3 These are official agencies supported by tax dollars.
35. Knowledge (a)
    2 The LP/VN is accountable for own actions.
    1, 3, 4 May be included in suit.
36. Knowledge (a)
    2 Health care delivery is a provincial responsibility in Canada.
    1 Federal health legislation applies to matters of national or international nature, for example, testing new drugs.
    3 Regulatory bodies are provincial, not local.
    4 Professional associations are provincial, not local.
37. Knowledge (a)
    4 All are included for the reasons listed below.
    1 Admission requirements vary from province to province.
    2 Each province designates a body to approve and review nursing schools.
    3 Certification, registration, and licensure assure the public of a minimum standard of safe nursing care.
38. Comprehension (a)
    2 This answer is correct.
    1 An RN has responsibility for the nursing team in institutional-type settings.
    3 The RN is responsible for the direction, not the supervision, of the practical/vocational nurse.
    4 The practical/vocational nurse cares for a variety of patients with different degrees of responsibility, depending on the complexity of care needed.
39. Knowledge (a)
    3 This answer is correct.
    1 The standards of care set by the regulatory bodies protect the public.
    2 Each registrant is responsible for his or her own practice.
    4 Licensure protects the actual acts within the practice of nursing.
40. Knowledge (a)
    3 This is the correct answer.
    1 Other than in Alberta and Quebec, certification, registration, licensing examinations are set by the Canadian Nurses Association Testing Service in Ottawa.
    2 Laws are passed by the provincial legislature.
    4 Regulatory bodies decide whether there is negligence in the individual practice of nursing, and are completely autonomous from the criminal court system.

ANSWERS AND RATIONALES FOR COMPREHENSIVE EXAMINATIONS

Comprehensive Examination 1: Part 1

1. Comprehension, assessment, environment (b)
   4 The right eye will have a dressing after surgery; nursing care plan will consider sight (or limitations) in left eye for the immediate postoperative period.
   1 Will not alter nursing care.
   2, 3 While these are considerations in care, sight should be restored after surgery.
2. Comprehension, assessment, physiologic (a)
   1 Usually the only symptom of a tumor in the GU tract.
   2, 3, 4 Frequent problems related to aging.
3. Application, implementation, physiologic (a)
   2 Assists in preventing hypostatic pneumonia.
   1 Turn only when there is a medical order.
   3, 4 Coughing is to be avoided after eye surgery.
4. Comprehension, assessment, physiologic (b)
   3 Vomiting must be avoided.
   1 Physician's preference will determine length of bed rest.
   2 The patient may eat as tolerated.
   4 With lenses (glasses or contact lenses) the patient will be able to see and resume activities.
5. Knowledge, assessment, environment (a)
   2 Usual patient description.
   1 There are no halos (glaucoma).
   3 Vision is not blurred (glaucoma).
   4 There is no exudate (conjunctivitis).
6. Comprehension, assessment, physiologic (b)
   3 In skim milk much of the fat has been removed. Lean fish and fruit contain little fat.
   1 Whole milk and pastry contain considerable fat.
   2 Fried potatoes and avocado contain fat.
   4 Ham and creamed peas are high in fat content.
7. Comprehension, planning, physiologic (b)
   1 Fresh or frozen beef is permitted. Also fresh fruits and vegetables have very little sodium.
   2 All smoked, processed, and canned meats are high in sodium. Most frozen foods have sodium added.
   3 Corned beef and dill pickles are high in sodium.
   4 Ham, cheeses, and regular bread are high in sodium.
8. Application, implementation, physiologic (b)
   4 The fall in blood sugar decreases available glucose for cell metabolism, causing the motor and sensory symptoms; because the brain does not store glucose, a depletion of available glucose for metabolism affects the brain cells, rapidly causing the CNS symptoms: irritability, confusion, etc.
   1 Symptoms of hyperglycemia.
   2 Symptoms of thyrotoxicosis.
   3 Symptoms of hypovolemic shock.
9. Comprehension, assessment, physiologic (a)
   2 Insulin overdose, excessive exercise, illness, or insufficient food intake may cause insufficient glucose to be available, causing abnormally low blood sugar.
   1 Produces diabetic coma or acidosis.
   3 Excessive insulin causes shock.
   4 Produces diabetic acidosis.
10. Comprehension, implementation, physiologic (b)
    3 The discarded specimen consists of urine produced before 8 AM of the first day. Urine produced and voided within 24 hours is necessary for the specimen.
    1 Collecting urine from only two voidings during a 24-hour period does not constitute a 24-hour collection.
    2 Discarding the urine produced at 8 AM of the second day would mean that some urine produced within the 24 hours would not be included in the specimen.
    4 Including the first day's 8 AM urine would mean that the specimen included urine produced during more than a 24-hour period.
11. Comprehension, assessment, physiologic (a)
    3 These signs are normal for a 2-day-old newborn.
    1 This is a full-term infant, so she cannot be premature.
    2 There is no indication in the situation that the infant is immature.
    4 Nothing abnormal is reported in the situation.
12. Comprehension, assessment, physiologic (b)
    2 The sperm no longer has an outlet from the body; thus the male can no longer reproduce.
    1 A vasectomy does not change the man's ability to have an erection or an ejaculation.
    3 Cryptorchidism is a developmental defect of failure of the testes to descend into the scrotum.
    4 Epididymitis is the inflammation of the epididymis.
13. Comprehension, assessment, physiologic (b)
    1 The gland surrounds the urethra and when inflamed and enlarged squeezes on the urethra and causes constriction.
    2 Cryptochidism is a developmental defect, failure of the testes to descend into the scrotum.
    3 Sperm is produced in the seminiferous tubules of the testes.
    4 Semen is produced in Cowper's glands.
14. Knowledge, assessment, physiologic (b)
    2 Correct; drainage is white or yellow and curdlike.
    1 Discharge is white or yellow, frothy, and malodorous.
    3 Discharge is profuse, yellow, and mucoid.
    4 Discharge, if noted at all, is puslike and yellow.
15. Knowledge, planning, physiologic (b)
    3 Usual medication for this condition.
    1 Acetic acid douches would be used, not alkaline douches.
    2 Flagyl is used in treating *Trichomonas vaginalis*.
    4 Penicillin is used in treating gonorrhea.
16. Knowledge, implementation, physiologic (b)
    2 Priority action is always airway, breathing, and circulation.
    1 Tourniquet is used only as a last resort.
    3 Appropriate, but not the first nursing action.
    4 Not an appropriate emergency measure.
17. Knowledge, assessment, physiologic (b)
    2 Hypovolemic shock results from decreased circulating blood volume.
    1 Cardiogenic shock is caused by reduced cardiac output from faulty pumping.
    3 Neurogenic shock results from decreased circulating blood volume due to disruption of vasomotor tone.
    4 Septic shock results from bacterial infection.
18. Knowledge, assessment, physiologic (a)
    4 Shallow, rapid respirations are a sign of shock.
    1 Decreased systolic and diastolic blood pressure is a sign of shock.
    2 Decreased urine output is a sign of shock.
    3 Feeble, weak, or thready pulse is a sign of shock.

19. Knowledge, implementation, physiologic (a)
    3 Pressure applied for at least 6 minutes is the first measure of control.
    1 Tourniquets are not recommended unless an extremity is amputated or severely mutilated.
    2 Done only if application of direct pressure does not control the bleeding.
    4 Tourniquets are not recommended unless an extremity is amputated or severely mutilated.
20. Comprehension, planning, physiologic (c)
    3 Brachial artery is the supplying artery; this is done when application of direct pressure does not control bleeding.
    1 Tourniquets are not recommended unless an extremity is amputated or severely mutilated.
    2 Direct pressure has already been applied unsuccessfully.
    4 Not the immediate supplying artery.
21. Comprehension, planning, physiologic (c)
    4 Tourniquet is removed only by a physician and under conditions where emergency medical support equipment is available.
    1, 2, 3 Once applied, a tourniquet is removed only by a physician.
22. Knowledge, assessment, physiologic (b)
    4 The hemoglobin is decreased, not increased, in sickle cell crisis.
    1, 2, 3 Common symptom of sickle cell crisis.
23. Knowledge assessment, health (a)
    2 Sickle cell disease is caused by a hereditary trait that occurs primarily among the black race.
    1 It is not a viral disease.
    3 It is not a bacterial disease.
    4 It is not caused by a mismatched blood transfusion.
24. Knowledge, assessment, health (b)
    2 School-age children are in this stage of development.
    1 Toddlers are in this stage of development.
    3 Preschoolers are in this stage of development.
    4 Infants are in this stage of development.
25. Knowledge, assessment, physiologic (a)
    2 Caused by ulcerated mucosal lining.
    1 Pancreatic symptoms.
    3 Not associated with ulcers.
    4 Symptoms of appendicitis and peritonitis.
26. Knowledge, assessment, physiologic (b)
    1 Ulcer erodes through blood vessel(s); can erode through all the gastric layers; scarring can cause obstruction.
    2 Pancreatitis is not associated with ulcers.
    3 Jaundice and anemia are not associated with ulcers.
    4 Hepatitis and cholecystitis are not associated with ulcers.
27. Comprehension, assessment, physiologic (b)
    4 An overabundance of parietal cells could cause overproduction.
    1 Not picked up on anaylsis; cause of diarrhea.
    2 Not picked up on analysis; cause of nausea and ileus.
    3 Associated with cancer of the stomach.
28. Comprehension, planning, health (a)
    3 Drugs and diet are needed long after the symptoms have ceased.
    1 Physical and emotional rest are needed with a gradual return to activity.
    2 Bland diet is usually prescribed.
    4 Use could lead to metabolic imbalances.
29. Comprehension, assessment, physiologic (a)
    4 Result from mechanical barrier to gastric flow usually caused by scarring.
    1 Gallbladder disorder does not occur as a result of peptic ulcers.
    2 Coffee ground emesis would be a key symptom.
    3 Signaled by fever and abdominal rigidity.

30. Knowledge, planning, physiologic (b)
    3 Protein sources (meat, fish, poultry, and eggs) are often restricted for a person with liver disease in order to limit the end products of protein metabolism.
    1 Fruits are not protein.
    2 Vegetables are not protein sources.
    4 Carbohydrates are not protein.
31. Knowledge, planning, physiologic (a)
    3 A person with a duodenal ulcer is often advised to avoid all food that could be irritating to the intestinal mucosa. This would include all raw foods, which are generally high residue and therefore more irritating.
    1 Refined cereals are lower in residue as a result of processing.
    2 Protein in most cases is not contraindicated.
    4 Broiling is an acceptable way to prepare foods for an ulcer patient.
32. Comprehension, planning, health (b)
    2 One egg is equivalent on the exchange list to 1 ounce of fish.
    1 Bacon is a fat exchange.
    3 Pumpkin is on the vegetable exchange.
    4 Milk is on the milk exchange.
33. Comprehension, implementation, environment (b)
    2 Moisture carries organisms by capillary action, thus rendering the field contaminated.
    1 Sterile sponges placed on a wet area of the field would be contaminated.
    3 Drying would be impossible.
    4 Removing would be impossible. Whatever would be used to cover the area would also become moist, thus contaminated.
34. Knowledge, assessment, physiologic (a)
    4 After injury to tissues there is a dilation of small blood vessels, bringing an increased amount of blood flow to the area, resulting in redness and heat.
    1 Bleeding is not an indication of inflammation.
    2 Bruising is not an indication of inflammation.
    3 Coolness is not an indication of inflammation.
35. Application, implementation, environment (a)
    2 Isolation keeps pathogens confined to a specific area, thus reducing transmission to others.
    1 Mere isolation does nothing to destroy or reduce the numbers of microorganisms.
    3 Isolation helps protect other patients and all members of the health care team.
    4 Would be provided only by reverse isolation.
36. Application, implementation, health (b)
    4 Contaminated gown and gloves cannot be worn outside the isolation unit.
    1 Would need to be done before removing gown and gloves so that hands and arms are not exposed to contaminated linens.
    2 Thermometer would be left in the patient's room until patient is discharged or isolation discontinued.
    3 Tray would be handled while the nurse was still gowned and gloved.
37. Knowledge, assessment, environment (a)
    1 Nosocomial infections are acquired in the hospital.
    2 Local infections are confined to a specific location.
    3 Systemic infections have spread throughout the body.
    4 Infections producing septic shock are those generally caused by gram-negative organisms.
38. Comprehension, assessment, physiologic (a)
    1 May reduce circulation.
    2, 3, 4 Contributes to healing.
39. Comprehension, assessment, health (b)
    3 It is not possible to feel more beats at the radial artery than are originating from the heart.
    1, 2, 4 This is possible.

40. Knowledge, assessment, physiologic (a)
    1 Bradycardia is a heart rate under 60 beats/min.
    2 Normal range.
    3 Higher rate than bradycardia.
    4 Tachycardia.
41. Knowledge, assessment, psychosocial (b)
    1 Anxiety is a manifestation of conflict.
    2 Homeostasis is a steady state unrelated to conflict.
    3 Panic is usually not seen in conflict unless anxiety is extreme.
    4 Motivation: conflict may motivate, but this is not always present.
42. Knowledge, assessment, health (b)
    3 Oral, because most therapeutic communications have this component.
    1 Written communication is infrequently used in patient-nurse interactions.
    2 Although nonverbal is very important, it is almost always accompanied by verbal communications.
    4 Proxemics are another form of nonverbal communications.
43. Knowledge, assessment, psychosocial (a)
    2 Everyone uses defenses at times.
    1 May not be pathologic.
    3 Usually are effective.
    4 Are not rewarding in that they are unconscious.
44. Knowledge, planning, health (a)
    1 Evaluation includes new problem identification.
    2 Is usually informal.
    3 Frequently involves family.
    4 Requires no special staff.
45. Comprehension, implementation, psychosocial (a)
    3 To allow feedback is essential.
    1 Logical argument may block communication.
    2 Questioning may block communication.
    4 Advising may block communication.
46. Comprehension, assessment, psychosocial (a)
    3 Relatively fixed over time.
    1 Potentially true; may be combined with statement 2.
    2 Potentially true; may be combined with statement 1.
    4 Is consistent over time.
47. Comprehension, assessment, psychosocial (b)
    1 Freudian theory defines three parts.
    2 Stress is not particular to this theory.
    3 All theories have statements about mediation of reality.
    4 Personality is relatively consistent.
48. Knowledge, assessment, psychosocial (a)
    4 A myth.
    1, 2, 3 Not true.
49. Analysis, assessment, psychosocial (b)
    2 Projection is assigning one's feelings to others.
    1 Repression pushes material out of consciousness.
    3 Displacement places angry feelings onto a safer object.
    4 Rationalization applies logical reasons to guard against feelings.
50. Comprehension, assessment, psychosocial (b)
    4 Sublimation channels unacceptable drives into socially acceptable behaviors.
    1 Projection is placing one's feelings onto others.
    2 In conversion, physical symptoms replace feelings.
    3 Intellectualization is the process of applying intellect to cover feelings.
51. Knowledge, evaluation, health (a)
    2 Best possible answer.
    1 Both Sally and Bob are at an ideal age.
    3 Nothing in the situation or question itself suggests this.
    4 The length of time between pregnancies does not alter the ability to conceive in this case.

52. Knowledge, assessment, physiologic (a)
    2 Correct.
    1 Wrong; she has been pregnant twice and has delivered one child.
    3 Wrong; pregnant twice.
    4 Wrong; pregnant twice but has only delivered one child.
53. Comprenension, assessment, physiologic (a)
    4 Nägele's rule: subtract 3 months and add 7 days to LMP.

    $$\begin{array}{cc} 4 & 24 \\ -3 & +7 \end{array}$$

    Answer: 1   31 (January 31)—correct.
    1 4 + 9 = 13 = January
    24 − 7 = 17
    Answer: January 17—wrong.
    2 10 lunar months—February
    February does not have 31 days, so 24 + 7 = 31
    Answer: March 3—wrong.
    3 Using 10 lunar months:
    4 + 10 = 14 or February 24 − 7 = 17
    Answer: February 17—wrong.
54. Application, implementation, environment (a)
    4 Best response: explanation and valid reason given; kind and courteous.
    1 Wrong. No solids given during active labor; prevents vomiting and thus aspiration, especially if anesthesia is necessary.
    2 Too technical and flippant; no jokes.
    3 Abrupt; no compassion; no explanation.
55. Knowledge, implementation, physiologic (a)
    2 First priority.
    1 Not first priority.
    3 Physician knows; not necessary to do test unless you are asked.
    4 Pads not used during labor and delivery.
56. Comprehension, assessment, physiologic (b)
    2 Correct.
    1 Transition occurs between 8 and 10 cm, not 6.
    3 These are some common symptoms of transition.
    4 Oxytocin (Pitocin) never given with titanic contractions.
57. Knowledge, assessment, physiologic (a)
    3 Most desirable.
    1, 2 Too low.
    4 Too high.
58. Knowledge, planning, psychosocial (a)
    4 Lets him share, yet gives him his own special time
    1 Don't separate him from the major activity (newborn) at this time; poor timing of such a plan.
    2 Presents will not substitute for presumed neglect or inattention.
    3 Never force a child to cuddle and kiss someone he feels is threatening.
59. Knowledge (a)
    4 All are included for the reasons listed below.
    1 The physician and nurse coordinate the total care.
    2 The patient and his or her family are active participants and consumers of care.
    3 Total care involves all health providers and skills.
60. Knowledge (a)
    1 This response is correct.
    2 Another reason was to provide for better use of all nursing personnel, not only RNs.
    3 An aspect was to augment health care providers, not to eliminate them.
    4 Better educated nursing personnel was another reason for LP/VNs.

61. Knowledge (a)
    2 In-service programs help maintain level of competency.
    1 All health-related journals do not provide nursing continuing education units.
    3 Simply paying dues does not provide a means of continuing education.
    4 Courses in other disciplines do not necessarily maintain competency in nursing.

62. Knowledge (a)
    3 Best response based on patient rights and patient expectation of nurse. Patient should know who you are and what your position is.
    1 Not considered a professional attitude.
    2 Empathy not sympathy encourages a good nurse-patient relationship.
    4 The nurse should explain all nursing procedures; however, in some cases may be called on to explain some medical procedures. Such explanation is the responsibility of the physician.

63. Knowledge (a)
    1 NLN (established service in 1949) accredits nursing programs.
    2 AMA (American Medical Association) national organization for physicians.
    3 NFLPN, national organization for practical nurses.
    4 ANA, national organization and official spokespersons for RNs.

64. Knowledge (a)
    3 One of many duties of board of nursing.
    1 Each state mandates size and participants.
    2 Retirement benefits.
    4 Also educators, consumer members, government members; physicians are also included on most boards.

65. Knowledge, implementation, environment (a)
    3 Virus is found in blood and feces; primary mode of spread is by food, drink, or water.
    1 Associated with HBV.
    2 Associated with HBV, non-HAV, and non-HBV.
    4 Associated with toxic hepatitis.

66. Comprehension, planning, physiologic (a)
    1 Promotes liver regeneration and increased blood filtration through the liver.
    2 Enteric precautions and proper hygiene prevent the spread of the virus.
    3 Cardiac effort is reduced, but the primary aim is to rest the liver.
    4 Will not reduce the risk of hepatic coma.

67. Comprehension, planning, environment (a)
    1 Spread through the fecal-oral route.
    2 Mask alone will not stop the spread.
    3 Spread through the fecal-oral route primarily.
    4 Will not destroy the virus.

68. Knowledge, assessment, health (a)
    2 Primarily associated with contaminated needles and syringes.
    1 Spread primarily through fecal-oral contamination.
    3 Spread primarily through multiple transfusions.
    4 Spread through drugs and chemical misuse.

69. Knowledge, assessment, physiologic (b)
    4 Early symptoms resemble cold or flu.
    1 Symptoms of cholelithiasis/cholecystitis.
    2 Symptoms of pancreatitis.
    3 Symptoms of MI.

70. Knowledge, assessment, environment (a)
    3 Slows pulse rate and lowers blood pressure.
    1, 2, 4 Not applicable.

71. Application, assessment, physiologic (c)
    3 One of its actions.
    1, 2, 4 Not applicable.

72. Application, evaluation, environment (b)
    2 Early signs of digitalis toxicity.
    1, 3, 4 Not applicable.

73. Application, implementation, physiologic (a)
    3 Determine drug effectiveness.
    1, 2, 4 Not applicable.

74. Knowledge, assessment, psychosocial (b)
    2 Principal agent used in acute depressive states.
    1, 3, 4 Not applicable.

75. Application, assessment, psychosocial (c)
    3 Antianxiety drugs decrease physiologic manifestations of anxiety such as elevated blood pressure, pulse, respiration.
    1 Signs of anxiety.
    2 Paradoxical reactions.
    4 Signs of anxiety.

76. Application, assessment, physiologic (a)
    1 The patient has little or no renal function; most of the fluid intake is retained and will be indicated in the weight; after the procedure, fluid removed will be reflected in the weight.
    2 Visits from people with infections must be avoided; others are allowed.
    3 The patient may eat; meals are served in the dialysis unit.
    4 A catheter will not be in place; there is no (or scant) urine output to measure; voiding is not the problem.

77. Knowledge, implementation, physiologic (c)
    4 This dissolves uric acid crystals; specific for pruritus in uremia.
    1, 2 Nursing intervention for dry skin.
    3 Water should be tepid in the bath; hot water is drying.

78. Comprehension, planning, health (b)
    3 Has increased susceptibility to infection; may be life threatening.
    1 Important but not first priority.
    2 Goal of the dialysis procedure, not the nurse.
    4 Only for immobile (comatose) patient.

79. Application, implementation, environment (c)
    1 Bleeding gums would be a major patient problem.
    2 Rest periods are provided, not complete bed rest.
    3 Protein is restricted in renal failure.
    4 Injections are avoided when a patient has a bleeding tendency.

80. Knowledge, assessment, physiologic (a)
    2 Urinary tract and GI system are frequent sites of internal bleeding.
    1, 3, 4 Would not give information concerning bleeding.

81. Knowledge, assessment, physiologic (a)
    3 Glomerulonephritis frequently follows a strep throat that has been inadequately treated.
    1, 2, 4 Noncontributory.

82. Knowledge, assessment, physiologic (b)
    4 Patient problems are related to glomerulonephritis.
    1 Pyuria and hypotension are not problems; hypertension is a problem.
    2 Polyuria is not a problem.
    3 Hypotension is not a problem; hypertension is.

83. Application, evaluation, physiologic (c)
    3 Not oriented to general season (Thanksgiving being in November).
    1 Not significant; he may not be closely familiar with the hospital.
    2 Orientation to person must be someone he is familiar with.
    4 Amnesia concerning the accident is common.

84. Comprehension, evaluation, physiologic (b)
    1 A change in level of consciousness (LOC) may be one of the first signs of increased intracranial pressure.
    2 Not associated; GI symptoms are nausea and vomiting.
    3 Pulse rate and respirations are decreased.
    4 Problems related to glaucoma.
85. Knowledge, implementation, environment (a)
    4 Correct description.
    1 Frequent and severe headaches follow.
    2 Angiography.
    3 Isotope not used.
86. Application, planning, physiologic (c)
    3 Fluids help absorption of air.
    1, 2 After nausea, may resume previous diet.
    4 See rationale for statement 3.
87. Comprehension, planning, physiologic (b)
    1 Bowel retraining is easier, and success is usually met in a much shorter period of time.
    2 Both are demoralizing.
    3 Bowel retraining does not solve urinary incontinence.
    4 Patient cooperation does not usually vary.
88. Knowledge, implementation, physiologic (b)
    2 Suppository insertion for bowel retraining is done 1 to 2 hours before the scheduled training time and after a meal.
    1, 3, 4 Suppository insertion for bowel retraining is done 1 to 2 hours before the scheduled training time and after a meal.
89. Knowledge, implementation, physiologic (b)
    2 Obtain bowel history; assess evacuation pattern; plan program; implement program; evaluate program.
    1 Part of assessment is obtaining a bowel history.
    3, 4 Follow steps of the nursing process.
90. Comprehension, planning, physiologic (a)
    1 Pattern is essential with retraining.
    2 Not necessary for the patient to understand the program for the program to be successful.
    3 Laxatives never used with bowel retraining.
    4 Regular days and times must be strictly followed to establish a pattern.
91. Knowledge, assessment, environment (b)
    1 Never use a suppository directly from refrigerator, because cold causes constriction.
    2 Lubrication ensures easy, painless insertion.
    3 Ineffective when inserted into a bolus of stool.
    4 Glycerin suppositories are inserted after 20 minutes if patient has not had a bowel movement.
92. Knowledge, assessment, environment (a)
    2 Cholesterol is found in blood and body cells, especially brain and nervous tissue.
    1 It should not nor can it be eliminated totally from the diet.
    3 It is necessary for normal body functioning.
    4 It is mainly through animal sources—meat, eggs, and saturated fats.
93. Comprehension, planning, environment (a)
    4 Hemorrhage could occur within 12 to 24 hours. The risk of bleeding and edema makes it necessary that a tracheostomy tray be available at the bedside.
    1 Not a classic intervention.
    2, 3 Would not prevent bleeding or edema.
94. Application, evaluation, physiologic (b)
    2 Postural drainage helps drain sections of the lung, aids in coughing and removing secretions, and improves breathing.
    1 High-Fowler's position (45- to 90-degree elevation) is most effective in relieving dyspnea.
    3 Fluids should be forced to liquefy secretions.
    4 Patient should have rest and conserve energy.

95. Comprehension, planning, health (b)
    3 Common side effect in long-term therapy.
    1, 2, 4 Are not characteristic side effects.
96. Knowledge, assessment, physiologic (a)
    1 Principal action of the drug.
    2, 3, 4 Not applicable.
97. Knowledge, assessment, physiologic (a)
    2 Increases heart contraction.
    1, 3, 4 Not applicable.
98. Knowledge, assessment, environment (a)
    2 Produces depression of respiratory center in medulla oblongata.
    1 Produces depression of brain's vasomotor center, causing hypotension.
    3 No significant effect on gastrointestinal tract.
    4 No significant effect on urinary system.
99. Knowledge, assessment, physiologic (a)
    1 Definition of adrenergic drugs.
    2, 3, 4 Not applicable.
100. Knowledge, assessment, physiologic (a)
    4 Aids arterial blood flow.
    1, 2, 3 Not applicable.
101. Knowledge, implementation, health (a)
    3 Any type of constriction about the lower extremities will decrease venous return.
    1 Not most appropriate response.
    2 Not necessary.
    4 Incorrect information.
102. Comprehension, assessment, environment (c)
    3 Size, location, and character of drainage should be noted on the chart; provides a reference for future evaluation of wound progress.
    1, 2, 4 Description lacking adequate information.
103. Knowledge, assessment, physiologic (c)
    2 Trophic change indicates circulation is poor.
    1 Not symptoms of diabetes.
    3 Edema may be present secondary to poor circulation.
    4 Incorrect symptoms for a positive Homans' sign.
104. Application, implementation, environment (a)
    1 Assisting with the use of the bedpan to collect admission urinalysis would be the most appropriate answer.
    2 BUN not routinely done on admission.
    3 Nursing actions not appropriate.
    4 Nursing actions not appropriate; see rationale for statement 2.
105. Application, assessment, environment (c)
    3 Absence of the pedal pulse on the affected leg indicates lack of circulation: FBS above 120 mg/L is high and should be reported immediately to the physician.
    1, 2, 4 Situation should be noted but does not require immediate physician response; compromised circulation has been noted.
106. Application, implementation, environment (a)
    4 Appropriate nursing intervention; bed cradle to prevent sheets from irritating injured area and heel protectors to prevent friction from sheets and eventual heel breakdown.
    1, 2, 3 Inappropriate nursing interventions.
107. Knowledge, assessment, physiologic (b)
    2 Diabetic ketoacidosis is manifested by elevated blood glucose levels; deep, blowing, rapid respirations (Kussmaul's respirations); and excessive protein and fat metabolism, which results in acidosis: fruity breath odor results when excessive acetones are excreted during respiration.
    1, 3, 4 Not correct symptoms for diabetic ketoacidosis.
108. Application, implementation, environment (a)
    2 To resuspend the solution and distribute evenly.
    1 Insulin protein molecules damaged by this action.
    3, 4 Extremes in temperature should be avoided; store at cool room temperature.

109. Application, assessment, health (b)
    3 Increase insulin requirements because of metabolic changes that occur specific to these factors.
    1, 2, 4 May decrease insulin requirements or have no effect on insulin requirements.
110. Knowledge, assessment, physiologic (b)
    2 Rapid-acting insulin.
    1 Slow-acting insulin.
    3, 4 Intermediate-acting insulin.
111. Knowledge, assessment, physiologic (a)
    2 Insulin is a protein that is destroyed by enzymes in the GI tract.
    1, 3, 4 Not appropriate response.
112. Knowledge, assessment, physiologic (a)
    2 Peak action from NPH insulin is 8 to 12 hours.
    1 Before peak action time.
    3, 4 After peak action time.
113. Comprehension, assessment, physiologic (a)
    2 Objective data noted relevant to patient's leg.
    1, 3, 4 Objective data, but not specifically relevant to the deterioration of patient's leg.
114. Knowledge, assessment, physiologic (a)
    3 Excessive fat metabolism causes changes in the arterial walls (atherosclerosis), inhibiting their ability to dilate and constrict, and arteriosclerosis, which is narrowing of the lumen through which blood must pass to nourish distal tissues.
    1, 2, 4 Incorrect information.
115. Application, implementation, psychosocial (a)
    4 Crying is normal and patients need to vent their grief. Holding her hand is a nonverbal means of communicating understanding and empathy.
    1, 2, 3 Inappropriate actions.
116. Knowledge, planning, environment (a)
    1 Pillows for elevating residual limb and positioning patient on side; IV fluids will be ordered; tourniquet as a safety measure, in case of hemorrhage from the residual limb.
    2 Inappropriate equipment.
    3 Sandbags not necessary.
    4 Booklet and elastic bandages not needed at this time.
117. Comprehension, assessment, environment (b)
    1 Indicative of shock—an emergency situation requiring prompt attention.
    2, 3, 4 Do not indicate an emergency situation.
118. Knowledge, implementation, health (a)
    2 This prevents hip flexion contracture.
    1, 3, 4 Not appropriate position to prevent hip contractures.
119. Knowledge, planning, physiologic (b)
    1 Stressful events (surgery) are likely to increase blood glucose levels, thus requiring higher insulin dosages.
    2, 4 Incorrect response as surgery is a stressful situation.
    3 Insulin is not usually given intravenously (in some cases regular insulin can be administered intravenously).
120. Application, implementation, psychosocial (a)
    3 An accepting nonjudgmental attitude by the nurse will often facilitate resolution of the situation.
    1, 2, 4 Inappropriate response.
121. Application, implementation, physiologic (b)
    1 Exercises will strengthen muscles necessary for walking; elastic bandages will help develop a cone shape that prevents prosthetic pressure at the distal end of the residual limb.
    2, 3, 4 Actions not relevant to prepare residual limb for the prosthetic device.

122. Comprehension, planning, health (a)
    1 Essential because of vascular changes that occur secondary to diabetes as well as past history.
    2 Not appropriate planning.
    3 Not necessary; has been insulin dependent.
    4 Not appropriate planning.
123. Comprehension, planning, physiologic (a)
    3 Response indicates nurse's knowledge of exchange list as well as patient's need for further explanation of foods on the list; dietitian is appropriate team member to provide information.
    1 Incorrect information.
    2 Not best response; only partially correct because this indicates nurse is not aware of patient's need for additional information.
    4 Inappropriate response altogether.
124. Knowledge, assessment, physiologic (a)
    1 Increased blood pressure; increased pulse rate.
    2 May have elevated temperature.
    3 Unrelated.
    4 Opposite.
125. Knowledge, implementation, health (a)
    2 Chlorpromazine makes skin sensitive to sunlight.
    1 Related to monoamine oxidase (MAO) inhibitor.
    3, 4 Not related.

Comprehensive Examination 1: Part 2

1. Knowledge, assessment, environment (b)
    3 These are all common symptoms of acute glomerulonephritis.
    1 Severe edema and proteinuria are symptoms of nephrotic syndrome.
    2 These are symptoms of nephrotic syndrome.
    4 These are not symptoms of acute glomerulonephritis.
2. Comprehension, assessment, environment (b)
    1 Acute glomerulonephritis usually occurs as a reaction to infections, especially streptococcal infections.
    2, 3, 4 This does not lead to acute glomerulonephritis.
3. Knowledge, implementation, environment (b)
    3 Corticosteroids are used to reduce the edema seen in nephrotic syndrome, not acute glomerulonephritis.
    1, 2, 4 This is commonly used in the treatment of acute glomerulonephritis.
4. Knowledge, implementation, psychosocial (b)
    2 This is the correct rate of infusion.
    1 This rate is too slow.
    3, 4 This rate is too fast.
5. Comprehension, assessment, physiologic (b)
    1 Swelling appears in the dependent parts of the body.
    2 See rationale for statement 1.
    3, 4 Not classic presentations for CHF.
6. Comprehension, assessment, environment (c)
    4 The port on drainage tubing is specifically designed for obtaining specimens.
    1 Attaching a new drainage bag requires opening the closed system, which is to be avoided.
    2 This would require opening the closed system, which is to be avoided.
    3 On most catheters, inserting a needle would leave a hole, which would then leak urine.

7. Comprehension, implementation, physiologic (a)
   3 Greg is old enough to understand and follow instructions you may give him.
   1 Rapid assessment emphasizing airway, breathing, and circulation is the first priority.
   2 Greg should be with you in the event you need assistance.
   4 Both you and Greg should go outside to Johnny. After you have done a rapid assessment emphasizing airway, breathing, and circulation, give Greg instructions to assist you.
8. Knowledge, implementation, physiologic (a)
   2 Prevents edema, facilitates vasoconstriction, increases blood viscosity, acts as local anesthetic.
   1 No indication for an eye patch.
   3 Inappropriate to promote vasodilation and reduce blood viscosity at this time.
   4 No indication for irrigation.
9. Comprehension, planning, health (b)
   2 Medical care should be sought for all childhood injuries.
   1 Rest and quiet is appropriate but not the first priority.
   3 Opticians make optical apparatus and is an inappropriate answer choice.
   4 The major priority is medical care.
10. Knowledge, assessment, environment (c)
    2 Symptom of intraocular hemorrhage.
    1 Not a symptom of intraocular hemorrhage. Such activity could, however, precipitate eye hemorrhage in this case.
    3, 4 Not a symptom of intraocular hemorrhage.
11. Knowledge, implementation, psychosocial (a)
    2 Promotes vasodilation, reduced blood viscosity, and increased tissue metabolism.
    1 Contraindicated after 24 hours.
    3 Covers ecchymosis; does not hasten absorption.
    4 No credence to this answer choice.
12. Knowledge, assessment, psychosocial (b)
    3 Behavior, because behavior ultimately defines health.
    1 Scientific studies in psychiatry are often inconclusive.
    2 Culture plays a role but is not an overriding factor.
    4 Feelings are not observable; therefore they cannot be used to define.
13. Knowledge, assessment (a)
    2 Included exorcism, because mentally ill were considered possessed.
    1 Treatment was often inhumane.
    3 Did not appear in general hospitals until recent times.
    4 Scientific principles are modern concepts.
14. Knowledge, assessment, psychosocial (a)
    2 Correct because tranquilizers do make patients more amenable to other forms of therapy.
    1 The incidence of mental illness has remained about the same.
    3 While there were some reductions in patient populations, few institutions were closed.
    4 Untoward reactions are not the prime consideration in the use of tranquilizing drugs.
15. Knowledge, assessment, psychosocial (a)
    2 A goal of community mental health is to maintain patients in the community.
    1 Some patients are hospitalized.
    3 Usually treated in general hospital units in the community.
    4 Hospitalizations are usually short term.
16. Knowledge, assessment, physiologic (b)
    4 Classic symptoms of hypothyroidism.
    1 Symptoms of Cushing's disease.
    2 Seen in diabetes mellitus.
    3 Frequency is not a classic symptom.

17. Comprehension, implementation, health (b)
    4 May indicate too much thyroid hormone is in the system.
    1 Not a standard aspect of teaching for a thyroid medication.
    2, 3 See rationale for statement 1.
18. Knowledge, assessment, physiologic (b)
    1 Correct response.
    2, 3, 4 Incorrect responses; there are inflammatory conditions; statements 2 and 3 are related to the female, and statement 4 to the male.
19. Comprehension, planning, physiologic (b)
    2 A wet dressing must be changed as soon as possible because it will be a source of infection and is irritating.
    1, 4 Not specifically related to question.
    3 The patient should be ambulatory before removal of tube.
20. Knowledge, planning, health (b)
    1 The most common problem after TURP.
    2, 3, 4 These are nonspecific, common postoperative problems.
21. Application, implementation, health (a)
    3 Can be detected in early stages only by examination; there are no early symptoms.
    1 Applies to VD.
    2 Usually without symptoms until there is metastasis.
    4 Not related to detection of prostatic cancer.
22. Application, implementation, health (b)
    4 Vital to reducing risk of lung cancer.
    1 Early detection practically impossible.
    2, 3 Should be included in teaching plan, but not the best answers.
23. Knowledge, planning, health (a)
    1 Angina may be brought on by the four *E*s: exercise, excitement, eating, and environment.
    2 Smoking and heat are not associated with precipitating angina; the act of eating, regardless of amount, may precipitate angina.
    3 Caffeine ingestion is not associated with precipitating anginal pain; anxiety is only one form of emotion that can bring on an attack.
    4 Lying supine is not associated with precipitating angina.
24. Comprehension, assessment, physiologic (a)
    4 There is an increased demand for oxygen in light of a diminished oxygen supply.
    1, 2 Increased flow will not cause angina.
    3 Angina is precipitated by reduced oxygen to the myocardium.
25. Knowledge, evaluation, physiologic (a)
    4 The smooth muscle relaxant action causes dilation of the coronary arteries, and this action provides blood and oxygen to the heart muscle.
    1 Has no effect on the pumping mechanism.
    2 Has no effect on cardiac output.
    3 Dilates the arteries.
26. Knowledge, implementation, health (b)
    2 Common side effect at the onset of therapy and usually subsides in time.
    1 The nitrates tend to cause headaches because of their vasodilation effect; changing drugs will not help.
    3 Symptoms do not subside with a reduction in the dose.
    4 Aspirin may not relieve the headache and could cause other problems.
27. Knowledge, assessment, physiologic (b)
    1 An objective symptom of rheumatoid arthritis.
    2 An objective symptom of gout.
    3 An objective symptom of scleroderma.
    4 An objective symptom of polyarthritis nodosa.

28. Knowledge, evaluation, physiologic (b)
    3 The WBC count would be slightly elevated and the ESR would be elevated because of the inflammatory process present in rheumatoid arthritis.
    1, 2, 4 Incorrect.
29. Knowledge, planning, physiologic (b)
    4 Uricosuric drugs are used in treatment of gout.
    1, 2, 3 All used in treatment of rheumatoid arthritis.
30. Knowledge, implementation, health (b)
    2 Correct; such activities would include combing hair, feeding self, and brushing teeth.
    1 Periods of undisturbed rest should be provided.
    3 A firm mattress is recommended for proper body alignment.
    4 ROM exercises should not exceed limit of pain tolerance.
31. Knowledge, implementation, health (a)
    4 Alcoholics Anonymous–type organization is most successful.
    1 Electroconvulsive therapy not usually used.
    2 May cause cross addiction.
    3 Usually not used.
32. Comprehension, implementation, psychosocial (b)
    4 The demands of the nurse lead to increased anxiety rather than a reduction of it.
    1 Ms. Jones may not be aware of her limitations.
    2 Not specifically related to the situation.
    3 Not related to situation.
33. Knowledge, evaluation, psychosocial (b)
    1 This is privileged communication.
    2 Refers to release from hospital, not relationship.
    3 No special malpractice laws.
    4 Not related.
34. Knowledge, planning, psychosocial (a)
    2 Touch, because of relational losses.
    1 May be deprived, but not the most correct answer.
    3, 4 May or may not be true.
35. Comprehension, implementation, environment (b)
    4 Memory is usually disturbed.
    1 Not a nursing responsibility.
    2, 3 Not necessarily needed.
36. Knowledge (c)
    3 1923; first to organize and to promote and distribute materials on contraception to the public.
    1 This was a bill (1922) to promote health and welfare of mothers and children.
    2 Established after the Margaret Sanger Research Bureau.
    4 Established by the United States government in 1912 to address problems regarding children (mostly dealt with problems of the industrial revolution, age, working conditions, abuse, and so on).
37. Knowledge, planning, physiologic (a)
    2 Absence of prenatal care precludes early detection so that condition may be watched and controlled.
    1 Hyperintensive drugs were discovered and used for primary hypertension and were adopted for use by obstetricians; poor answer.
    3 Controversial; recent studies reveal may have no effect.
    4 PIH may occur at any age; number of pregnancies is of more concern, that is, whether first baby; although PIH is more likely in teenagers or older women, not best possible answer.
38. Comprehension, implementation, physiologic (b)
    2 Uterus at umbilicus at 24 weeks or 6 months.
    1 Fundal height at 12 to 13 weeks (3 months) is just above symphysis pubis.
    3 At 16 to 20 weeks mother first experiences fetal movement.
    4 Engagement occurs about 2 weeks before EDC in nullipara; not before labor in parous woman.

39. Knowledge, comprehension, psychosocial (b)
    2 True statement.
    1 Though highly contagious, there must be direct bloodstream contact with the HIV virus.
    3 The fetus of an HIV-infected pregnant mother is likely to become infected.
    4 It is important that all nursing personnel familiarize themselves with all aspects of AIDS.
40. Comprehension, implementation, environment (c)
    3 This is the guideline from the CDC.
    1 Must have gown as well, not just mask and gloves.
    2 Must have gown besides.
    4 The AIDS victim needs as much protection as the caretaker.
41. Comprehension, assessment, health (c)
    2 You comprehend the CDC statements and analyzed and chose this correct answer.
    1 Pregnant nurses are not known to be at greater risk than any other nurse.
    3 False. Strict adherence to precautions should protect you from contracting the infection.
    4 The first part is true, but the second part is not based on any medical or scientific proof.
42. Knowledge, assessment, environment (a)
    2 Hearing impairment common with advancing age.
    1 Personality and reality contact alterations.
    3 Loss of visual accommodation in advancing age.
    4 Cognitive dysfunction characterized by disorientation and confabulation.
43. Application, implementation, psychosocial (a)
    4 Reality orientation—only response that does not reinforce confusion and disorientation.
    1, 2, 3 Reinforce disorientation and confusion.
44. Knowledge, assessment, physiologic (b)
    2 Elderly have a decreased need for calories.
    1, 3 Caloric needs are decreased.
    4 Nutritional needs are the same as those for other adults.
45. Comprehension, planning, health (b)
    3 Good source of iron with a texture appropriate for an 8 month old.
    1 Good source of iron, but an 8 month old could choke on the tiny pieces.
    2 Source of vitamin A but not iron.
    4 Provides calcium and protein but not iron.
46. Knowledge, assessment, physiologic (a)
    1 Vitamin A deficiency is manifested by dry, scaly skin and dry mucous membranes.
    2 Deficiency of vitamin D.
    3 Anemia may be the result of a deficiency in vitamins E, C, and B_6 or of iron deficiency.
    4 Vitamin C deficiency causes easy bruising.
47. Knowledge, planning, physiologic (a)
    3 Toddlers enjoy eating finger foods. Many nutrients can be added to a child's diet in this way.
    1 Large servings discourage a child from eating.
    2 Coaxing or bribing a child to eat places unnecessary attention on not eating and may lead to more serious problems later.
    4 A child should be allowed to choose between several foods with none being forced on him or her.
48. Knowledge, evaluation, health (a)
    4 Additional protein and calories are needed for the overall lactation process including milk content and production.
    1 Increased fluids are needed to produce milk, a fluid tissue.
    2 Maintenance of sodium intake and fats is needed.
    3 Additional carbohydrates are needed to provide the additional calories necessary for lactation.

49. Knowledge, assessment, physiologic (a)
   1 Breast milk is severely lacking in iron; and by the time a child is 8 months of age, all prenatal reserves of iron would be used up.
   2 Milk is a good source of calcium.
   3 Milk is one of the best sources of protein.
   4 Breast milk contains adequate amounts of vitamin C.

50. Knowledge, implementation, physiologic (b)
   2 When vitamin C and iron are ingested simultaneously, vitamin C increases the amount of iron absorbed.
   1 Regulates calcium and phosphorus absorption.
   3 Necessary for synthesis and metabolism of proteins.
   4 Many of its functions are unknown, although there is no evidence to suggest a connection with iron absorption.

51. Knowledge, implementation, environment (c)
   3 Strict isolation is used for diseases like chickenpox, which are transmitted through the air.
   1 Drainage/secretion isolation is used only to prevent contact with infected drainage.
   2 Respiratory isolation is used for diseases spread by air droplets.
   4 Universal blood and body fluid isolation is used to prevent contact with infected body fluids or blood.

52. Knowledge, implementation, physiologic (a)
   1 High-Fowler's position allows better lung expansion, thus promoting better oxygenation.
   2 Oxygen therapy would require a physician's order.
   3 Vital sign frequency is determined by a complete assessment of the patient.
   4 Log-rolling technique is used to turn a patient whose back cannot be flexed.

53. Application, assessment, physiologic (b)
   4 Touching the uvula causes the patient to gag or vomit.
   1 The nasal turbinates are located in the nasal passages, not the throat.
   2, 3 The posterior pharynx and tonsils are areas where throat microorganisms are located.

54. Knowledge, planning, physiologic (b)
   2 Emergency nursing care of the CVA patient includes placing the patient on the affected side to promote drainage of saliva, elevating the head slightly to promote venous drainage, and keeping the patient as quiet as possible.
   1, 3, 4 Opposite actions of what should actually be done.

55. Knowledge, assessment, physiologic (a)
   2 High blood pressure is a hereditary disease in which increased stimulation of sympathetic nerve fibers leads to greater vasoconstrictor activity.
   1, 3, 4 Incorrect response.

56. Knowledge, assessment, health (a)
   2 The normal blood pressure range is 100/60 to 140/90.
   1, 3, 4 Abnormal blood pressure reading.

57. Comprehension, planning, health (a)
   4 Prevention of contractures, decubitus, and other physiologic complications will speed up the eventual rehabilitation process.
   1, 2, 3 This is not an *immediate* goal.

58. Application, planning, environment (b)
   3 Expressive aphasia results from damage to Broca's speech area. The patient understands what is said to him and knows the words he wishes to say, but he cannot form the words verbally. Many times he may still be able to write words.
   1, 2 See rationale for statement 1.
   4 Not necessary.

59. Knowledge, implementation, environment (a)
   2 Dysphagia is defined as difficulty in swallowing. If the patient has lost the gag reflex, he may easily aspirate oral fluids.
   1, 3 Not applicable to situation.
   4 Means of assessing the gag reflex.

60. Application, implementation, physiologic (b)
   3 Elevation of the arm helps prevent edema and fibrosis, which will interfere with normal range of motion.
   1, 2, 4 Inappropriate position that will promote, not prevent, edema/fibrosis.

61. Application, planning, physiologic (a)
   1 These activities will put the arm through range of motion (ROM) as the patient assumes some responsibility for personal care.
   2 Part of daily routine in rehabilitation.
   3 Inappropriate activity.
   4 Too fine a movement and one that does not allow full ROM.

62. Comprehension, evaluation, psychosocial (a)
   2 Depression is a natural response to catastrophic illness. Other psychologic problems manifested by cerebral damage include emotional lability, hostility, frustration, and noncooperation.
   1, 3, 4 Inappropriate nursing response showing clearly that the nurse lacks understanding of the disease process.

63. Knowledge, planning, physiologic (a)
   3 An increase in fruits in the diet will increase bulk in the intestines. Increasing bulk and fluids in the intestines will promote normal elimination.
   1, 2 Not appropriate means of encouragement as a routine to follow.
   4 This may or may not be possible.

64. Knowledge, planning, physiologic (a)
   3 Ingestion of dairy products increase calcium intake. Excessive calcium in the body during periods of decreased mobility increases the chance of kidney stone formation.
   1, 2, 4 Incorrect response, not applicable to kidney stone formation.

65. Comprehension, planning, physiologic (b)
   2 Quadriceps setting exercises improve the strength of muscles needed for walking.
   1, 3, 4 Actions will not strengthen muscles as indicated above.

66. Application, implementation, physiologic (b)
   3 Best and simple nursing measure for comfort and relief.
   1, 2, 4 Inappropriate nursing action that is unnecessary and would not correct situation.

67. Application, evaluation, environment (b)
   2 Major adverse reaction.
   1 Unlikely to occur.
   3, 4 Complications that should be the concern with every patient in labor.

68. Comprehension, implementation, environment (a)
   3 Because there is danger of bladder rupture if the bladder is full, it is important to be sure the bladder is emptied.
   1 Expected in this situation.
   2 Physician's responsibility.
   4 Assessing FHS is a normal nursing responsibility before any delivery.

69. Knowledge, assessment, physiologic (a)
   4 Transient ischemic attacks (TIAs) are temporary neurologic disturbances, manifested by sudden loss of motor, sensory, or visual function and lasting a few minutes to several hours. The cause is a temporary lack of blood flow to the area.
   1 Indicative of a CVA.
   2, 3 Not necessarily applicable to situation.

70. Knowledge, planning, environment (a)
   2 Coumadin interferes with blood-clotting mechanisms by blocking the synthesis of vitamin K in the liver. Even minor injuries may result in hemorrhage in the patient taking Coumadin.
   1 Counteracts purpose of drug.
   3 Light exercise is fine; no massage.
   4 Counteracts purpose of drug, and patients are never to take medications unless ordered by the physician.

71. Knowledge, assessment, physiologic (a)
    2 Coagulation factor II (prothrombin) is dependent on the adequate synthesis of vitamin K. The one-stage prothrombin time test is used to monitor Coumadin therapy. The usual aim of therapy is to maintain prothrombin time 1 to 1½ times normal.
    1 Often used to monitor heparin therapy.
    3 Not a test of choice.
    4 Basic test used to measure specific factor activity and to detect hemophilias.
72. Knowledge, planning, physiologic (a)
    3 Patients taking Coumadin should be monitored for any signs of bleeding. The mucous membranes, intestines, and urinary tract are common sites.
    1 Inappropriate unless necessary.
    2, 4 Actions do not allow total observation for signs of bleeding.
73. Comprehension, assessment, physiologic (a)
    4 Correct—subjective is how the patient perceives the symptom.
    1, 2 Not applicable.
    3 Incorrect—objective is how an observer perceives the sign.
74. Application, implementation, environment (c)
    4 Correct.
    1, 2, 3 Not correct—do not pertain to eye surgery.
75. Comprehension, assessment, physiologic (c)
    1 This could be a manifestation of increased intracranial pressure.
    2 No reason to restrict self-care; can be accomplished when restricted to bed rest.
    3 A patient has the legal right to refuse medication.
    4 Appropriate to show emotional reaction when separated from children.
76. Application, implementation, health (c)
    3 Uninterrupted patching of one eye may lead to blindness in that eye.
    1 Sterility not necessary.
    2 Appropriate when there is no blink reflex.
    4 Safety requires the patch to be used when patient is awake.
77. Comprehension, assessment, environment (c)
    4 Patients with uremia are confused; safety is the priority.
    1 No need demonstrated for this patient; it may be contraindicated.
    2, 3 Essential, but not *first* priority.
78. Application, implementation, environment (a)
    3 Prevents aspiration of saliva and vomitus.
    1, 2, 4 Not best responses.
79. Knowledge, assessment, physiologic (b)
    2 Potassium affects muscle tissue, specifically cardiac muscle.
    1, 3, 4 Imbalance not as life-threatening.
80. Application, implementation, environment (a)
    1 Nearby furniture that a patient might hit during a seizure should be removed.
    2 A patient's extremities should not be restrained during a grand mal seizure. An attempt to restrain them might cause a fracture.
    3, 4 If not already on the floor, the patient should be eased gently to the floor.
81. Comprehension, planning, psychosocial (c)
    1 Modesty and sensitivity are of prime importance to this age group.
    2, 4 This is part of the normal admission procedure for any age group.
    3 Not so for this age group.

82. Comprehension, assessment, psychosocial (b)
    2 Patient's way of expressing anxiety.
    1, 3, 4 Not best response.
83. Application, planning, psychosocial (a)
    2 Behavior indicative of anxiety; verbalization of feelings will help decrease level of anxiety.
    1, 3, 4 Not appropriate action because it totally disregards patient's feelings.
84. Comprehension, planning, physiologic (b)
    2 General anesthesia decreases the gag reflex.
    1, 4 Not a true statement.
    3 True, but not the reason for an NPO order before surgery.
85. Comprehension, assessment, physiologic (a)
    2 High in protein as well as calcium.
    1 Provides protein but little else.
    3, 4 Does not provide any protein.
86. Application, implementation, psychosocial (b)
    3 Allows patient to maintain some independence and dignity while ensuring procedure is done properly.
    1, 2, 4 Inappropriate nursing action.
87. Application, implementation, environment (c)
    2 Response allows patient to express her feelings.
    1, 3, 4 Inappropriate response that does not react to patient's need.
88. Application, implementation, environment (b)
    4 First nursing action, because patient had been fitted by a qualified individual.
    1 Inappropriate response—assessment not carried out.
    2, 3 Not a *first* response.
89. Application, implementation, health (b)
    2 Best response; presenting and reinforcing information already given patient.
    1, 3, 4 Contradicting information given; offering incorrect information.
90. Knowledge assessment, physiologic (b)
    4 Urate crystals deposit in joints as a result of excessive serum uric acid levels.
    1, 2, 3 Are not classic precipitating factors in gout.
91. Knowledge, planning, physiologic (a)
    4 Has a metabolic effect, blocking the formation of uric acid.
    1 An analog of gold, used in treating arthritis.
    2 Urinary antiseptic used to treat urinary tract infection.
    3 An antiinflammatory used in arthritis.
92. Application, planning, health (a)
    1 Forcing fluid minimizes precipitation of uric acid; limiting fluids may lead to precipitation and stone formation.
    2, 3, 4 Weight loss reduces pressure on joints. A diet that decreases urate formation and increases urine alkalinity is desirable.
93. Comprehension, planning, physiologic (b)
    1 Used to immobilize the leg when internal fixation is to be done within a short time.
    2 Pediatric traction used in femoral fractures.
    3, 4 Similar traction devices used for providing balanced traction in injuries where internal fixation cannot be performed within a short time period.
94. Comprehension, assessment, environment (a)
    4 Defeats the purpose of the traction. Weights should clear the floor and hang freely.
    1, 2, 3 Actions are appropriate.
95. Comprehension, planning, physiologic (a)
    2 Thromboembolic problems are a postoperative complication of hip surgery. Low-dose aspirin reduces the risks of this complication.
    1 Dose is too low for an antiinflammatory effect.
    3, 4 Not the primary purpose behind such an order.

96. Application, implementation, health (b)
    1 Unless the physician provides orders to the contrary, the hips may be flexed to 45 degrees.
    2, 3, 4 These activities could pull the head of the femur out of the acetabulum.

97. Comprehension, assessment, environment (a)
    2 The *foremost* complication is hemorrhage.
    1 Is possible during the postoperative period.
    3 Is possible if an exercise regimen is not adhered to.
    4 Is possible after any surgery.

98. Comprehension, implementation, health (b)
    3 Hip and knee contractures can occur after surgery.
    1, 2, 4 Not generally the prime consideration for the identified nursing measure.

99. Comprehension, assessment, physiologic (a)
    4 Phantom limb sensation sometimes occurs after this type of surgical procedure.
    1, 2, 3 The sensation is not imaginary, it is not related to a side effect of medication, nor is it a reflection of the grieving process.

100. Application, implementation, environment (a)
    2 Correct.
    1 Homosexuals and heterosexuals who practice safe sex are at equal risk.
    3 Indicated where the organism or amount of secretions is yet unknown.
    4 Safe precautions and medical asepsis in care are indicated.

101. Knowledge, assessment, physiologic (a)
    4 Correct.
    1 Hyperventilation.
    2 Bradypnea.
    3 Cheyne-Stokes.

102. Application, implementation, environment (a)
    3 Local anesthesia is given before bronchoscopy. During the procedure the gag reflex is absent and may not have returned when the patient is admitted back to his room.
    1 Activity is not restricted.
    2 No dye used in procedure.
    4 NPO until gag reflex returns.

103. Comprehension, implementation, environment (a)
    4 These are the modes of transmission.
    1, 2, 3 Not necessary to contain the virus.

104. Comprehension, assessment, psychosocial (c)
    3 The first stage toward final acceptance.
    1 Second stage.
    2 Third stage.
    4 Fourth stage.

105. Application, evaluation, psychosocial (b)
    2 The finding of antibodies means that the person has been infected with the HIV at some time, but may not have the disease.
    1 Not correct.
    3 No immunity known.
    4 No prevention after exposure; only to prevent exposure.

106. Comprehension, evaluation, health (b)
    3 A malignancy rare and low growing in general population, highly malignant in patients with AIDS.
    1 Hives in an allergic reaction are not purple.
    2 Internal bleeding would be demonstrated as petechiae.
    4 No evidence of self-injury.

107. Comprehension, planning, environment (a)
    1 The AIDS virus attacks the immune system.
    2 His age, 37, would not be a factor—immunity is lessened in the elderly.
    3 Immunity has no relationship to one's sexual preference.
    4 No medication given to this patient with bone marrow suppression.

108. Application, implementation, health (b)
    4 A major aspect in care is to prevent additional infections.
    1 Ideally the patient can and should return to the community and can have a productive lifestyle.
    2 The patient can only be of danger through the exchange of body fluids.
    3 Health care is provided by third-party payments and community agencies. The expensive drugs are those specifically for AIDS.

109. Comprehension, implementation, health (a)
    4 Will encourage circulation and alleviate pain; symptoms may be indicative of a femoral vein thrombus.
    1 This treatment has not been ordered.
    2 An unauthorized treatment.
    3 Should be aware of possibility of thrombus in postpartum patient; should not move leg until the physician examines it.

110. Knowledge, implementation, health (a)
    2 True; includes all pertinent phases of childbearing.
    1 Untrue; drugs may be requested or even given when necessary, such as with dystocia.
    3 Preparation for labor and delivery; not necessarily "young" parents; does not include child-rearing classes.
    4 This is more a description of the Bradley method.

111. Knowledge, planning, health (b)
    4 Ideal time.
    1 Too early; would not retain instructions.
    2 Too early; may forget or become bored if too early.
    3 Too late; classes are usually once a week for 5 to 6 weeks.

112. Comprehension, implementation, environment (b)
    2 Best response; facts are true, and you are suggesting alternatives.
    1 Giving only partial response is not advisable.
    3 Have not answered anxieties regarding IUDs.
    4 Unwarranted criticism; unanswered question.

113. Knowledge, implementation, health (b)
    3 True and best response.
    1 The physician or nurse should instruct the woman how to determine time of ovulation.
    2 Several days of abstinence are suggested, not 10.
    4 Cycle must be regular, not necessarily every 30 days; could be every 26 days; the key word is *regular*.

114. Knowledge, implementation, health (a)
    1 Massaging the area and avoiding repeated pressure will enhance circulation.
    2, 3, 4 Inappropriate nursing action for pressure areas.

115. Comprehension, implementation, health (a)
    3 Artificial tears and a patch will protect the cornea from drying, trauma, and ulceration.
    1, 2, 4 Action will not protect cornea over long period of time.

116. Knowledge, implementation, health (c)
    3 Injection of human immune gamma globulin provides already formed antibodies; there is no active production of antibodies on the part of the recipient.
    1 Acquired active immunity occurs after the recipient receives an injection of a vaccine made up of living or killed organisms.
    2 Acquired immunity occurs naturally after a disease such as chickenpox.
    4 Passive immunity occurs naturally when the fetus receives antibodies from the mother in utero.

117. Comprehension, assessment, environment (c)
    2 Upper respiratory infection (URI) occurs frequently in children with cleft palate.
    1 Urinary tract infection.
    3 Of or pertaining to fat.
    4 Shortness of breath.

118. Comprehension, implementation, environment (c)
  3 Patient scheduled for OR with an elevated temperature; admitting physician should be notified.
  1 Respirations are within normal limits; physician should be notified of abnormal vital signs, not anesthesia.
  2 Pulse is within normal limits; physician should be notified of abnormal vital signs, not anesthesia.
  4 Blood pressure is within normal limits.
119. Application, implementation, psychosocial (b)
  1 The mother needs support to help replenish her emotional strength and to know she is helping her baby.
  2, 3 Inappropriate action.
  4 Can be done at a later time.
120. Application, planning, environment (b)
  2 Elbow restraints keep hands out of mouth yet allow for a degree of mobility.
  1, 3 Restraints permit no mobility.
  4 Not appropriate response.
121. Knowledge, planning, environment (a)
  4 If a baby vomits water, it is less likely than other choices to cause aspiration pneumonia.
  1, 2, 3 Inappropriate *first* foods.
122. Comprehension, implementation, psychosocial (b)
  2 Baby may eat readily if fed by his mom and not the nurse.
  1 Not necessary/indicated.
  3 Not best response.
  4 Inappropriate response.
123. Knowledge, implementation, environment (b)
  1 Placement of NG tube is checked in all patients. Food could go into lungs if placement is incorrect.
  2, 3, 4 Not relevant to situation (this is a given).
124. Comprehension, planning, environment (b)
  4 Before removing NG tube, make sure baby retains Asepto feeding and do not stimulate vomiting with tube removal.
  1 See rationale for statement 4.
  2 If done, and the feeding was not tolerated, Kevin would have to have the NG tube reinserted.
  3 See rationale for statement 4.
125. Comprehension, planning, environment (a)
  3 Mobile is suitable for age and patient with wrist restraints.
  1, 2, 4 Inappropriate for age and diagnosis.

Comprehensive Examination 2: Part 1

1. Application, planning, environment (b)
  1 A victim suspected of having an injury to the spine is never moved because of the risk of causing paralysis.
  2, 3 Any movement may cause further damage.
  4 This is not the proper procedure for assessing pulmonary status.
2. Comprehension, assessment, physiologic (b)
  3 Paraplegia is paralysis of the lower extremities.
  1 Quadriplegia is paralysis affecting all four extremities.
  2 S_1 injury causes paraparesis (partial paralysis of lower extremities).
  4 C_7 injury causes paralysis of the trunk and all four extremities.
3. Application, implementation, health (c)
  4 Treatment for shock is a priority life-sustaining emergency measure.
  1, 2, 3 Appropriate but not the highest priority.

4. Knowledge, evaluation, physiologic (a)
  1 Cardiac output is not adequate in relation to venous return and the body's needs.
  2 The left ventricle is not pumping out enough blood to meet the body's needs.
  3 CHF is a result of ventricular failure.
  4 Blood pooling in the heart does not occur in hypovolemia.
5. Knowledge, planning, physiologic (a)
  2 Improves the pumping action of the heart.
  1 Used in treatment of dysrhythmias.
  3 Vasoconstrictor, is not a drug of choice.
  4 Vasodilator, is used in angina.
6. Comprehension, planning, environment (b)
  3 Patient may fatigue easily; skin is fragile; sodium and fluid may be restricted to reduce blood volume.
  1 Sodium is restricted; there is gradual return to activity, and rest periods are a consideration.
  2 Fluid may be limited; there is a gradual return to activity along with rest periods.
  4 Rest and activity are balanced; fluids and dietary sodium may be restricted.
7. Comprehension, planning, physiologic (b)
  1 Blood return to the right atrium is delayed.
  2 Blood return is delayed.
  3 Will not directly affect either.
  4 Positioning has no effect on dysrhythmias.
8. Knowledge, assessment, physiologic (b)
  4 Symptoms of pulmonary edema are the result of pulmonary congestion and fluid in the interstitial spaces and alveoli.
  1 May have chest pain, not necessarily angina; nausea and vomiting are not usually associated symptoms; there is dyspnea not necessarily associated with exertion.
  2 Patient is restless but not necessarily confused; tachycardia and hypertension are usually present.
  3 Angina and bradycardia are not associated symptoms.
9. Comprehension (a)
  4 Licensure is granted to individuals who have met predetermined standards by means of education and examination (licensing).
  1 Individual does not have to have a nursing license to render first aid.
  2 Not necessary to have a nursing license to recommend a physician. Ethically, an LP/VN should recommend the names of three physicians when asked.
  3 The LP/VN provides nursing care to patients under the supervision of a registered nurse or physician.
10. Comprehension (a)
  2 The board of nursing implements the laws governing the practice of nursing.
  1 Defines the practice of nursing; does not establish nursing procedures.
  3 Accredits schools of nursing based on predetermined established standards.
  4 Does not oversee in-service programs. Documentation of continuing education required in some states for license renewal.
11. Knowledge (a)
  2 Possession of a nursing license means the LP/VN has met the requirements of minimal safe practice, which primarily protects the public and nursing practice.
  1 Employer required to employ only licensed nurses or new graduate scheduled to take next exam.
  3 See rationale for statement 2.
  4 Nursing malpractice is failure to possess and exercise the knowledge and skills of a reasonable and prudent nurse.

12. Knowledge (a)
    1 LP/VN must bring the matter to the attention of supervisor, since the supervisor is responsible for the patient's welfare.
    2 The LP/VN must inspire the patient to have confidence in his physician and must never advocate dismissal or replacement of a physician.
    3, 4 Not LP/VN chain of command.
13. Knowledge (a)
    4 All are included under the Patient's Bill of Rights.
    1 The right to refuse treatment to the extent permitted by the law.
    2 To know by name the physician responsible for coordinating his care.
    3 To considerate and respectful care.
14. Application, implementation, environment (b)
    2 She should be ready to push and should be assisted to do so effectively.
    1 Primipara with infant's head at station 0 does not have to be wheeled into the delivery room stat unless there is a problem; better to push several times in bed.
    3 Offer bedpan and see if bearing down can be relieved by emptying bladder; do not catheterize without trying that first.
    4 Primiparas may take anywhere from 20 minutes to an average of 1 hour to push the infant out. Transfer to delivery room should be accomplished without undue haste.
15. Comprehension, implementation, psychosocial (a)
    1 Increased flow progressive; reaches peak about transition.
    2 Physician has just examined patient; unnecessary to call. Abruptio placentae is accompanied by pain.
    3 Normal sequence of bloody show; not necessary to take blood pressure for that.
    4 Pads rarely used; source of discomfort and contamination.
16. Application, planning, environment (c)
    2 Sarcoidosis is an infrequently seen disease process.
    1 Medication regimen is not needed for the nursing care plan initially.
    3 Information about the process cannot be given until the nurse is familiar with the disease process.
    4 Sarcoidosis is not contagious; list of contacts is not pertinent.
17. Comprehension, planning, physiologic (b)
    4 There is no specific treatment; the disease runs its course.
    1 Sarcoidosis is not contagious; no isolation is needed.
    2 No specific treatment; bed rest restriction is unnecessary.
    3 Direct sunlight can cause vitamin D sensitivity, which may increase calcium in the blood and cause kidney damage.
18. Comprehension, implementation, health (a)
    3 Lymph node biopsy is the most definitive diagnostic procedure for sarcoidosis.
    1 Would give patient false sense of spreading disease.
    2 The question was not understood properly.
    4 Swollen glands are symptomatic of sarcoidosis.
19. Application, implementation, health (a)
    2 Smoking decreases pulmonary function; sarcoidosis compromises lung capacity.
    1 Focus treatment on healing; patient cannot assess pulmonary function.
    3 Physician will monitor any increased involvement; too involved for patient.
    4 Focus treatment on positive aspects of healing because course of disease is to resolution.

20. Knowledge, planning, physiologic (a)
    3 When the baby is stable, which is frequently moments after birth.
    1, 2, 4 Parental contact should not be on a schedule.
21. Comprehension, implementation, environment (b)
    4 Urine voided at 2 PM was produced during the 24-hour period and needs to be included in the collection.
    1 If patient voids urine produced after 2 PM, the collection would cover more than 24 hours.
    2, 3 If 2 PM voiding is not included, the collection would not include all urine produced in the 24-hour period.
22. Application, assessment, environment (c)
    2 May indicate change in condition, requiring further assessment.
    1 Normal range.
    3 Not a priority.
    4 With no indication of heart failure; would not be a priority.
23. Knowledge, assessment, physiologic (b)
    1 Orthopnea indicates that the patient breathes best when sitting upright.
    2 Periods of apnea.
    3 Stertorous breathing.
    4 Tachypnea.
24. Knowledge, assessment, environment (a)
    4 Cooling of their environment may destroy ova and parasites.
    1 Although changes may take place in bacteria if specimens are held at room temperature, they may be stored in the refrigerator before being sent to the laboratory.
    2, 3 Presence of blood in a stool specimen is not altered by cooling.
25. Knowledge, implementation, environment (a)
    2 Most likely time to obtain a good specimen.
    1, 3 Not a good time.
    4 Not the best time.
26. Comprehension, evaluation, environment (c)
    2 Goals/objectives are the expected results of nursing actions.
    1 Nursing measures other than those assigned are often necessary to meet patient needs.
    3 In many situations, nurses provide excellent care, yet the patient may not feel better.
    4 At times, good nursing care may not make the patient happy.
27. Knowledge, implementation, physiologic (b)
    3 Slowly rotating the catheter ensures that all areas are reached by the suction.
    1 Suction is *not* applied while the catheter is inserted to prevent unnecessary trauma to the mucous membranes.
    2 Each suction attempt should last no more than 15 seconds. While suctioning, you are preventing the patient from inhaling any oxygen.
    4 Most suctioning requires surgical asepsis.
28. Comprehension, implementation, physiologic (a)
    1 A spark caused by friction can be enough to cause an explosion if it comes in contact with oxygen.
    2 Some gases, when mixed with oxygen, can cause an explosion.
    3 An airtight enclosure is not necessary for the use of oxygen.
    4 A self-contained ventilation system is not required for the use of oxygen.
29. Knowledge, implementation, physiologic (b)
    1 Ambulation requires a written order.
    2 Should be done but after seeing the order.
    3 Not before seeing the order.
    4 Should be done, but the order should be seen.

30. Knowledge, assessment, physiologic (a)
    4 Normal range for rectal temperature is 98° to 100° F.
    1 Would not be indicative of an error.
    2 Perhaps, but not immediately.
    3 100° F rectal temperature is normal.
31. Knowledge, assessment, physiologic (c)
    2 Cardiac dysrhythmias are associated with hypokalemia.
    1 Tendency toward bleeding is not associated with hypokalemia.
    3 Nausea and vomiting are associated with hyperkalemia.
    4 Thirst is not associated with hypokalemia.
32. Knowledge, assessment, physiologic (a)
    4 Tachycardia is a heart rate greater that 100 beats/min.
    1 Bradycardia.
    2 Normal rate.
    3 Higher than bradycardia; lower than tachycardia.
33. Comprehension, assessment, environment (b)
    3 It is not possible to feel more beats at the radial artery than are originating from the heart.
    1, 2, 4 This is possible.
34. Comprehension, assessment, environment (a)
    2 These are symptoms of chickenpox.
    1 Symptoms of measles include a red, slightly raised rash with no itching.
    3 Symptoms of scarlet fever do not include reddish blisters on the trunk.
    4 Symptoms of rubella do not include a fever or reddish blisters on the trunk.
35. Comprehension, implementation, environment (a)
    4 The pinworms lay their eggs near the anal opening during the night, so they are most easily captured in the early morning hours.
    1, 2 This would be too late in the day.
    3 Any eggs near the anal opening would probably be expelled along with the stool.
36. Knowledge, assessment, environment (a)
    1 Tinea capitis is a fungal infection found on the scalp.
    2, 3 Tinea corporis is a fungal infection on the body.
    4 Tinea pedis is a fungal infection on the feet.
37. Comprehension, assessment, physiologic (b)
    3 Cerebral palsy is caused by a lack of oxygen to the motor centers of the brain.
    1, 2 This is a hereditary disease.
    4 Crohn's disease is a chronic, recurrent inflammatory disease of the intestines.
38. Comprehension, assessment, psychosocial (b)
    3 Erikson's theory is based on the child's psychosocial development.
    1 This is Freud's theory.
    2 This is Piaget's theory.
    4 This is a portion of Piaget's theory.
39. Knowledge, assessment, psychosocial (a)
    4 Freud's theory states that infants are in the oral stage.
    1 Toddlers are in the anal stage.
    2 Preschoolers are in the oedipal stage.
    3 Adolescents are in the genital stage.
40. Comprehension, assessment, environment (b)
    2 These are classic signs and symptoms of the condition known as failure to thrive.
    1 These are not symptoms of celiac disease.
    3 These are not symptoms of Hirschsprung's disease.
    4 These are not symptoms of pyloric stenosis.
41. Knowledge, assessment, environment (a)
    1 Impetigo can be caused by streptococcal or staphylococcal infections.
    2 It is not the same as pinworms.
    3 Impetigo is not caused by an allergic reaction.
    4 This is called pediculosis.

42. Knowledge, assessment, physiologic (a)
    4 The specific cause of SIDS is presently unknown.
    1 SIDS is not caused by a respiratory virus.
    2 SIDS is not caused by an obstruction of the airway by a foreign body.
    3 SIDS is not caused by hypertrophy of the larynx.
43. Knowledge, assessment, physiologic (b)
    4 This is the definition of nephrotic syndrome; the damaged glomeruli cause the symptoms of the syndrome.
    1, 2, 3 This is not the cause.
44. Comprehension, assessment, environment (b)
    3 Edema is the most common symptom of nephrotic syndrome. Anorexia and varying degrees of diarrhea are also common.
    1, 2, 4 Not a symptom of nephrotic syndrome.
45. Application, implementation, physiologic (b)
    3 Use of diuretics is necessary because of the patient's edema.
    1 Semi-Fowler's is the most comfortable position to facilitate respiration.
    2 The normal diet for a child with nephrotic syndrome is a high-protein diet.
    4 Sodium and potassium supplements are not usually given; sodium is limited.
46. Comprehension, assessment, environment (b)
    2 This is a symptom of the condition.
    1 Amenorrhea, not dysmenorrhea, is commonly seen in these patients.
    3 Bradycardia and hypotension are common, probably because of the state of starvation.
    4 Constipation, not diarrhea, is a symptom of anorexia nervosa.
47. Application, implementation, psychosocial (b)
    1 The nurse should promote a positive self-image in a patient with anorexia nervosa because her present self-image is a negative one.
    2, 3, 4 Current measure used in the treatment of a patient with anorexia nervosa.
48. Application, implementation, environment (b)
    4 Unrecognized airway closure can be fatal, therefore this position is recommended if no trauma to the spine is suspected.
    1, 2, 3 Not a recommended position in this type of situation.
49. Application, implementation, physiologic (b)
    2 Correct rate of rescue breathing for a child.
    1 Incorrect; one breath every 2 seconds was never a recommended rate for rescue breathing.
    3 Incorrect; this was the recommended rate of rescue breathing for a child before the changes implemented early in 1993.
    4 This is the recommended rate of rescue breathing for an adult victim.
50. Knowledge, assessment, health (a)
    4 Correct assessment.
    1 Not likely to be delusions.
    2 Unlikely.
    3 Incorrect; symptoms may worsen.
51. Comprehension, evaluation, psychosocial (b)
    2 Suits may be brought by patients who believe they have not been actively treated.
    1 Legal competency does not alter patient's rights to treatment.
    3 Nurses may be called to testify.
    4 Patients retain civil rights.
52. Knowledge, assessment, health (a)
    2 All persons have ongoing sexual needs.
    1 Children are sexual.
    3 Homosexuality is not considered a disease.
    4 Minor dysfunctions are relatively easy to treat.

53. Knowledge, assessment, environment (a)
    1 Increased blood pressure; increased pulse rate.
    2 May have elevated temperature.
    3 Unrelated.
    4 Opposite.
54. Application, implementation, physiologic (b)
    3 Correct per the 1993 changes instituted by the American Heart Association.
    1 Incorrect; eight back blows and eight chest thrusts were never a recommended sequence for obstructed airway in an infant.
    2 Incorrect; six back blows and six chest thrusts were never a recommended sequence for obstructed airway in an infant.
    4 Incorrect; four back blows and four chest thrusts were the recommended sequence for obstructed airway in an infant *before the changes instituted early in 1993.*
55. Knowledge, implementation, environment (a)
    1 Electrocardiogram, because imipramine (Tofranil) may have cardiac side effects.
    2 Not especially related.
    3 IQ is irrelevant.
    4 Not especially related.
56. Application, implementation, psychosocial (c)
    1 Concrete, short-term solution may resolve crisis.
    2 Long-term therapy not indicated.
    3, 4 Long-term solution not indicated.
57. Comprehension, planning, environment (b)
    4 Correct per the changes instituted in 1993 by the American Heart Association.
    1 Too fast; see rationale for statement 4.
    2 Too fast; compressions on an adult victim are administered at the rate of 80 compressions/minute.
    3 Too slow: see rationale for statement 4.
58. Application, implementation physiologic (b)
    3 The most common cause of arrest in the pediatric age group is primary respiratory arrest or an obstructed airway; it is thought that this age group will benefit from 1 minute of rescue support before entry into the EMS.
    1 This is only partially correct; it is also necessary that the rescuer activate the EMS.
    2 This is only partially correct: it is also necessary that the rescuer perform 1 minute of CPR before entry into the EMS.
    4 Both are correct, but in the wrong order; see rationale for statement 3.
59. Comprehension, assessment, environment (b)
    2 Not oriented in time, because he thinks it's 1886.
    1 Not oriented in time.
    3 Although confused, not oriented better describes John's state.
    4 Dishonest may or may not be true but is not relevant.
60. Comprehension, assessment, environment (b)
    4 Pressured is the word used to describe rapid speech patterns.
    1 Not unintelligible; he was understood.
    2 Disorganized may be true, but irrelevant.
    3 Variable, not true; described as rapid.
61. Comprehension, assessment, environment (b)
    1 Scattered thoughts are indicated by rapid frequent topic changes.
    2 Rapid speech may or may not indicate scattering.
    3 Physical appearance is only a general indicator.
    4 History is only a general indicator.
62. Knowledge, implementation, physiologic (a)
    1 All are good sources of potassium.
    2 Good sources of iron.
    3 Good sources of vitamin C.
    4 Good sources of vitamin D.

63. Knowledge, assessment, health (b)
    4 Home-canned, low-acid foods such as meats, peas, corn, and green beans are frequent culprits.
    1 Salmonellosis is caused by a *staphylococcus* organism.
    2 This is true of salmonellosis and perfungens.
    3 Also true of salmonellosis and perfungens but does not affect botulism.
64. Knowledge, planning, physiologic (b)
    1 Small, low-carbohydrate meals are often prescribed for dumping syndrome to decrease the amount of glucose released all at once into the small intestine.
    2 High-calorie diet is often used in hyperthyroidism.
    3 Low-protein diet for liver diseases.
    4 Low-protein diet for kidney diseases.
65. Knowledge, implementation, environment (b)
    4 The RDA are suggested levels of nutrients known from research to meet dietary needs of most healthy individuals.
    1 Individuals with nutritional deficiencies may need amounts above what the RDA suggest.
    2 The four basic food groups were developed by the U.S. Department of Agriculture and are another guide to proper nutrition.
    3 This pertains to the U.S. Dietary Goals, another set of guidelines to proper nutrition.
66. Knowledge, planning, environment (a)
    2 Fasting plasma glucose is measured after 12 to 14 hours of fasting, during which plasma glucose levels should fall.
    1 The blood sample must be drawn after a complete fast.
    3 These are instructions for a postprandial plasma glucose test.
    4 A regular breakfast is given after the blood is drawn.
67. Comprehension, assessment, physiologic (b)
    4 During fasting, blood sugar levels should fall, stimulating release of glucagon; glucagon acts to raise plasma glucose levels by increasing glycogenolysis and glyconeogenesis and inhibiting glycogen synthesis; insulin checks this rise in plasma glucose levels in nondiabetic patients; a deficiency in insulin allows the glucose to persist at high levels.
    1 The blood glucose level should be low or normal, not elevated.
    2 Normal plasma glucose levels range between 60 and 110 mg/dl blood, depending on the laboratory method used.
    3 Plasma glucose levels would be decreased.
68. Knowledge, planning, environment (a)
    1 Correct procedure for GTT.
    2, 4 Not a procedure for any test.
    3 Not a procedure for any test, although these are essentially postprandial blood samples.
69. Comprehension, assessment, physiologic (b)
    2 Normally the plasma glucose level will rise sharply in 30 minutes, then fall to normal in 2 hours as the pancreas responds to the increased glucose level by secreting more insulin.
    1 Insulin is omitted before the test.
    3 Not specific enough: a reiteration of the root statement; she may tolerate taking the glucose but not metabolize it.
    4 No ketones are produced in the presence of excessive glucose in the blood.
70. Knowledge, assessment, physiologic (b)
    3 These are three elements to score in obtaining total for Glasgow Coma Scale.
    1, 2, 4 All of these are part of a complete neurologic assessment but not specific for Glasgow Coma Scale.

71. Application, implementation, physiologic (a)
    3 Primary intervention to maintain muscle tone.
    1 Inappropriate to transfer to chair in unconscious state; does not relate to increasing mobility.
    2 Necessary, but not the best.
    4 Inappropriate position and will promote skin breakdown.

72. Application, implementation, health (a)
    2 Correct; most appropriate response; putting paralyzed arm through sleeve first facilitates the dressing process.
    1, 3, 4 Incorrect; may be possible, certainly more difficult.

73. Knowledge, assessment, physiologic (a)
    1 Correct definition of expressive aphasia.
    2 Receptive aphasia indicates lack of comprehension or understanding verbal or written messages.
    3 Dysphagia means difficulty swallowing.
    4 Hemiphagia—meaningless term.

74. Application, implementation, health (a)
    1 Weakened cognitive skills need stimulation.
    2, 3 Incorrect, unrelated to cognitive skill improvement.
    4 Opposite to the goal of cognitive stimulation.

75. Application, planning, environment (b)
    1 ADLs before admission can be used as a baseline for ADLs in the hospital and to measure change.
    2, 3, 4 Not relevant in development of nursing care plan.

76. Application, evaluation, environment (b)
    2 Common adverse reactions.
    1, 3, 4 Not applicable to situation.

77. Application, assessment, physiologic (b)
    4 Increases cardiac output.
    1 Not primary action of drug.
    2, 3 Incorrect response.

78. Knowledge, assessment, environment (a)
    1 Average adult dosage.
    2, 3, 4 Incorrect dosage.

79. Application, assessment, environment (a)
    2 Pulse rate is below 60 beats/min.
    1, 3, 4 Could lead to adverse reactions.

80. Comprehension, planning, environment (c)
    3 Abrupt onset of confusion relates to side effects of antihistamine, benzodiazepine, beta blocker, and cardiac glycoside combination.
    1 Would not resolve situation.
    2 Would not resolve situation and is not necessary.
    4 Not necessary.

81. Application, implementation, environment (b)
    4 Immediate action is required for choking.
    1, 2, 3 Situation is an emergency—these are not relevant emergency actions.

82. Application, evaluation, psychosocial (b)
    4 Because of impaired excretion, combined medications have a greater cumulative effect in the elderly, making them confused.
    1, 2, 3 Response does not relate cause clearly in terms that patient would understand.

83. Comprehension, assessment, psychosocial (c)
    3 The nurse challenges without collecting additional data.
    1, 2 This is a therapeutic technique.
    4 Not related to the situation.

84. Comprehension, assessment, physiologic (c)
    2 Drug users, especially cocaine users, are often in financial difficulty and may be in realistic danger from dealers and others.
    1 One cannot conclude that he is delusional from the data given.
    3 Faulty statement.
    4 This is not a specific legal requirement.

85. Comprehension, assessment, physiologic (a)
    4 The gallbladder secretes bile to emulsify dietary fat.
    1, 2, 3 Not classically associated with pain precipitation in gallbladder disease.

86. Comprehension, assessment, physiologic (a)
    3 With blockage by a stone, little or no bile passes into the small intestines. Bile gives stool its classic color.
    1 May indicate upper GI bleeding or a normal change if the patient is on iron therapy.
    2, 4 Not characteristic of a gallbladder dysfunction.

87. Comprehension, planning, physiologic (a)
    4 When the bile duct is explored for stones, edema could ensue and block the duct, hindering bile flow. The T-tube maintains patency.
    1, 3 The tube is not placed in the abdominal cavity nor in the intestines.
    2 Not the primary purpose of the tube in this situation.

88. Knowledge, evaluation, physiologic (a)
    3 Causes venous stasis.
    1, 2, 4 A preventative measure.

89. Comprehension, planning, environment (b)
    1 Causes vasodilation and reduces edema.
    2, 3 Inappropriate treatment for this patient because this would aggravate the condition.
    4 Coumadin does not dissolve clots, but prevents their formation; may not be an initial treatment.

90. Comprehension, planning, health (b)
    3 In case of an emergency a medical identification tag can inform of the anticoagulant and the dosage being taken.
    1 Not without first consulting with the physician.
    2 Stockings are to be removed for bathing and at night when retiring; they are to be reapplied after bathing and upon awakening in the morning.
    4 Incorrect since restrictions will apply.

91. Application, planning, psychosocial (a)
    2 Reassuring; understanding patient's concern; reiterating routine of nursery procedure for cesarean babies.
    1 Not reassuring; unsympathetic; not answering her question.
    3 Not answering mother's concern; passing "the buck"; curt and not helpful.
    4 Not helpful. You have suggested another question from the mother: "What's going to happen to my milk?"

92. Comprehension, implementation, psychosocial (a)
    2 This is true. Section babies are more prone to RDS than vaginally delivered babies are, because gravity and pressure of delivery help rid the baby of mucus.
    1 Babies delivered by cesarean may be postmature, premature, normal, or immature; the reason for a section is not necessarily because the baby is immature.
    3 Vaginally delivered babies may also suffer from RDS, so "never" is not correct; that is, premature babies delivered vaginally may exhibit RDS.
    4 Cephalohematoma is rarely evident in a section baby; the process of vaginal delivery and the mechanisms of descent often put pressure on the caput, producing a cephalohematoma, whereas in a section the caput may not undergo such pressure.

93. Comprehension, implementation, physiologic (a)
    3 Discharge materials are from the uterine wall and are the same for vaginal delivery as for cesarean delivery.
    1, 2, 4 False. Because lochia is the discharge from the uterus after delivery of its contents, the lochia would be different only if there were internal hemorrhage or some untoward complication.

94. Comprehension, planning, environment (b)
    2 Stimulates circulation and prevents the formation of thrombi, besides aiding in breaking up clots.
    1 This is to relieve pain, promote healing, and prevent infection.
    3 Helps to diminish pain and discomfort.
    4 Keeping urinary functions at a maximum aids in promoting involution, and offering stool softeners relieves initial pain and discomfort during the postpartum period.

95. Knowledge, assessment, environment (a)
    2 Indicate obstruction to blood flow.
    1 Not all objective data.
    3 Not indicative of diagnosis and decreased circulation.
    4 Not all objective data.
96. Comprehension, planning, health (b)
    2 Injury could lead to infection. The tissues are already compromised of oxygen and nutrients; certain positions (legs crossed, knees flexed) hamper circulation.
    1, 3, 4 Measure could lead to greater compromise in circulation and burns.
97. Comprehension, planning, physiologic (b)
    2 Principal action.
    1, 3, 4 Incorrect response.
98. Application, assessment, environment (a)
    1 Monitor for possible adverse reaction.
    2, 3, 4 Not relevant to situation.
99. Knowledge, assessment, physiologic (a)
    4 Correct response.
    1 Depletes catecholamines in sympathetic postganglionic fibers.
    2 An adrenergic blocking agent prescribed for vasodilation in peripheral vascular disease.
    3 An anticholinergic drug used in treating peptic ulcers to decrease gastric secretions and delay gastric emptying.
100. Knowledge, planning, health (a)
    1 Increased weight in childhood and middle age predisposes a person to the disorder; high salt intake also increases the risk.
    2, 3, 4 Not totally correct response, although smoking and age are considered risk factors.
101. Application, planning, physiologic (b)
    1 The tracheostomy tray is obtained in the event that Bill develops an obstructed airway. Tracheal edema results from the inhalation of smoke and heat.
    2, 3, 4 Routine for any emergency.
102. Application, implementation, physiologic (b)
    3 In assisting the physician you would prepare an IV fluid administration set and fluids (as ordered) for the immediate replacement of fluids lost from the burn site(s).
    1, 2, 4 Yes, but not vital at this point in time.
103. Comprehension, assessment, physiologic (a)
    4 An immediate physical observation of a person burned in the area of the face is assessment of respiration (difficulty, rate, sound).
    1, 2, 3 Not immediate physical observation during an emergency.
104. Application, planning, environment (a)
    3 Reverse isolation protects the patient and the burn areas from infections transmitted by others.
    1, 2, 4 Not applicable to situation at hand.
105. Comprehension, assessment, physiologic (b)
    1 Urine specific gravity is monitored to assess filtration capabilities of the renal glomerulus. Urine output and urine specific gravity provide data to determine fluid replacement needs and the status of renal function.
    2, 3, 4 Done, but does not effectively monitor fluid replacement.
106. Application, planning, psychosocial (a)
    1 Nurturing and spending time with him will decrease his fears of the unknown, anxiety about separation from his parents, and pain (injury).
    2, 3 Inappropriate nursing action.
    4 Inappropriate for this age group.
107. Application, planning, physiologic (a)
    2 To help him cope with immobility, you can use play therapy and diversional activity to decrease his anxiety. Preschoolers describe objects as real, and by simulating application of Russell traction on his favorite toy you can lessen his feelings of aloneness.
    1 Short-term diversional activity.
    3, 4 Inappropriate to situation.
108. Comprehension, assessment, physiologic (a)
    1 Circulation and sensation are periodically assessed to determine the presence of pressure areas that may obstruct circulation and nerve pathways.
    2, 3, 4 Inappropriate action.
109. Comprehension, implementation, psychosocial (a)
    2 Informing the patient of what is expected of him during the procedure will lessen his anxiety and increase his capability to control his feelings.
    1, 3, 4 Inappropriate response indicating lack of understanding and concern.
110. Knowledge, planning, physiologic (b)
    1 The diet provides essential nutrients that encourage tissue repair and replacement, energy for increased metabolic demands, and carbohydrates to prevent utilization of protein for energy.
    2, 3, 4 Inappropriate diet for situation.
111. Comprehension, assessment, physiologic (a)
    2 A preschooler enjoys the close family relationship of mealtimes. Parents are usually the significant persons during the preschool years. Since his parents are dead, his grandmother will become the significant person in his life now.
    1 Not for his age group.
    3, 4 Inappropriate before attempting above.
112. Knowledge, implementation, physiologic (a)
    2 Increasing fluids, cellulose, and bulk in the diet will facilitate bowel elimination.
    1 Not appropriate foods.
    3, 4 Lacks fluid, bulk and/or cellulose.
113. Comprehension, assessment, physiologic (b)
    3 The grandmother should try to determine how much information he has and build on that.
    1, 2, 4 Inappropriate response for this age group.
114. Comprehension, implementation, physiologic (a)
    3 Physical contact offers much needed security at this time.
    1 Inappropriate—see above.
    2 Inappropriate to do so at this time.
    4 He needs to cry at this time; inappropriate to say everything will be all right.
115. Knowledge, assessment, environment (a)
    3 All foods on a soft diet have limited fiber; therefore they are easily digested and require less work of the heart.
    1 Soft diets have no specific caloric restrictions and, in fact, may have more calories.
    2 Although many protein foods can be included in this diet, that is not its primary reason for being given.
    4 Bland diets are used for gastrointestinal disturbances.
116. Knowledge, planning, health (a)
    1 Meats and milk products are high in sodium.
    2 Fruits contain little sodium.
    3 Most vegetables contain little sodium unless they are in packaged form.
    4 Legumes and root products contain little sodium.
117. Knowledge, planning, physiologic (a)
    4 All organ meats (including liver), egg yolks, and shellfish are high in cholesterol.
    1 Good sources of calcium, not cholesterol.
    2 Good sources of vitamin C.
    3 Good sources of potassium.

118. Knowledge, planning, environment (a)
     3 Polyunsaturated fats, because they have several places for additional hydrogen to be added, are usually liquid and are recommended in a diet to lower blood lipid levels.
     1 Saturated fats are from animal sources and contribute to higher blood lipid levels and consequently to development of atherosclerosis.
     2 Usually liquid at room temperature.
     4 From animal sources and tend to raise blood lipid levels.
119. Analysis, implementation, physiologic (b)
     2 Of the choices given, this is the lowest in both cholesterol and sodium.
     1 Smoked sausage and milk are both high in sodium.
     3 Liver is extremely high in cholesterol.
     4 Eggs are high in cholesterol; cheese and milk are high in sodium.
120. Knowledge, assessment, environment (a)
     4 Water-soluble vitamins are not stored in the body and must be resupplied each day.
     1 Fat-soluble vitamins A, D, E, and K are carried and absorbed along with fat in the diet.
     2 Fat-soluble vitamins are stored in the body.
     3 Also applies to fat-soluble vitamins.
121. Knowledge, assessment, environment (a)
     4 Thiamine is necessary for proper muscle and nerve functioning.
     1 Good sources of vitamin C.
     2 Vitamin C aids in absorption of iron.
     3 This is a function of vitamin C.
122. Comprehension, implementation, health (c)
     4 Passive natural immunity is received by the fetus from mother and lasts about 6 months.
     1 Active acquired immunity results from administration of live or killed vaccines or toxoids.
     2 Active natural immunity results from having had a specific disease.
     3 Passive acquired immunity results from administration of immune serum or gamma globulin.
123. Application, implementation, environment (b)
     4 Respiratory isolation prevents transmission of disease through air droplets. A gown would usually not be required.
     1 The glass thermometer should be left in the room to prevent its use by any other patient.
     2 Hands should be washed before caring for any patient.
     3 A mask is always worn while caring for any patient in respiratory isolation.
124. Comprehension, assessment, environment (b)
     3 Palpation reveals the amount of pitting involved.
     1 No sounds are produced by ankle edema.
     2 Evaluation is a step in the nursing process.
     4 Percussion is used to assess masses, organs, and body cavities.
125. Comprehension, assessment, physiologic (b)
     2 An error has been made. The number of beats felt at the radial site cannot be greater than the number of beats heard at the apex.
     1 The patient needs no care—an error has been made.
     3, 4 An error has been made—results should not be reported.

Comprehensive Examination 2: Part 2

1. Comprehension, assessment, psychosocial (a)
   1 Repression is unconsciously pushing something from one's conscious awareness.
   2 Projection is the assignment of one's feelings to others.
   3 Displacement is the acting out of feelings on a less threatening object.
   4 Rationalization is finding explanations for one's behavior.
2. Comprehension, assessment, psychosocial (b)
   4 Ms. Smith must know behavior is meaningful regardless of how apparently insignificant.
   1 The situation does not describe the nurse's behavior.
   2, 3 Nurse's reactions are not described.
3. Knowledge, assessment, psychosocial (b)
   4 Trust vs. mistrust is Erikson's first stage.
   1 Appropriate for a later stage.
   2 Sullivan's theory not Erikson's.
   3 Freudian theory.
4. Comprehension, evaluation, environment (c)
   3 The goal is inappropriate and too difficult for the type of patient.
   1 See rationale for statement 3.
   2 The goal itself is not too broad, just unrealistic.
   4 It is not long term as stated (24 hours).
5. Knowledge, planning, environment (a)
   3 First level of the hierarchy.
   1, 2 High level of the hierarchy.
   4 Second level of the hierarchy.
6. Comprehension, implementation, environment (b)
   2 Markings must remain as guides to therapy.
   1 The region can be cleansed as long as the markings remain.
   3, 4 The markings must remain.
7. Comprehension, implementation, environment (a)
   1 May interfere with surgery.
   2, 3, 4 Should have rectal thermometer.
8. Knowledge, assessment, physiologic (b)
   3 Antibodies must be present to have immunity.
   1 Inflammatory diseases do not produce antibodies.
   2 Exposure to organisms causing contagious diseases does not necessarily lead to production of antibodies.
   4 Resistance is unrelated to immunity.
9. Application, implementation, environment (c)
   3 Irrigation solution flows into drainage container and must be subtracted from total drainage to calculate actual urine output.
   1 Nurse needs not only to measure and record but also calculate actual urine output.
   2 Nurse's responsibility, not the laboratory's.
   4 Incorrect means of calculating.
10. Knowledge, implementation, environment (a)
    1 The AIDS virus is transmitted via blood and body fluids.
    2 Used for pathogens spread through feces.
    3 Used for pathogens spread through air, droplets.
    4 Used for pathogens spread through air, contact.
11. Knowledge, assessment, environment (b)
    4 Common indication.
    1 Body temperature is often elevated.
    2 Respirations are often rapid and shallow.
    3 Skin is often cool and clammy.
12. Knowledge, implementation, physiologic (a)
    2 Suspected spinal cord injuries should be handled with care to prevent further damage to the spinal cord.
    1 Spinal cord injury is main concern; fractures of extremities are secondary.
    3, 4 Not relevant to situation.

13. Knowledge, assessment, physiologic (b)
    2 Frequent or improper handling may result in further spinal cord damage.
    1, 3, 4 These are major concerns; however, a conclusive diagnosis of SCI can only be made by x-ray examinations.
14. Knowledge, assessment, environment (a)
    2 Injury at the cervical level causes paralysis of all four extremities and the trunk. Respiratory failure and death may result.
    1 Injury at the sacral level results in paralysis of lower extremities.
    3 Injury at the lumbar level results in paralysis of lower extremities.
    4 Injury at the thoracic level results in chest, trunk, bowel, bladder, and lower extremity muscle losses.
15. Comprehension, planning, physiologic (b)
    2 Respiratory assistance is required because of lack of diaphragm innervation.
    1 Pain is not usually an early problem.
    3, 4 These actions are relevant to any emergency, especially a suspected spinal cord injury.
16. Knowledge, assessment, physiologic (b)
    2 Crutchfield tongs lessen pressure on the spinal cord.
    1, 3 Type of stabilization used for fractures of the extremities.
    4 Used in treatment of scoliosis.
17. Application, implementation, environment (c)
    2 Correctly positioned sandbags prevent the patient from slipping, thus assuring effectiveness of the traction. Slipping of patient renders traction useless.
    1, 3, 4 Inappropriate nursing action that would negate purpose of traction.
18. Comprehension, implementation, environment (b)
    4 Fluids tend to flow into the nasopharynx easily, with the danger of aspiration.
    1 Not necessary—inappropriate.
    2 See rationale for statement 4.
    3 Inappropriate action.
19. Knowledge, assessment, environment (b)
    2 Pain is caused by contraction of the gallbladder, which has been stimulated by fat in the duodenum and is having difficulty releasing bile because of obstruction.
    1, 3, 4 Response does not reflect cause of pain of the disease process.
20. Knowledge, planning, environment (b)
    3 Lima beans, cabbage, and onions are gas-forming foods.
    1, 2, 4 Because flatulence is also common with this condition, these foods are usually permitted for this condition.
21. Knowledge, evaluation, environment (a)
    3 This procedure is the correct technique to ensure that the nasogastric tube is in the stomach.
    1, 2, 4 Incorrect technique.
22. Application, implementation, environment (a)
    4 $\dfrac{50 \text{ mg}}{1 \text{ ml}} = \dfrac{75 \text{ mg}}{x \text{ ml}}$
    $50x = 75$
    $x = 1.5 \text{ ml}.$
    1, 2, 3 Incorrect dose.
23. Application, implementation, environment (a)
    3 $\dfrac{60 \text{ gr}}{1 \text{ ml}} = \dfrac{1/100 \text{ gr}}{x}$
    $60x = \dfrac{1}{100}$
    $x = 0.6.$
    1, 2, 4 Incorrect dose.
24. Comprehension, assessment, environment (b)
    2 Collection of fluids in the stomach may cause nausea and vomiting.
    1 Inappropriate immediate action.
    3 Not relevant to situation.
    4 Not an immediate response.
25. Knowledge, assessment, physiologic (b)
    3 Penrose drains are used to remove bile and blood from the operative area.
    1, 2, 4 Incorrect response.
26. Comprehension, planning, environment (a)
    4 Location of the incision associated with cholecystectomy makes the patient prone to pulmonary complications.
    1, 2, 3 Routine postoperative nursing action.
27. Knowledge, implementation, environment (a)
    1 Bile is irritating to the skin.
    2, 3, 4 Inappropriate response.
28. Knowledge, implementation, environment (b)
    2 $\dfrac{125 \text{ ml}}{60} \times 10 = 21 \text{ gtts}.$
    1, 3, 4 Incorrect drip rate.
29. Knowledge, implementation, environment (a)
    4 Insert at a 90-degree angle.
    1, 2, 3 Incorrect angle for IM injection.
30. Comprehension, planning, physiologic (b)
    3 Irrigating the tube will ensure patency.
    1, 2 Inappropriate first action.
    4 Inappropriate action.
31. Comprehension, implementation, environment (a)
    1 Stop the flow of the IV fluids to prevent further swelling and report to charge nurse.
    2, 3, 4 Inappropriate responses that will not correct the stated situation.
32. Knowledge, implementation, environment (a)
    2 A principle of surgical asepsis states sterile objects only touch sterile objects.
    1 Forceps can be used but they must be sterile. Response does not indicate if forceps are sterile.
    3, 4 Response not relevant to dressing change procedure.
33. Comprehension, assessment, environment (a)
    1 A temperature may be indicative of a postoperative infection, which requires initiation of treatment.
    2, 3, 4 Expected occurrence in this situation.
34. Knowledge, evaluation, health (b)
    3 Following cholecystectomy, most patients can return to a normal diet as long as they avoid excessive fat intake.
    1, 2, 4 Incorrect response related to diet as indicated above.
35. Comprehension, planning, environment (a)
    2 Many states have Good Samaritan laws to encourage medical aid at the scene of an accident by limiting the legal liability that might arise.
    1 It is not mandatory for nurses or physicians to render emergency aid.
    3 It is expected that the person rendering aid will act as a reasonable, prudent person would act under similar circumstances. A higher standard of medical aid would be expected of a nurse, physician, and members of a first-aid squad than that of the average general public.
    4 Laws vary in each state.
36. Application, implementation, environment (a)
    2 Only exception.
    1 All surgical procedures must have signed consent.
    3 X-ray procedures using dye must have signed consent.
    4 Written consent by patient unless under age or incapacitated; then need written consent of next of kin.

37. Knowledge (a)
    2 Each state has its own laws pertaining to nursing.
    1 Laws are passed by the state's legislature.
    3 The laws regulate nursing practice and standards.
    4 The laws define the qualification and fees required of the applicants for licensure.

38. Comprehension, assessment, environment (a)
    3 Failure to do what a reasonable and comparably trained person would or would not do.
    1 Unauthorized bodily contact with another person.
    2 Responsible for own actions.
    4 Breach of duty caused harm.

39. Application, implementation, environment (a)
    4 Proper procedure.
    1, 2, 3 Improper procedure.

40. Knowledge, assessment, physiologic (a)
    3 Principal action of sedatives.
    1 Principal action of hypnotics.
    2, 4 Not an action of the drug.

41. Knowledge, assessment, environment (a)
    3 Action depends on dosage.
    1, 2 Not true.
    4 Hypnotic drugs as well as sedative drugs cause depression of the CNS but in varying degrees.

42. Knowledge, planning, physiologic (a)
    4 24-hour evaluation of the heart pattern; patient may need assistance documenting the log that accompanies this test.
    1 Not a 24-hour evaluation.
    2 A study of the brain waves.
    3 An invasive study of the heart and vessels.

43. Knowledge, assessment, physiologic (b)
    2 Plaque formation in coronary vessels diminishes blood flow and oxygen supply to the myocardium, which, carried by the blood, is also reduced.
    1 Plaque reduces vessel size and reduces the capacity to carry blood.
    3 The diminished supply is to the myocardial tissue.
    4 Ballooning is more descriptive of aneurysms.

44. Knowledge, assessment, physiologic (a)
    3 Increases myocardial demand for oxygen.
    1 Does not precipitate chest pain, but in severe angina, the patient may awaken with chest pain.
    2 Not an associated factor in chest pain.
    4 See rationale for statement 2.

45. Comprehension, assessment, environment (b)
    4 Chest pain that radiates is a significant finding.
    1 Not associated with chest pain.
    2 Increases in respiration caused by anxiety is common.
    3 Not associated with chest pain.

46. Application, planning, health (a)
    1 In primary hypofunction (not the result of a pituitary disturbance), the therapy is lifelong.
    2, 3, 4 Hormonal therapy is not classically adjusted on a day-to-day basis, nor is hormonal therapy, in this case, temporary or intermittent.

47. Comprehension, planning, environment (a)
    2 All are foods included on a clear liquid diet, one that is nonirritating and easily digested and absorbed.
    1 Cream of tomato soup would be on a full liquid diet.
    3 Sherbet and strained cereal are on a full liquid diet.
    4 Custard and cocoa are on a full liquid diet.

48. Knowledge, assessment, physiologic (a)
    1 Dietary requirements for a diabetic patient are calculated on the basis of age, sex, body build, weight, and activity. They should be the same as those of a nondiabetic patient.
    2 Diet will be lower in calories only if the diabetic patient is overweight.
    3 Diabetic diet contains approximately 50% to 60% carbohydrates, equal to a well-balanced diet of a nondiabetic patient.
    4 Should be equal in protein to that of a nondiabetic patient.

49. Knowledge, implementation, environment (a)
    4 Oranges, bananas, dried apricots, whole grain cereals, meat, fish, and poultry are all good sources of potassium.
    1 Good sources of calcium.
    2 Good sources of iron.
    3 Sources of vitamin C.

50. Comprehension, implementation, physiologic (c)
    2 Airway is compromised; administer oxygen to prevent shock.
    1 Not the priority.
    3 Should be done but not the first priority.
    4 Not the priority, and vital signs should be taken before placing patient in high-Fowler's position.

51. Comprehension, planning, environment (b)
    1 Expedient examination and treatment are appropriate for an already traumatized victim.
    2 Inappropriate, because victim should never be left alone and if left to own devices may not seek needed medical care.
    3 Privacy should be provided but victim should not be left alone.
    4 Accommodations for bathing and douching should not be offered until examination and treatment are completed.

52. Knowledge, assessment, environment (b)
    4 State Good Samaritan Act will provide information on the extent of protection and legal limitations of practice under emergency medical circumstances.
    1 Civil Defense Laws are also known as Disaster Relief Laws. An MVA is not a disaster by definition.
    2 State nurse practice act speaks to scope and focus of general nursing practice.
    3 ANA Code For Nurses speaks to nursing ethics.

53. Application, implementation, environment (b)
    3 Roll victim in carpet or blankets to extinguish fire or use water.
    1, 4 Victim is screaming hysterically and should not be relied on to hear or follow instructions.
    2 Extinguish the fire and have someone call the fire department.

54. Knowledge, assessment, environment (b)
    1 Follow rule of nines.
    Left leg = 18%
    Right leg = 18%
    Right arm = 9%
    Total = 45%
    2, 3, 4 Does not follow rule of nines.

55. Comprehension, evaluation, environment (b)
    1 Victim should be observed for laryngeal and tracheal edema because the degree of inhalation burns is unknown.
    2, 3, 4 Characteristic of second-degree burns; previously determined that victim has second-degree burns.

56. Application, implementation, physiologic (a)
    2 Early access, early defibrillation, and early advanced care is necessary for all patients in cardiac arrest. Studies confirm that survival of the adult victim is strongly linked to early system access.
    1 As of early 1993 this was changed by the American Heart Association as described above.
    3 Such action would not be appropriate in this type of situation.
    4 Such action was never deemed appropriate to such a situation.

57. Application, implementation, physiologic (b)
    2 Studies have confirmed that ventilations given over a longer period help to minimize gastric distention.
    1 This was the length of time recommended for administration of ventilations before the change in early 1993.
    3, 4 Too long; does not fall within the time recommended in the guidelines.

58. Knowledge, assessment, environment (b)
    2 True labor is characterized by regular, forceful contractions, dilation and effacement of the cervix, and descent of the presenting part into the pelvis. Other options refer to signs of impending labor and possible complications (abdominal pain).
    1, 3, 4 Incorrect—see rationale for statement 2.

59. Knowledge, implementation, environment (a)
    3 Fetal heart tones are most accurately measured between contractions. During the early stages of labor, monitoring is generally done every 30 minutes.
    1 True rate not attainable since FHTs normally decrease during contractions.
    2 Inappropriate—need to be taken more often as indicated above.
    4 May be necessary especially closer to delivery.

60. Application, assessment, environment (b)
    2 This patient is now in the second stage of labor. All options listed include nursing responsibilities done during this time. Increasing the frequency of monitoring FHTs and maternal vital signs is most critical to maternal-infant well-being.
    1, 3, 4 See rationale for statement 2.

61. Knowledge, assessment, environment (b)
    2 The gestational age of the premature newborn is 37 weeks or less.
    1 A normal newborn may be large for its gestational age.
    3 Low–birth-weight newborn is 5½ lb (1500 g) or less at birth.
    4 Newborn with respiratory distress syndrome (RDS).

62. Comprehension, assessment, environment (b)
    2 The appearance of jaundice at birth or soon after is usually the initial sign to support suspected diagnosis of erythroblastosis fetalis.
    1, 3, 4 See rationale for statement 2.

63. Knowledge, assessment, environment (b)
    4 The premature newborn is covered with lanugo (fine downy hair), and eyelashes and eyebrows may be thin or absent at birth.
    1, 2, 3 Typical characteristics of premature newborn.

64. Knowledge, planning, environment (a)
    4 Oxygen therapy for the newborn must be administered with great caution to prevent retrolental fibroplasia. This condition is caused by high levels of oxygen concentration and may result in blindness.
    1 Purulent gonococcal conjuctivitis.
    2 Hemolytic disease, which is hereditary.
    3 Acute lung disease of newborn, caused by deficiency of pulmonary surfactant.

65. Comprehension, assessment, physiologic (a)
    4 Refers to something that occurs "in several forms."
    1, 2, 3 Increased glucose accumulation in the bloodstream caused by a lack of insulin, starts a chain of events. Polyphagia occurs when cells are in need of glucose. Polyuria occurs as the result of an osmotic diuresis when renal threshold is exceeded. When the body loses excessive amounts of fluid, the symptom of polydipsia (thirst) develops.

66. Comprehension, planning, health (b)
    1 Exercising muscle does not require the presence of insulin to take up glucose.
    2 "Reduces" the need for insulin in a sense.
    3 Not the prime reason to take precautions.
    4 Enhances muscle uptake of glucose, does not decrease it.

67. Comprehension, implementation, health (a)
    3 Not a classic complication of the disease. Diabetes is associated with microvascular and macrovascular changes that may affect the heart, retina, kidney, and nerves.
    1, 2, 4 Classic complications of uncontrolled diabetes.

68. Comprehension, implementation, environment (a)
    3 Regular insulin, a rapid-acting insulin, is classically the only insulin given in a sliding scale.
    1, 2, 4 Incorrect.

69. Knowledge, planning, environment (b)
    4 Any trauma to the meningocele sac can cause further neurologic damage and infection.
    1 Nursing action for meeting nursing goal.
    2 A nursing observation specific to an infant with a myelomeningocele.
    3 Not applicable at this time.

70. Application, implementation, environment (b)
    3 The meningocele sac is kept moist to prevent drying of the meninges from exposure to air.
    1, 2, 4 Incorrect means to keep meningocele moist.

71. Comprehension, assessment, physiologic (b)
    4 Hydrocephalus results from the obstruction in cerebrospinal fluid caused by the myelomeningocele. Increasing size of head circumference indicated by daily measurement, bulging fontanelles, and high-pitched cry is a symptom of increased intracranial pressure.
    1, 2, 3 Would not clearly indicate signs of increased intracranial pressure.

72. Knowledge, assessment, environment (b)
    2 As the cerebrospinal fluid accumulates, the neonate's or infant's head increases in size (noted by separation of cranial sutures and increased head circumference), and intracranial pressure increases.
    1, 3, 4 Not all reflective of signs and symptoms of increased intracranial pressure.

73. Knowledge, assessment, physiologic (b)
    1 These are signs and symptoms of heat exhaustion.
    2 These are signs and symptoms of heat stroke.
    3, 4 These are signs and symptoms of second-degree burns.

74. Knowledge, planning, physiologic (a)
    4 A diet high in proteins decreases the incidence of pressure sores.
    1 A diet high in calories is inappropriate for an immobilized patient.
    2, 3 Necessary, but not in excessive amounts.

75. Comprehension, planning, environment (b)
    1 High fluid intake and intermittent catheterizations keep the kidneys active and initiate voiding.
    2 Not the best to keep kidneys active, because of continuous irrigations.
    3, 4 Incorrect response.

76. Comprehension, planning, physiologic (a)
    1 These help to prevent pressure sores and contractures and can be done without danger of further injury.
    2, 3, 4 Exercises not the best to begin early in the treatment process.
77. Knowledge, planning, physiologic (a)
    1 Decubiti form easily if proper care is not given to patient.
    2, 4 Not necessarily specific to a spinal cord injured patient's treatment program.
    3 Not necessary.
78. Comprehension, implementation, psychosocial (a)
    3 You should offer Sal the opportunity to verbalize his feelings rather than internalize them. Depending upon a patient's adjustment process, this response can happen even years after the injury.
    1, 2, 4 Response shows lack of nurse's understanding of the situation and the patient's feelings.
79. Knowledge, assessment, environment (c)
    2 Autonomic dysreflexia may occur in 85% of all spinal cord injured patients with lesions at T6 level or above.
    1, 3, 4 Given symptoms do not describe this condition.
80. Comprehension (b)
    1 Atrophy means wasting or decrease in size.
    2 Muscle not used tends to grow smaller and shorter, not longer.
    3 Hypertrophy means to increase in size.
    4 Twitch is a quick, jerky contraction.
81. Analysis (b)
    3 The cerebellum regulates coordination, balance, and muscle tone.
    1 Breathing is regulated by the medulla.
    2 Hearing is regulated by the midbrain.
    4 Vision and hearing is regulated by the midbrain.
82. Comprehension (b)
    2 The hypothalamus contains cells that control appetite.
    1 The medulla regulates respiration, heart rate, and blood pressure.
    3 The cerebellum regulates coordination, balance, and muscle tone.
    4 Cerebral cortex is the outer nerve tissue, grey matter, of the cerebral hemispheres.
83. Knowledge (c)
    3 Vagus regulates swallowing, speaking, and peristalsis.
    1 Trigeminal regulates pain, touch, and temperature in face, scalp, and teeth.
    2 Hypoglossal regulates the muscles of the tongue.
    4 Glossopharyngeal regulates sense of taste, secretions of saliva.
84. Application, implementation, environment (a)
    2 DD = 4 mg
    DH = 10 mg
    V = 1 ml
    $$\frac{DD}{DH} = \frac{4 \text{ mg}}{10 \text{ mg}} \times 1 \text{ ml} = 0.4 \text{ ml}.$$
    1, 3, 4 This is not the correct amount.
85. Application, implementation, environment (a)
    1 $\dfrac{\text{Child's age (5)}}{\text{Age (5)} + 12} \times$ Average adult dose (500 mg)
    $$\frac{5}{17} \times 500 \text{ mg} = \frac{2500}{17} = 147 \text{ to } 148 \text{ mg}.$$
    2, 3, 4 This is not the correct answer.
86. Application, implementation, environment (a)
    2 $\dfrac{\text{Weight in pounds (30)} \times \text{Adult dose (10 mg)}}{150} =$
    $$\frac{300}{150} = 2 \text{ mg}$$
    1, 3, 4 This is not the correct answer.

87. Knowledge, assessment, physiologic (a)
    1 The most common classic sign of pyloric stenosis is projectile vomiting.
    2, 3, 4 This is not a common symptom of pyloric stenosis.
88. Application, implementation, environment (a)
    3 After repair of a pyloric stenosis, the infant is started on a schedule of frequent (every 2 hours) feedings of glucose water. This usually starts approximately 6 to 8 hours after surgery.
    1 The infant should be positioned on his side or abdomen.
    2 This is not a routine measure of treatment.
    4 The infant is only kept NPO for a few hours after surgery.
89. Knowledge, assessment, environment (b)
    1 Sucking chest wound is a direct threat to airway, breathing, and circulation.
    2, 3, 4 Not immediately life threatening.
90. Application, planning, physiologic (c)
    2 Vitamin K promotes hepatic formation of active prothrombin.
    1, 3, 4 Not applicable.
91. Application, planning, environment (b)
    3 Correct response.
    1, 2, 4 Not applicable to situation.
92. Comprehension, planning, environment (a)
    1 Correct calculation.
    2, 3, 4 Incorrect dose.
93. Comprehension, planning, environment (a)
    4 Correct dose.
    1, 2, 3 Incorrect dose
94. Application, planning, environment (b)
    1 An accurate culture is not possible once antibiotics have been started.
    2, 3, 4 Not applicable.
95. Application, planning, environment (a)
    2 60 mg = 1 gr
    $60 \times 5 = 300$ mg/tablet: 2 tablets = 600 mg
    1, 3, 4 Incorrect dose.
96. Knowledge, planning, environment (a)
    4 Cellulose is found in the stalks and leaves of plants and in the skins of fruits and vegetables.
    1 Refined cereals have most of the fiber removed.
    2 Milk products are low in cellulose.
    3 Tender meats are low in cellulose.
97. Knowledge, assessment, physiologic (a)
    1 Frequent diarrheic stools result in loss of essential electrolytes, especially potassium.
    2, 3, 4 Not relevant assessment for stated situation.
98. Knowledge, assessment, physiologic (b)
    1 Normal serum potassium level is 3.5. Symptoms of hypokalemia are muscle weakness and paralysis.
    2 Normal serum sodium concentration: 135 to 145 mEq/L.
    3 Normal serum potassium concentration.
    4 Serum sodium concentration low; edema would not be present.
99. Knowledge, assessment, environment (a)
    2 Vaginal or hidden bleeding and fetal distress are problems seen in patients with placenta previa.
    1 Abdominal rigidity is common to abruptio placentae.
    3 Symptoms of a ruptured uterus.
    4 Not symptomatic of placenta previa.
100. Knowledge, planning, physiologic (a)
    2 All are good sources of complete protein.
    1 Good source of carbohydrate and vitamin A.
    3 Carbohydrate source.
    4 Good source of carbohydrates, iron, and vitamin A.

101. Comprehension, planning, physiologic (b)
    3 Good sources of vitamin D, which aids in the absorption of calcium and phosphorus.
    1 Good sources of vitamin A.
    2 Good sources of vitamin E.
    4 Good sources of water-soluble vitamin C.
102. Knowledge, planning, physiologic (a)
    1 Fluids, if not contraindicated, help to prevent several complications of immobility, including constipation, urinary infection, and urinary calculi.
    2 Too high a calcium diet may predispose a patient to urinary calculi.
    3 Adequate but not high fats are recommended.
    4 Adequate amounts but not high sodium is recommended for the diet.
103. Application, planning, environment (b)
    1 Color coding has been successful in helping the elderly identify locations they cannot remember.
    2 Reminiscence therapy assists one with adaptation to the aging process.
    3 Reality orientation emphasizes orientation to time, place, and person.
    4 Key components of remotivation therapy are stimulating participation and interest in the environment and the reinforcement of normal behavior.
104. Knowledge, assessment, environment (a)
    3 Correct definition.
    1, 2, 4 Incorrect definition for this condition.
105. Comprehension, assessment, health (a)
    2 Developed in the 1960s and routine in most public schools.
    1, 3, 4 Not relevant diagnostic tests for scoliosis.
106. Knowledge, assessment, environment (a)
    2 Normal hemoglobin level for women: 12 to 16 g/100 ml.
    1, 3, 4 Normal values.
107. Application, implementation, environment (b)
    1 To be adhesive and to seal, the self-adhesive plastic bag must be applied to a clean, dry area.
    2, 3, 4 Incorrect procedure for obtaining urine specimen from infant.
108. Knowledge, assessment, health (c)
    1 All three foods are high in tyramine and should be avoided.
    2 Only beer is high in tyramine.
    3 Only liver is high in tyramine.
    4 Cheese and wine are high in tyramine.
109. Comprehension, assessment, environment (a)
    4 Puncture wounds are those created by a sharp, pointed object (e.g., nail).
    1 A closed wound (bruise) is caused by a blow from a blunt instrument or object.
    2 A cut is an open wound caused by a sharp instrument (e.g., scalpel).
    3 A laceration is an open wound caused by objects that produce a jagged tear (e.g., broken glass).
110. Knowledge, assessment, environment (b)
    1 During talking, sneezing, and coughing, microorganisms easily leave the mouth.
    2 Although the skin harbors and is a means of spreading microorganisms, it is not considered a portal of exit.
    3, 4 Common portal of *entry* for microorganisms.
111. Knowledge, assessment, environment (a)
    3 Disease is passed from parents to children through the genes.
    1 Disease is not caused by chemical factors.
    2 Congenital refers to conditions present or occurring at birth but not passed to children from parents.
    4 Disease is not caused by physical factors.

112. Comprehension, implementation, psychosocial (a)
    4 Response shows understanding and allows patient to verbalize feelings.
    1, 2, 3 Clichés, advice, and excuses that do not reflect understanding and empathy by the nurse.
113. Knowledge, planning, physiologic (a)
    2 Because of the removal of important muscles the patient must keep remaining muscles active.
    1 Does not apply to situation.
    3, 4 Eventual goal, but not primary reason for exercises.
114. Knowledge, planning, environment (b)
    2 The esophagus is close to the chest and becomes irritated during this treatment.
    1 Occurrence not specific to irradiation.
    3 Common side effect of chemotherapy.
    4 Complication not specific to irradiation.
115. Knowledge, assessment, health (a)
    3 About 95% of women discover this condition through breast self-examination.
    1, 2, 4 Diagnostic tool also used for breast cancer detection.
116. Knowledge, assessment, health (a)
    3 Most recognized, because most lesions occur in this quadrant.
    1, 2, 4 Not most recognized procedure to follow.
117. Knowledge, planning, health (a)
    2 Most growths occur during the active ovarian period.
    1 Not the best time.
    3 Not often enough.
    4 Incorrect statement.
118. Application, implementation, health (a)
    2 Drawing blood could lead to serious infection.
    1, 3, 4 Appropriate instructions allowing blood pressure (not pulse) to be taken on affected side.
119. Knowledge, planning, health (a)
    2 A woman who has experienced anxiety, disabilities, and pain associated with surgical intervention usually can anticipate a patient's needs more effectively than one who has not.
    1, 3, 4 Incorrect response.
120. Comprehension, assessment, psychosocial (a)
    4 Causes of mental illness are considered to be multifactorial.
    1 There is incomplete evidence of the biochemical basis of mental illness.
    2 There is incomplete evidence that developmental conflicts are the only causative agents.
    3 Although true, it does not sufficiently explain the causes of mental illness.
121. Comprehension, planning, environment (a)
    1 A necessary part of the care of an anorexic.
    2 Frequently offering food may increase anxiety and have a negative effect.
    3 Pressuring the patient to eat is usually what she has experienced from her family, and has a negative impact.
    4 Medications may have only a limited effect.
122. Knowledge, assessment, psychosocial (a)
    3 Freud believed the struggle between internal forces to be the basis of human behavior.
    1 Freud theorized that there are three stages of ego development.
    2 Freud did not take environmental factors into consideration to any great extent.
    4 Freud did not give much consideration to interpersonal conflict.

123. Comprehension, assessment, environment (a)

    3 Exaggerated ideas of one's power or influence are usually delusions of grandeur.

    1 Tactile hallucination refers to the false sense that there is something on one's skin.

    2 Flight of ideas refers to scattered thoughts, which are manifested by illogical connections made during verbalization.

    4 Neurosis is not usually characterized by delusion.

124. Comprehension, assessment, psychosocial (a)

    3 Denial is indicated by Jim's inability to recognize the seriousness of his act, and his belief that he can go home.

    1 Sublimation is the process by which negative impulses are channeled into more acceptable outlets.

    2 Projection is the placing of unacceptable impulses onto another person.

    4 Regression is the moving back to an earlier time or developmental level during periods of stress.

125. Comprehension, assessment, psychosocial (a)

    2 Flight of ideas refers to scattered thoughts, as evidenced by illogical connections made during verbalizations.

    1 Confusion is usually a matter of being disoriented as to time, place, or person.

    3 Delusions are fixed false beliefs.

    4 Hallucinations are the perceptions of sensory stimuli when no external objects are present.

Index